1 MONTH OF
FREE
READING

at

www.ForgottenBooks.com

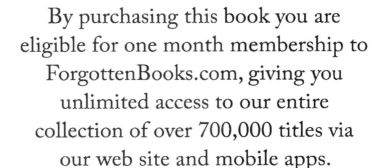

By purchasing this book you are
eligible for one month membership to
ForgottenBooks.com, giving you
unlimited access to our entire
collection of over 700,000 titles via
our web site and mobile apps.

To claim your free month visit:

www.forgottenbooks.com/free144069

ISBN 978-0-428-92973-2
PIBN 10144069

THE

CLINICAL JOURNAL

CLINICAL RECORD, CLINICAL NEWS, CLINICAL GAZETTE, CLINICAL
REPORTER, CLINICAL CHRONICLE AND CLINICAL REVIEW

*A WEEKLY RECORD OF CLINICAL MEDICINE AND
SURGERY, WITH THEIR SPECIAL BRANCHES.*

IN TWO VOLUMES ANNUALLY.

VOL. XXVII.

OCTOBER 18, 1905—APRIL 11, 1906.

FOURTEENTH YEAR.

EDITED BY

L. ELIOT CREASY, M.R.C.S.Eng., L.R.C.P.Lond.

THE MEDICAL PUBLISHING COMPANY, LIMITED,
22½ BARTHOLOMEW CLOSE, LONDON, E.C.

Supplement to the Clinical Journal, April 18, 1906.

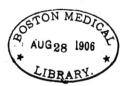
ADLARD AND SON

LONDON AND DORKING

LIST OF CONTRIBUTORS.

THE CLINICAL JOURNAL,

CLINICAL RECORD, CLINICAL NEWS, CLINICAL GAZETTE, CLINICAL REPORTER, CLINICAL CHRONICLE AND CLINICAL REVIEW.

EDITED BY L. ELIOT CREASY.

No. 677.   WEDNESDAY, OCTOBER 18, 1905.   Vol. XXVII. No. 1.

CONTENTS.

* *Specially reported for the Clinical Journal. Revised by the Author.*
ALL RIGHTS RESERVED.

NOTICE.

Editorial correspondence, books for review, &c., should be addressed to the Editor, 51, *New Cavendish Street, W., Telephone No.* 904, *Paddington; but all business communications should be addressed to the Publishers,* 22½, *Bartholomew Close, London, E.C. Telephone* 927, *Holborn.*

All inquiries respecting Advertisements should be sent to MESSRS. ADLARD & SON, *Bartholomew Close, E.C. Telephone* 927, *Holborn.*

Terms of Subscription, including postage, payable by cheque, postal or banker's order (in advance): for the United Kingdom, 15s. 6d. *per annum; Abroad* 17s. 6d.

Cheques, &c., should be made payable to THE PROPRIETORS OF THE CLINICAL JOURNAL, *crossed* "*The London, City, and Midland Bank, Ltd., Newgate Street Branch, E.C. Account of the Medical Publishing Company, Ltd.*"

Reading Cases to hold Twenty-six Numbers of THE CLINICAL JOURNAL *can be supplied at* 2s. 3d. *each, or will be forwarded post free on receipt of* 2s. 6d.; *and also Cases for Binding Volumes at* 1s. *each, or post free on receipt of* 1s. 3d., *from the Publishers,* 22½, *Bartholomew Close, London, E.C.*

A CLINICAL LECTURE

ON

THE PARAMOUNT IMPORTANCE OF THE LOCAL CONDITIONS IN SURGICAL DIAGNOSIS.

Delivered at St. George's Hospital.

By SIR WILLIAM BENNETT, K.C.V.O., F.R.C.S.,

Senior Surgeon to St. George's Hospital, etc.

GENTLEMEN,—In the diagnosis of disease I do not think it can be too fully understood that a point of great importance is the general impression which you form of a case when it first comes under observation. In order that such an impression may be of real value it is essential that the case be approached in a mental mood which is altogether free from bias. The ordinary academic method of taking notes, as you know, is that in which the history of the patient comes first. The history of the patient is often taken without any special regard to the local condition of the disease as it presents itself to the observer; the history having been taken, the examination of the diseased part follows. If you consider the details of such a method, you will see at once that the examination of the actual disease is not approached with quite a free mind, because you will have been biassed, more or less, by what the patient has told you with regard to the history of the complaint. Now, if too much importance is attached to the history in certain conditions of disease, you are very liable to be misled in the matter of diagnosis, because, as I have just said, of the bias which you are apt to get from the account which the patient gives. It is necessary to bear in mind that patients, in giving the history of their own diseases, very frequently include in it the details or recollections of other cases of the same kind of which they have heard, either from their doctor or from friends as the case may be. It is very easy to illustrate this fact, and I will relate a case or two to show you what I mean in a moment. The method of taking notes to which I have referred tends frequently to very imperfect results from a clinical point of view. Here is a very exaggerated example of the effect which the academic teaching has upon some people. A candidate at one of the examining bodies had placed before him for diagnosis a case of perfectly obvious sebaceous cyst of the scalp, a thing which any senior student or junior practitioner could ordinarily diagnose without any difficulty. The candidate, who was already qualified to practise, after having regarded the patient critically, but without having touched the tumour, put to him the somewhat crucial question : " What did your mother die of ? " That is the tendency of this method, which, in my opinion, is altogether faulty. Here was an apparently intelligent man so impressed with the importance of obtaining a " history " of the case that he could make no attempt to diagnose such a simple condition as sebaceous cyst of the scalp without having first ascertained the cause of the parent's death. It is a good illustration of the faulty tendency of this traditional method of teaching. The sound method in the making of a diagnosis is to examine the diseased part first and take the history afterwards. A very practical example in that relation is shown by a case which I have only recently admitted into the Fitzwilliam Ward. The patient is a man beyond middle age who has a tumour of the thigh, or at all events a swelling above the knee. The aspect of the swelling is clear enough. It is large and rounded, its edges are well-defined, there are large veins running over it, it is inseparable from the bone, and, as a matter of fact, any ordinary person upon examining the tumour would conclude that the man is the subject of malignant disease. But supposing a not particularly skilful person in the matter of diagnosis were first of all to investigate the man's history and so were to approach the case prejudiced by what he had been told by the patient, it is more than likely that a mistake would be made, and, as a matter of fact, a mistake was made in this way some time since in this case. The history is as follows : Some twenty years ago or thereabouts the patient dislocated his knee or knee-cap. Some little pain and swelling followed, but he soon recovered. Two or three years after that a painful swelling appeared on the inner side of the thigh, which, he says, disappeared upon taking · medicine, and he thought nothi rg more of it until four or five years ago, when he says he again put his knee out. A couple of years later the knee was dislocated once more, and finally in July, 1904, he met with an accident which put his knee out for the last time ; then again he was able to reduce the displacement himself, as he had generally been able to do. Asked whether there was much continuous swelling between these accidents, he replied, " Nothing worth mentioning." Now, the whole tendency of that history is to lead to the inference that this man's trouble was a purely traumatic one, and that, perhaps in consequence of the frequent dislocations or injuries to the knee-joint, the swelling above and to the inner side of the knee was, in all probability, a tense bursa or something of that kind, and therefore a matter of very little consequence, especially as there was not very much pain in it, and as he was in perfectly good general health. He had suffered a good deal of pain, but the pain was in the joint, below the swelling. You see how a story of that kind might have puzzled any person who had gone into the history before examining the case, whereas by examining the local condition unprejudiced by a deceptive history a faulty diagnosis would hardly be possible. The case is also a good one to show how little the history of some of these cases can be relied upon. By a curious coincidence it happens that I saw this man seventeen years ago, when there was a swelling in the same place as the one he shows us now, although it was not so large ; under treatment it diminished, but it did not disappear by any means, and as a matter of fact from that date until the time he came into the hospital he has had, I have no doubt, a tumour on the inner side of his thigh, just above the knee, although he considered that this tumour had only appeared last July. It is at first sight a curious fact that a man could have had for sixteen or seventeen years a considerable lump on the inner side of the thigh and yet only have become fully alive to its existence about six months ago. There is, however, nothing very remarkable in the matter ; for the tumour was, in fact, an endosteal sarcoma which had remained quiescent until the accident in July last, which no doubt caused a partial fracture of the femur, and broke down the bony capsule of the tumour and so led to its "sprouting" and rapidly increasing in size. Behaviour of this kind in the case of endosteal sarcoma is not very uncommon. In another instance with which I was concerned a tumour of the same nature remained apparently quiescent for twelve years and then after an accident sprouted with great rapidity.

Let us take another example. There is a woman in Drummond Ward who came to the hospital with a story that six weeks ago she first noticed a tumour on the inner side of her leg. It was then about the size of a filbert, and since that time had been rapidly increasing in size. It had been painful and sometimes very tender on pressure, hot, and altogether distressing—just the sort of history that would point as clearly as possible, especially as the temperature had been as high as 101°, to the existence of an abscess, coming forward, perhaps, from the deeper parts, and indicating that the increase in size was due to rapidly progressing suppuration. I first saw this patient outside the hospital, and following my usual habit, I looked of course at the leg first, and there I found a tumour the size of an orange, with some discoloration over the surface of it. It was softish, appeared as if it might be fluctuating, but was rather suggestive to me of a soft solid structure. It was not tender in the way that an abscess would be tender which had come on so quickly as this was said to have done, there was no material swelling of the limb around, and there was no œdema of the ankle below. There were two degrees of fever, but the woman appeared to be, as far as one could tell, in good health. On handling this tumour rather carefully it appeared to cling a little to the bone, and it certainly came up from the deeper parts. Taking the age and general condition of the patient into consideration, I concluded that this, again, was most likely some form of malignant disease, in all probability sarcoma, which had existed very much longer than she had any idea of. Going into the history subsequently, which was something like that which I have just mentioned, corresponding pretty accurately with the formation of a somewhat acute abscess, I found there were certain other points which led one to think that my impression with regard to the nature of this tumour was right, namely, that it was not an abscess, as it had been thought to be up to this

time in consequence of the story of the rapid growth, the tenderness, the heat which was sometimes felt about it, and the general symptoms which were described. When I came to inquire a little further into the case, following the lines of my primary impression with regard to the nature of it, I found that for some eighteen months or two years there had occasionally been certain crampy uncomfortable pains in the calf of the leg, and that she had also from time to time suffered from attacks of what she called "blue-foot." The leg had never swelled, but from time to time her foot, after she had been taking much exercise, got very blue and congested, becoming quite unlike the other. She could not understand this herself, but she had been told that the condition was due to a blocked vein in her calf. This, as I say, was some two or three years previously. That was more or less of a revelation with regard to the inaccuracy of her history. She had in her mind merely the prominent points in the history, in the same way that the man I mentioned just now had the prominent points of his history in his mind. And in this case, again, anyone approaching it from the evidence afforded by the history would hardly have suspected the existence of a malignant growth, and being biassed in that way before examining the case, might easily have been led to the conclusion that an abscess existed. But the evidence elicited in consequence of inquiries *following upon an examination of the part* showed clearly that there had been developing for a long time some abnormal condition in the deeper part of the leg, which led occasionally, under certain conditions of engorgement and so forth, to this peculiar discoloration and alteration in the normal condition of the foot which had attracted her attention at an early period of her complaint. It was clear that the condition was not likely to be thrombus because there was no pain associated with it, excepting the little crampy pains which she sometimes felt, and they were too slight to be of importance. This case, again, shows well what I mean with regard to the importance of taking into consideration first, *not the history of the patient, but the aspect of the disease from which the patient suffers.* In the usual way in which a student is taught to take notes of a case the cart is placed before the horse in a very unfortunate way, and I am certain that this method of investigating cases is sometimes the cause of mistakes in diagnosis which should easily be avoided.

Leaving the consideration of the fallacies which may arise from placing too much reliance upon the history of the patient, let me impress upon you the importance in diagnosis of a proper estimation of the aspect of the disease from which the patient suffers as compared with any evidence of other disease from which he is or has been suffering. The following is a good example to illustrate my meaning :

A man, aged about 28 or 30 years, was sent home from one of our possessions beyond the seas in consequence of what was called a multiple arthritis, and as sometimes happens in these cases of multiple arthritis, which in people of that time of life may be of an osteo-arthritic kind occurring in young subjects, the so-called arthritis disappeared from the majority of the joints, and settled itself in two of them—the knee on one side of the body and the elbow on the other. By degrees the elbow lost its disability to a great extent, although it remained somewhat stiff, leaving us to deal with the knee-joint. Following up the idea that this was one of those cases of osteo-arthritis or whatever it is correct to call it, occurring in a comparatively young subject, I had formulated a definite line of treatment which I thought would meet the case. But incidentally this patient, having seen several authorities, was finally seen by some one who directed that a very careful investigation of the urine should be made, with the result that gonococci were said to be present. This at once seems to have led to the conclusion by those who had the case in hand at that time that the case was one of gonorrhœal arthritis, although it was many years since the patient had suffered from gonorrhœa. Here, then, was a man with a chronic effusion in his knee : he had had an effusion in some other joints, but all had got comparatively well except one elbow and this particular knee. Gonococci are found in the urine, therefore it is concluded that the case is of gonorrhœal origin, an entirely unnecessary deduction. It so happened in this instance that it was a very unfortunate diagnosis for the patient, because it affected to a very large extent, or threatened to affect, his future prospects. In spite of the evidence of the gonococci I could not myself believe that it was a case of gonorrhœal rheumatism. The aspect

of the case was quite unlike gonorrhœal arthritis, whilst it exactly, as I said just now, resembled osteo-arthritis, following the ordinary course which that disease so frequently takes. Moreover in this knee, which was stated to be in the condition of what is known as gonorrhœal rheumatism, there were gratings and cracklings and rubbings, and pedunculated bodies could actually be felt in the joint, a condition which I have never met with in connection with gonorrhœal arthritis. The aspect of the case appeared to me to be quite characteristic. But, you see, these other people, not content with taking the local conditions at their true value and exercising their clinical acumen in the diagnosis of the case, placed so much reliance upon the discovery of these gonococci—if they were gonococci—that the local signs were ignored, and a diagnosis made solely upon the evidence of the existence of gonococci, forgetting this one very important fact—a fact that you should never forget—that the evidence of the previous existence of specific disease, such as gonorrhœa, for example, or enteric fever, does not necessarily either give rise to, modify, or influence any pathological condition from which the patient may suffer afterwards. Let me make my meaning clear. Here was a man who had gonorrhœa eight or nine years ago—the attack, he said, being so slight that he did not bother very much about it. Many years after this attack he develops a form of arthritis ; there are found in his urine evidence of his having had at some time or another gonorrhœa, therefore it is concluded that this arthritis must be gonorrhœal in origin. A more faulty reasoning, having regard to the local condition, it would be difficult to find ; and it is a most excellent example to show how you may be misled by having your attention taken away from the actual disease itself—and this is what I want to particularly impress upon you—by the discovery of some accidental evidence of previous disease in the way I have mentioned. Taking the matter a little further, you must remember that the evidence of pre-existing disease (in the shape, say, of the presence of gonococci in the case of gonorrhœa, or in the response to certain tests after enteric fever) may very long outlive the activity of the specific element itself, and you may get, for example, in the case of a man who has had at some time or another enteric fever, some condition long after that illness which you may think to be associated with enteric fever, if you attach too much importance to any evidence of its former occurrence. Here is an example in illustration. A man was invalided home during the South African war. He had had enteric fever in South Africa, as well as another attack some years previously. He had had, in fact, two attacks of enteric fever in the course of his life. He was invalided home in consequence of a large swelling on the inner end of his clavicle, a situation in which, as you who have been in the out-patient room know, gumma is common. Gumma at the inner end of the clavicle, involving to some extent the sterno-clavicular joint, is not an uncommon affection. Taking this case in the way of which I am speaking, i. e. by regarding the local condition as the paramount factor in making a diagnosis, I concluded, and should always conclude under the same circumstances unless I had a very distinct evidence that I was wrong, that it was in all probability one of syphilitic gumma. The paramount factor in this case was the existence of this tender swelling, painful at night, at the inner end of the clavicle, with some involvement of the sterno-clavicular articulation, the whole sequence of symptoms being as clear as it well could be. Upon examining this man's blood after hearing that he had had enteric fever, it was found to respond to one of the tests that the blood of people who have suffered or are suffering from that disease do respond to, and therefore it was very strongly suggested, because there was evidence in this man's blood that he had been the subject of typhoid fever, that the disease was not gumma, but post-enteric osteo-myelitis, not because the local condition looked like it, but because there was evidence in his blood that he had suffered from typhoid fever. It is an exactly parallel sequence of evidence, you see, to that which occurred in the case of the man who had an osteo-arthritic joint which was concluded to be gonorrhœal because the gonococcus had been found in his urine. In both of these cases I operated. In the case of the man with the supposed gonorrhœal knee I opened the joint, and took out a large number of pedunculated and one or two loose bodies. The whole of the inside of the joint had the ordinary aspect of osteo-arthritis in the early stage, tending towards the production of pedunculated and loose bodies, as these cases

sometimes do in young people. The younger the subject at the time of the onset of the osteo-arthritis the more rapidly do pedunculated and loose bodies form. In fact, they show the specific signs of the case being osteo-arthritis much earlier than any lipping or any other change in the articular ends of the bones. In the case of the man with the swelling at the inner end of his clavicle I operated because the swelling was breaking down and I should have had to operate under any circumstances. But when I came to operate, the abscess was on the surface of the clavicle, it was not in its substance. Now, these bone abscesses after enteric fever are a local osteo-myelitis, and therefore in opening the abscess cavity of that type in a case like this you would at once go into the interior of the bone. The ordinary syphilitic node, on the other hand, so far as any evidence when it forms an abscess is concerned, lies on the bone surface, and the bone is solid beneath it. Such was the condition which I found in this particular case. Moreover, the wound which resulted from my operation did not heal until the man had a course of iodide of potassium. And seeing the rapidity of the healing which followed the use of the drug, it was not surprising to learn that two other small nodules, one on a rib on each side of the chest, also disappeared, thereby negativing for practical purposes the possibility of the disease being anything in the nature of a post-enteric condition.

These four cases illustrate very clearly, then, the point I am trying to impress upon you—that in the matter of diagnosis and a proper estimate of cases the great point is to keep your mind on the disease that the patient is suffering from, and not to be misled by all sorts of collateral and curious evidences which may be brought into the case as a result of very careful and thorough examination of the secretion in the chemical or clinical laboratory; such examinations very properly are as thorough as possible, and produce results which are always interesting and sometimes of value. It is well, however, to remember that if these investigations are sufficiently thorough there will be found in a considerable number of apparently healthy people some deviation from the normal condition, hence the value attached to such findings should be relative rather than absolute. Here is a good illustration of this point : A man, æt. 30 years, as robust a specimen of humanity as could well be imagined, broke his knee-cap.   The question of operation naturally arose, the operative treatment being welcomed by the patient without hesitation. As a matter of routine the urine was subjected to an exhaustive examination, with the result that with a specific gravity of 1030 it contained a considerable percentage of sugar, a condition of things which would—supposing the patient to have been a diabetic—have made the operation unjustifiable. But the aspect of the man and the rudeness of his health made it practically, for clinical purposes, almost impossible that he could be the subject of diabetes. As a sound knee was of vital importance to him I, therefore, ignored the apparently grave condition of the urine and operated. All went well and a second examination of the urine ten days after the operation showed a perfectly normal secretion.   Had the evidence afforded by the examination of the urine been taken at its face value, without regard to the clinical and general aspects of the patient, he would have been condemned by the nature of the fracture to permanent crippling, since this could only have been prevented by operation.

Thus far I have only dealt with the fallacies which may arise in connection with collateral evidence of the positive kind ; the following case teaches the same lesson in connection with negative evidence. A soldier, æt. about 30 years, nine years before coming under observation was crushed by his horse falling upon him ; the main damage was on the left side of the abdomen and he was laid up for some six or seven weeks. He apparently recovered, but for four years had frequently been attacked by acute abdominal pain, referred principally to the left side.   There was usually vomiting and constipation, which was sometimes extremely difficult to overcome.   He had not noticed any irritability of the bladder or other urinary inconvenience either before or during the attacks.   Two years before I saw him he had married, with the result that the attacks became more frequent and intense — the pain at times concentrating itself about the navel above and the inner side of the thigh below. Taking the general aspect of the case into consideration and judging from what I had seen in similar cases before, I came to the conclusion that the symptoms from which he suffered were probably due to one of two conditions—either (1) a band,

the result of some peritonitis which had followed upon his accident, or (2) a stone in the ureter. That being my impression and knowing that in a general way the existence of a stone in the kidney or in the ureter is easily determined by the intelligent use of the X rays, I had this man skiagraphed very carefully by the most skilful man of the time in this particular line of investigation, with the result that no stone was visible in any part of the urinary tract.   The result of the examination at once threw me back upon the possibility that the cause of the trouble might be a band resulting from the crush, followed, as it might- have been, by peritonitis—a possibility quite consistent with the story which he told, especially considering that these attacks of pain were preceded by sudden and acute constipation.   I was on the point of making an exploratory operation, on the strength of there having been no stone found in the urinary tract by means of the X rays, but after seeing him again two or three times, I could not, although I made several careful examinations, get away from my first impression that he had a stone in his ureter. He had no sign of it in his urine, there was no blood or anything abnormal to be found, but stone in the ureter may exist without any abnormality of the urine.   There were one or two things about the man which inclined my views in the direction I have mentioned, and in spite of the negative result of the X rays examination I hesitated about making an abdominal section, for which, by the way, he was extremely eager.   The attacks continued to occur ; I saw him whilst one of them was in progress. He was curled up, lying on his left side in acute pain, his muscles were as hard as a board, and you could see a sort of attempt, apparently, at peristalsis in his intestine when he took a breath sufficiently deep to allow the muscles to relax a little.   Still I clung to my old idea in spite of the absence of stone as revealed by the X rays ; one morning a more acute attack than usual ceased suddenly and twenty-four hours later he passed a little stone from his urethra. The practical point about the case is this.   Had I relied implicitly upon the negative evidence in this instance afforded by the X-ray investigation, I should certainly have made an abdominal section with the idea of finding a band or something of that kind about the intestine to account for the symptoms—a reasonable thing to do under the circumstances, and therefore justifiable even in the absence of the X-ray evidence. But knowing that all these mechanical helps to diagnosis and treatment do sometimes fail, especially if their evidence is negative, I preferred the evidence of my powers of observation and clung to my impression about the stone. Of course in this particular instance the evidence of the X rays ought to have been conclusive, but it was not. The stone, no doubt, was lying about the edge of the pelvis, and being of a not very·opaque kind, it showed no shadow apart from the shadow which the pelvis itself gave, therefore it escaped our notice. But in spite of that, by the exercise of a little shrewdness in dealing with the case, an unnecessary operation was avoided because I felt that the conclusions I had come to, apart from and in spite of mechanical aids, were correct. Speaking generally, I do not attach any importance to the evidence afforded by the X rays in a case of this kind unless they are applied by a person of singular skill and experience, because it is extremely difficult sometimes to show stones in the kidney, or in the ureter, or in the bladder by means of the X rays. When the rays are applied by people of great skill they are rarely overlooked, but as it is clearly possible that they may in some instances escape detection, there is every reason, in spite of having such an admirable mechanical help at your disposal, to cultivate your own acuteness in diagnosis to the very utmost in order to meet those cases in which mechanical help entirely fails, as it will sometimes do. It is the case with the cystoscope and other apparatus of the same type. There are, in fact, certain fallacies connected with the evidence of nearly all mechanical contrivances which, as a rule, can be avoided if you have the aptitude and take the trouble to exercise your ordinary acumen sufficiently. This brings me to the point which I particularly wish you to understand, viz. that in the diagnosis of disease the most important thing of all is the aspect which the disease itself presents to your eyes and to your touch. That is the first and most important thing. The second point I would have you bear in mind is the fact that evidence of the previous existence of any specific disease need not lead to the conclusion that the pre-existing disease has caused, or has in any way influenced disease arising subsequently; and again, that all these evidences of specific diseases, like gonorrhœa, enteric fever, and conditions of that sort, may so very long outlive the active period of the disease that they exist in very many instances as quite independent factors, and therefore should not mislead you sufficiently to make you come to a wrong diagnosis when the aspect of the case with which you have to deal is obvious so far as you can tell under the circumstances in which you meet it. These three points in connection with diagnosis are, I think, very important, because we undoubtedly are inclined to rely too much in these times upon the evidence of the clinical laboratory and the physiological chemist, to the detriment of the cultivation of our powers of observation; and it behoves us, I am sure, to hold fairly closely to the old-fashioned plan of diagnosing by observing a disease from its purely clinical standpoint if we are to avoid, as far as possible, the occurrence of grievous errors in the treatment.

October 16th, 1905.

A LECTURE

ON

EXOPHTHALMIC GOITRE.

Delivered at University College Hospital.

By H. BATTY SHAW, M.D., F.R.C.P.,
Assistant Physician to the Hospital and to the Hospital for Consumption, Brompton; Lecturer on Therapeutics, University College, London.

GENTLEMEN,—I have chosen this subject for the clinical lecture to-day for several reasons, and chief amongst them has been the question raised by one of your number as to the apparent great rarity of the disease. If this were really the case, there would be little excuse for choosing it as a subject for a clinical lecture; but the fact that during the last five years thirty-four cases have applied for relief as out-patients under my care alone justifies the belief that probably the disease is not so rare as would be thought judging from the comparatively few cases admitted to the wards for treatment; Dr. Bown, our Resident Medical Officer, tells me that during seven years, 1894–1901, 12 men and 31 women have been admitted as in-patients; of the total number, 43, 3 cases (women) have proved fatal. Another reason for bringing this subject before your notice is that it is a common experience that such cases come as out-patients for a few months and then appear no more. I find on communicating with these patients that the reasons for this are that some are so comparatively well that they do not need further help; others, who are very candid, express their conviction that the various forms of treatment advocated have not proved of much value, or that their improvement does not seem to depend upon any particular plan of treatment; some cases have wandered off to other hospitals; a few have been lost sight of as they have changed their addresses; of the 34 cases there is but 1 recorded as dead.

Etiology.—You are well aware that this disease is more common in women, the proportion being roughly 4 to 1 compared with men (Ehrhardt), though other observers find the proportion as much as 48 to 1; in the present series there are 31 women to 3 men—about 10 to 1; taking the average of various collections of cases the proportions work out to about 8 to 1. The disease declares itself between 16 and 40 years, but it has been known to develop within the first ten years of life; it is very exceptional for it to begin in advanced age. The oldest patient in my series is 50 years of age; it is impossible to say, however, that she has not had evidence of the disease longer than the six or seven months before she sought relief.

It is well recognised that exophthalmic goitre appears to be closely associated occasionally with sudden emotional disturbance, shock, etc., and one of our cases showed the first signs after a motor accident. The great majority, however, do not give any account of a shock, and it really is a matter for careful consideration and inquiry to settle this point; for .it quite well might be that exophthalmic goitre existed prior to the sudden shock or fright which served merely to call attention to the condition; such an opinion would be attacked by many authorities, but I want you, as far as possible, to derive your impressions of the disease and its etiology, etc., from the cases actually under your own notice. The collected experience of different writers in different countries may be very valuable, but it has drawbacks; the picture may be very representative, but it is a blurred one, and I cannot but consider that the effect of fright, etc., is one of the false elements in the composite picture of the etiology of this disease.

Another matter of interest which the present series proves to be worthy of close consideration is the occurrence of the disease in the ascendants, descendants, or collaterals. The series includes examples of the disease in a father and his son, in two sisters, and in a mother and daughter; but probably what will prove most interesting of all to you is the study of a family consisting of a mother and her six children, all of whom you will be able to examine, and so will be able to check for yourselves the observations made.

Mrs. T—, æt. 45 years, has an obvious tremor of the hands, a pulse rate which varies from 104 to 120 to the minute, and an enlargement of the thyroid gland involving especially the right lateral globe and the isthmus; there are, however, none of the eye phenomena visible in some cases of Graves' disease. Her eldest daughter, M. T—, æt. 22 years, also an out-patient of the hospital for the last two years, has a goitre, tremor of the fingers and hands, and a pulse rate of 120: the second daughter, D. T—, æt. 16½ years, has had for the last year enlargement of the thyroid gland, forming an obvious goitre; she has also slight tremor, but there is no tachycardia, for the pulse rate is only 80-90, nor are there any signs of exophthalmos; a third daughter, E. T—, æt. 14 years, has slight tremor, well-marked general enlargement of the thyroid gland, and an excitable heart, the rate varying from 84 to 124 per minute; she is, as you will see, rather emotional, has recurring hot flushes and a very moist skin. This, however, does not complete the account of this goitrous family, for the next two children in point of age are two boys, H. T— and S. T—, æt. 12 and 9 years respectively; they have a slight tremor and general enlargement of the thyroid, · which is especially obvious when the profile of the neck is examined; the youngest child of the family, a girl, æt. 8 years, has no evidence of tremor, goitre, or heart hurry. I do not want to insist too much on the tremors of the two boys, but they must be taken into consideration, and I think they may be looked upon as possibly early cases of exophthalmic goitre; the same may be said of the third daughter; the mother and two eldest daughters must, however, be considered cases of developed Graves' disease, for they have enlargement of the thyroid, tachycardia and tremor. It is certainly curious that there is no exophthalmos in any of the members of this goitrous family. Interesting as this account is, there is a much more remarkable family described by another observer. There were ten children the offspring of hysterical patients; eight of these children had Graves' disease, and one of these, a daughter, had three descendants who also suffered with the same malady. A fallacy is, however, apt to occur in the study of such cases as form the family I have shown, for it is known that the thyroid gland may be enlarged at the time of puberty in both sexes, and it is also enlarged in chlorotic subjects, so that it is not correct to conclude that exophthalmic goitre is certainly developing merely because the thyroid enlargement is so obvious. There must, as in these cases, be other signs. Your suspicions may be aroused, but that is all. It must also be remembered that the thyroid enlarges in pregnancy, at the monthly periods, and as a result of infectious diseases.

One other matter of great interest is that exophthalmic goitre has been noticed in horses, dogs, and cattle. A racehorse after a severe gallop was noticed to lose its appetite, and later on it developed marked pulsation of the thyroid as well as enlargement of the organ; eventually œdema of the lids, sleeplessness, and exophthalmos developed, and the animal died within two months of the onset of the malady.

Pathogeny, etc.—When we attempt to come to closer quarters with the causation of this curious disease we find that so far as morbid anatomy is concerned there is practically nothing to discuss beyond the very characteristic changes met with in the thyroid gland itself, such as reduction in colloid and proliferation of the lining epithelium of the alveoli, as well as degenerative changes in the cardiac muscle and hæmorrhages into the medulla and other parts of the central nervous system; some inconstant changes have been described in the vagus and its endings in the heart, but it must be admitted that the study is disappointing because of the paucity of demonstrable change. When we turn to the evidence afforded by experimental pathology, a very great diversity of opinion is found to exist. Many observers have been struck by the very marked nervous character of the symptoms of Graves' disease. The general appearance of the patient suggests terror, and from this rather slender evidence it has been considered that disturbance of the nervous system is a very important etiological factor in the causation of the malady. For various reasons the sympathetic nerve has been singled out as the actual element the disturbance of which causes the symptoms; irritation of its centres of origin or of its nerve-fibres is considered to be responsible for the retraction of the upper lid by irritating the muscle of Müller and to cause heart hurry, but the same irritation should cause contraction of the blood-vessels generally, and there is reason to believe that the vessels are rather dilated than contracted, though evidence on this point even is not conclusive, for some observers find a rise of blood-pressure by sphygmometric observations and others a fall.

One great objection to this theory is that of all the methods of active treatment which appear to influence the disease, direct removal or suppression of part of the gland appears to be followed by the most markedly favourable effects; though it must be remembered that " thyroid collapse," as it is called, supervenes in many of the cases which are so treated,

and robs the surgeon of all claims to advance this procedure as a good method of treating exophthalmic goitre.

Much of modern thought inclines to the view that exophthalmic goitre is due to disturbance of the thyroid gland; it is considered by some that there is an excessive activity on the part of the thyroid gland, and that the system is flooded with an excess of colloid—a view which is supported by the observation that many symptoms analogous to those of Graves' disease can be produced by the internal administration of thyroid gland, even to the production of exophthalmos. Such observations must be accepted with some reserve, because when the thyroid gland of sheep is administered, probably parathyroidal substance is also given; so far, however, the specific effects produced by administering pure parathyroid substance have been demonstrated only in the laboratory; the few alleged beneficial results of its clinical use require more confirmation; it is stated by some observers that they were unable to detect any effects resulting from the administration of parathyroids in cases of myxœdema, insanity, etc.

Amongst the more recent views of the cause of exophthalmic goitre must be mentioned the one according to which Graves' disease is due to suppression of the parathyroid body, just as myxœdema is due to the suppression of the thyroid. This ingenious theory derives considerable support from the fact that tetany and other allied nervous disturbances which are met with in exophthalmic goitre can be induced experimentally by ablation of the parathyroids and be dispelled by the administration of parathyroidal tissue or by the removal of the thyroid. It thus appears likely that the thyroid gland produces substances which excite metabolic change, and that the parathyroids secrete material which neutralises the by-products of such activity; such metabolites if not neutralised are considered to be the cause of various nervous disturbances, such as tremors, tetany, etc., symptoms which are met with in exophthalmic goitre.

There remains another theory which cannot be put aside without due consideration, and that is that exophthalmic goitre is due rather to a qualitative change of the thyroidal secretion, a theory which can claim much more consideration than the hyperthyreic or parathyroidal causation of the disease, for the anatomical picture of the thyroid gland is more suggestive of quantitative change of the thyroid secretion than of excessive function of the organ, and, so far as observation in man is concerned, of absence of parathyroidal activity. This disturbed activity of the thyroid gland may conceivably pass on to depression of function altogether—a sequence which is as' natural, if not more so, as a transition from excessive function to depressed activity. Clinical experience shows how possible it is for exophthalmic goitre to pass into myxœdema. One of the present series is a case in point, and forms a very interesting clinical illustration. Mrs. D—, æt. 38 years, applied for relief as an out-patient, and it was found that she had albuminuria and also ascites, as shown by movable dulness in the abdomen. She was admitted to the wards, with the diagnosis of albuminuria and ascites, and you can guess my chagrin on hearing from Mr. A. M. H. Gray, Dr. Bradford's house-physician, that the signs of ascites and other abnormal symptoms had cleared up very largely under the internal administration of thyroid gland. There is still slight albuminuria. You will see her presently, and will be able to hear her favourable estimate of the improvement under such treatment, and she will show her photograph as a young woman, æt. 23 years, when she attended St. Bartholomew's Hospital for prominent eyes, palpitation, and " trembling."

One other view remains to be mentioned, and one which is allied to the explanation for the occurrence of acromegaly, viz. that the goitre or change in the thyroid gland met with in Graves' disease—for the gland is not always *enlarged*—as well as the other signs, are merely part of the result of a general toxic condition which is at present unknown to us. That there is such a toxic agency is supported by the occurrence of localised œdema, pruritus, sclerodermia, leucodermia, and melanodermia, and by the existence of excessive perspiration and general pigmentary changes in the skin, also by the occurrence of diarrhœa and vomiting, and in some cases by albuminuria, and even by albumosuria, all symptoms suggestive of disturbances of three important eliminative tissues. Unfortunately, the experimental observations made on the toxicity of the urine in this malady are so far unconvincing.

Reviewing the question of the cause of this disease, a few facts and theories stand out in prominence. It is a disease more common during the period of greatest sexual activity, and is more ·frequent in women. There is considerable evidence for believing that simple goitre and exophthalmic goitre may occur in the same family, and that exophthalmic goitre may occur in two or more generations. Further, there is considerable evidence to support the view that the disorder is due to excessive function of the thyroid gland,. though there is probably more reason for the opinion so well maintained by Moebius that the disease is due to dysthyrea, meaning by that term that there is a qualitative rather than a quantitative perversion of thyroidal activity; the evidence in favour of the disease being due to depressed activity of the parathyroids is not sufficiently convincing. That the disease is due to perversion of some kind or another of the thyroid gland is indirectly supported by the fact that although myxœdema may occur subsequently to exophthalmic goitre, it is never succeeded by the latter malady, the cases which have been recently described by certain French observers as examples of this sequence being merely examples of the existence at the same time of myxœdemic symptoms and some signs of exophthalmic goitre. In such cases myxœdema is presumably developing, but is not completely established, or it may be that symptoms of Graves' disease are developing in cases of myxœdema as a result of thyroid medication.

Symptomatology.—I do not propose to rehearse the symptoms and signs which are so well described in your text-books, but it is well to insist again that in the ordinary descriptions of this disease the principle of the multiple photograph is apt to lead us astray; we hesitate too much to label a case as one of Graves' disease, because we are unable to establish all the cardinal signs, which in the present series show the following order in point of frequency—first *tachycardia*, then *goitre* and *tremor*, and, finally, *exophthalmos*. It is really necessary for you to learn all the possible signs of the disease, because one or other may precede for months the complete manifestation of other stigmata. One of the best marked cases to be presently shown to you appeared at the Brompton Hospital because she was wasting; her facial aspect was rather comical, for one palpebral fissure was held widely open—the condition known as *lagophthalmos* or hare's eye. There were no other signs of Graves' disease ; but Mr. Flemming, who was good enough to see the case for me in the early days, confirmed my suspicions—she now shows delay in descent of the upper eyelids when the eyes are turned downwards, tachycardia, double proptosis and tremor.

Another case which is worth while relating to you is that of a young man afflicted with mitral disease. He developed *tetany*, which involved not only the arms and legs but even the face ; he was found to have von Graefe's sign and tremor but no marked goitre and no proptosis, merely some retraction of the upper eyelid. He died shortly after, and his thyroid gland showed microscopic appearances similar to those found in exophthalmic goitre. The occurrence of tetany in a case of exophthalmic goitre need not, however, presage death, for Dr. Hector Mackenzie has shown that this group of symptoms may be present for twenty years. Another difficulty is the occurrence of *joint pains* and of other symptoms, such as *chorea*, which are usually associated with the acute infectious diseases; the youngest of the series, a girl, æt. 9 years, who I am bound to admit is merely a "suspect" case—an example, in fact, of incomplete Graves' disease—has irregular choreic movements rather than fine tremor, the pulse rate is 96-160 and the thyroid is distinctly enlarged ; in one other case " rheumatic pains " in the small joints of the hands are marked features occurring periodically. *Paralyses* of various kinds are common towards the end of the disease, including monoplegia, paraplegia, or the so-called " giving way " of the legs, and even hemiplegia. Amongst other phenomena which may suddenly appear are paralyses of the *external* ocular muscles ; curiously the internal muscles of the eye do not appear to be affected or but very rarely : *epileptiform* attacks also occur and Bristowe records a case in which this development was combined with external ophthalmoplegia and hemiplegia. Sudden attacks of *hurried breathing* are well known and may usher in the final scenes. Mental changes, such as *mania*, *melancholia*, acute *delirium*, and excessive *sleeplessness*, are also met with. Rise of *temperature* may occur and persist till death ; *dermatitis* and even *icterus* has been recorded. Exophthalmos may be so great as to lead to the *dislocation* of the eye from the orbit ; corneal ulcers do occur but are rare. *Vomiting* and *diarrhœa* may persist till the end. One of our series caused much difficulty because of the marked dulness to percussion of

the right apex of the chest, but tubercle bacilli were unable to be discovered, for there was no cough or expectoration ; possibly the dulness was due to an enlarged *thymus*, persistence and enlargement of the thymus being met with in Graves' disease, or it may have been due to *thoracic goitre*, such cases having been described.

Clinical types.—Various simple clinical types are recognised in this disease. There are *chronic* cases which constitute the large majority of the out-patients suffering from Graves' disease; they may last for years. On the other hand, there are some cases which develop the recognised signs and even end fatally within a few months, constituting a group of *acute* cases ; such cases should not be confused with those of acute exacerbations occurring in the chronic form. One of the present series died within a fortnight after seeking relief for weakness of the hands, having been ill altogether for three to four months. *Transitory* cases are also recorded in which some of the more well-recognised signs of the disease develop and disappear quite rapidly even in a few days. Marie has described a form " fruste " or *incomplete*, in which exophthalmos is absent and the malady is declared by tachycardia and tremor. When exophthalmic goitre occurs in *children*, palpitation is less marked, the pulse rate rarely exceeds 120, the ocular signs are often absent, but thyroid hypertrophy is common. The tremors are in children frequently replaced by choreic movements such as are described in the child already referred to.

From what you have seen of the cases shown, I am sure the question will have occurred to you, Do cases of simple goitre ever become cases of exophthalmic goitre ? This is, a very important matter, but unfortunately is a very difficult one to settle. It is well known that many cases of simple goitre continue as such and never show signs of Graves' disease ; but it must also be admitted that enlargement of the thyroid may be the first and only sign of Graves' disease, and that some of the cases in which the thyroid gland is attacked surgically for the relief of apparently simple localised enlargement of one or other lobe or of the isthmus, succumb in a most curious fashion. Such a case occurred not long ago in this hospital, the patient developing aphonia and dying comatose shortly after the operation of excision of a part of the thyroid gland. It has been suggested that some of these cases are really cases of *latent* exophthalmic goitre and that the operation has been sufficient to provoke acute and fatal symptoms, according to some observers, by facilitating the process of intoxication by abnormal thyroid secretion which escapes into the tissues during operation.

French writers have endeavoured to separate a special group of cases of exophthalmic goitre, which they speak of under the rather clumsy title of " *Basedowified goitre* " or "*false surgical exophthalmic goitre.*" You will remember that Basedow shares with two British physicians, Parry and Graves, the honour of first recognising the disorder. The group includes those in which the symptoms of Graves' disease develop in cases of simple goitre often of very many years' duration. According to Dr. Paul Sainton. tachycardia is often the first symptom to develop, and dyspnœa is more marked than in simple goitre; the goitre is voluminous and is less vascular and less expansive than in primary Graves' disease. Such cases are usually much older than ordinary cases of Graves' disease, and the symptoms occur as long as twenty-two to twenty-five years after the onset of the goitre.

It is important to recognise this last group of cases, which may also be described as *secondary* Graves' disease, because it appears that they are more amenable to treatment by means of the thyroid gland or by partial or complete thyroidectomy than are the cases of *primary* Graves' disease.

Prognosis.—There can be few more distressing disfigurements to a woman than the exophthalmos and goitre of Graves' disease, and you will be constantly met with the question, " Is the, disease curable ?" So alarming are the symptoms at times that you must be prepared with answers to the question, " Is it fatal ?" According to the statistics of Sallten, of von Graefe, and of von Dusch, 25 per cent. of the cases get quite well, and 46 per cent. can be made much better. The mortality varies according to different observers, and includes extremes of 11·6 per cent. (Buschan) and 25 per cent. (Charcot) ; an average of a number of observations gives a mortality of about 15·3 per cent.

Diagnosis.—Seeing how common it is to meet with a fine tremor of the fingers, and the readiness with which in women the upset of examination causes tachycardia, it is not to be wondered at that

it is necessary to make repeated examinations before the "incomplete form" of Graves' disease, in which these two symptoms predominate, is diagnosed. "Paroxysmal tachycardia" is a well-known phenomenon, but it occurs quite independently of other signs met with in Graves' disease. Tremor of the hands is common in cases of alcoholism, in many women suffering from debility, and in cases of rheumatoid arthritis ; it is known to be inherited and to occur in families quite independent of any disease.

The difficulty of diagnosis is greatly increased when the following diseases or groups of symptoms which have been found to occur with Graves' disease are remembered: hysteria, epilepsy, chorea, paralysis agitans, tabes dorsalis, syringomyelia, myxœdema, osteomalacia, disseminated sclerosis, and acromegaly.

The best advice to give in the management of cases which show tachycardia and tremor is to keep them under observation and treat so far as is practicable as if they were cases of exophthalmic goitre.

Treatment.—Probably no disorder pursues its course more independently of our efforts to check it than does Graves' disease. The particular nostrum which is being administered at the time when one of the favourable periods of improvement occurs, such as often happens in the disease, gets the credit for improvement, but frequently fails on another occasion. There is no doubt, however, that much can be done in the way of judicious management of the malady. Of all remedies, there is none to compare with rest in bed ; you should advise your patients who have to work for their living to go to bed early during the week and, if possible, to stay in bed on Sundays. In extreme cases ice-bags may be applied to the precordium and to the goitre. A milk dietary is to be preferred to an ordinary one, and where possible faradic and galvanic currents may be applied to the gland and to the neck. Patients who can afford the luxury of quiet travel and residence in high altitudes should be advised to follow this treatment ; of late years residence in Alpine resorts has been reported upon most favourably. Various drugs have been credited with success, such as digitalis, arsenic, nux vomica, iron, belladonna, potassium iodide, and phosphate of soda. Iodine has been injected locally as well as applied externally in the form of lin. potassii iodidi cum sapone, and with beneficial results in some cases. Saline infusion has also been found useful in overcoming the more grave symptoms of intoxication.

Attempts have also been made to treat cases of primary Graves' disease by means of thyroid gland and with thymus, but the results are contradictory ; the serum, milk, and flesh of thyroidectomised animals have also been introduced recently and are on their trial ; use has been made, too, of the serum of animals which have been fed upon thyroid gland or have had preparations of the gland injected subcutaneously, but here, again, it is too early to express an opinion on the value of the remedy. No practical results have been obtained from the use of sera cytolytic against the thyroid gland, for it has been found in this as in other similar sera that the cytolysis is not specific, and leads to the dissolution of the tissues other than the thyroid. The practice of sympathectomy or of exothyropexy has been discontinued by many surgeons ; the statistics of the results following complete or partial thyroidectomy do not encourage such an operation, for the mortality is as much as 10 per cent. or 16 per cent. according to different authors : conservative treatment appears to produce as good results, the mortality amongst such cases being 11·6 per cent. (Buschan). At the hands of certain enthusiasts thyroidectomy has produced much better results ; e.g. Allan Starr has secured 74 cures out of 190 cases, Buschan 51 satisfactory results in 80 cases, Briner 24 successes in 29 cases, and Heydenreich 82 per cent. of cures (Sainton). The uncertainty of avoiding the very tragic fatalities which are known to follow some cases of thyroidectomy for exophthalmic goitre is sufficient to exclude this method of treatment; e.g. sudden death may occur during or shortly after the operation, and tetany, fever, and severe hæmorrhages may occur some time later.

In conclusion, it may be said that the cure of this disorder forms one of the greatest difficulties in practical therapeutics : there are so many remedies that suspicion is at once aroused that the cure has yet to be found. Some good purpose will have been served if this series of cases familiarises you with some of the more important problems associated with the study of this disease, and makes you more acquainted with the very odd ways in which the disease may begin and end.

October 16th, 1905.

THE RELATION BETWEEN CERTAIN PHYSICAL SIGNS AND SYMPTOMS IN "MOVABLE KIDNEY." IN WOMEN.

By VICTOR BONNEY, M.S., M.D., B.Sc.Lond., F.R.C.S.Eng., M.R.C.P.Lond.,
Lecturer on Practical Midwifery, Middlesex Hospital: Physician to Out-Patients, Chelsea Hospital for Women.

In the 'Edinburgh Medical Journal' of December, 1902, I published the results of an examination of the kidneys of 100 consecutive out-patients at the Chelsea Hospital for Women, and I endeavoured to show from those results and from the examination of the cadaver that degree of descent should not in itself be taken as the only standard whereby pathological mobility of the kidney is to be estimated.

I showed that the symptoms associated with pathological, or, as I preferred to call it, "injurious" renal mobility, bore a striking relation to the presence of two signs.

The first and least important of these is absence of "expiratory return"; the second and more important is the rotation of the kidney on an antero-posterior axis, whereby the organ comes to lie obliquely or even transversely across the posterior parieties with its hilum upwards.

Since writing that paper a large number of women have been examined by me, and my opinions on this subject have been greatly strengthened.

The Method of Examination.

I would premise my remarks by restating what I have already laid stress on in the article I have mentioned—namely, the importance of two things in the examination of the kidneys for injurious mobility.

The first of these is, that patients must be examined *in the standing posture*, since the defect is one caused by gravity, and can, therefore, be only properly estimated when that force is allowed to act on the organ ; secondly, that the best method to examine the kidney is by means of the manœuvres collectively termed "*palpation nephroleptique*" by Glenard.

I shall not in this short communication describe this method, as I have already done so in my previous article, but a glance at Fig. 1 will sufficiently indicate its application. How far it applies to men, with their broader loins, I cannot say, as these patients do not come under my observation.

The Normal Support of Pedunculated Organs.

In nature no pedunculated organ is suspended by means of its neuro-vascular pedicle ; that is to say, that there is always some device to prevent abnormal tension upon the nerves and vessels constituting it. Thus, the liver is suspended by the coronary ligament, the ovary by the ovarian and ovarico-pelvic ligaments, the testicle by the

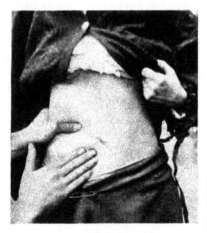

FIG. 1.—"Palpation nephroleptique " in the standing posture.

cremasteric fascia and the other coverings of the cord, and so on. The kidney is no exception to this rule. Its principal support is the perinephric fascia, which passes inwards from the kidney in two layers, one in front of and one behind the renal vessels and nerves which constitute its neuro-vascular pedicle. This fascia is very strong between the kidney and middle line, where it blends with the fascia in front of and behind the aorta. Outwardly it becomes much thinner, blending with the renal capsule and the loose perinephric tissue. Above it is connected with the fascia covering the diaphragm. This fascia supports the kidney after all the other structures

surrounding the organ have been cut away, and it does so in such a way that no tension or supporting function is thrown upon the renal vessels and nerves. If in the cadaver a small hole be made in the anterior layer of the perinephric fascia, the renal vessels be then divided on an aneurysm needle, and the hole sutured up, no increase in the mobility of the kidney is apparent. This fascia, then, maintains the organ in its normal position on the muscles of the posterior parieties and the diaphragm. Relaxation of it is the cause of injurious renal mobility (" movable kidney ") because the kidney then comes to hang by its neuro-vascular pedicle, a condition of things which, when occuring in any pedunculated organ, gives rise to pain invariably. The two physical signs to which I wish to call attention depend upon the relaxation of this fascia.

Loss of Expiratory Return.

As is well known, the kidney has a normal range of mobility over an extent of from 1 to 1½ inches, which is dependent on the movement of the diaphragm. As I have pointed out, this excursion is apt to be exaggerated in women possessing a large extent of diaphragmatic movement ; and it is for this reason that in persons with *post-partum* flaccidity of the abdominal wall the kidney is often (wrongly) held to be injuriously movable, because on account of the lax anterior abdominal parietes the diaphragm is able to descend much lower than normal. But on examining these patients in the upright position, it will be found that the kidney recedes with expiration like a normal organ, and the natural inference that its supports are intact is confirmed by the absence of symptoms in such cases. Indeed, in these patients the kidney often descends during respiration much lower when they are recumbent, because the abdominal wall is then more lax than in the standing posture, and the diaphragmatic excursion consequently greater. The loss of expiratory return, then, is an important sign, pointing to a relaxed condition of the perinephric fascia, which allows the kidney to slip down on the quadratus lumborum muscle off the diaphragm, and, therefore, to be independent of its movement. It is obviously impossible to demonstrate it, except by examination in the standing posture.

Renal Rotation.

There is, however, a second and still more important physical sign which when obtained is, I believe, a certain proof of injurious traction upon the renal pedicle, and that is the oblique or transverse position assumed by the organ in all the worst cases of "injurious" mobility. It must be searched for with the patient in the standing position, and it is here that the method of "palpation nephroleptique" has such advantages over the ordinary bimanual method, since it permits of a much more thorough examination to be made of the organ. My practice is to pass the kidney backwards and forwards underneath my thumb by

apparent; inward rotation of its lower pole is resisted by the very dense and strong perinephric fascia, which, passing behind and in front of the renal vessels, anchors the kidney in its normal position. Division of all the tissues above and below the organ does not make the artificial production of this displacement possible. To effect it, it is necessary to divide the perinephric fascia in front of the renal vessels, and if after this the kidney be forcibly pushed down into the loin, the displacement at once occurs. The further you push the organ downwards, the more its inner pole rotates inwards until its long axis comes to lie more or less horizontal, and the same result occurs if, instead of pushing the kidney, you elevate the

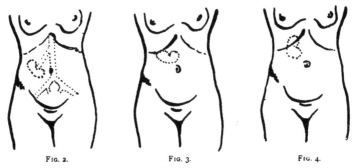

Fig. 2.   Fig. 3.   Fig. 4.

Fig. 2.—Illustrating the occurrence of "renal rotation"
Fig. 3.—Illustrates the right kidney lying *transversely* under the costal margin.
Fig. 4 shows the right kidney in the position often assumed normally in full inspiration.

Note that the abnormal organ in Fig 3 descends no lower than the normal organ in Fig. 4.

means of the hand not engaged in compressing the loin. The direction in which the long axis of the kidney lies as it passes under one's thumb is then very readily appreciated. In many cases, of course, the contour of the organ can be easily defined with the lower hand alone, and this manœuvre is then not required, but it is useful in fat patients.

The Anatomical Explanation.

If in the cadaver one attempts to thus displace the kidney, it will be found to be impossible. I have tried it many times, and never succeeded, except once, and that patient almost certainly had had during life a movable kidney. The reason that you cannot thus displace the organ is very

cadaver into the upright position. On examining the parts to see what compels this movement, it is obviously the traction exerted by the kidney on its neuro-vascular pedicle, which causes the organ as it descends to rotate round the circumference of a circle of which the renal vessels are the radius (Fig. 2). The discovery of this inward displacement of the lower pole of the kidney in a case of suspected injurious mobility is, I believe, an absolute sign that the organ is being suspended in a manner which is grossly abnormal, and against the occurrence of which Nature, as we have seen, has guarded all the pedunculated organs of the body.

It is often said that many or all of the symptoms in a case of "movable kidney" are neurotic in origin, and there is no doubt that in certain persons a hypersensitive condition is induced thereby. But when one considers that the anatomical condition which exists in these patients causes an unnatural tension on a structure containing many nerves, one must admit, I think, that the basis of their aches and pains is very real indeed.

A kidney exhibiting rotation always exhibits loss of expiratory return as well, but loss of expiratory return often exists without rotation.

Probably the relaxation of the perinephric fascia at first simply allows the kidney to slide down off the diaphragm, but without permitting of abnormal tension on its neuro-vascular pedicle. At a later date the stretching of the fascia causes the organ to be arrested in its descent by this pedicle itself with its contained vessels and nerves.

I analysed in my previous paper the relation that symptoms bore to these two physical signs; and I found that whereas in cases exhibiting lost expiratory return alone symptoms were absent or slight, in those in which renal rotation existed as well symptoms, often severe, were always present.

Since then I have examined, as I have said, a large number of fresh cases, and my earlier results have been absolutely confirmed.

It should be remembered that the statements of out-patients are very unreliable, especially on their first visit, and that they often omit to mention or even deny symptoms of which at a later date they may be most communicative, and for that reason it is wise to postpone an estimation of the relation of symptoms to physical signs until they have been seen several times.

"Movable Kidney" without Abnormal Range of Descent.

There is a further point to which I would strongly call attention. I have within the last two years had some half-dozen cases, in which the kidney was lying transversely, immediately under the costal margin; all these cases exhibited the typical backache and frequency of micturition which are the earliest signs of injurious mobility (Fig. 3). Such cases are probably accounted for by abnormal shortness of the renal vessels, which results in their being dragged upon sooner than they otherwise would be when the perinephric fascia becomes stretched.

Now, if the question of pathological mobility had been decided upon by mere extent of descent, then none of these cases would have been diagnosed as "movable kidney," and their symptoms would

have been attributed to some other organ, or to neurosis (Figs. 3 and 4).

It is possible that some of the obscure pains complained of in the region of the kidneys may be due to a kidney lying transversely above the costal margin, and therefore not detectable. The importance, then, of "renal rotation" is manifest, and that its occurrence may be looked upon as a much greater abnormality than unusual extent of descent both anatomical considerations and post-mortem experiment demonstrate.

When found in a patient detailing symptoms possibly referable to the kidney, it most strongly suggests that such symptoms are of renal origin, and is an indication for nephropexy.

The backache complained of by these women strongly suggests both to the medical and lay mind some pelvic disorder, and gynæcological operations are not infrequently undertaken for their relief.

In cases where abnormal renal mobility and uterine displacement are present in the same patient the presence or absence of the signs I have detailed will assist in making the diagnosis (often not easy) as to which organ these symptoms may be due, and consequently in determining our curative measures.

October 16th, 1905.

The Hæmorrhagic Form of Cirrhosis of the Liver.—v. Aldor groups under this name those cases of hepatic cirrhosis in which the most prominent symptom is recurrent hæmorrhage appearing in the preascitic stage. In two of the cases reported by the writer the bleeding proceeded from the stomach, in a third from the intestine, in the fourth from the nose. A hepatic and a splenic tumour were present in all the cases, but the symptoms of the later stages of cirrhosis—ascites, diarrhœa, meteorismus — were lacking. The hæmorrhages appeared without premonitory symptoms, or were preceded by mild digestive disturbances. The amount of blood lost may be sufficient to cause exitus, or, as in v. Aldor's intestinal case, small amounts of blood may be constantly present in the fæces. A rapid recovery after the hæmorrhage is characteristic, but a high grade of anæmia persists. Owing to the obstruction in the liver a collateral circulation is established between the portal system and the vena cava inferior through the œsophageal and gastric vessels. These vessels are in a varicose condition, and the sudden hæmorrhage is due to rupture of such a varix. In the intestinal hæmorrhage the blood probably proceeded from a hæmorrhagic erosion following inflammation and neurosis. The anatomical lesions are identical with those in the ordinary form of cirrhosis and in the so-called Banti's disease. v. Aldor believes it not impossible that his cases may be a form of the latter.— *Medical Record*, vol. lxviii, No. 13.

THE CLINICAL JOURNAL,

CLINICAL RECORD, CLINICAL NEWS, CLINICAL GAZETTE, CLINICAL REPORTER,
CLINICAL CHRONICLE AND CLINICAL REVIEW.

EDITED BY L. ELIOT CREASY.

No. 678.   WEDNESDAY, OCTOBER 25, 1905.   Vol. XXVII.   No. 2.

CONTENTS.

* Specially reported for the Clinical Journal. Revised by the Author.

ALL RIGHTS RESERVED.

NOTICE.

Editorial correspondence, books for review, &c., should be addressed to the Editor, 51, New Cavendish Street, W., Telephone No. 904, Paddington ; but all business communications should be addressed to the Publishers, 22½, Bartholomew Close, London, E.C. Telephone 927, Holborn.

All inquiries respecting Advertisements should be sent to MESSRS. ADLARD & SON, Bartholomew Close, E.C. Telephone 927, Holborn.

Terms of Subscription, including postage, payable by cheque, postal or banker's order (in advance) : for the United Kingdom, 15s. 6d. per annum; Abroad, 17s. 6d.

Cheques, &c., should be made payable to THE PROPRIETORS OF THE CLINICAL JOURNAL, crossed " The London, City, and Midland Bank, Ltd., Newgate Street Branch, E.C. Account of the Medical Publishing Company, Limited."

Reading Cases to hold Twenty-six numbers of THE CLINICAL JOURNAL can be supplied at 2s. 3d. each, or will be forwarded post free on receipt of 2s. 6d. ; and also Cases for binding Volumes at 1s. each, or post free on receipt of 1s. 3d., from the Publishers, 22½ Bartholomew Close, London, E.C.

A LECTURE

ON

FLOATING KIDNEY AND ITS SURGICAL TREATMENT.*

By J. HUTCHINSON, Junr., F.R.C.S.,
Surgeon to the London Hospital.

GENTLEMEN,—There were recently, and I have no doubt there exist still, a Society and a Journal in Germany devoted to the study of subjects which lie on the borderland between medicine and surgery. The subject now to be discussed is eminently one of that kind, one in connection with which strong differences of opinion may be found between surgeons and physicians. First, attention should be called to the views held by some prominent physicians in their writings with regard to floating kidney, views which a surgeon may hold require modification. Dr. J. F. Goodhart, than whom one could quote no keener observer and higher authority, fully discussed in 1891 the subject of floating kidney in his Harveian Lectures (on Common Neuroses). He declared that all the subjects of floating kidney, whether male or female, were of neuropathic or neurotic disposition. He urged that the surgeon who undertook to treat a floating kidney by operation with the idea of curing the symptoms that attended it was foolish, to say the least of it. Another authority, Sir James Sawyer, who has written much about floating kidney, sums up by stating that the diagnosis of floating kidney is important only because you can assure the patient that she has a trivial complaint and need take little or no notice of it. So shrewd and accurate a teacher as the late Sir William Roberts held very much the same view and expressed it in his book on ' Diseases of the Kidneys.' He did not even mention surgical interference, but wrote

* Delivered at the Medical Graduates' College and Polyclinic.

that you might if you liked apply a belt, and that such an appliance was sometimes useful. Although he admitted the condition of floating kidney was occasionally accompanied by serious symptoms and led to pathological changes in the organ itself, he regarded it on the whole as a matter of little importance.

I venture to think, gentlemen, that surgeons have largely modified these views. To assure a patient with marked symptoms due to floating kidney that she is suffering from a condition of no importance is but cold comfort. Suppose that you or I had a condition which prevented our taking active exercise, which caused symptoms which in their severity and kind were like those of gastric ulcer (for which indeed the condition has been frequently mistaken), which was characterised by paroxysmal attacks of abdominal pain, and which sometimes led to serious changes in an important organ, if we were told by our physician that it was a matter of no significance, we should consider that such an opinion was almost an insult.

It is, of course, necessary to discriminate. The term "movable kidney" means very little if taken in the ordinary literal sense, for slight up and down movement is normal with respiration, and even much more vertical displacement is of no practical importance since it causes no symptoms. But when a kidney really "floats" it comes forward amongst the intestines, its lower end often touching the anterior abdominal wall. A "floating kidney" therefore is one which can wholly leave the lumbar regions at times. Sir William Jenner, and others following him have attempted to confine the term to those cases in which there is a mesonephron—i. e. in which both surfaces of the kidney are covered with peritoneum. Out of forty cases of nephrorrhaphy I have only once come across a kidney in which there was a true mesonephron. How rare it is may be judged from the fact that Dr. Newman of Glasgow, who has had much experience of kidney work, lately published "An Unique Case of Nephrorrhaphy for Floating Kidney," unique because there was a mesonephron. What is the use of limiting a term which has been widely used such as "floating kidney" to the almost unique cases, which can moreover only be distinguished in the course of an operation? A floating kidney, then, is one which falls forwards or floats in the abdomen, a satisfactory and simple definition, which has the

support of Mr. Henry Morris. A few words may be given to the problem of the frequency of the condition on the right side of the body. In 80 per cent. of the cases it is the right kidney alone which floats, in ten per cent. the left one only, and in ten both organs. (I have operated on one case of floating horse-shoe kidney, a particularly rare and interesting condition. I fixed the right half of the single kidney in place, thinking this would suffice. The operation entirely relieved the patient's symptoms so far as the right side was concerned, but three years later she came up again for increased trouble on the left side which was cured by operation on the corresponding half of the kidney.)

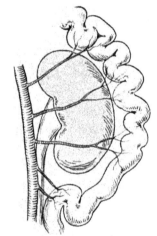

Fig. 1.—The left kidney and ureter in a fœtus at nine months.

The problem has been much discussed and various reasons assigned. That it is due to "the liver pushing down the right kidney" seems unreasonable. Mr. Lane ('Brit. Med. Journ.,' April 1, 1905) attributes it to the effects of constipation, the distended colon causing a greater drag on the right than on the left kidney. I incline to attribute it partly to the different anatomical relations between colon and kidney on the two sides. These are illustrated best by dissections on a fœtus of nine months (Figs. 1 and 2). It is of interest to note that a floating right kidney has occasionally been observed in childhood.

The splenic flexure lies at the top of the kidney, the descending colon astride it ; both are firmly anchored by peritoneum. The mesocolon and branches of the inferior mesenteric cross the kidney and keep it in position.

On the right side the cæcum lies just below the kidney and at first the ascending colon runs to the inner side. Although the colon subsequently lies more in front of the kidney, the hepatic flexure never anchors it in the way the splenic flexure does the left kidney.

On the front of the left kidney, especially fixing its lower half, is the "fascia of Toldt," which is supposed to be formed from fusion of two layers of peritoneum originally belonging to the descend-

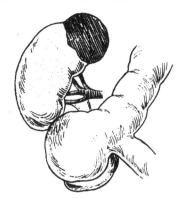

Fɪɢ. 2.—The right kidney and supra-renal capsule.

ing colon. On the right side there is no corresponding fascia. It will be seen from the foregoing that there are developmental reasons why the right kidney is loosely secured to the posterior abdominal wall, and why the left kidney is more fixed. In adult life additional causes account for the floating condition, such as repeated pregnancies, abdominal strain, and the rapid absorption of peri-renal fat.

Turning now to the various symptoms which may attend floating kidney, we note that the organ is provided with nerves which differ from the ordinary sensory nerves of the skin. Whilst incapable of appreciating slight tactile stimulation, the kidney, like other viscera, will be sensitive to coarse or rough stimuli such as sudden change of

position, or vascular tension, compression and the like. The pain felt will be imperfectly localised and is apt to be referred to the peripheral distribution of the spinal nerves giving branches to the renal plexus. Dr. Henry Head's recent researches throw an interesting light upon the symptoms of such a condition as floating kidney, confirming the view that the nerve symptoms attending it have a real physical basis and that they are to be relieved by correcting the latter.

To illustrate it we may refer to one of the grave complications described, namely, that of torsion of the pedicle of the kidney, which is sometimes referred to as strangulation. You know that in floating kidney the renal vessels become greatly elongated. The right renal vein is only a couple of inches long normally, but yet the kidney often travels six inches out of its ordinary place ; therefore, this vein must stretch two to three times its normal length, and the artery with the abundant sympathetic plexus around it must undergo a similar degree of elongation. This elongation being gradual, as a rule, may not be of much more importance than the extraordinary elongation of the spermatic vessels, for instance, in varicocele, or the tortuosity of varicose veins of the leg. Still, it is a point to remember. In cases where there are attacks of very severe lumbar pain with temporary anuria followed by hæmaturia, attacks which are known as strangulation or incarceration of a floating kidney, the view is held that the whole pedicle gets twisted on itself. That is, no doubt, correct, but one must not imagine it is anything like that which occurs in twisting of an ovarian pedicle. I have operated upon many cases of twisted ovarian pedicle, and in nearly all of them the twist was at least two or three times upon itself—that is to say, it was twisted through first one complete circle, and then another (i. e. 720 degrees). The result of this is, of course, that the circulation is absolutely stopped. The same extreme degree of torsion cannot possibly occur in "strangulation of the floating kidney." In true floating kidney the lower end comes forward and is generally situated just beneath the liver, sometimes opposite the umbilicus, or even down in the iliac fossa. In either case the lower end projects forwards in front of the ureter. This relation is, I think, invariable, for I have not been able to find any case recorded where, in an operation or dissection, the ureter was seen in front of the lower end of the floating kidney. The axis of the kidney, instead of being vertical, becomes roughly horizontal (see Fig. 3.) The ureter obviously tends to be kinked, instead of running straight down, but there is no chance of the twisting of the vessels two or three times as there is in cases of ovarian cyst. There may be a rotation of the renal vessels through an angle of 90°, but that is all, and such rotation is unlikely to do more than temporarily impede the renal circulation. The symptoms may, no doubt, be accounted for in another way. Whilst there is a twist of a quarter of a circle with regard to these vessels the ureter may be obstructed by kinking or it may be bent sharply over an aberrant inferior

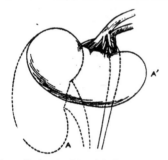

Fig. 3.—To show the tilting of the floating kidney, the lower end of which (A) becomes anterior (A'). The ureter, passing behind this end, is liable to be kinked. The simultaneous descent of the organ is not shown.

renal artery, as Dr. Newton Pitt actually verified in a post-mortem examination. "Strangulation of the kidney" by torsion of the pedicle is comparatively rare, and is one of the most severe accidents that can happen to the organ when floating. Probably its chief feature is a temporary obstruction to the ureter which leads to backward pressure, temporary anuria, and may if repeated produce intermittent nephritis or hydro-nephrosis. There may be albuminuria for several days after the attack. Secondly, attention may be drawn to the close connection that exists between the renal plexus of sympathetic nerves and the solar plexus—in other words, the nerves of the kidney and those of the stomach. The last dorsal nerve gives an important branch to the renal plexus, and the same nerve also gives branches to the cutaneous supply over

the iliac crest, the buttocks, and the great trochanter. Hence the fact that pain connected with floating kidney is often referred over the iliac crest ; indeed, it may be referred to almost any branch of the lumbar plexus. Just as the pains of renal calculus may be experienced in the heel, so the pain of floating kidney is sometimes felt low down in the leg as well as round the abdomen. The pain may be referred, again, to the lower inter-

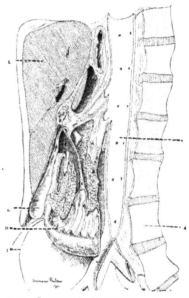

FIG. 4 —Section made obliquely downwards in a subject with nephro- and hepato-ptosis, to show the displacement of the duodenum and sharp bend of the bile-ducts L, The liver ; A, the aorta slit open ; G, the gall-bladder ; I, iliac bone ; D, duodenum ; 4, the fourth lumbar vertebra.

costal nerves which communicate with the renal plexus. And the fact that the renal plexus may be considerably dragged upon every time the floating kidney comes forward explains to some extent the reflex vomiting which is such a marked symptom in certain cases of floating kidney. Thirdly, of considerable importance is the relation of the floating kidney to the duodenum and to the biliary passages, the common bile-duct, and the gall-bladder. Undoubtedly in many cases of floating kidney this organ and the liver have first been displaced downwards by corset-pressure. Fig. 4 is taken from a case where the kidney had been forced down with the liver, so that the latter touched the iliac crest, entirely concealing the intestines or forcing them down below into the pelvis, and the top of the kidney was below the tip of the last rib. The specimen, which was prepared by Dr. Arthur Keith, is in the London Hospital Museum. It will be seen that the gall-bladder formed with the ducts an angle of only about 30 degrees. So the mere vertical displacement of the kidney and liver (nephro- and hepato-ptosis) may interfere with the escape of the bile. This, however, refers simply to the downward displacement of the kidney, and not to the true floating condition. But in a forward tilting of the floating kidney there is another explanation—that it displaces the vertical part of the duodenum, or presses on it, and thus interferes with the escape of bile. In not a few cases of floating kidney symptoms exist of supposed biliary obstruction. I have now operated on at least six cases of this kind, all of which were referred to me by the physicians as either gall-stones or cholecystitis. Sir Frederick Treves has published instances, and several others, including Dr. Habershon, have drawn attention to it. Probably a good many patients vainly seek relief at Carlsbad for symptoms of stomach or biliary trouble which are really due to the existence of a floating kidney, which "a course of the waters" can hardly be expected to cure. Floating kidney may possibly so interfere with the escape of bile as to cause gall-stones, or it may lead indirectly to cholecystitis. In one of the cases operated on I found that the gall-badder had been inflamed and the cavity almost obliterated by thickening of its wall ; in two there were a few gall-stones. It should be noted that in these cases of biliary obstruction due to floating kidney the jaundice is never of a high grade. There have been several cases in which intermittent hydronephrosis has been ascribed to the floating condition of the kidney, and it is at least suspicious that hydronephrosis is many times more frequent in women than it is in men. On the other hand, if it were a frequent cause, one would expect to find that hydronephrosis is much commoner on the right side than on the left ; this, however, is not the case. The great majority of cases of hydronephrosis are due to pressure on or stricture of the ureter, and have nothing to do with floating kidney.

An interesting case was sent to me by Dr. Colmer of Yeovil. He had diagnosed a floating right kidney, but said it was something more, that it was a tumour of the kidney as well ; and so it proved to be. On operating from in front I found a floating kidney, the lower half of which was greatly enlarged and converted into multiple cysts, with a collection of yellow fluid in the cystic part, the upper part being healthy. This was, no doubt, a congenital condition. I excised the lower half of the kidney, fixing the upper half, which was absolutely healthy, by some stitches at the back. The wounds healed perfectly well without any urinary fistula. The wound made in the kidney was wedge-shaped, and the edges of it were carefully sutured.

With regard to the gastric symptoms, which are of importance, a case was brought before the annual meeting of the British Medical Association about two years ago, in which fatal obstruction of the pylorus had been produced by the dragging of a floating kidney on the peritoneal band which goes from the gastro-hepatic omentum down in front of the first part of the duodenum ; a sort of adventitious band of peritoneum seemed to have been formed and the patient had obstruction from pressure on the duodenum, the stomach became enormously dilated, and the patient ultimately died, the cause not having been detected. This is one of the few cases of death from floating kidney recorded, the possible occurrence of which is denied in most books.

To take the more usual cases, it may fairly be said that the gastric symptoms due to or associated with floating kidney are readily mistaken for those of chronic ulcer of the stomach. In the case of a lady upon whom I operated gastric ulcer had been diagnosed by a first-rate physician, who had gone carefully into the case, and it was a question whether the stomach should be operated upon or not. However, floating kidney was fortunately detected, and she has been entirely cured of her gastric symptoms. It is not improbable that gastro-jejunostomy has been occasionally performed for the relief of symptoms really caused by floating kidney.

Other symptoms are described, of more doubtful nature. A recent work on medicine describes cardiac neuralgia and cardiac palpitation as frequent reflex symptoms of floating kidney. One may doubt the connection between floating kidney and cardiac neuralgia and palpitation, except a very indirect one such as a general feeling of ill-health.

As to the engorgement and swelling of a floating kidney at each menstrual period which is supposed to have been observed by the late Sir William Roberts, and others, I am entirely sceptical.

Our credulity is also tested with regard to the treatment of floating kidney. You may have noticed an advertisement of a company calling itself by a well-known and a very taking name. They undertake to treat floating kidney by a small pad, which is applied with a belt, and they say that without the slightest difficulty floating kidney can be kept in its place by its means. I have seen that pad; it is a small thing about three inches by two inches. It might make an indentation in the skin if it were fixed on very tightly, but I cannot imagine it doing anything else. They say " the support retains the kidneys in their natural position without injury or troublesome pressure, and with immediate cessation of pain. All that is necessary is for the sufferer to state if the displacement is on both sides or on only one." Now, that apparatus pretends to do what a vigorous and skilful assistant in the operating theatre may find considerable difficulty in effecting whilst the patient is under an anæsthetic. Of course the contention of the above Company is merely childish. Some members of our own profession are also guilty of exaggeration in this matter. I read lately a long paper written by a Scotch physician which affirmed that he cured every case of floating kidney by means of a large lead pad—it must be pure lead—placed in front of the abdomen and retained there by a belt. There is an example of "scientific" imagination. Another physician published in the 'Lancet' not long ago five cases of floating kidney cured by massage and the wearing of a belt, combined with slight exercise. He laid especial stress on the massage. That reminds one of Sir Frederick Treves' story, who once came across a vigorous-handed nurse endeavouring to massage a floating kidney along the colon under the impression that it was impacted fæces; she was chagrined at her failure. We cannot expect massage to be of much value in cases of floating kidney. We may

also frankly admit that of all the surgical apparatus for the replacement and fixation of floating kidney, there is hardly one that truly answers the purpose for which it was devised.

I have seen several instances in which such apparatus with levers and springs and pads for pressing the kidney back into the loin have been applied, and in which the result has been complete failure. It should be noted, however, that Mr. Ernst has made for Sir Frederick Treves a very light and simple form of truss which seems to have had far more success in cases of floating kidney than previous experience of similar devices would have led one to expect (see ' Practitioner,' vol. lxxiv, p. 1). That a freely floating kidney can be restored to and retained in its normal lumbar position by means of this truss may be questioned, but that it relieves the symptoms in many cases is undoubted. But just as a radical cure of a hernia is often done to prevent the necessity for wearing a truss, so nephrorrhaphy could be justified on similar grounds.

To refer now in a spirit of due respect to one or two strange methods of treating floating kidney by operation. " Senn's method " consists in exposing the kidney very freely by a lumbar wound, clearing it on both surfaces, passing two large bands of iodoform gauze around it, and leaving these bands, which sling the kidney back, with their ends coming out of the wound. The patient is kept in bed four weeks, and the band of gauze is removed at the end of the third week. The method was only published two or three years ago, so one may fairly quote it as modern. It has, I believe, been frequently followed in this country as well as in the United States. The idea is to fix the kidney in place by a firm scar all round the organ. This implies, of course, healing by granulation, which is closely related to suppuration. You can hardly get healing by granulation without suppuration. Would you have an organ of such importance as the kidney fixed by any method which implied free suppuration round it? The question answers itself. Moreover, I do not believe that keeping the gauze there for twice three weeks would fix the majority of such kidneys. The method therefore seems to me awkward, risky, and probably inefficient.

There is another method which is amusing. Importance is attached to the capsule of the kidney in the matter of fixation, and it was recommended by one surgeon that the capsule should be divided into a series of eight or ten little ribbons, each of them to be tied to a silk thread, and each of these threads was to be brought through the muscles and so secured. If some of these ten little ribbons gave way, of course others would be left. The description of this method is not quoted from a book of fairy tales, but from the ' Clinical Society's Transactions.' More recently methods have been published which rely solely on a single flap of kidney capsule brought through the muscles. One feels that much ingenuity has been wasted in surgery, and that some methods of treatment recommended ought to be carefully held back for a few years before publication.

In nephrorrhaphy or nephropexy we aim at restor-

exposed and cleared over the whole of its posterior surfaces, working round its outer edge on to the anterior surface. This exposure extends to the capsule, which need not be divided. Four or five kangaroo tendon sutures are then passed, traversing the capsule and the cortex and also through the muscles forming the abdominal wall in that position. This will be understood by reference to Fig. 5. The stitch traverses the abdominal muscles, goes into the cortex as near the outer border as possible, passes out towards the inner border, through the muscle again, and four or five of them are applied but not tied until they are all in place. The ends of each suture are held in a pair of Wells' forceps until they are ready to be tied. By gentle trac-

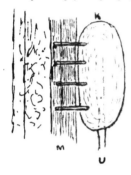

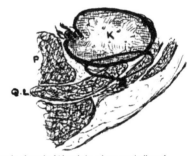

Fig. 5.—Diagrammatic representation of the tendon sutures in place, the kidney being shown vertically and in transverse section. K, the kidney; M, muscles of lumbar region; Q.L., quadratus lumborum; P, psoas.

ing the kidney to its original position as nearly as possible ; but its exact level cannot matter much so long as it is well fixed to the posterior abdominal wall. It is almost impossible to give it as high a position as it occupies in many subjects with the upper half of the organ above the last rib. The important thing is to prevent the possibility of the true dislocation forwards, the real floating condition. '

In performing nephrorrhaphy, an oblique incision is made from the angle of the last rib and the erector spinæ, downwards and forwards towards the iliac crest, going through all the muscles. The aponeurosis of the transversalis is easily recognised and divided, then the transversalis fascia. The ascending colon is often in the way, and should be drawn outwards ; the kidney is then thoroughly

tion on these stitches you can ascertain that the posterior surface of the kidney is held evenly in contact with the muscles by their means. The highest of the three or four stitches is near the summit of the organ, the second and third about the centre, the lowest at the lower end of the kidney (see Fig. 5). With ordinary care there is no risk of passing any of the sutures near the calyces. I always use an ordinary curved needle with an ordinary holder, as there is no necessity for any special form of holder. Care should be taken to avoid including either of the lumbar nerves in the grasp of the sutures, which may well be tied after the patient has been moved towards the supine position. The hæmorrhage varies considerably ; it is chiefly venous, oozing from the points of suture in the kidney. It will be found that the cortex of the kidney and the capsule give a very good hold for the sutures, though it is possible to tie these too tightly. It is unnecessary to use any drain. The patient is kept on her back for a fortnight or three weeks. Perhaps one is apt to overdo the time of confinement in bed. I have always employed kangaroo tendon, fairly stout, for the sutures, and I attach the greatest importance to the use of this material for the reason that the use of stout silk is almost certain to result in sinuses and its ultimate elimination. In fact, the employment of silk has brought the operation into discredit. Kangaroo tendon, how-ever, hardly ever works out; it is in every way as good as human tendon (from the erector spinæ), which has been advised for use in this particular operation. Indeed, I think it is a good deal better. I have had occasion twice to dissect down on to kidneys which I had fixed by kangaroo tendon two and four years previously, and both times I found the tendon stitches practically as they were put in, forming a white fibrous band. Many surgeons have the idea that kangaroo tendon when aseptic and buried in the tissues is absorbed in two or three weeks. This false idea can only arise from complete want of experience in the use of the tendon.

In nearly all the cases of nephrorrhaphy the patient complains of considerable pain during two or three days succeeding the operation. Back pain is of common occurrence after any abdominal operation, but it is especially noticed after nephrorrhaphy and its cause is difficult to explain. It is certainly not due to nipping of any important nerve within the sutures, and the sensitiveness of the kidney is exceedingly slight. It occurs when the wound heals perfectly; in fact, it disappears before many days have elapsed. There is hardly ever the slightest leakage of urine through the wound, and hæmaturia is practically never met with. It is interesting to note that these thick tendon sutures may be passed through the cortex of the kidney without producing temporary albuminuria or any other disturbance of function.

I have had two examples of suppuration of the wound in a long series of nephrorrhaphy cases. One of them occurred recently; I could not discover any cause for it. It may have been an accidental inoculation with one's fingers, or it may have been a case of infection through the urine itself; but I regard this last suggestion in the light of a handy excuse. The suppuration entirely ceased in a fort-night, the tendon sutures did not come away (as silk would certainly have done), and the patient left the hospital at the end of three weeks none the worse, the kidney being certainly fixed. The other case was more protracted and serious, but the patient was extremely neurotic, and the anæsthetic seemed to throw her completely off her balance. She became one of the most troublesome persons I have ever had to deal with. She tore the dressings off the first night, and was, indeed, maniacal for a time. You know the type of " strong-minded " woman, who surprises you after an operation by the most outrageous behaviour. I had also, on another occasion, to operate on her gall-bladder. She was one of those patients who combine floating kidney and gall-stones (with cholecystitis). She behaved as badly after the gall-bladder operation as she did after the kidney one. I have seen her several times since during the last few years, and am glad to say she is now in very fair health. She has got back to household work after being a chronic invalid before the operations, but is still neurotic. I doubt if she will ever be wholly free from discom fort in some part of her body.

It is useless to contend that nephrorrhaphy always results in a cure. Every surgeon admits that in some of his cases the operation proves a failure. The proportion of failures in selected cases is about 20 to 30 per cent. (in this I am quoting M. Tuffier, with whose experience my own agrees) ; that is to say, in every ten cases of true floating kidney nephrorrhaphy will probably succeed in curing or much relieving the symptoms in eight, in two the operation apparently does no good. In some of these instances the failure is probably due to imper-fect methods of fixation. In some it is due to the patient violently wrenching the loin, as happened in one of my cases, the patient six months after the operation falling from a ladder to the floor ; the symptoms relapsed from that day. Probably at the time of the accident the kidney was wrenched away from its attachment. Neither explanation accounts for every instance of failure to relieve. Those patients in whom the abdomen is pendulous and there is marked enteroptosis should, as a rule, not be operated on, however floating their kidney may be. This, at any rate, is the dictum of many writers.

But I suggest that we possibly exaggerate the importance of displacement of intestines or stomach. It is only the solid viscera which, as a rule, give trouble when they get loose from their moorings. I have seen, for example, a patient whose stomach was so displaced that the pylorus habitually touched the right anterior superior spine of the ilium. I came across this extreme displacement accidentally in a case in which there was pyloric cancer, for which I performed gastro-jejunostomy. But though the pylorus had evidently been displaced for long, her gastric symptoms were quite recent. The transverse colon is often found down by the pubes, and yet this does not seem to cause any trouble. As a general rule where there is enteroptosis with floating kidney it is advisable to order an abdominal belt and not to operate. But now and then in cases where the indications for operation seem clear the result is disappointing, for no reason that we can ascertain. I will quote two of my own. One was that of a young woman who had been under one hospital physician after another for the relief of abdominal pain, one-sided and coming on after the least exertion. I found that the patient had a floating right kidney, which had not, apparently, been detected previously. I thought we had found the cause of all her trouble, and performed nephrorrhaphy. The kidney was undoubtedly fixed, but I received a letter three months afterwards from her mother inviting me to attend her daughter in a distant suburb, because since the day she left the hospital she "had been queer in her head," that she was sure the stitches which had been put into the abdomen were doing harm, and would I come and take them out. It is hardly necessary to say that no further operation was performed.

The physician's view is, of course, right, that many of the subjects of floating kidney are abnormally neurotic ; but with sufficient cause (acting for a sufficient time) we should all be neurotic. If we suffered from a condition which prevents healthy exercise, hinders digestion, causes vague abdominal discomfort, with frequent attacks of spasmodic pain, which of us would not be neurotic? Yet genuine floating kidney is just such a condition, and it is reasonable to suppose that if such cases were treated early and the kidney properly fixed these patients would be cured and prevented from developing the neurotic habit.

Another case I quote as an instance of failure was that of a man who undoubtedly had floating kidney. His chief symptoms were attacks of pain in the right loin and the front of the abdomen. These attacks were always worse during exercise and greatly hindered him in doing his work. He did not look neurotic ; he was quiet and almost sullen in his answers, there was every inducement for him to keep at work, and no reason for malingering. I found a floating kidney, which did undoubtedly come forwards at times, and I fixed it in the loin. He was sent to me as a renal calculus case. I examined the kidney at the time of operation but could find no calculus (this was before the X rays were introduced.) He was relieved by the operation for a time but afterwards the symptoms returned as badly as before. He was convinced that the kidney had got loose again. He was not a thin patient, and therefore not easy to examine in this respect. It seemed advisable to have the kidney explored again. I accordingly cut down, and found it securely fixed in position. He was no better after the second operation, he went to several other surgeons, and ultimately settled down in the Middlesex Hospital, where the surgeon said the whole trouble was due to the vermiform appendix. He removed this organ and told the man he would be cured. So far from being that, he expressed himself as in no way relieved. He came back to me and we had him radiographed very carefully. There was no stone. His pain (which had now lasted three years) was worse than ever. It was chiefly lumbar, and he asked to have that kidney removed. This, however, I absolutely refused to do. The case remains unsolved, though it may conceivably be one of latent gall-stones. Cases like this may now and then discomfort and discredit any surgeon.

One word in conclusion. It is by no means always easy to diagnose a floating kidney. Increasing experience only leads to a more frank recognition of this fact. The misplaced organ often lies just under the liver in the position of a distended gall-bladder, it often causes "biliary symptoms", it may suggest a pyloric tumour and cause the symptoms of pyloric obstruction. As Prof. Rose Bradford observes ('Brit. Med. Journal,' June 10, 1905), "Strange as it may seem, movable kidney is often confounded with new growth."

Above all, it should be remembered that a floating kidney does not constantly float. In several cases I have known the organ to be back in the loin one day when no effort could induce it to come forwards, whilst on another occasion it was found freely floating under the anterior abdominal wall. Repeated examination is essential in a doubtful case.

The chief points which I have endeavoured to make clear are the following :

(1) The important symptoms which floating kidney may produce, symptoms having a real physical explanation, of which interference with the gastric and hepatic functions are especially noteworthy.

(2) That the "neurotic condition" which is so often found in the subjects of floating kidney is largely the result of such symptoms long continued, and is to be avoided in many cases by early fixation of the organ.

· (3) That whilst a truss or belt pressure may undoubtedly suffice in slight cases, nephrorrhaphy is the most certain method of treatment.

(4) That nephrorrhaphy is superior to "Senn's gauze method," being safer, more effectual, and involving a shorter period of convalescence.

(5) That kangaroo tendon is admirably adapted for nephrorrhaphy, the use of silk being attended with the risk of causing tedious sinuses.

October 23rd, 1905.

Influence of Alkalies on Degree of Acidity of Urine in Anæmia.

—Sodium citrate and sodium bicarbonate are able to render the urine alkaline in anæmia. In some instances, however, especially in cases in which there is enlargement of the liver, this alkalinising action is retarded for several days. On suspension of the alkali the urine becomes excessively acid, with increased secretion of ammonia and oxalic acid. Anæmias without enlargement of the liver are accompanied by normal relations between the nitrogenised elements.—*Jour. A.M.A.*, vol. xlv, No. 12.

BORACIC acid is the most practical urinary preservative that we possess when used in the proportion of five grains to four ounces of urine. Formaldehyde should be used only by a responsible person. One drop of the solution will preserve a pint of urine for about a week.— *Monthly Cyclopædia*, vol. viii, No. 8.

WITH DR. G. A. SUTHERLAND AT THE PADDINGTON GREEN CHILDREN'S HOSPITAL.

LOBAR PNEUMONIA IN CHILDHOOD.

LOBAR ór croupous pneumonia is one and the same disease in early years and in adult life, and yet the clinical manifestations are in many respects very different. In order to obtain a correct impression of the clinical course and symptoms one must study pure pneumonia—that is to say, uncomplicated attacks of the disease in previously healthy patients. Fortunately, these are not particularly rare, and possibly the virgin soil of childhood is, in some respects, better suited for this study than that of adult life, furrowed by former habits and diseases.

CLINICAL SIGNS AND SYMPTOMS.

In the early stages the diagnosis is by no means always easy, and yet I believe if we carefully studied the history of the onset and the appearance of the patient, and were not in such a hurry to make a physical examination of the chest, we should more easily and more frequently arrive at a correct conclusion. Especially is this the case in infants ; for an infant lying quietly in its mother's arms may show definite and unmistakable signs of pneumonia, while the same infant after being undressed may be such a terrified, shrieking, kicking mass of humanity that one can learn nothing. While a physical examination may be useful to ascertain the exact condition of the lungs, we shall probably learn more, as our fathers used to do, before proceeding to auscultation and percussion. Lobar pneumonia begins as well as ends with a crisis. The sudden onset, with the development of acute symptoms, is quite as striking as the sudden termination, with the cessation of acute symptoms. A child has been apparently in good health, when suddenly or after slight malaise an attack of vomiting comes on, he shivers or complains of feeling cold—rigors are not characteristically present in childhood—and there may be superadded epistaxis, or severe headache, or convulsions, or diarrhœa. But the important thing to note is that from the onset the child is definitely and visibly ill, and that within a few hours the skin is pungently hot, the face is flushed, the temperature has risen considerably, and the breathing is increased in frequency. According to the nature of the infection and the state of the system he may become restless and delirious, or may be plunged into a drowsy or stuporous condition. The early stage is not usually under medical supervision and it is, therefore, important to get a statement as to the exact condition at the onset and for the following twelve hours, as observed by the mother.

The breathing is specially worthy of study, as it presents many changes which are more characteristic than in the pneumonia of adult life. It is very important to observe it when the child is lying quietly, as the least emotion or physical disturbance brings in voluntary movements of respiration which alter the character. Pure pneumonic breathing in childhood presents the following characteristics in the early stages :

(1) The breathing is very frequent from the onset of the illness, increasing in rapidity out of proportion to the rise in temperature. The number of respirations may reach 40, 50, 60, or even more per minute.

(2) In character the breathing is shallow or superficial, and from this fact the increased frequency may be easily overlooked. The bystander sees nothing in the face or in the chest movements of the patient to suggest tachypnœa, but if he places a hand on the abdomen the rapid shallow breathing will be at once detected.

(3) The breathing is chiefly abdominal, slightly lower costal, and scarcely at all upper costal. In other words, it is natural breathing accelerated. If upper costal movement is at all marked, one may be quite sure that there is some other cause than a patch of pneumonic consolidation.

(4) An inverted type of respiratory rhythm is frequently present. The normal respiratory cycle is inspiration, expiration, pause, the pause being the imperceptible termination of the expiration. Very frequently in pneumonia this cycle is inverted, and becomes expiration, inspiration, pause. There is a distinct abnormality about this process, both the expiration and the pause being accompanied by muscular action, and not merely passive as in ordinary breathing. During expiration the air is forcibly driven out of the chest, a rapid inspiration follows, and during the pause the air is, as it were, held up in the chest, the vocal cords being closed.

The phenomenon may occasionally be seen in children in other conditions, as, for example, after a fit of crying, but in pneumonia it may persist for hours or days. It is by no means, however, a constant symptom either in all cases or in any individual patient, but when present it is of very great diagnostic value in at once suggesting pneumonia in a case which may have been obscure. In many cases of this inverted rhythm the breathing is quite quiet, but if the expiration is specially forcible there may be audible " panting," or " grunting," or a nasal " whiffle." This inverted type of breathing may be noticed on inspection of the patient, or it may first attract attention during auscultation. If one is auscultating a consolidated part of the lung, one may be struck by the fact that the bronchial or tubular element is louder during inspiration than expiration—the reverse of what usually occurs. The fact, of course, is that with the inverted type of breathing the apparently inspiratory sounds are really expiratory, and one has been misled by the altered position of the pause in the respiration.

Associated with this inverted rhythm is a peculiar action of the alæ nasi, which I have not seen in any other affection. We all recognise a slight inspiratory dilatation of the nares in early childhood, and a marked increase of this dilatation when any obstruction of the respiratory passages is present. This is characteristically seen in catarrhal pneumonia. In all writings on lobar pneumonia one finds mentioned " an exaggerated movement of the alæ nasi," and when this is described it is stated to be an inspiratory dilatation. My own observation has led me to believe that there is no such inspiratory dilatation of the nares in uncomplicated pneumonia, because there is no pulmonary obstruction. Nevertheless there is in pneumonia an exaggerated movement of the alæ nasi, but it consists of an *expiratory* dilatation. It is not the exaggerated physiological movement, but an exactly reverse condition. It occurs during or at the end of expiration, and it occurs only in association with the inverted type of respiration to which reference has been made. When the breathing is very rapid, the timing of the nasal movement is very difficult, but in ordinary cases with a little patience one can easily determine the correspondence between expiration and alar expansion. The method of its production is probably as follows. In the inverted type of breathing the expiration is forcible, and air is driven out with a certain explosive force, so that the air rushing through the nose distends the lax alæ nasi. Exactly the same action of the alæ nasi is produced in blowing the nose, if carried out in the proper manner—that is, without compressing the nares.

(5) In rare cases there may be observed irregular cerebral breathing. Some ten or twelve rapid respirations are taken and then comes a complete pause, or a temporary slowing, followed by rapid respirations again. This is sometimes described as "cyclic" breathing.

(6) There is a complete absence of that distressed and anxious look on the patient's face which is usually seen associated with very frequent breathing. The child may be sitting up in bed, breathing sixty to the minute, with a perfectly placid expression of face, and evidently not suffering from orthopnœa. Or the child may be lying down, looking ill, looking as if suffering from severe toxæmia, but not presenting that anxious and distressed look which is so marked a feature in pulmonary obstruction, as, for example, in catarrhal pneumonia.

(7) The signs of obstructed breathing are entirely absent. You will find in this stage of pneumonia that the inspiratory dilatation of the alæ nasi is not exaggerated, that the sterno-mastoid and the scalene muscles are quite slack, and that there is no supra-sternal or infra-costal retraction.

(8) The pulse-respiration ratio which is so characteristic of pneumonia in adult life is not so well marked in early life. The pulse-rate is usually high, running up to 120, 140, or 160 per minute. But even in infancy one can determine that the respiratory rate has increased out of proportion to the number of cardiac pulsations. With a respiratory rate of 60 per minute, one would expect, under normal relations, a pulse rate of 240 per minute, which of course is never seen. So that even in infants there is a certain *retardation* of the cardiac rate. In older children the characteristic pulse-respiration ratio of pneumonia in adult life may be exactly reproduced.

These different characteristics of the breathing —increased frequency, shallowness, absence of distress, inverted rhythm, and inverted action of the alæ nasi—are so valuable in the diagnosis of pneumonia, that one naturally goes a step further and seeks for an explanation of them.

The explanation usually given is that they are dependent on the pulmonary condition of consolidation and congestion. There are many difficulties in the way of accepting this view. The alterations in the breathing may be fully developed long before there are any recognisable pulmonary changes ; they may persist unchanged while rapid advances in pulmonary consolidation are going on, and they may disappear more or less abruptly at the crisis, while the pulmonary condition is still unaltered. In pneumonia a small amount of pulmonary engorgement may be accompanied by great respiratory disturbance, while, on the other hand, a large area of consolidation may be accompanied by slight respiratory disturbance. Rapid shallow breathing does not meet a demand for more oxygen, and abdominal respiration *per se* does not suggest pulmonary distress.

Pain, the pain of pleurisy, has been suggested by Dr. Eustace Smith and others as the cause of the "panting" or "grunting" breathing, with the inverted type of respiration, to which reference has been made. The child, it is said, holds its breath and lets go with a "pant" or a "grunt." This type of breathing will be found to be present characteristically when there is no pleurisy and no pain. If there is one thing one can tell decidedly about a child from the appearance, it is the presence or absence of pain, and in no condition is this more clearly shown than in pneumonia.

It has also been suggested that the inverted rhythm is really an improvement on the normal type of breathing, in that it allows of the patient's retaining a larger quantity of fresh air in the lungs during the respiratory pause for the purpose of oxygenating the blood. The pause coming at the end of inspiration allows of a more prolonged and active interchange of gases. This explanation is, at first sight, rather plausible, but if it were correct in all probability Nature would have made physiological breathing to be of this character. I have found by experience that it is a most uncomfortable form of breathing to carry out voluntarily for any length of time, and yet in pneumonia it appears as an easy and natural action. I have failed, as regards this and the other characteristics of pneumonic breathing, to find a satisfactory explanation in the objective changes in the lungs and pleura.

Some of the facts which I have brought before

you as to the nature of the breathing in pneumonia have attracted the attention of various writers, as the following quotations show. Dr. Walsh, on the subject of pneumonia in adult life, wrote as follows: "The amount of subjective distress varies inexplicably ; not uncommonly 30 to 40 respirations per minute may exist without the patient becoming conscious of particular dyspnœa—whereas, if they reach 70 to 80, speech is obstructed and suffocation may appear imminent ; but, on the other hand, a man breathing 60 to 70 times in a minute may be wholly unconscious of dyspnœa."

Sir William Gairdner has written : " The dyspnœa of *pure* pneumonia is a mere acceleration of the respiration, without any of the heaving or straining inspiration observed in bronchitis, or in cases where the two diseases are combined. So much is this the case, that I have repeatedly observed patients affected with a great extent of pneumonia in both lungs, and in whom the extreme lividity and the respirations, numbering 50 to 60 in the minute, showed infallibly the amount to which the function of the lung was interfered with, and who, nevertheless, lay quietly in bed breathing without any of the violent effort, or the disposition to assume the erect posture, so constantly accompanying the more dangerous form of bronchitis."

Dr. Hughlings Jackson has kindly referred me to a paper of his on some curious nervous phenomena in a case of "latent pneumonia." In that paper there occurs the following suggestive passage : " I suggest that the central lesion is the cause of the non-pulmonary symptoms of pneumonia, the high temperature, rapid respiration, and infrequent pulse (infrequent, I mean, only in relation to the respiration rate). I do not think the local pulmonary inflammation would produce such symptoms in such relation." He has not, however, pursued his investigations into this subject, and so it wants the full illumination which Dr. Hughlings Jackson alone could give.

What we desire in connection with these respiratory conditions in pneumonia is a theory which, while explaining them, is also in accordance with the accepted pathology of the disease, and, more important still, will be a safe guide as to its proper treatment. As a useful working hypothesis I suggest to you that the respiratory and cardiac phenomena of pneumonia are not primarily pulmonary or cardiac, but are due to a disturbance of the respiratory and cardiac centres in the medulla. You will remember that these centres are in close relation to each other, and also to the nuclei of the vagi nerves. Branches of the vagus—afferent and sensory—pass from each lung to the medulla and convey to the centre those impulses which regulate the respiratory movements in accordance with the requirements of the lungs. Other branches of the vagus — efferent and inhibitory—pass from the medulla to the heart and control the rapidity and strength of its movements. This has been demonstrated by the following physiological experiment : If one vagus be divided and the central end be stimulated, two results will follow—(1) an increase in the frequency of the respirations, which at the same time become more superficial, and (2) a slowing of the heart's action.

Now, we have in pneumonia a local irritant present in the lungs, and we have also proceeding from this source toxins which enter the blood and reach the respiratory and cardiac centres in the medulla. Will these factors serve to explain the respiratory phenomena which we have been considering? Let us take them in the same order as before.

(1) The increased frequency of the respirations. This would follow directly from the stimulation of the respiratory centre, as in the physiological experiment referred to above. Instead of the stimulation of the central end of the divided vagus, we have in the lung the stimulation of the terminal branches of the vagus. We can also understand, on this theory, why it is that the increased frequency of breathing is present from the onset, is quite irrespective of the extent of lung involved, and is out of proportion to the rise in temperature when compared with other pyrexial affections.

(2) The shallow, superficial breathing is similarly explained.

(3) The respirations are abdominal in character. This is a very interesting point, for marked diaphragmatic breathing is not common in pulmonary affections. In healthy children breathing is abdominal and lower costal, but in the case of any respiratory obstruction, as in catarrhal pneumonia, it at once becomes costal as well as abdominal. This difference was noted long ago by Walshe, who wrote : " The adult male seems to the eye to breathe with the abdomen and the lower ribs, the adult female with the upper third of the chest alone.* " The sexual differences disappear

in *forced* breathing : in both sexes the pectoral movement is, out of all proportion, greater than the abdominal, and even in the male the expansile action, if abrupt, commences superiorly." The explanation of these different forms of breathing, as given by Dr. Hughlings Jackson, is that automatic (medullary) breathing is, certainly in males, chiefly abdominal, while voluntary (cortical) breathing is chiefly upper costal. This would explain why it is that in pneumonia the disturbance of the respiratory centre in the medulla produces exaggerated abdominal breathing, and why thoracic breathing is not apparently altered in any way.

(4) The inverted type of breathing.

(5) Irregular or cyclic breathing.

I do not know of any explanation which will account for these types of breathing, save that which assumes a disturbance of the respiratory centre. The difficulties which exist in the way of tracing the inverted type of respiration to the pulmonary condition have already been considered. Under the term "cerebral breathing" there are classed various abnormal types of respiration, such as Cheyne-Stokes' breathing, uræmic breathing, etc., and the types under consideration may be entered in the same class.

(6) The absence of a distressed expression, and the patient's unconsciousness of any alteration in the breathing. I must emphasize again that I am referring to pure pneumonia in the early stage. For an explanation of the facts I have to turn again to Dr. Hughlings Jackson's theory as to the nervous mechanism in respiration. His view is that the medullary respiratory centre presides over involuntary and unconscious breathing, while in voluntary and conscious breathing the cortex cerebri comes into action, as, for instance, preparatory to lifting a weight or when a person is told to draw a breath. Accepting this view as to the difference of the two movements, I suggest that it explains why in pneumonia the patient is unconscious of distress or alteration in the breathing, because the disturbance is in the medulla. A comparison may be made with the condition of paroxysmal tachycardia, where, although the heart may be beating at the rate of 200 per minute, the patient may be unconscious of any alteration in the cardiac pulsations or of any distress. In this case also the explanation is that the seat of the disturbance is in the medullary cardiac centre.

(7) The signs of obstructed breathing are absent and the dorsal decubitus is maintained. This is not to be wondered at, as there is no obstruction present and no cause for respiratory distress.

(8) The altered pulse-respiration ratio. According to the physiological experiment referred to above, the effect of stimulating the central end of a divided vagus is to increase the frequency of the respirations, and at the same time to slow the action of the heart. In pneumonia there is an actual increase in the number of the respirations and a relative decrease in the number of the heart-beats—relative, that is, in reference to the rise in the temperature. Thus, in pneumonia it would appear that there is an exact reproduction of the results of the physiological experiment referred to. These results can only follow from excitation of the cardiac and respiratory centres in the medulla, which may be produced by the local lesion in the lung either directly through the vagus, or indirectly through the poisoned blood reaching the medulla.

In older children this altered pulse-respiration ratio may be as well manifested as in the case of adults, but in infants the holding back or inhibitory action on the heart is less marked. This may be explained by the fact that in infants the inhibitory centres, and consequently inhibitory actions, are not fully developed (Hughlings Jackson).

Pain in the chest is not so frequent or so severe a symptom of pneumonia in children as it is in the case of adults. When present the symptom is, of course, of great value as suggesting the situation and nature of the trouble. If the child has a pained expression, one must not conclude too readily that the cause is pleuritic. Young children have great difficulty in localising pain, and the strained expression may be from the pain of acute otitis or headache. Sometimes the definite rub of pleural friction will be found at or near the painful spot, but as frequently there will be no characteristic signs of pleurisy. It will not infrequently be found that the only complaint of the patient is of pain in the abdomen, and on examination this may be found to be accompanied by tenderness and rigidity of the muscles in the area affected. This is at first sight distinctly misleading, and I suppose most of us have met with such cases, and overlooked the real disease because we forgot the golden rule to examine the chest in all cases of acute abdominal pain. I do not know if such things have happened in this country, but I am told that many a healthy appendix has been removed in America because the patient, suffering from unsuspected pneumonia, complained of pain in the right iliac region. No doubt the surgeon in such a case would ascribe the pneumonia to the ether given at the operation.

Coughing is not usually a troublesome symptom in uncomplicated lobar pneumonia. Many children pass through the whole illness, including complete resolution, with only a slight occasional cough. If catarrh of the larger bronchial tubes is present, as often happens, then coughing is more frequent and troublesome. The temperature chart may be the typical one, the fever soon rising to 103° or 104° F., and oscillating but slightly along the line until the crisis occurs. On the other hand, a diurnal range of two to three degrees is not uncommon, and this is more frequently the case during the first two years of life than later. One must also be prepared to meet with cases of pneumonia in which the temperature oscillates from day to day in a most uncharacteristic way, and makes the diagnosis uncertain until there occurs a sudden cessation of all fever at some period, usually between the fifth and seventh days. A pseudo-crisis is a very common prelude to the real crisis in childhood, and is accompanied by a lull in the severity of the symptoms, which, however, return in full force with the subsequent rise in temperature. A crisis in two stages, as this may be called, is probably better for the patient than a sudden drop of from seven to nine degrees in temperature, as one sometimes sees. Such a drop may be accompanied by considerable prostration, although as a rule the crisis is not followed in children by such collapse as one often sees in adults. The crisis occurs in the majority of cases between the fifth and the seventh days of the illness. It may occur as early as the second day or as late as the fourteenth. An abortive attack of pneumonia is one in which the crisis occurs on the second or third day, and this early cessation of all acute symptoms is sometimes ascribed by the physician to the result of his active treatment. The cases of this nature which have come under my own observation have had no treatment at all, so that I am inclined to think that Nature, not Art, decides the date of the crisis. The prolongation of the illness to the fourteenth day naturally increases the gravity of the patient's con-

dition, and yet here we may meet with a natural crisis and a rapid recovery.

TYPES OF PNEUMONIA.

While in most cases of pneumonia, even in those in which the objective pulmonary signs are quite latent for some days, it is possible for the unbiassed observer to diagnose with considerable accuracy the nature of the disease at an early stage, there occur others in which the poison seems to attack with virulence some other organ than the lung. The result of this is that we are apt to concentrate our attention on the organ chiefly affected, as regards physical signs, and miss the real disease in the background. More especially is this the case in the cerebral type of pneumonia. Certain nervous phenomena are common in all cases of pneumonia in children. Amongst these are vomiting, headache, delirium, or convulsions at the onset. In some cases these symptoms do not subside, but become more aggravated day by day. Hence the term "cerebral pneumonia" is in common use. The child may from the onset continue in a drowsy, lethargic state, crying out when disturbed, and wishing only to be left alone. I have often been struck by the drowsy languor or complete apathy which may persist all through an attack of pneumonia, and how, after the crisis, the child seems to wake up as from a long dream, a wide-awake being again. Extreme tremulousness of the hands and of the tongue is often a marked feature. In other cases the nervous symptoms are of a more active type. There may be screaming and delirium at night. Headaches may be severe, and convulsions, head retraction, opisthotonos, and rigidity of all the limbs may be present. In short, the clinical picture of meningitis may be so exactly reproduced that one does not hesitate to make a diagnosis of that affection. As a matter of experience, we find that the above symptoms may be produced by (1) the poisoning of the cerebral tissues by the pneumococcus or its products; (2) an acute inflammation of the middle ear, frequently suppurative, and also pneumococcal in origin; or (3) actual pneumococcal meningitis. This last is extremely rare. As regards the first, the condition known as meningism, if it is not recognised before the crisis, it will be very apparent soon after, since the symptoms, as a rule, cease abruptly with the fall in temperature. The second condition, namely, inflammation of the middle ear, may be suggested by the pain in the ear and head complained of by the patient, but in the majority of cases in young children there is no such localising symptom. Consequently, I have made it a rule in all cases of pneumonia with cerebral symptoms to examine the ears, and if the membrane is bulging to have it freely incised. By this means the speedy disappearance of all cerebral symptoms has frequently followed. In some cases, at a later stage, when after the crisis the temperature continues to fluctuate, and the patient does not seem to be progressing satisfactorily, the condition will be found to be due to middle-ear inflammation.

Another puzzling form of pneumonia is that in which the gastro-intestinal canal is the seat of great disturbance, probably from direct infection. Vomiting is present, the tongue rapidly becomes inflamed, all appetite is lost, the abdomen becomes distended and hard and sometimes tender, and rather severe and intractable diarrhœa sets in. When these signs are obtrusive, in a child manifestly ill, with continued fever, and when the signs of pulmonary disease are more or less latent, it is easy for the medical attendant to be led astray for a time, and a diagnosis of typhoid fever is sometimes made. The symptoms themselves do not call for any active treatment, save when tympanites is marked, and the pressure upwards of the diaphragm seriously impedes respiration in the later stages of the disease.

A third type of pneumonia in which the symptoms may at first puzzle one is that in which a condition of nephritis is present from the beginning of the illness, and the striking symptoms are hæmaturia, albuminuria, and dropsy. These are not common cases, but I have met with three, in two of which advice was sought because of hæmaturia and in the third because of general dropsy. If the signs of pneumonia are present and are recognised the question will at once arise, Is this a case of pneumonia complicated with nephritis, or of nephritis complicated with pneumonia? If the signs of pneumonia are latent, one is easily led to make a diagnosis of nephritis only. Perhaps the chief diagnostic point in these cases is the elevated temperature, because a continued temperature of 103° or 104° is not common in acute nephritis. The course of the pneumonia is entirely unaffected by this complication, and with the crisis comes a rapid disappearance of the renal signs. In all of my own cases the hæmaturia, the albuminuria, the dropsy, the tube casts, and the oliguria disappeared within three days of the crisis. I have read recently, however, of a case of pneumonia in an infant which terminated fatally from acute nephritis.

It is to be noted about these special types—the cerebral, the gastro-intestinal, and the renal—that the symptoms may persist right up to the crisis, and may be to such a degree the striking symptoms of the illness that the real underlying disease may not even have been suspected. This may appear difficult of belief to some, but I do not think my own experience or my own faulty diagnosis is unique. At the same time, looking back on these cases, I find that there was always sufficient evidence, had one but observed carefully, to enable one to make a correct diagnosis at a much earlier stage.

PHYSICAL SIGNS.

The physical signs in the lungs are very important, are very characteristic, and are very fully described in the text-books. In many cases, however, their appearance is delayed for some days, and in others they never appear at all. I do not go the length of saying that pneumonia may run its course without any pulmonary exudation at all—a local exudation in the lungs is probably the primary source of irritation and the seat of toxin-production in all cases—but certainly one meets with cases in which a slight impairment of resonance or a few crepitations are all the physical signs recognised in the lungs. In some cases it may be necessary to adopt special measures in order to elicit the physical signs of pneumonia. If the child is breathing in a rapid or shallow manner, we may hear nothing but vesicular breathing without accompaniments ; but if he is made to breathe deeply, as on coughing, or laughing, or crying, one can often hear a burst of crepitations or the high-pitched tubular breathing which clinches the diagnosis. Another method of securing the same result is to lay the child on one side of the chest and examine the lung which is uppermost. The air will be found to enter this lung more freely than when both lungs are acting equally. The child is then turned on the opposite side for the examination of the other lung. A change of position from lying down to sitting up, and *vice versâ*, may so increase the depth of the breathing that latent signs are elicited. These points may seem of small moment, but all who engage much in work amongst children must have recognised frequently the difficulty in auscultatory examination. It is easy to tell an adult patient to breathe deeply, but with a young child both precept and example are frequently of no use. In the examination of the chest in children the bases of the lungs are usually fully examined, but it is well also to remember the three apices—the apex of the upper lobe, the apex of the lower lobe, and the apex of the axilla ; for in these places evidences of pulmonary consolidation are often found when they are absent elsewhere.

(To be concluded.)

October 23rd, 1905.

THE CLINICAL JOURNAL,

CLINICAL RECORD, CLINICAL NEWS, CLINICAL GAZETTE, CLINICAL REPORTER,
CLINICAL CHRONICLE AND CLINICAL REVIEW.

EDITED BY L. ELIOT CREASY.

| No. 679. | WEDNESDAY, NOVEMBER 1, 1905. | Vol. XXVII. No. 3. |

CONTENTS.

NOTICE.

*Editorial correspondence, books for review, &c.,
should be addressed to the Editor, 51, New
Cavendish Street, W., Telephone No. 904, Paddington ; but all business communications should
be addressed to the Publishers, 22½, Bartholomew
Close, London, E.C. Telephone 927, Holborn.*

*All inquiries respecting Advertisements should be
sent to MESSRS. ADLARD & SON, Bartholomew
Close, E.C. Telephone 927, Holborn.*

*Terms of Subscription, including postage, payable
by cheque, postal or banker's order (in advance) : for
the United Kingdom, 15s. 6d. per annum ; Abroad
17s. 6d.*

*Cheques, &c., should be made payable to THE
PROPRIETORS OF THE CLINICAL JOURNAL, crossed
"The London, City, and Midland Bank, Ltd.,
Newgate Street Branch, E.C. Account of the
Medical Publishing Company, Ltd."*

*Reading Cases to hold Twenty-six Numbers of
THE CLINICAL JOURNAL can be supplied at 2s. 3d.
each, or will be forwarded post free on receipt of
2s. 6d. ; and also Cases for Binding Volumes at 1s.
each, or post free on receipt of 1s. 3d., from the
Publishers, 22½, Bartholomew Close, London, E.C.*

TWO LECTURES

Delivered at St. Bartholomew's Hospital.

By C. B. LOCKWOOD, F.R.C.S.,
Surgeon to the Hospital.

LECTURE I.

SWELLINGS ABOVE, BELOW, AND WITHIN THE NECK OF THE SCROTUM.

GENTLEMEN,—Almost the commonest clinical case
that you will be called upon to diagnose is one in
which there is a swelling in the neighbourhood of
the inguinal canal, of the scrotum, or of the neck
of the scrotum. I have observed that this class of
case is exceedingly difficult. Many mistakes are
made concerning them, mistakes which are often
very serious as regards the patient, and also as regards the reputation of the man who makes them.
You may remember, if you attended the first
clinical lecture which I gave, that I attach far more
importance to methods of thinking and methods of
seeing than to anything else. The sense of touch
affords information, but it is not of a very reliable
character. Still, with regard to the diagnosis of
the tumours which we are about to consider to-day,
the sense of touch forms an important part, and it
has to be used methodically. Before I proceed
further, I want to draw your attention to the parts
which are concerned. First of all, I would ask you
to pay especial attention to the part which I will
call the neck of the scrotum—that is, the constriction where the scrotum joins the trunk. It is
situated just below the external abdominal ring
and near the root of the penis. The neck of the
scrotum is not an anatomical landmark mentioned,
as far as I am aware, in any book on surgical
topography. Nevertheless, it is one of the most
important landmarks in the whole of this region.
Obviously, if there is a tumour in this region it
must be either above the neck of the scrotum, in
the neck of the scrotum, or below it. We will

begin to consider the tumours which are situated above the neck of the scrotum. Clearly, the moment you cast your eyes upon a swelling in this region, you can say whether it is or is not above the neck of the scrotum, and you know then fairly well the class of tumours which you have to investigate. If it is in the neck you have further information, and if it is below it you have still further information. Not only is the neck of the scrotum to be looked at, but it is also to be felt. What constitutes a normal neck of the scrotum? Observe I use the word "normal," and I did it intentionally. I know there are many who use the word "normal" and have no clear idea in their mind as to what the word really means. Now, what constitutes the normal neck of the scrotum? There *is* a neck at all events, and you notice that the scrotum on one side appears the same as it does on the other; the skin is not red, it is not inflamed, it is not apparently altered. When you feel the normal neck of the scrotum you feel in it the spermatic cord and nothing else. How often have I asked gentlemen to feel a cord and they have not known the proper way! Observe how you proceed and practise doing it. Stand upon that side of the patient on which you are going to feel; that is to say, if you are going to feel on the right side, stand on his right side. Pass the index finger underneath the neck of the scrotum, opposite the root of the penis, and pinch the thumb down upon it, and slip the constituents of the scrotum through your finger from within outwards. You ought to feel the vas deferens, which is hard like whipcord. If the sense of touch is good, you feel the spermatic artery beating. You will feel a number of other small cords, and strings, and fibres, which you cannot define. The veins and lymphatics I do not think you can feel. You possibly may be able to feel the nerves of the cord, more especially the genito-crural and branches of the ileo-inguinal, but I think the fibres which you feel are probably the fibres of the cremaster muscle. Unless you can feel those things clearly and accurately, you are not feeling a normal spermatic cord. What constitutes a normal inguinal canal? First of all, the inguinal canal is situated opposite the inner third of Poupart's ligament. You find the most extraordinary differences of opinion as to the exact extent of the inguinal canal. It is limited above by the so-called internal

abdominal ring (which I have never seen), below by the external one, which everyone knows and is familiar with. The internal abdominal ring is outside the epigastric artery. The term "internal abdominal ring" is merely the name of a locality. The inguinal canal ought to have no impulse in it. I am now going to tell you something which, to my mind, is of the very gravest importance for you to realise. It may not be true, so accept it critically. I am strongly of opinion that impulses can be better seen than felt. If you see an impulse, be very cautious what you say about that patient. If you do not feel an impulse, do not attach too much importance to your failure to do so. In the normal inguinal you cannot see any impulse. When a patient stands in front of you in a good light, you should see no impulse. Of course, the whole abdominal wall may heave, but there should be no localised impulse in the inguinal canal. Next pass your finger towards the inguinal canal by tucking up the scrotum. When the tip of the finger is near the neck of the scrotum, feel for the spine of the pubes. The external abdominal ring is situated inside the spine of the pubes; perhaps it is more correct to say that it is above the spine of the pubes. What ought a normal external abdominal ring to be like? I cannot tell you. As a rough standard, it should barely admit the tip of your index finger. When a patient coughs it should close, and squeeze out the tip of your finger, which means that its boundaries are strong and taut, and not weak and flaccid. You can infer from what I have said that if you pass your finger up the external abdominal ring into the canal, that that is an abnormal canal. Well, I have explored canals of that sort and found nothing in them, but I am always very suspicious when the external ring is large enough to admit the index finger and enable me to explore freely with my finger the inguinal canal. The next structure which you ought, I think, to be clear about after the inguinal canal is the contents of the scrotum. What should you feel in the scrotum? Sometimes the scrotum contains swellings which are not testicles, but which are mistaken for testicles because the examiner is careless. But unless you can feel the spermatic cord coming down to join the epididymis, and unless in front of the epididymis you can feel the elastic body of the testicle, you should be careful what you say about it. Also, in the scrotum you may be able to feel the pampiniform plexus with a certain amount of ease. But, because you can feel the veins, it does not necessarily follow that you should diagnose a varicocele. Where the normal pampiniform plexus ends and varicocele begins I cannot tell you. But you must not condemn everybody as having varicocele if their pampiniform plexus is fairly easy to feel. Assuming that that is clear in our minds, I will proceed to consider some swellings above the neck of the scrotum. The patient having been stood up in a good light and told to cough, we will assume that you see a swelling in the region of the inguinal canal ; that is to say, it is opposite the inner third of Poupart's ligament. When the patient coughs there is a sharp, distinct impulse. The probabilities in your mind in a case of that sort would be that the tumour is a hernia. But I advise you not to put that proposition first. I advise you to say to yourself that there is a swelling above the neck of the scrotum and in the region of the inguinal canal, and then say to yourself, I will now try to ascertain whether that swelling is outside or inside the inguinal canal. You will be very puzzled some day with a swelling in that region which is not in the inguinal canal, but outside it. It is, of course, a foolish mistake to begin to operate on a supposed swelling in the inguinal canal and to find that after all you are dealing with, say, a chronic abscess over the inguinal canal, or an enlarged gland. There may be other things over the inguinal canal. For instance, besides the tumours I have mentioned, a femoral hernia, not infrequently after leaving the saphenous opening, turns up over Poupart's ligament and lodges over the inguinal canal. Another structure which sometimes passes over the inguinal canal is the testicle itself. You may have seen a boy operated upon last week in whom we thought this had happened. On the left side his scrotum was empty. In the left inguinal region he had a swelling, and the question was, Is that swelling inside or outside the inguinal canal? We suspected it was a testicle. I guessed it was outside the inguinal canal. We thought we could feel the aponeurosis of the external oblique underneath the swelling. At the operation this proved to be the case. Whether the testicle had ever passed into the scrotum I cannot tell, but it had turned back over the aponeurosis of the external oblique, and covered over the inguinal canal. As you may be aware,

the first step in the transition of the testis is the passage of a sort of test-tube of peritoneum down from the abdomen into the scrotum, and then the testicle follows that, descending into the test-tube. Sometimes the test-tube, or processus vaginalis, passes back over the external oblique without the presence of the testicle at all. For instance, on Monday I operated on a small boy who had his testicle in the abdomen, but the processus vaginalis had passed down the inguinal canal, and turned up again in the external oblique towards the anterior superior spine of the ilium. To revert to the question of femoral hernia over the inguinal canal, a condition which is not always very easy to diagnose. In a thin person it may be easy, because you can feel the neck of the hernia running outside the spine of the pubes and below Poupart's ligament into the saphenous opening and towards the femoral canal. But if you cannot feel the neck you must be exceedingly cautious in your diagnosis. I have seen the late Luther Holden begin to operate on a case of supposed inguinal hernia in the female, and before he had proceeded far with his operation find that he was dealing with a femoral hernia which had passed upwards. A few years ago I began to operate on a female patient for the radical cure of an inguinal hernia, and found the sac of a femoral hernia over the inguinal canal. In fact, I had mistaken a femoral hernia for an inguinal hernia. How shall you avoid such mistakes ? I will tell you how you can easily find out whether a tumour is outside or inside the inguinal canal, if you are able to perform the manœuvre. You cannot always do it on fat people or on females, but if you can pass your finger through the external abdominal ring and feel the tumour above the external oblique, you need have no doubt about your diagnosis. I daresay there are other structures which may be discovered outside the inguinal canal which I have not mentioned to you. I do not think it would be right for you to endeavour to carry in your minds a list of the structures which might be found outside the inguinal canal. The thing to carry clearly in your mind is this : that when you are confronted with a swelling in the neighbourhood of the inguinal canal, your first thought should be, Is it inside or outside the inguinal canal? Let us proceed a little further with the diagnosis of tumours which may be met with inside the inguinal canal. There is a swelling in the neighbourhood of the inguinal canal which has a sharp impulse when the patient coughs. The finger passed up the scrotum passes into the external abdominal ring, which is loose, and when a cough is given something is felt to be striking against the finger. This something comes down when the patient stands up, and goes back when the patient lies down. That, I suppose, would be the simplest possible case of an ordinary inguinal hernia. If, in addition, you felt it gurgle as it went back, you would think it was probably intestine containing air. With the exception of the case in which it gurgles, I have seen those signs over and over again simulated by a condition which is common, but I think seldom talked about or recognised. The condition I refer to is that which I have called an inguinal varicocele. In future do not speak of varicocele as I did at the beginning of this lecture, but speak of two kinds, scrotal varicocele and inguinal varicocele. When once you have realised that the veins in the inguinal canal may be very greatly enlarged and varicose, and bulge out the canal there is no difficulty in understanding that that is very frequently indeed associated with ordinary scrotal varicocele. I do not think a case of varicocele in which you could feel the enlarged veins passing up into the neck of the scrotum, in which you could feel them passing through an enlarged inguinal canal, and in which you saw a large swelling in the inguinal canal corresponding to its boundaries, would be a source of difficulty to your mind. You would say such a man had got a varicose condition of the veins in the neck of the scrotum and in the inguinal canal.

Now, consider another condition which I have often seen. I have seen many times no scrotal varicocele, no varicocele in the neck of the scrotum, but a marked varicose condition of the spermatic veins in the inguinal canal. And that is a very puzzling condition, and the diagnosis of it is exceedingly difficult. The possibility of its presence is not recognised, and I suppose, therefore, it is not diagnosed. I wonder how many people are wearing trusses upon an inguinal varicocele, and I further wonder how many people are complaining of the pain and discomfort which that entails. It is of the greatest importance

to diagnose inguinal varicocele for many reasons. For instance, I remember seeing a patient who had an inguinal varicocele. I guessed that he had inguinal varicocele for these reasons. First of all, he had a little swelling in the region of his inguinal canal. This swelling became greater when he stood up and coughed. Next, that swelling had an obvious impulse when he coughed, so that it was in that respect very like a hernia. Next, the swelling went away when he lay down, but slowly. Next, he had a dilated inguinal canal. I might have said it was an inguinal hernia, but he had some slight dilatation of the veins of the neck of the scrotum and, I think, also in the veins of the pampiniform plexus. The advice given was to have the inguinal canal opened and the veins removed. I attach the greatest importance to opening the inguinal canal when a patient has got an inguinal varicocele. Over and over again when we open these canals in which there is an inguinal varicocele we find that the patient has got a small hernial sac there. Perhaps it is an inch long, and, as a rule, there is something very curious about the sac ; it is rather pointed. In the last ten days a man has been operated upon by me in the theatre. On the left side he had a large varicocele and dilatation of the veins in the neck of his scrotum, also an impulse and swelling in the left inguinal canal, with dilatation of the external abdominal ring. Obviously an operation done on the scrotum would not have cured him. I can tell you of an instance of that. The patient I was telling you of a moment ago had almost a similar condition, and was advised to have his inguinal canal opened and the veins removed. He was operated upon some time later, and the operation was done in the ordinary manner through the scrotum. I remember seeing him a year later. He said : " I have come to see you again because I have had my operation done, but I have still got my pain and discomfort." " What operation have you had done ? There is a scar upon your scrotum. You have not had the operation done which you required, which should have been done higher up, where there is still a swelling, and an impulse on coughing, and enlarged veins." I might have added that the surgeon who did it ought to have looked for a hernial sac, which is so frequently present. The man you have seen in the ward had on the left side a huge dilated vein and a small sac. On the right side, when he stood up in a good light, he had also a faint impulse on the upper part of the right inguinal canal. I said that that side also ought to be explored, because he had either got some dilated veins on that side or possibly a hernial sac. When we explored we did not find dilated veins, but a hernial sac at least one and a quarter inch long by more than three quarters of an inch in diameter, and the condition necessary for him to get a rupture. I am very suspicious of inguinal varicocele. I cannot help thinking that when the veins in the inguinal canal are varicose they dilate and weaken the canal, and that they are an advance guard for the hernial sac which you will so frequently find there. Inguinal varicocele, when it is present, is often accompanied with fat in the inguinal canal, which also bulges it out, and has an impulse. When the testicle makes its transition out of the abdomen into the scrotum it is preceded by the processus vaginalis, or test-tube of peritoneum, to which I have just referred. But peritoneum has fat upon it, and therefore it is easy for you to understand that in infants you find about the processus vaginalis some lobules of this so-called subperitoneal fat. That fat accompanying the testicle in its transition does not always wither away or remain small, but sometimes grows, so that I have removed fatty tumours of considerable size from the inguinal canal, and also occasionally from the upper part of the scrotum. Now I am going to tell you a very curious thing about these fatty tumours of the spermatic cord. You may observe I myself attach a good deal of importance to that which I can see ; it is quite natural for anybody to think when he has seen fat in the inguinal canal that he has seen fat—in other words, that fat can always be recognised with the naked eye. Well, I know that very strange things are found in the inguinal canal, and I have been in the habit of having what I have removed from the inguinal canal examined microscopically whenever I could ; and I confess I was decidedly surprised when one day, after saving up some fat for examination the pathologist sent me back a specimen of suprarenal body. If you are interested in the matter, you will find a photograph of the section in the Pathological Society's 'Transactions' of about seven years ago. And you will also find the photograph of a human embryo which throws some light on the point. In the human embryo in one complete section there is at the top of the

abdomen the proper suprarenal body, and there is passing over the front of the embryo kidney the lower part of the suprarenal body, becoming continuous with its epididymis. In other words, the top part of the Wolffian body has become suprarenal body, the lower part has become epididymis. Now I shall set you thinking, be-cause there must be men who have got, or will soon acquire, inquiring minds. Why does not some-body investigate the fate of the part of the Wolffian body which lies between the suprarenal body and the epididymis ? I very strongly suspect, first of all, that the part in the hilum of the kidney accounts for those curious malignant adenomata of the kidney which are exactly like pieces of Wolffian body. Next proceed along the course of the ureter. I have removed curious cysts which otherwise appeared to be unaccountable. They are very like ovarian cysts, but they occur along the ureter and almost in the flank. I believe they are to be found also in males, though the two I have seen have been in females. This is a branch of pathology which is worth working up, and which I am sure will afford valuable results for any man who will pursue it. There are other things to be found in the inguinal canal besides fat. I have spoken of males so far, but I might have mentioned a case of lipoma in the female. The female has a smaller inguinal canal than the male, and it is less liable to disturbances, I think. But occasionally odd things are found in the inguinal canal of the female. For instance, I remember a lady who complained of pain in the top part of the inguinal canal. When she stood up before a good light—and a good light is essential for the diagnosis of these conditions— the first thing that could be seen was a minute elevation of the skin at the upper part of the inguinal canal. When she coughed there was an impulse at that point. The opinion was expressed that she had something in her inguinal canal, and that as she had a pain there, and it was interfering with her comfort, and she hated wearing trusses, it was better that it should be explored. The result was that a lipoma of some size was found in the top part of the inguinal canal, and it was removed. She then dispensed with the truss which she had worn for some time. Another tumour which is sometimes found in the inguinal canal of females is constituted by the ovary and Fallopian tube. I have twice met with an ovary and Fallopian tube in supposed inguinal hernia of females. One was in a child, and I remember it very well; it is very vivid in my mind. It was a child who was thought to have a strangulated inguinal hernia in the right inguinal region. It had a swelling which was tense, red, exceedingly painful, and would pass very well for strangulated hernia. But the child was not vomiting and its bowels acted, so that was out of the question. When this swelling was examined, I found an intensely inflamed ovary and Fallopian tube. The reason they were inflamed was that they had become twisted and full of blood. That case had been described somewhere, and others have been met with since, but the condition is one of extreme rarity. The presence of the ovary and tube in the inguinal canal is not particularly rare, but still it is far too rare for you to diagnose. Supposing you make up your mind that a patient had got a rupture; do not make up your minds that you know what is inside the sac. I think it was Petit who, about two centuries ago, said no wise man pretends to know what is inside a hernial sac. I remember hearing a surgeon make a speech when he was going to operate upon a female to remove the ovary, which had (he said) descended into her inguinal canal. I watched to see what did come out, and the thing which came out was a lump of hard, inflamed omentum. It is hopeless to guess what is inside hernial sacs; if you do you are almost certain to be wrong.

Another structure which is met with inside the inguinal canal is hydrocele of the cord. The processus vaginalis ought to be closed from the so-called internal abdominal ring down to the head of the epididymis; but its closure is often incomplete. Fluid may collect in a piece which has failed to close. If this be situated in the inguinal canal, a small globular tumour results. This may be taken for a rupture, for when the patient coughs there is an impulse. When you put your finger up the external abdominal ring, which is usually dilated, you feel a swelling and impulse. There is a great temptation to call that hernia, and you are apt to do that unless you pull it down by pulling on the cord below it. You will observe then that it moves completely with the cord. If you can pull it down sufficiently far to get your fingers above the top part of the globular swelling, you are reasonably sure of your diagnosis. If you were to get one of those lamps which are used for the diagnosis of fluid in the frontal sinus, you would see that the swelling in the inguinal canal is not opaque, but translucent. The treatment of hydrocele of the inguinal canal is simple : you perform an ordinary radical cure of hernia and get quit of it.

I will very briefly recapitulate the points to which I have drawn your attention, and to which I believe I draw your attention in the wards once a week, and that is the various steps in the diagnosis of tumours in the region of the neck of the scrotum and of the inguinal canal. First of all, inspection. The fault often committed is that the patient is not put in a proper light. I do not know of any class of case which wants more careful visual inspection than these tumours in the inguinal region. So the patient is put in a strong light, and the swelling is seen. Mark its position. If it is above the neck of the scrotum in the region of the inguinal canal, you have to proceed to investigate the inguinal canal and its surroundings. Do not assume that the swelling is inside the inguinal canal. Your first instinct must be to say, " I see a swelling in the neighbourhood of the inguinal canal, and I am going to ascertain whether it is inside or outside the inguinal canal." Swellings outside the inguinal canal may be exceedingly misleading. But if you can pass your finger into the canal and get behind the swelling you cannot have any doubt that the tumour is outside the inguinal canal. If it is a tumour outside the inguinal canal, it may be an inflamed gland or an abscess, or it may be that most misleading thing—a femoral hernia which has ascended. If it is a tumour inside the inguinal canal and you are sure of it, begin to try to diagnose the different possibilities. Do not be led away by that dreadful fallacy of diagnosing what is commonest. I cannot imagine anything more silly than that. Unfortunately for you, there is no " common " case ; every case is one for original observation and will necessitate an original conclusion on your part ; otherwise you may find you are very wrong. The thing most apt to mislead you is, I think, an inguinal varicocele. If you mistake an inguinal varicocele for a hernia, you may condemn your patient to wear a truss. If you do not condemn him to that, you permit him to go on with these dilated veins, perhaps in pain, perhaps in discomfort, till at last he develops a hernial sac which he should not have developed. The proper course is to open the inguinal canal and to get rid of the veins.

The other things in the inguinal canal which I have mentioned are rarer, but still they are of importance. Fatty tumours of the canal are occasionally found. When you meet one in operating, explore the interior of it and then very likely you will find a hernial sac. When the inguinal canal contains the testicle a number of questions will arise.

The following is a by no means unusual state of things : A child has a testicle undescended. What is to be done? He is sure to have communication with the abdomen. It is so rare not to have a communication between the processus vaginalis and the abdomen that it is hardly worth while taking it into consideration. If he has a communication with his abdomen, he may develop a hernia. If he does the condition is rather dangerous. The processus vaginalis often has a very tight neck. On the whole, therefore, it is by far the best to operate. That will prevent or cure the hernia. What is to be done with the testicle when it is in the inguinal canal? Is it to be taken away? It may have to be, and you ought to have permission to do that before you proceed. Or is it to be pushed back into the abdomen? Why not? I have seen more than one patient who has had a testicle pushed back into the abdomen. One complained of pain in the iliac fossa and others did not. If you push a testicle back into the abdomen it will never grow—it will remain half its proper size ; and if you were to examine it microscopically you would find that it contained no spermatic cells. Why not put the testicle down into the scrotum? You cannot always promise to do that. I think you could promise to put it outside the abdominal ring, but it is not a very satisfactory place to put it into. But often you can put it down into the scrotum. When the testis is turned back over the external oblique it goes into the scrotum well. What becomes of the testicle when it is put into the scrotum? If the testicle is in the inguinal canal, it never develops spermatic cells. If it is put down into the scrotum, what happens to it? I have got this far, that I have seen such a testicle grow bigger ; of this I am sure. But that is very different from saying it develops and contains spermatic cells and spermatozoa. To settle the question would be very difficult. To do so some-

body would have to put the testicle down into the scrotum without tension, and see it grow larger, and then remove it, and see if it contains spermatic cells and spermatozoa. And that I am afraid will not be done. Observe this is a very important problem, and that practically a great many questions will turn upon it. For instance, there was an heir to a very fine estate and title, whom it was discovered had both testicles in the abdomen. He was a cryptorchid. First of all the question arose, If his testicles remained in the abdomen could he beget children? That is an important matter for one who is going to succeed to a title and estate. As long as the testicles are in the abdomen he will certainly not beget children. I know that cryptorchids have claimed to have begotten children, but it depends on your frame of mind as to whether you believe it or not. I am rather sceptical, so I disbelieve it.

Next, cannot the testicles be brought down? It is highly improbable, because if they are in the iliac fossa the cord is too short. If they were in the inguinal canal, the cord might be long enough to let them come down into the scrotum. If that were to be done, if they were to be got down in that way, would the testicles then develop? Nobody can answer that. But there are a great many curious, interesting, and important questions which arise concerning tumours and swellings in the inguinal canal such as we have been considering to-day.

I think next week I will proceed to consider with you the swellings in the neck of the scrotum, and the swellings in the scrotum itself, because quite recently we have had some swellings in the scrotum and in the neck of the scrotum, which have been of the most perplexing and curious character ; and as you, gentlemen, are attending the Out-Patients' Department and the wards you will be constantly brought into contact with cases such as those we have been considering. I shall be interested to know from any of you whether I am correct in my statement that that important disease inguinal varicocele is not mentioned in the text-books. And if not, you may take it as a warning and remember that the best text-books are the patients in the out-patient rooms and wards of the hospital.

October 30th, 1905.

THE
TREATMENT OF GONORRHŒA.

Abstract of a lecture delivered to the Medical
. Graduates' College.

By J. ERNEST LANE, F.R.C.S.,
Surgeon and Lecturer on Surgery, St. Mary's Hospital;
Surgeon to the London Lock Hospital.

THE treatment of gonorrhœa may at first sight appear to be hardly of sufficient importance to be dealt with in a post-graduate lecture, but when you come to consider the possible sequelæ and complications of the disease the importance of efficient treatment will be recognised. It cannot be too emphatically insisted upon at the outset that gonorrhœa must not be looked upon as an easy disease to cure, but that, on the other hand, it is one which may sorely tax the resources and try the patience of the practitioner, and the failure to give relief for what is so often considered to be a trivial disease may bring the surgeon into disfavour and disrepute, and may entail the loss of a lucrative patient. The great prevalence of the disease appears to me to be a sufficient justification for bringing the subject before you, for it has been computed by an American observer that 20 per cent. of males and 5 per cent. of females of the community have at some time been infected with gonorrhœa ; and Neisser has stated that next to measles it is the most prevalent of all diseases.

In comparison with syphilis, the disease may appear trivial, but on comparing the effects of the two diseases with one another, you will find that there is not much to choose between them in respect of their deteriorating influence on the human organism. I will not detain you by enumerating all the possible complications and remote effects of gonorrhœa, but will mention a few of them which occur to me. In the first place, urethral stricture, almost invariably due to gonorrhœa and its dire consequences and often fatal issue from renal complications, epididymitis, and orchitis may be productive of the gravest consequences, and ultimately be the cause of the greatest social misery. How many homes are rendered unhappy by the absence of children ! and to what disease is that occurrence mainly to be attributed ? A German observer has stated that 90 per cent. of all cases of sterility can be directly traced to

gonorrhœa. Then, again, endometritis, pelvic peritonitis, pyosalpinx, pyelitis, and nephritis from direct microbic extension, general peritonitis due to the same cause ; endocarditis and pericarditis ; prostatitis and its frequent companion hypochondriasis ; gonorrhœal ophthalmia, and ophthalmia neonatorum (responsible for a large proportion of the cases of blindness in children) ; gonorrhœal arthritis, possibly crippling the patient for life— these are only a few of the remote effects of the disease, but they are quite sufficient to cause the surgeon to reflect and ponder as to whether there is any other disease, except, possibly, syphilis, with such far-reaching consequences and fraught with such possible danger. And yet the disease is treated by the general public, and even by some of the medical profession, in a spirit of unseemly levity, ignoring the fact that in no case can an absolute cure be guaranteed, and overlooking its remote consequences and the indirect mortality for which it is responsible.

The efficient treatment of gonorrhœa is almost as important as is that of syphilis ; and as in the latter disease the whole aim of our treatment is to avert the tertiary stage by ridding the patient of the syphilitic virus, so in gonorrhœa our object should be to minimise its ill effects, and to prevent, if possible, the occurrence of its complications. On examining the principal text-books in use amongst medical students I find that the subject of treatment of gonorrhœa is compressed into a very small compass ; instructions are given as to the early administration of alkalies, aperients, sedatives, simple diet during what is called the first stage, and on its subsidence the administration of the customary oleo-balsams, whilst later the use of astringent injections is advocated. The so-called abortive treatment is alluded to, and amongst the topical applications mentioned are solutions of argent. nit. 1 per cent., sol. hydrarg. perchlor. 1 ad 1000, protargol 1 to 2 per cent., and mercurol ½ to 2 per cent. During this course it is recommended that the patient should remain in bed, but that if that is impracticable some milder form of treatment should be adopted. Not much incentive is given to the employment of active early measures, but a palliative and expectant treatment is rather advocated, and on the subsidence of the acute symptoms the use of astringent injections. The scanty encouragement to employ these so-called abortive measures was due to the intense inflammatory reaction produced thereby giving rise to such tumefaction of the urethra as to cause retention of urine, prostatic and perineal abscess, cystitis, and as a later consequence stricture of the urethra. The early employment of local applications has also been deprecated, since it is said that thereby the gonococcus is washed back to the deeper parts of the urethra, and a posterior gonorrhœa is the result. But if the patient is instructed to urinate before using the injection, and to retain the injection for a longer space of time than was formerly considered advisable this proceeding is more likely to avert a posterior gonorrhœa than to produce one. The ordinary hand injection does not reach the posterior urethra, being prevented from so doing by the contraction of the compressor urethræ unless great force is used in introducing it, so the effect of an early injection is merely to disinfect the anterior urethra, to destroy or hinder the proliferation of the gonococcus. The pain caused by the abortive treatment as formerly carried out was often so acute as to be prohibitive, but the employment of less irritating applications, and the use of cocaine if necessary, has overcome to a great extent that objection. The treatment of gonorrhœa as indicated above is almost precisely as it was taught when I was a student, and from the text-books it would appear that not much advance has been made since that remote era. But if the treatment recommended nowadays remains much where it was twenty-five years ago, our knowledge of the pathology of the disease has made a distinct advance since the discovery of the gonococcus by Neisser in about the year 1878. We know that it is an infective process due to a specific micro-organism, the gonococcus, one of the characteristics of which is the readiness with which it extends and proliferates, and invades the epithelial cells, reaching ultimately into the deepest layers of the urethral mucous membrane, and spreading backwards to the posterior portions of the urethra and even the bladder. It has further been pointed out that gonorrhœa is not merely a localised infection of the urethral mucous membrane, but that it causes a generalised infection of the blood by means of a poison, which has been denominated the gonotoxin, which poison is the direct cause of many of the phenomena of the disease. In all cases it is

absorbed into the system, where its presence gives rise to systemic degeneration of varying degrees of severity. Gonorrhœa is thus a general toxæmic affection, but the microbes which produce the toxin are usually localised on or around a mucous tract. The microbic invasion may extend to the organs communicating with the infected tract, or it may reach the interior of the body either directly through the Fallopian tubes, or by penetrating the mucous membrane affected and gaining the submucous spaces. Thence it invades the lymphatics, the glands, and the vascular system, and growing locally, produces the toxin which sets up local inflammations. Thus the joints may be invaded by the organisms, which may also be found in the pleura and pericardium. The gonococcus could be cultivated in certain media, and the culture when it arrived at its maturity possessed remarkable toxic properties ; applied locally, it produced an acute inflammation, followed by suppuration, and when injected into the veins or subcutaneous tissue it produced a general toxæmia, characterised by emaciation, fever, and in large doses causing the death of the inoculated animal. Applied to the mucous membranes of animals, it produced only slight irritation, but if injected into the human urethra it produced a discharge resembling gonorrhœa, but of only twenty-four to forty-eight hours' duration. Attempts at immunising against the gonotoxin had been successfully employed with goats, and though the process took about two years to complete, at the end of that time they were refractory to the poison. The serum obtained from these immunised animals prevented the development of the morbid phenomena which were produced by the injection of the gonotoxin. I am not aware of any experiments having been performed upon man with a view of testing the efficacy of injections of this anti-gonorrhœal serum, but it is quite possible that it might exercise a favourable influence in cases of general gonococcic infection by neutralising the toxic products, and that it might hasten the cure of cases of gonorrhœal arthritis, salpingitis, and other chronic inflammations due to this toxin which have hitherto obstinately resisted treatment. At the present moment, then, this anti-gonorrhœal serum cannot be included amongst practical therapeutic measures at our disposal.

The palliative treatment just alluded to will encourage and promote the gonococcic invasion, and will entail the infection of the whole urethra down to its prostatic portion, and the absorption or production of a larger amount of the toxin. As long as the gonococcus is limited to the anterior part of the urethra, it does not, as a rule, give rise to any serious complications, but when it reaches the prostatic urethra, and becomes a posterior gonorrhœa, then the surgeon may begin to anticipate some of the sequelæ and eventualities before enumerated.   The rational and scientific treatment then would appear to be to attack the gonococcus *at the first possible opportunity*, with some substance that will destroy its virulence and prevent its spread and that of its toxin.   Unfortunately, the youth of the present day, from motives of economy and secrecy, too often resorts at first to the prescribing chemist, whose ideas of the treatment of the disease are somewhat behind those which appear in surgical text-books.   The victim will first be dosed with alkalies and balsams; his gonorrhœa will spread down his urethra, he will then be advised to use injections, and on the appearance of some painful and disquieting complication he will consult a surgeon.   It is then a matter of regret that so often the patients through ignorance and neglect have given the gonococcus such a scope for the exercise of its baneful proclivities, for if these cases could be taken in hand early much might be done to mitigate the evil consequences of the disease.   The principal desideratum is to discover some non-caustic or corrosive application which will destroy the gonococcus without injuring the mucous membrane of the urethra, and without giving rise to an acute inflammatory reaction.   It has long been known that weak solutions of nitrate of silver are destructive to the gonococcus, but the irritating properties of this substance were such as to preclude its use.   Recent research in the therapeutics of gonorrhœa have evolved various compounds of nitrate of silver, which, whilst retaining its gonococcidal properties, are non-irritating to the urethral mucosa, but are capable of penetrating into its deeper layers.   Mention may be made of a few of these compounds and of the different proportion of nitrate of silver contained in each :

Argyrol, containing 30 per cent. of argent nit., a combination of silver and vitellin.

Ichthargan, containing 30 per cent. of argent nit., compound of ichthyol and silver.

Albargin, containing 15 per cent. of argent nit., compound of silver and gelatose.

Nargol, containing 10 per cent. argent nit., compound of nuclein and silver.

Protargol, containing 8 per cent. of argent nit., compound of proteids and silver.

Argonin, containing 4 per cent. of argent nit., compound of casein and silver.

Argentamine, containing 2 per cent. of argent nit., compound of ethylene diamine and silver.

In all these preparations the irritating effect of the nitrate of silver has been to a great extent abolished ; for the most part they do not coagulate albumen or precipitate chlorides, so that they are not chemically altered by contact with mucous membranes and their secretions.   Through the agency of these preparations we are enabled to attack the gonococcus in the early stages of the disease, and to prevent its extension to deeper and inaccessible regions.   Directly the case comes under observation, and the presence of the gonococcus has confirmed the diagnosis, the treatment should be commenced, and its success will depend to some extent upon the thoroughness with which it is carried out.   Minute instructions should be given to the patient as to the technique of injections, and no reliance should be placed on his representation that he is familiar with their use. By means of one of the forms of urethral syringe in common use the solution should be introduced into the urethra so as thoroughly to distend it, and there retained for a period varying from five to thirty minutes, its retention for this prolonged period obviating the frequent repetition of the process, and insuring its penetration into the deeper layers of the urethral mucous membrane. The pain resulting from this process is not, as a rule, severe, but does occasionally necessitate the introduction of a few drops of a cocaine solution.   The result of this treatment is that a profuse purulent discharge will be considerably modified at the end of a week or ten days, after which time it gradually becomes muco-purulent or watery ; this condition will probably subside and disappear altogether with the use of an astringent injection.   The gonococci usually disappear after a fortnight's treatment, but are apt to reappear if the silver applications are not continued for three weeks.   If the treatment is begun sufficiently early and carried out efficiently, there is a probability that the disease will be confined to the anterior urethra, but if it does reach the posterior urethra the method will have to be considerably modified. The preparations of which I have had the most experience are argyrol, nargol, and protargol, with all of which I have obtained satisfactory results. Argyrol, though possessing a greater strength of argent nitrate than any of the other substances except ichthargan, is the least irritating and can be employed at a strength of 2 per cent. to commence with, increased gradually up to 5 per cent. ; with nargol and protargol, a strength of $\frac{1}{2}$ to 1 per cent. is sufficient to begin with. It is well that the first injection should be introduced under the supervision of the surgeon ; but since this is often not practicable, clear instructions should be given as to the manner in which the injection treatment should be carried out. To all my patients, whether hospital or private, I give a printed slip, informing them as to the nature of the disease. In the treatment of gonorrhœa, as in that of syphilis, the surgeon owes a responsibility to the community at large, and not the least important part of the treatment should be to thoroughly enlighten the patient as to the nature of his disease, and its possible consequences to himself and to those with whom he is brought into contact.

Hitherto I have only alluded to gonorrhœa of the anterior urethra ; but when, owing to delay in commencing treatment, or when in spite of the measures I have indicated it has spread to the prostatic portion of the urethra, then other means must be adopted to rid the patient of his microbic infection. First, though, it would be well to describe the symptoms of a posterior gonorrhœa (though they are generally sufficiently obvious), and the means of diagnosing this condition. The ordinary two-glass test, as advocated by Sir H. Thompson, affords the requisite information if the discharge is copious, but is not absolutely reliable when the discharge is subsiding, and is limited, possibly, to an inspissated thread from the prostatic urethra. In such a condition the anterior urethra down to the triangular ligament should be well irrigated to get rid of any secretion, when any discharge present in the prostatic urethra will be manifest when the patient empties the bladder into a urine glass. One of the first symptoms of involvement of the posterior urethra is increased frequency of micturition with spasmodic pain in

the perineum and at the end of the penis following the act, and leading the patient to think that there is still some urine left in the bladder, and following urination there may be a drop or more of blood ; the cardinal symptoms then are frequency of micturition, pain in the perineum and penile urethra, and slight hæmaturia. In this condition the ordinary method of injection fails to afford relief or amelioration of the symptoms, since the fluid does not reach that portion of the urethra which is principally involved. To reach the posterior urethra either deep irrigations must be practised, or instillations of a limited amount of one or the above-mentioned silver compounds by means of a Guyon's syringe. Irrigation is particularly indicated when both the anterior and posterior urethra are involved, and is best carried out by passing into the prostate a urethral irrigating tube such as that shown, attaching to it an india-rubber tube connected with a glass funnel, and passing in a pint or half a pint of $\frac{1}{2}$ per cent. solution of one of the silver preparations, and allowing it to flow back and escape by the side of the tube from the meatus. Guyon's syringe acts in much the same manner, only here a very small amount, $\mathfrak{m}$ v- $\mathfrak{m}$ x, of a more concentrated solution is introduced into the prostatic urethra and allowed to remain there till expelled by the next act of micturition.

Time at my disposal will not admit of my discussing the general treatment of the disease, nor can I deal with its many complications. One adjunct to local treatment may be mentioned, viz. the internal administration of copaiba, cubebs, or sandal-wood ; of these remedies the former two are useful in the early stages of the disease, while sandal-wood is more effective when the discharge is subsiding. A preparation which I have found most effective is called "gonosan," which is prepared by extracting from the root of Piper methysticum its essential resins, which are then dissolved in pure East Indian sandal-wood oil ; it is given in capsules containing 5 minims, and the dose is from eight to ten capsules, given daily. Their effect on the urinary tract is somewhat anæsthetic, so that they diminish the ardor urinæ and the painful erections ; they are diuretic and modify the amount of the urethral discharge, without in any way disturbing the digestive functions.

October 30th, 1905.

WITH DR. G. A. SUTHERLAND AT THE PADDINGTON GREEN CHILDREN'S HOSPITAL.

LOBAR PNEUMONIA IN CHILDHOOD.

(*Concluded from p.* 32.)

THE SECOND STAGE AND THE MODE OF DEATH IN PNEUMONIA.

Whether in infancy, in childhood, or in adult life the most common cause of a fatal termination in pneumonia is cardiac failure. It is rather a curious fact that in what is often regarded as a pulmonary affection without any cardiac lesion the chief danger to life should be cardiac failure. Some have explained this on the ground that the heart is unable to carry on the circulation owing to the pulmonary obstruction. But the cutting off a part of the lung from the circulation, as happens in pneumonia, does not necessarily produce cardiac stress or cardiac failure, provided that, as usually happens, there is enough of sound pulmonary tissue left to keep up the oxygenation of the blood. At necropsies in fatal cases of pneumonia one will usually find quite enough of acting lung-tissue for respiratory purposes, and will not find evidence of pulmonary obstruction sufficient to cause cardiac failure. The purely pulmonary theory as to the cause of a fatal issue in pneumonia, which assumes a mechanical failure on the part of the heart to carry on the pulmonary circulation, is not justified either by the clinical conditions or by the post-mortem findings.

We pass from this to the other theory which regards pneumonia as a profound toxæmia, producing disturbances through the system generally, and selecting more especially certain nervous centres. In these respects the disease may be compared with diphtheria, which is first of all a general toxæmia, and, secondly, shows a special affinity for certain nerve-centres. In pneumonia a patient may die from the profound toxæmia, being in a prostrate condition from the onset, and never showing any signs of rallying. This is not a common mode of death in childhood, although it may occur. We have already considered the clinical phenomena in the first stage of pneumonia, and have associated the respiratory and cardiac phenomena with a stimulation of the respiratory and cardiac centres in the medulla. But over-stimulation or prolonged stimulation of these centres will tend to induce a condition of paresis or even paralysis. Further, the toxins may be expected to attack more especially those centres which have already been weakened in any way. The second stage in pneumonia is reached when, instead of increased activity of these medullary centres, we find signs of weakness beginning to appear.

Let us consider first the effect on the respiratory centre in the medulla when the second stage is reached. Were the medullary centre the only available means of carrying on the respiration, death would in many cases follow from paralysis of this centre, but you will remember that we have already referred to another centre in the cortex cerebri. We have in this cortical centre a second source of nervous energy for respiratory purposes when the medullary centre fails. We have also a second mechanism for expanding the lungs when abdominal (diaphragmatic) breathing fails, namely costal breathing by means of the intercostal and accessory muscle of respiration.

Clinically, the onset of cortical, as contrasted with medullary breathing is marked by certain definite changes in the respiration, which are easily recognised. We described the breathing in the first stage of pneumonia as being rapid, shallow, abdominal, without distress, and without any laboured action of the chest. The picture is changed in this, the second stage, for cortical breathing is conscious, voluntary, and under pneumonic conditions, laboured. I have drawn up here in parallel columns the differences which are seen clinically.

PNEUMONIC BREATHING.

Stage I.	Stage II.
1. Increased frequency.	Not so frequent.
2. Shallow.	Deeper.
3. Abdominal chiefly.	Upper costal chiefly.
4. No evident difficulty or distress.	Evident difficulty and distress.
5. Not laboured.	Laboured.
6. Accessory muscles of respiration not acting.	Accessory muscles of respiration acting.

The excessive frequency disappears and the breathing becomes slower, the shallow abdominal breathing is replaced by deeper breathing in which the upper thoracic region takes the chief part; the placid expression of the patient's face changes to one of anxiety and distress, and the over-action of all the muscles of respiration shows a laboured action in the breathing which did not formerly exist. These conditions may be entirely due to a failure of the medullary centre to carry on the work, or they may be aggravated still further by extensive consolidation of the lung, or by the supervention of cardiac weakness, with defective circulation. In most cases the respiratory powers will be sufficient to carry the patient safely through the crisis, in others cardiac failure supervenes before the respiratory powers are exhausted, and in some cases it may happen that death ensues directly from respiratory failure

Consider next the effect on the heart of failure of the cardiac centre. We have here no auxiliary mechanism, central or peripheral, to call into play as in the case of respiration. The inhibitory action of the vagus is diminished or cut off, and this second stage is marked clinically by an increased rate in the cardiac pulsations. If relief is not secured, either through the natural termination of the disease or through artificial aids, the result will be that the heart runs on, and finally runs itself out. Hence we can understand why it is that a fatal issue is much more common in pneumonia from cardiac than from respiratory failure.

I think that the two stages in the course of pneumonia are mixed up together in the text-book descriptions of the disease, but their recognition is of importance. In some cases only the first stage is present, the crisis supervening before the second is reached. The second stage begins as a rule about the fifth or sixth day of the disease, and may be termed the precritical stage. The symptoms may be alarming, and the condition of the patient may cause anxiety for a day or two, but as a rule recovery takes place.

In the case of a child, previously healthy, who is suffering from uncomplicated lobar pneumonia the prognosis is always good. A fatal issue in lobar pneumonia can almost always be traced to impaired health or impaired nutrition in the child, or to the presence of some complication.

THE TREATMENT.

In an ordinary case, in the majority of cases, if we put the patient under favourable conditions as regards rest in bed, fresh air, and suitable diet, the disease will run its course to a favourable termination without any active interference on our part. No treatment of pneumonia has yet been devised which will shorten or influence the natural course of the disease, and many forms of treatment have fallen into well-merited discredit. Nevertheless it is necessary that every case should be carefully watched by the physician, for two reasons : (1) to relieve troublesome and weakening symptoms, and (2) to treat complications if they arise.

We shall suppose that, the diagnosis having been made, the patient is put in bed, clothed in a flannel nightdress, with or without some extra flannel or cotton-wool round the chest ; that the bed-clothes are sufficiently thick to preserve warmth but not to be a burden or cause sweating ; that any chilling of the extremities is guarded against by the use of hot bottles ; that the bed is not placed in a corner, or close to the fire, or covered with a tent, but in an open part of the largest available room, where fresh air can play freely about it (without draught), so that the lungs may have a plentiful supply of cool fresh air ; that a diet of milk and barley-water, with some mutton or chicken soup has been ordered, and that a febrifuge mixture containing citrate of potash and acetate of ammonia has been prescribed. In many cases the above, with the help of good nursing, and the treatment common to all acute specific fevers, will carry the patient safely through the illness.

Certain symptoms may call for treatment.

(1) *Pain about the chest.*—If the pleuritic pain is manifestly causing the child suffering, a local application in the shape of a turpentine fomentation or linseed poultice may be applied over the painful area for half an hour, or until the skin is thoroughly reddened. This may be repeated some hours later if necessary. The practice of poulticing or fomenting the whole chest continuously throughout an attack of pneumonia and irrespective of definite symptoms, as was common when I began the study of medicine, has now fallen into disuse. It was based on a wrong pathology, it had no beneficial effect on the course of the disease, and it distinctly did harm by disturbing the patient, interfering with the freedom of the respiratory movements, and depressing the heart. On the other hand, the interrupted use of hot moist applications, for the relief of special symptoms, is, I

believe, of great value. These local measures will usually serve to relieve the patient, except in that very painful variety associated with diaphragmatic pleurisy. In this condition the application of a few leeches (two or three) over the affected area, combined with strapping of the affected side, may secure relief and rest. But if they fail to do so then opium or morphia must be given. Opium is distinctly contra-indicated in pneumonia because of its toxic effect on the respiratory centre, and as I believe that centre is always affected to a greater or less extent in pneumonia, I should refrain from giving it for any symptom save very severe pain. We have to consider whether the patient will not be more weakened by the pain and restlessness than by the opium, and decide accordingly.

(2) *Coughing* may at times disturb the patient. The amount of coughing probably depends on the extent of lung involved. If there is a whole lobe involved, there will probably be a good deal of coughing from the irritation of the exudation. If only a small focus is involved, the irritation will be slight and the coughing trifling. It may be either of the short hacking pneumonic type, or bronchial, from the presence of catarrh. In both of these the interrupted use of hot local applications, as described above, will be beneficial. The position of the patient in bed must also be attended to, as frequently the coughing only occurs in certain positions, and is relieved by a change. The use of steam inhalations may also check an irritable condition of the bronchi. Here again the old practice of continuous steaming in a tent must be avoided, as it produces a most depressing and uncomfortable atmosphere. If steam is used, it should be turned on for from ten to fifteen minutes at a time, and at intervals of some hours. For the relief of persistent coughing, with or without much secretion, belladonna in doses of ♏v–x of the tincture, or ♏¼ to j of the liquor atropinæ, will be found advantageous. It is especially indicated in pneumonia because (1) of its checking secretion, (2) dulling the sensory branches of the vagus throughout the lungs, and (3) stimulating the respiratory centre. One can also safely and beneficially give five to ten minims of paregoric occasionally for a hacking cough.

(3) *Pyrexia.*—The ordinary temperature of pneumonia, averaging from 103° to 104·5° F., requires no treatment. In children the height of the temperature is not an indication of the gravity of the disease, and the rapid recovery after the crisis shows that the pyrexia is not *per se* a source of weakness or danger. Prolonged continuous pyrexia, say after the seventh day, is probably weakening, but should not be interfered with by drastic measures, as the pyrexia may directly bring the crisis nearer. I think that for once the medical profession is quite unanimous in deprecating the use of antipyretic drugs in pneumonia. In some cases the temperature rises to 105° F. or 106° F. without the patient showing any signs of distress. Here, again, no treatment is called for. But if great restlessness supervenes, with sleeplessness, symptoms which we trace to the presence of hyper-pyrexia, then some interference is called for. In the case of infants, the employment of a hot bath, which is rapidly cooled to 85° F., will frequently be followed by a fall of temperature of from 1° to 2° F., and the restlessness will disappear. In older children sponging in bed with hot or tepid water is the corresponding treatment and if extreme nervous disturbance is present the temporary application of cold water cloths or Leiter's tubing to the head. It will often be found also that the application of a hot fomentation, combined with drachm doses of liquor ammoniæ acetatis, has a distinctly antipyretic effect. An ice bag to the chest has its advocates, but my own experience has led me to avoid extremely cold applications in childhood and infancy. When confronted with a rise of temperature amounting to hyperpyrexia one must not assume at once that this is due to the pneumonia. Disturbances of an entirely different kind may be present in other parts of the system, and may be sufficient to raise the temperature by a few degrees. I believe that such a disturbance will frequently be found in the gastro-intestinal tract, and consequently, in the absence of other definite cause, I am in the habit of ordering a couple of grains of calomel or grey powder in cases of hyperpyrexia, with restlessness. Another possible source of hyperpyrexia is acute otitis media.

(4) *Sleeplessness.*—Pursuing our plan of securing rest to the patient, we shall find it necessary to take action if sleeplessness occurs. Probably there is nothing more exhausting to the child's whole system than want of sleep. Delirious sleep is very common in pneumonia, and is probably not in-

jurious. On the other hand, sleeplessness is often accompanied by active delirium and marked prostration follows. I have already referred to the presence of middle-ear inflammation, and this condition should always be looked for, and if necessary treated, when delirium and sleeplessness are present. Cold water to the head or hot applications to the chest may produce relief of these symptoms, but constant fussing about the patient with local applications is apt to increase the condition. Probably the free use of bromide of ammonium, in ten-grain doses, or bromidia in ℥xv doses, is at once the most effective and the least harmful treatment. Sulphonal or veronal may be used, but not opium. A dose of brandy, ℥ij to ℥ss., in hot water, will often act like a charm. As a matter of clinical experience I believe there has been far less delirium and sleeplessness in pneumonia since we dropped the "active treatment" of the disease, and simply kept the patient quiet and comfortable in bed.

(5) *Symptoms preceding the crisis.*—The symptoms of pneumonia are as a rule most pronounced and most threatening for the twenty-four or forty-eight hours preceding the crisis, and possibly for a short time after it. This is very strikingly shown in hospital practice, where so many pneumonia patients are admitted shortly before the crisis. The explanation would seem to be that the condition of the child in mild cases of lobar pneumonia does not appear to the lay mind to be very serious until this pre-critical stage has been reached. The breathing and coughing may then have been observed to get worse, the restlessness greater, or the lethargy and prostration more profound. Sometimes an increase in the nervous symptoms may have excited alarm, sometimes blueness of the face or a tendency to faint may have been noticed. These or other signs have led the parents to seek medical advice for the first time. The same conditions are often present in cases which have been carefully treated from the first, and therefore it is important to be on the watch for the symptoms of the pre-critical or second stage of pneumonia. The longer the crisis is delayed, the more severe will the symptoms of the pre-critical stage become. This is the stage at which the active treatment of pneumonia should commence, as contrasted with our previous treatment for the relief of symptoms. Not that even at this stage do we actually treat the

disease, but only certain results of it which are of vital importance.

Signs of cardiac weakness are to be carefully watched for, and we have to note whether the failure is primarily in the left or in the right ventricle. There are many elaborate methods described for determining these points, but clinically the simplest method is best. If dilatation of the left ventricle is taking place, as the result of cardiac failure, we shall find the apex beat extending outwards to the left, the first sound at the apex becoming weaker, the pulse tension falling and the rate increasing, and a tendency to faintness and pallor appearing. At the onset of these signs the use of brandy, strychnia, and ether is indicated, in doses increasing in amount until we get a definite improvement. If the condition is more serious or is rapidly advancing, the hypodermic injection of strychnia is as serviceable in children as in adults. The injection causes little discomfort to the patient, and the only remark I have to make about the dose is that enough is not usually given. For an infant one year old in the precritical stage of pneumonia, liquor strychninæ in one-minim doses by the mouth and half-minim doses hypodermically, every four hours, will produce good results. The reaction of the system to strychnia is much less easily induced in the profound toxæmia of pneumonia than under normal conditions. Consequently the drug should be pushed until we get the desired improvement, or until some symptoms of the physiological action, such as twitching, have been produced. If dilatation of the right ventricle is present, with cyanosis, dyspnœa, and over-action of the right side of the heart, then some depletion of blood is called for. A very useful test as to the presence of this condition is the gradual enlargement of the liver, and clinically the increase in size of the liver will be found to be a very exact guide as to the degree of embarrassment of the right side of the heart. This may be accompanied by signs of œdema in the affected lung or the sound lung. The application of three or four leeches over the hepatic region, followed by a hot fomentation to encourage further bleeding, will usually be found to produce marked relief. This treatment is further aided by a dose of calomel (two or three grains) followed by a saline, and by the use of alcohol and strychnine as cardiac tonics. Instead of the leeching we may employ dry cupping over the bases of the lungs posteriorly, especially when pulmonary engorgement is present. It is also when cyanosis and right-sided enlargement of the heart occur that the use of oxygen inhalations, or better of a hyperoxygenated atmosphere about the patient, may be of distinct service. In the treatment of pneumonia generally I have not been able to convince myself of the benefit of oxygen inhalations, and the patient does not appear to be suffering from a defective supply of oxygen ; but in cyanotic conditions oxygen certainly gives relief in some cases and presumably benefits the patient.

We shall sometimes find that there is an increasing amount of respiratory distress, with dyspnœa and rapid breathing, which does not appear to depend directly on the pulmonary or the cardiac condition. We have here probably to deal with a failure of the respiratory centre from toxæmia. In such cases atropine, as a direct respiratory stimulant, may be combined with the strychnia, in doses of $\frac{1}{100}$th grain hypodermically every four hours, for a child of five years.

October 30th, 1905.

Operative Injury of Thoracic Duct.—Vautrin

has observed four cases of operative injury of the thoracic duct during an operation. The results were insignificant in three of the cases, but in the other they were so serious that he writes to protest against the optimism which prevails in regard to injuries of this nature. He reviews the various methods of caring for such an injury in vogue, preferring himself to ligate the vessel after exposing it and testing the condition of its walls. This ligature may prove very difficult when the duct has to be sought behind the blood-vessels, in the retro-sternal region. This should be done at once, instead of waiting until the patient has become so much debilitated from the loss of lymph from the duct that he is scarcely able to bear any surgical intervention. In his fatal case the patient had had congestion of the lungs, dyspnœa, and tachycardia on previous occasions, which made him hesitate to resort to general anæsthesia and to ligate the thoracic duct when it could have been done on the exposed, easily accessible portion. When he was finally compelled to this course, ligation was no longer possible except at a more inaccessible part of the duct, rendering the operation so grave that the patient finally succumbed. He advises ligature from the first, without wasting time on compression, if the walls of the duct are not too friable. It is a dangerous procedure in case of the absence of collaterals. When both these conditions are encountered the prognosis is necessarily bad.—*Journ. A. M. A.*, vol. xlv., No. 15.

THE PRACTICE OF MEDICINE : A Text-book for Practitioners and Students, with Special Reference to Diagnosis and Treatment. By JAMES TYSON, M.D. Third edition, with 134 illustrations. London : REBMAN, Ltd.

This book has now reached its third edition, and forms a handsome, well-printed volume of 1240 pages. Well arranged and concisely written, it constitutes one of the best one-volume text-books of medicine in the English language. Being written with special reference to diagnosis and treatment, it is eminently practical in its scope. Another factor which the reader will appreciate is the judicious use of heavy type and italics for head-lines and important facts, by means of which a readier grasp is obtained of the subject-matter.

This edition has been thoroughly revised. The alterations and additions have been so numerous that the whole book has been re-set. The sections on Dysentery and on Diseases of the Nervous System have been subjected to the greatest alterations, the former with the collaboration of Dr. Simon Flexner and the latter with that of Dr W. G. Spiller, names which are a guarantee for the thoroughness with which the revision has been made. Both sections are thoroughly well up to date.

The systematic descriptions of the most important diseases are prefaced by a brief historical note, printed in smaller type, so that the volume is not appreciably increased in size. Many instructive charts or diagrams also add to the usefulness of the work, among the best being the three coloured plates showing respectively Koplik's spots, which are stated to be pathognomonic signs of measles ; the different forms of malarial organism, with their stages of development, and the varieties of the colourless corpuscles of the blood in leukæmia.

We have no hesitation in declaring that, armed with a good knowledge of the contents of this volume, the student can face the ordeal of his examination with equanimity and with every assurance of success.

WE have received from BURROUGHS, WELLCOME & Co. specimens of pleated compressed bandages and dressings. In the country and in emergency cases these should quickly establish their popularity, as their compactness enables a practitioner to carry in a minimum of space all the necessary dressings in a day's routine practice.

THE CLINICAL JOURNAL,

CLINICAL RECORD, CLINICAL NEWS, CLINICAL GAZETTE, CLINICAL REPORTER, CLINICAL CHRONICLE AND CLINICAL REVIEW.

EDITED BY L. ELIOT CREASY.

No. 680.   WEDNESDAY, NOVEMBER 8, 1905.   Vol. XXVII. No. 4.

CONTENTS.

. * *Specially reported for the Clinical Journal. Revised by the Author.*

NOTICE.

Editorial correspondence, books for review, &c., should be addressed to the Editor, 51, New Cavendish Street, W., Telephone No. 904, Paddington ; but all business communications should be addressed to the Publishers, 22½, Bartholomew Close, London, E.C. Telephone 927, Holborn.

All inquiries respecting Advertisements should be sent to MESSRS. ADLARD & SON, *Bartholomew Close, E.C. Telephone 927, Holborn.*

Terms of Subscription, including postage, payable by cheque, postal or banker's order (in advance) : for the United Kingdom, 15s. 6d. per annum ; Abroad, 17s. 6d.

Cheques, &c., should be made payable to THE PROPRIETORS OF THE CLINICAL JOURNAL, *crossed " The London, City, and Midland Bank, Ltd., Newgate Street Branch, E.C. Account of the Medical Publishing Company, Limited."*

Reading Cases to hold Twenty-six numbers of THE CLINICAL JOURNAL *can be supplied at 2s. 3d. each, or will be forwarded post free on receipt of 2s. 6d. ; and also Cases for binding Volumes at 1s. each, or post free on receipt of 1s. 3d., from the Publishers, 22½ Bartholomew Close, London, E.C.*

TWO LECTURES.

Delivered at St. Bartholomew's Hospital.

By C. B. LOCKWOOD, F.R.C.S., Surgeon to the Hospital.

LECTURE II.

SWELLINGS ABOVE AND BELOW THE NECK OF THE SCROTUM—PARTICULARLY INGUINAL VARICOCELE AND HYDROCELE.

GENTLEMEN,—You will remember that last time we dealt with the methods of ascertaining what a particular patient was suffering from. We said that from each thing seen or felt something was inferred, so that at last you had in your possession several inferences, and from those you drew a conclusion which was your diagnosis. Now we will proceed. Last time I essayed swellings above the neck of the scrotum, and naturally you might expect to-day that I should proceed with swellings in the neck of the scrotum. So I might, but instead I will proceed with swellings in the scrotum. And I do so for this reason : that most of the swellings which are in the neck of the scrotum either have descended into it from the inguinal canal or they have ascended into it from the scrotum. So obviously for the elucidation of swellings in the neck of the scrotum it is first of all necessary to pass in review the kind of swelling which may have descended and also the kind of swelling which may have ascended. Clearly, it is necessary to know both before you can proceed with the swellings in the neck of the scrotum. We will assume that the swelling is in the scrotum itself. You will begin with your eyes, and inspect the skin of the scrotum first. It is red, it is shiny, and from that fact you will infer that there is beneath the skin of the scrotum an inflamed structure of some kind. And that will make you exceedingly cautious ;

because the inflamed structures which are met with in the scrotum are often of exquisite sensibility, and if the unwary proceeds to feel incautiously, or squeezes the cord to see whether it ascends into the neck of the scrotum (and perhaps has not observed that there is a urethral discharge at the same time), he will probably make an enemy for the rest of his life. So it is, both to you and to the patient, of the very greatest importance that you should look at the scrotum as a beginning, with the view of seeing what after that you may venture to do. Let us suppose you have looked at the scrotal swelling, that the neck of the scrotum is the same on that side as the other; you will then see what shape and kind of swelling you have to deal with. Suppose that, at the bottom of the scrotum you see a globular swelling, perhaps lying horizontally or obliquely; you may assume that that is the testicle, and you will probably be right. You will then apply your test to it. If that swelling at the bottom of the scrotum is testicle, you will be able to feel the spermatic cord descending to it. You will recognise the cord because you will be able to feel the vas deferens, and perhaps the spermatic artery and those small cords will slip about in your fingers. Next, the swelling itself will have an epididymis which you can feel—and you ought to make yourselves quite familiar with the exact feel of those structures when they are healthy. Let us suppose that, in addition, there is to be seen above the testicle a pyriform swelling which is irregular in outline, which disappears when the patient lies down, and fills up again when he stands up, and can be felt to consist of thickened vessels; then obviously you have to do with varicocele of the scrotum. That ought to be very easy to diagnose. and very few people would fail in diagnosing a scrotal varicocele. This is where so many fail; they fail to observe that the scrotal varicocele is continued up into the neck of the scrotum, and thence into the inguinal canal, which is dilated, and exhibits a faint impulse on coughing. I mentioned such an one last time, and said that an unobservant surgeon operated upon the veins at the neck of the scrotum but omitted to observe that the external ring was dilated and there was an impulse in the inguinal canal. The patient afterwards came back, complaining bitterly that he had not been cured, and expressed great sorrow

that a further operation was necessary to put him right. That is a position in which anybody may be placed unless he is an observant person and unless he proceeds with his diagnosis in a methodical manner.

Now let us proceed to consider another swelling in the scrotum, which is almost always quite easy to detect with the naked eye, and that is an oval swelling in the scrotum covered by natural skin, and which in part of its length shows a slight broad constriction. Notice, I did not say it was a pyriform swelling, but an oval swelling which in some parts is slightly constricted. If I were to compare a jargonelle pear you might expect the constriction to be one third the distance from the thin end, but the constriction is often half-way down. Now, in making generalisations I would say that collections of fluid in the tunica vaginalis become constricted. If you go to the top gallery of the museum, you will see a specimen of hydrocele which has been dried and blown up, and if you look critically at it you will observe its shape and that there is a slight constriction, and I think you will agree that at the situation of the constriction there are a few transverse fibres in the processus vaginalis. What these fibres are I do not know, but they are always there in some part of the tunica vaginalis, and they are the fibres which produce this constriction. I have further evidence that it is so from my own experience, because over and over again when operating for the radical cure of hydrocele I have looked for these crossing bands and divided them, and as I have divided them I have observed the contsriction disappear. Now, I did not say hydrocele only: I said any collection of fluid in the tunica vaginalis, because I have seen hæmatocele—that is to say, a collection of blood—in which this applied. And when I saw patients in the Out-Patient Department, there were two cases of fluid which had all the appearance of pus when tapped. I think I remember that the Pathological Department reported to us that it was not actually pus. I confess I should have been surprised if it had been pus. Has anybody here seen pus come out of a hydrocele or tunica vaginalis? It must be of very rare occurrence. Why is hydrocele so little given to suppuration? I have seen dreadful trocars pushed into hydroceles, and I have known such hydrocele given every possible chance of suppurating and yet they have not. In fact, I suspect it is very hard to make them suppurate, because one of the old methods of treating hydrocele was to lay the sac open and fill it full of gauze, and another was to put setons in, and these hardly succeed. To proceed with the hydrocele, I should say it is full of traps for the unwary. Let me give you an instance. A Governor of this hospital sent his gardener to the surgery with a note from his doctor, saying : " I have attended this man for what I believe to be hydrocele, which I have tapped, and nothing but blood came out, and therefore I have sent him up in order that you may remove a malignant testicle." This is not exactly what he said, but it is the summary of it. That statement had also been imparted to the man. Now, these are the various false steps which were taken there. A hydrocele is translucent. Next, the vast bulk of hydroceles have a healthy spermatic cord above them. So when you have seen the shape of the tumour and felt the spermatic cord, and felt that it is all separate and distinct, you proceed to see whether the tumour is translucent. I have seen translucency looked for in all sorts of absurd manners, with wax matches, and I have seen a patient leap because the scrotum has been burnt. I have also seen the investigation made with tallow candles. I wonder the examiner did not ask for a rush-light. But if you resort to such medieval things as that you are sure to come to grief. My advice is that amongst your possessions you should include some sort of small electric light. You probably have one which is used as a head-lamp, and I strongly advise you to have a Hering's lamp which is used for illuminating the antrum of Highmore. You may go further and have an extra good one, and have a focussing lens upon it, which enables you to illuminate the frontal sinus. When you get a powerful light like that behind a hydrocele in a dark room, what was formerly difficult now becomes an easy matter. I am afraid our friend omitted to examine the case I have referred to with a proper light, though that is only a surmise of mine. He should have taken the patient into a darkened room, lifted up the scrotum, nipped the skin so as to make the hydrocele tight, and get every opaque structure out of the way—for instance, the penis and the thigh—and then examine it properly with his head-lamp or electric light. Had he done that, he would have found out something else, because he tapped it with what I call a cow-doctor's trocar—that is, one of those horrid medieval things which used to be put into all the instrument-cases. He might have used a trocar of one millimetre or one and a half millimetre, which is quite big enough to let the water out. The patient would not have felt any more than a mere prick, the fluid would have run out, and he would have felt so little inconvenience from the operation that he might have gone and bought a trocar and tapped himself in future, which is what I have known patients do. This doctor had used a cow-doctor's trocar, and out came blood. He had omitted, when he examined it with the light, to examine it with another definite intent in his mind, and that was to see where the testicle was. This patient had the testicle in front instead of behind. The rule is for the cord to be behind the hernial sac and the testicle to be behind the hydrocele, but you must not trust to such rules as that, because some people have got an inversion of the testicle : it is rotated upon its axis, the tunica vaginalis being at the back instead of in front. And that seems to have happened to this man. When he came here he was tapped behind with a minute trocar, the fluid was drawn off, and his malignant tumour was gone. That is an awkward position for any human being to place himself in, but all of you will do it unless you take the precautions I have mentioned. Supposing you agree, after examination, that a patient has got a hydrocele, you have observed its oval shape, have seen its translucency, and made up your mind that the testicle is behind ; do not be too sure, but examine the neck of the scrotum. If there is any thickening in the neck of the scrotum, be very, very cautious how you proceed. That is not a straightforward hydrocele. Now look at the inguinal canal and at the cord. If that thickening goes up through a spacious external abdominal ring into a dilated canal, be very, very careful. Hydrocele is not often unaccompanied by some form of hernia. One of the forms which accompany it is congenital hernia with epiplocele, the epiplocele being perhaps impacted in the neck of the sac, and the neck of the sac being, in a case of congenital hernia, exceedingly tight, with firm fibrous rings in it. That is not an imaginary danger, because within the last five years I have had a patient in the wards who was diagnosed by his doctor to have a hydrocele. He was tapped under that belief. Very little fluid came out, and when it was over the doctor got suspicious and came to the conclusion that the patient might possibly have a rupture. That is exactly what he had, a congenital hernia, with the neck full of impacted and adherent omentum, which was removed. He was a source of great anxiety to us, because his hernial sac, we thought, was in an inflamed and septic condition, and obviously to do the operation for the radical cure of hernia on a person with an inflamed hernial sac was to do it under circumstances of great additional danger. I may possibly have conveyed to your minds so far that I believe hydrocele to be a disease. Of course, it would be just as rational to tell you that I think a cough is a disease. As a matter of fact hydrocele is a sign of disease. As regards the ordinary common passive hydrocele I do not know what it is due to in the least, but I know that ordinary hydrocele is only part of a chronic inflammatory condition of the tunica vaginalis and of the testicle. Supposing you proceed to cure the hydrocele the cure would be, not tapping once, but to lay it open, remove the parietal layer of the tunica vaginalis, and perhaps drain it for a few hours, and in ten days' time it would be quite well. I advise you always to pay the greatest attention to the radical cure of hydrocele, as it is a simple operation and gives most admirable results, the patients are exceedingly pleased, and there is little anxiety. But, like all other operations, it requires to be exceedingly well organised and properly managed and to be founded upon a perfectly correct diagnosis. And that is my chief point. You have done this, but you have omitted before you began to say to the patient: "You know this hydrocele of yours is due to chronic inflammation, and it is due to chronic inflammation of your testicle; therefore after my operation you will find that that organ will remain rather large, rather hard, and perhaps occasionally tender." If you do not tell him that, I think he would blame you, and legitimately, for having produced those results. There is another thing I should like to mention, and that is that in a person who has had hydrocele for a great number of years the pressure of the fluid apparently spreads out the testicle and flattens it, so that at last it becomes an atrophied organ. But I will assume that the cases have been operated upon within a reasonable time.

Now let us consider some other causes of hydrocele. We will take tubercle next. In some cases of hydrocele the collection of fluid in the tunica vaginalis conceals the fact that the patient has behind it a tuberculous testis. Supposing you overlook a tuberculous testis, and you see it only at the operation, and you have proceeded to remove it without permission, then you have landed yourself into an uncomfortable place. Some hydroceles are associated with syphilitic disease of the testis, and they too ought to be considered and carefully diagnosed. And lastly, some hydroceles are associated with malignant disease of the testicle. I think, gentlemen, you should be very cautious how you approach any kind of hydrocele. I might mention other causes, but they are not active in this country. We seldom see those huge hydroceles which occur abroad and which are due to parasitic causes.

Before I leave the consideration of hydrocele I will mention one other cause of hydrocele, and that is traumatism. I have occasionally seen hydrocele follow accidental injuries and surgical injuries. For instance, I remember operating upon a gentleman for the radical cure of hydrocele who had had his testicle injured by a cricket ball, and when I came to operate there was the remains of a wide split in his testicle, which one could not help associating with the production of his hydrocele. As a further reason for that, I have at least on one occasion after operating for varicocele observed a certain amount of hydrocele appear. I have been under the impression that it has disappeared again, but I can remember one case in which it did not disappear. I recollect operating upon an officer for the radical cure of hernia. He was not a good case for radical cure, but he wished to remain in the army, and as a result of the operation a little fluid formed in his left tunica vaginalis. During the course of two years it very slowly increased, and ultimately, to enable him to ride and be more comfortable, the radical cure of the hydrocele was performed, and he remained well.

Lastly, I will draw attention to a class which are called congenital, and which are so important that I, perhaps, ought to have put them first. When we use the word "congenital" we simply mean that it is due to developmental defect. Congenital hydrocele in babies would be a source of great anxiety to you as medical men, for all sorts of reasons. There is a particular amount of terror which seems to attach to any swelling in the scrotum. These hydroceles in babies, I think, do not require to be complicated by the addition of words such as "infantile," and so on. They are associated with an open condition of the upper part of the processus vaginalis. Whether the fluid comes down out of the abdomen or commences round the testicle I do not know, but I think it must come down out of the abdomen. The treatment is very simple in these cases. First of all the infant should have a truss given it, because you must assume that its processus vaginalis has remained patent. Do not believe all that you are told about the inability of infants to wear trusses. I never yet met with a baby which could not wear an ordinary rubber truss, provided it was properly fitted. After the truss has been fitted you may take other steps, and one other step is to tap the hydrocele with a minute trocar, and the next is to apply a slightly irritating fluid, such as chloride ammonium lotion, and that results in the cure of the hydrocele. If the child grows up and is not cured, it would be desirable to perform an ordinary operation for the radical cure of hernia, and close the processus vaginalis high up in the inguinal canal. With regard to congenital hydrocele associated with hernia, I have told you about that, but I want to mention one other complication of congenital hydrocele which may shock you. Our rules are to look at the whole patient first, next look at the whole inflamed structure and compare it with the other side of the body if you can, and lastly, see it in a position of rest. Now, if you omit to look at the whole patient you may see a child—as I have—with a hydrocele of considerable size, and you may have omitted, from the lack of looking at the whole patient, to see that it had a large abdomen, and you would have been shocked when you tapped that case, having got an ounce glass ready to receive the hydrocele fluid, to collect a pint ; and then it would dawn upon your mind that that child had a collection of fluid in its tunica vaginalis, and that it communicated with its abdomen, and that the child had tuberculous peritonitis, with effusion of fluid. We had such a child in the wards here. I cannot tell you all the surgical details, but I remember part of the treatment, and the case resulted in a series of events such as those which I have mentioned to you. So when you are dealing with children with so-called congenital hydrocele, I advise you to approach them carefully.

Now I come to speak of another common affection of the testicle, and that is tuberculous testis. In my mind there are two kinds of tuberculous testis; one of them is the acute and the other the chronic. The acute tuberculous testis is, as the name implies, usually painful, rapid in its increase in size, and attended with considerable inflammation. It soon begins to soften in various parts and if left alone it begins to ulcerate. The swelling may ·be ovoid, but it is sure to be accompanied with considerable thickening and tenderness of the cord in the neck of the scrotum, perhaps passing up into the inguinal canal. When you operate upon such a case as that you will find that the spermatic cord, where you divide it, is œdematous, and perhaps has areas of caseous degeneration in it. The testicle itself is a huge inflammatory mass full of caseous lumps or nodules, and which are in the process of softening, also threatening the ulceration that I have mentioned, and so it becomes a question what you should do with such a testicle, because it is only a part of the general tuberculosis. Patients with that condition have got a high temperature and perhaps advanced tubercle in the lungs or elsewhere, and it is doubtful whether it is worth while to remove the testicle or not. I am in favour of removing such testicles on the ground of humanity. First of all, the removal of a testicle of that description causes singularly little shock or illness to the patients. They take the anæsthetic well if it is properly given. The removal of the testicle is a great mental and physical relief. You can imagine how painful it must be to possess a huge inflamed heavy testicle which is on the point of degeneration and ulceration. So that, contrary to the practice of some, I feel a tendency to get rid of such an encumbrance, although the operation may not in the slightest degree prolong the patient's life, as he is dying of tubercle in various tissues or organs.

The chronic tuberculous testis is a different matter. Think much about the nodule of chronic tubercle which the patient has got in the head or in the tail of the epididymis—because that is where it usually first appears—that nodule should excite in your minds a very strong suspicion. At that period it may have gone through the various changes which tubercle undergoes. The tubercle bacillus gets into the human body in some manner, through the tonsil or some wound or is inspired ; it then passes along the lymphatics and vessels, say into a gland near the tonsil where it perhaps began. The inflammatory products then undergo a curious change ; they become converted into what is usually called caseous material, because, I suppose, it resembles cheese, and perhaps it does a little. It may remain quiet for a long time, or it may even calcify, but the common course for that caseous material to pursue—so common is it that I would act upon it—is for it to soften, and there results a tuberculous abscess. Place this condition of things in the epididymis or in the testicle, and it will go through exactly the same course of events. It will inflame, and at that stage the epididymis is tender. You may say there is a slight attack of epididymitis. If you are a credulous individual, you might credit it to gout, or neurasthenia, or some rubbish of that sort. If you are not credulous, you will say that there is inflammation of the epididymis and will observe and see what happens. Next, in the course of weeks or months the tenderness will become less, but the nodule will be very hard. You will be suspicious. We will take it at that stage, because that is the one in which they are generally when you meet with them. But tubercle is not a disease of an organ, but a general disease. It will spread quickly, and it spreads up the vas deferens and up the lymphatics. Your mind should carry you from the beginning to the end of the genito-urinary tract. You feel the head of the epididymis, you feel the vas deferens which may have in or about it little nodules of caseous material. After the vas deferens has entered the pelvis at the so-called internal abdominal ring it passes down the pelvis towards the prostate. There you can begin to feel it again, rectal examination is an essential part of the examination of these cases of nodule in the testicle. If you do not make a rectal examination you will overlook the true cause of the disease. If it is tuberculous you will probably find small hard nodules in the prostate, close to the end of the vas deferens, on one side or the other. As a rule you feel these nodules on the side of the diseased testicle. Next, the finger is passed up the rectum beyond the prostate, and then you feel the ampulla of the vas deferens, and the vesiculæ seminales. They may have gone through exactly the same stages. They may be inflamed, and in that case you feel them thickened, tender, and hard. If it has gone on to caseation, you will feel a hard lump, with very little sensation of pain in it at all. Next you proceed one step further, and I have been rather astonished at the result of this manœuvre. The patient is supposed to have tubercle, and you have very strong reasons for thinking that he has tubercle of his genito-urinary tract. He is asked to pass his water into a glass, and that is held up to the light, and very likely it will contain blood, and I have seen it contain pus and muco-pus, and all sorts of shreds. In other words, the tuberculous disease may have begun close to the epididymis, passed along the vas deferens to the prostate and the vesiculæ seminales, and out of the ejaculatory ducts and have affected the neck of the bladder, where there is tuberculous ulceration, because as the tuberculous material softens it discharges into the bladder. When you look into the bladder with the endoscope you see it is tuberculous. How do you know ? You see the caseous material in the base of the ulcer. But you have not finished with your case yet ; your mind will still be prompting you to follow up the ureters. Tubercle may spread up the ureters, just as the sepsis does in the case of ascending pyelonephritis, and you should therefore examine the kidneys, to see if there is any suspicion of tubercle there, because it would be a great disaster to remove a tuberculous testis and then discover that there is tubercle of the prostate, tubercle of the vesiculæ seminales, and perhaps tubercle of one kidney—errors of diagnosis against which I am sure you must be most anxious to guard yourselves. Your best means of avoiding these mistakes is to pursue a proper method of examination, and that method really means that you are to get into the habit of thinking in anatomical order, just what I myself have been doing during the so-called diagnosis of a case of tubercle. I need hardly say that in any case which presents doubts to your mind you should proceed further in the diagnosis by seeing the tubercle bacillus, which is difficult in chronic cases. I think you should have a proper report from the pathologist, who should be able to tell you that he has produced tubercle in some animal with the fluid which you have sent to him.

I have not time to-day to say much about

syphilitic testicles, but there are two kinds of syphilitic testicles which may be a source of trouble to you. The first is that kind of syphilitic testicle which appears during the course of the general eruption of syphilis. I do not think that should be a source of trouble to you, because if the patient comes to you with a heavy, hard, round tumour of the scrotum, with but very slight inflammation or tenderness of the cord above, and perhaps on the other side a similar condition, you will naturally proceed to strip him and examine the whole of his body and see if he did possess at that time any of the ordinary signs of general syphilitic eruption. You would see that he had roseola or papules, or syphilitic ulceration of his throat, or perhaps syphilitic alopecia. Perhaps you might have suspicions that he had syphilitic anæmia. You should be on your guard about such a case and put him upon anti-syphilitic treatment. If the treatment were efficient and carried out in the right kind of way, you would produce a startling result. Then there is the gummatous testicle, which appears in the later stages, what may be called the fourth stage of syphilis. The gummatous testicle may be very much more difficult to diagnose. I will tell you what happened to me some ten years ago, and I remember it perfectly vividly. An old labourer was brought into the Great Northern Hospital, and I was told he had malignant disease of his testicle. He had a huge soft tumour, evidently solid, in the right side of his scrotum ; it tapered off up the cord in quite the proper manner, and he had evidently some thickening of the cord ascending into his inguinal canal, and he clearly, for that malignant disease, wanted a serious operation performed. We debated the point as to whether it could be got away ; it seemed to ascend so far in his inguinal canal. I was told he had had some iodide of potassium and mercury, and I think he had. I remember operating upon him and removing this huge malignant testis, and when I cut into it I still thought it to be malignant. I did not see any other syphilitic scars or gummata, such as are usual in these cases. But the case did not go on well afterwards ; the wound suppurated and the scrotum began to ulcerate. And it did not ulcerate in the usual way, because it was clear that something preceded the ulceration ; there was an inflammatory thickening of some sort, and it dawned upon

my mind that I had removed a gummatous testicle. But the wound got well quickly when he had had what he should have had before, namely full doses of mercury and iodide of potassium. Tumours of the testicle are very difficult to recognise and full of pitfalls, and therefore you should always be on the look-out for syphilis of the testicle, of the early or late kind, and if there is any possibility of it being syphilitic, you should give a strenuous course of treatment by iodide of potassium and mercury before you proceed to perform an operation. And under those circumstances these tumours not infrequently disappear in the most extraordinary manner.

But a greater pitfall than any is one which I now have to draw your attention to, and that is malignant disease of the testicle. I will not talk about sarcomas and carcinomas, which are refinements. It seems more rational that you and I should try to make up our minds whether it is malignant or not malignant before we try to label it as a hypothetical sarcoma or carcinoma. Because if you think of it you will admit that carcinoma and sarcoma are absolutely unknown diseases. Nobody knows anything about sarcoma or carcinoma, whatever they may like to say. Nobody can tell you their cause, or where they came from, nor can they even tell you what course they are certain to pursue. They may guess what course they are likely to pursue. And therefore I think it is irrational to proceed with the mysteries of histology and so forth until our minds are capable of looking at a clinical case and forming a fairly reasonable diagnosis as to whether it is malignant or not—a very difficult thing to do. I have brought down the notes of a case which was in our wards recently, and indeed the man is in there now. You cannot learn much from looking at him, I am afraid, but you can study his notes, and I have brought them here to see what is said about his previous history. Some of you are aware that I take a gloomy view of the truthfulness of histories, but I think we may take the broad facts of this case because they are so strange. He came in in May, 1904, and is said to have had influenza. I dare say he had—many people have. After that he had a very much inflamed testicle on the left side. It was so acutely inflamed that it was treated with antimony and sulphate of magnesia mixture. I do not think it ever got better. He went on to quinine and iodide of potassium, and it was assumed to be an inflamed testicle which did not get well and was apt to recur. The testicle itself had a peculiarity ; it had not descended properly into the scrotum, it remained near the root of the penis. When I saw him we came to the conclusion that the tumour was ovoid, and the cord and vas deferens and spermatic artery and the strings could not be felt. The cord tapered off gradually, becoming thinner as it went up the inguinal canal. It led to the belief that whatever was in the cord had grown up, and not down. It was obviously tender and inflamed, and therefore one had to admit it might be inflamed. But what a source of fallacy that is! I hesitated the other day to remove a tumour from a man's neck. First of all we concluded the tumour was in the lymphatic glands, next that it was inflamed, next that it was adherent to the sterno-mastoid, but not much to the carotid sheath. All that was true. It was in the lymphatic glands, it was inflamed, it was adherent to the sterno-mastoid and slightly adherent to the carotid sheath. It was an inflamed epithelioma of the glands. As regards the tumour of the man with a partially descended testicle. First, it was solid, next it was going up into the abdomen, next it was inflamed and yet I thought it ought also to be malignant. A portion of it was removed and examined microscopically and it was found to be malignant, and I proceeded to remove it as high as I could, and I think I got it all away. What a trap to fall into that was! Is it true that these partially descended testes are more prone to malignant disease than other kinds? Once I should have said no. But within the last year I have removed two. A man had both testicles retained in the inguinal canals, right and left. The right one became inflamed and was brought to me as an inflamed testicle. I said, "Yes, but we had better wait and see." And I said at the time, "I am suspicious about these inflamed testicles because it is a retained testicle and they sometimes become malignant." The man came back with it a little bigger and more painful, and exhibiting a little more anxiety. He probably derived the impression that it was malignant from one's look—human beings are very clever in this respect. I advised him to have it explored and removed. It turned out to be malignant growth, and I removed it. That is the history. I remem-ber a man was brought to me some years ago who was said to be suffering from a gouty inflammation of the testicle, and I examined him and came to the conclusion that he had a fluid swelling at one point. I advised him it should be tapped and some of the fluid withdrawn, so that we might see what it was. It might be tuberculous or an ordinary cyst. And out of it came blood when it was tapped. At the end of the trocar was adherent a piece of tissue, and this was sent to the pathologist and he sent back the report that it was malignant disease. The pathologist was not informed where it came from. The testicle was removed and was found to contain one or two nodules of malignant disease. I have told you that I am suspicious about all tumours about the testicle ; they require a great deal of thought and observation.

I will conclude by telling you of another case of malignant disease. A young gentleman had had a loose cartilage removed from his knee, and that is what first of all brought him within my circle. Two years afterwards he came, looking exceedingly thin and ill, and having a nodule in his epididymis, which I thought was tuberculous. I was very anxious about that, because tubercle of the epididymis, as you will have observed, is very serious. I asked Sir Thomas Smith to see the patient with me, so that we could tell him what should be done. Sir Thomas Smith agreed in the diagnosis of tubercle, and thought it was clear and advised removal. It was done. The testicle contained a malignant growth in the epididymis, consisting of a peculiar kind of malignant adenoma, which I thought to be like a developing Wolffian body. The history was curious. I advised him to leave this country and go to a better climate, where he would have a better chance of fighting the disease. He went to another country, and five or six years afterwards, I am told by a relative, he had his right testicle removed for a similar malignant growth. There is one more strange thing about him. I know his mother died of carcinoma of the liver, his father died of carcinoma of the larynx or œsophagus, and an uncle died of carcinoma of the tongue. And in cases of carcinoma you not infrequently come across rather startling histories of malignant disease such as that.

I am quite aware that in my brief remarks upon the tumours of the scrotum, the neck of the scrotum, and the inguinal canal, I have omitted a great deal, especially hæmatocele, and you may observe that I have omitted to deal with, or have only half dealt with, tumours of the neck of the scrotum itself, but that is because I have not had time to go into them. But you have not missed much after all, because these tumours nearly always ascend or descend, and those which originate in the neck of the scrotum are quite rare. My memory tells me of a few cysts or fatty tumours or varicoceles which did not go far down or far up, and a few tuberculous lumps, but tumours which originate in the neck of the scrotum are relatively unusual. If any one does me the compliment afterwards of thinking over what I have said, they will come to the conclusion that I have been telling them to pursue methods of diagnosis, and not to try to remember cases. I have told you about a few cases, but they were to exemplify my own errors. And after all, you cannot remember cases ; you can only remember startling cases, such as those I have related.

November 6th, 1905.

Potassium Permanganate as a Hæmostatic.

—Vörner has found in potassium permanganate an extremely efficient hæmostatic which, owing to its antiseptic nature, does not introduce the risk of infection, and does not, to any extent, destroy the tissues. He uses it either in strong solution, in powder form, or in a paste. He obtains a fine powder by triturating it with one half its weight of diatomaceous earth, after having first moistened and then dried the mixture. The paste is made with vaseline in the proportion of one part to three. This is most conveniently used in collapsible tubes. If there is bleeding to any extent after the excision of warts, condylomata, small tumours, etc., the bleeding surface is to be wiped dry with a piece of gauze, and the permanganate, in one form or the other, applied instantly. Usually a single application suffices, but occasionally more are necessary. Any discoloration of the skin about the wound, accidentally produced, is readily concealed by covering it with a piece of zinc plaster. About mucous membranes the paste is preferable, but epistaxis is well controlled with the solution. The patients complain of slight burning after the application of the permanganate.—*Medical Record*, vol. lxviii, No. 16.

WITH DR. FAWCETT AT GUY'S HOSPITAL.

CANCER OF THE STOMACH : ITS CLINICAL VARIETIES, DIAGNOSIS, AND TREATMENT.

I PROPOSE to deal with the subject of cancer of the stomach mainly from the clinical aspect, with special reference to some symptoms and signs upon which comparatively little stress is laid in the text-books. I also intend to deal later with the question of treatment. On inspecting specimens of malignant disease of the stomach, it is at once obvious that, for purposes of clinical classification, they may be grouped, more or less exactly, according to the part of the organ involved. I may perhaps be allowed to remind you of these by showing you specimens from the museum at Guy's Hospital.

(1) *The pyloric region.*—This is the seat of the disease in the largest number of cases. Drs. Perry and Shaw state its frequency as 70 per cent. ; Welch, out of a total number of 1300 cases, as 61 per cent.

In Specimen No. 685 you see a very good example of a typical pyloric carcinoma, and in Specimen No. 709 another preparation of the same condition.

(2) *The body of the stomach.*—Specimen No. 683. Here the greater part of the organ is thickened and infiltrated by new growth, but although the involvement of the organ is in this case so extensive, yet in many others it is strictly limited. As, however, I do not intend entering into an exact description of the different varieties, I would only here remind you that, after the pyloric region, the portion of the stomach most often involved is that in the region of the lesser curvature and its contiguous surfaces.

(3) *The cardia.*—Specimen No. 690 is a good example of a limited growth of the cardiac orifice, and another one that I show you (Specimen S. 05), exhibits a villous growth which not only obstructs the cardiac orifice, but has spread into the body of the organ, and upwards into the œsophagus.

(4) *The diffuse form.*—Specimen No. 703 is a good example, showing the extreme contraction that this form often undergoes so as to produce the so-called "india-rubber bottle stomach."

. The varieties in which the disease involves the pyloric and cardiac orifices have more or less well-defined symptoms and signs, while in those of the body of the organ the evidence is more often latent or indefinite. To the cases of "latent" cancer I shall refer later, but at the present time I should like to draw your attention to the history of one of the specimens (Specimen S. 05) that I have shown you, and also to another case, both of which illustrate certain features of disease of the cardiac orifice.

The patient (*vide* Specimen S. 05) was a woman, æt. 55 years, who was admitted under Mr. Symonds in 1904 for gastric pain and vomiting associated with dysphagia. For a few weeks previously she had been unable to take solid food, and even fluids were soon vomited. Obstruction in the lower part of the œsophagus was diagnosed. An œsophageal tube was passed and tied in position, but this operation was followed by repeated vomiting, and the patient, becoming progressively weaker, died two days later.

Another case in which the symptoms were mainly those of difficulty in swallowing was that of Alice M—, æt. 36 years, who was admitted under me early in this year. She stated that she had been losing weight for six to seven months and was unable to retain solid food, but that she could swallow fluids. An indefinite tumour was detected in the epigastric and left hypochondriac regions, and a mass could also be felt in the recto-vaginal pouch. It was thought that the patient had a carcinoma of the cardiac orifice spreading out into the body of the organ. The presence of an obstruction was confirmed by Mr. Steward, who passed a bougie, but no attempt was made to tie in a Symonds' tube in this patient.

The cardiac region is one of the parts of the stomach least often affected, but when it is so, it is important to remember that the œsophagus is involved in a large proportion of the cases, and that it may be this factor which adds to the difficulty in swallowing. Fagge used to teach that growths involving the cardia originated in the œsophagus. As pointed out by Drs. Perry and Shaw (1), this is probably incorrect ; and although I do not propose to enter into the histology of gastric growths, yet this point is one which needs correction and which it may be well to emphasize here. Growths involving the cardiac opening for the most

part arise in the stomach. Perry and Shaw (1) showed that of more than thirty specimens of malignant growths from all parts of the œsophagus, with the exception of two cases of sarcoma, every one was a squamous epithelioma. In a very large proportion of the growths of the cardiac end of the stomach the œsophagus is involved, and histologically these growths exhibit the structure of glandular carcinoma, and not epithelioma. If Fagge's view as to their origin in the œsophagus is the correct one, how is it, Perry and Shaw very pertinently ask, that they alone among such growths are spheroidal-celled carcinomata, while at every other part of the tube nothing but squamous epithelioma is found.

Having drawn your attention for a short time to the regions of the stomach which cancer may attack, I will now proceed to consider some of the facts connected with the incidence and course of the disease.

As a factor in its development we cannot, for the present, lay our hands upon anything definite. Chronic dyspepsia is too common to be regarded as of any importance, except that a prolonged history of such a condition may be looked upon as rather against than for a diagnosis of malignant disease. As to alcohol opinions are somewhat divergent. In some statistics recently quoted at a meeting of the Life Assurance Medical Officers Society, it was stated by one speaker that the death rate from cancer in abstainers and non-abstainers was as 70·19 : 100, or 29 per cent. less in the former, but this, of course, only applies to a comparatively small number of cases, all of whom have undergone a process of selection to start with.

With regard to its relation to simple ulcer we may say that there is nothing antagonistic between the two diseases ; possibly simple ulcer may even predispose to cancer. In the last 100 cases of Drs. Perry and Shaw's paper (5), 9 per cent. of them presented appearances which suggested a development of malignant disease upon a simple ulcer. I may refer you also for further particulars on this point to a paper by W. J. Mayo (6), 1904.

On the other hand, it has been suggested that simple ulcer has no direct relation to the development of a cancerous ulcer, in that in the former the region most frequently involved is the lesser curvature and the posterior surface, and that it is commoner in women, whereas in cancer the commonest seat of the growth is the pyloric region, and men are more often the subjects of it.

Age.—The variation in age is well seen in some of the cases to which I shall refer.. They are 37, 68, 42, 35, 50, 71, 67, 39, and 36 years.

These correspond very closely to the age limits stated by Drs. Perry and Shaw (5) as the most fatal years, viz. 40 to 70 years for males, and 30 to 60 years of age in females.

More than half of their cases died between 40 and 60 years of age, and rather more than a third between 40 and 50 years.

Up to 20 years of age cases of cancer are very rare, and even in the next decade infrequent, but from 30 to 40 the rise is considerable. In Osler's (2) cases 4 per cent. were between the ages of 20 and 30 ; this is a high figure. In Perry and Shaw's series it worked out at rather under 2·5 per cent.

What we have to remember is that although under 30 years of age cases are infrequent, and still more so under 20 years, yet gastric cancer cannot be left out of consideration at these early ages, as there is a very definite percentage of deaths from carcinoma during these periods. Of course, we have to bear in mind the possibility of the presence of sarcoma, which occurs, as a rule, at a somewhat earlier age than carcinoma.

There are two points of considerable interest which are drawn attention to by Osler and McCrae (2) in regard to the cases of cancer occurring between 20 and 30 years of age, viz. :

(1) The sudden onset of the disease. For example, in cases quoted by them it—

(a) "Began rather acutely four months before, with pain after eating" ;

(b) "Began suddenly, with vomiting after eating";

(c) " Pain came on after lifting a heavy weight, and he felt that something had given way inside."

(2) The rapid course. I have looked through Drs. Perry and Shaw's (5) paper, and find that in the 4 out of the 6 cases recorded by them in which the age of the patient was thirty years or under, the onset was sudden and the duration of the disease short, the longest being five months, the shortest five weeks after the first appearance of symptoms. The abstracted histories of these cases are as follows :

CASE 22.—Robert R—, æt. 28 years. Previously had been a patient in St. Thomas' Hospital for some months, suffering, as was thought, from a diseased liver. Died about three months from onset of symptoms.

CASE 97.—Rose T—, æt. 30 years. History of whole illness only about four months. Carcinoma of pylorus present, giving rise to a palpable tumour. Softening secondary deposits in cervical and gastric lymphatic glands and in liver.

CASE 120.—George D—, æt. 20 years. Had been healthy till four weeks before admission, when he noticed tightness of chest and gradual enlargement of abdomen. Death occurred six days after entering the hospital. At the autopsy a carcinoma of the pylorus was found, with secondary deposits in the peritoneum and the abdominal lymph glands.

CASE 240.—Ellen B—, æt. 29 years, was admitted for intestinal obstruction. She had been subject to attacks of indigestion and vomiting, with constipation, since 1888, the last attack occurring in October, 1893. Death took place on December 18th, nine days after admission. At the autopsy a carcinoma of pylorus was found, possibly arising from a simple ulcer, the intestinal obstruction being due to the contraction of secondary growths in the peritoneum.

CASE 266.—Alfred P—, æt. 24 years, was admitted for a popliteal aneurysm on July 23rd, 1896, and died on August 2nd, as the result of an ulcerative endocarditis. At the autopsy an early carcinoma of the lesser curvature was found, which apparently had never given rise to any symptoms.

CASE 287.—Catherine R—, æt. 30 years. Admitted August 10th, and died August 23rd, 1899. Her illness commenced in March, with vomiting after food and abdominal pain, and was therefore of five months' duration. Cancer of pylorus with carcinomatous peritonitis was found at the autopsy.

Duration of life after appearance of symptoms.—From a practical standpoint it is very important that you should remember what may be looked upon as an average duration of life after the appearance of symptoms.

Drs. Perry and Shaw (5) out of their 306 cases found that the greater number of the patients had been ill less than six months before admission, and that the average duration of life from the time at which symptoms were first noticed was eight and three quarter months. The cases in their series represented patients who had presented symptoms for periods varying from one to twenty-four months.

Mode of onset.—The suddenness of onset is, although more common at earlier ages, not confined to them. For instance, to take examples of one or two of the cases that have come under my notice in the past few years.

(1) Henry G—, æt. 37 years, was admitted, under Dr. Pitt, on December 30th, 1901. He first complained of indefinite pains in his legs after getting wet on December 11th. On December 23rd he had been standing on a chair to get something down from a shelf, when, on jumping down quickly, he felt a violent pain in his "stomach," which made him think he had "ricked" it. From that day till his admission to hospital he said the pain had become worse, and that his abdomen had been getting harder, and felt as if it were going to burst. He died in July, 1902, about six months after admission, and at the autopsy a diffuse carcinoma of the stomach was found.

(2) John B—, æt. 70 years, was admitted, under Dr. Perry, on October 7th, 1901. One day, some ten months before admission to hospital, he had had some bread and cheese and ale for lunch. Immediately after swallowing it he was sick, and since that time the sickness had continued. He died a month after admission to the hospital. This patient also had a small contracted stomach infiltrated throughout with growth.

(3) John L—, æt. 68 years, was admitted, under Dr. Perry, on May 21st, 1900. On the Sunday before Christmas-day, 1899, he found he could keep nothing down. Although he had since that time felt inclined to take solid food, and had made several attempts to swallow it, yet he had never succeeded in retaining it for any length of time.

I have quoted these three cases because they serve to show us that a sudden onset is not so uncommon as perhaps we are inclined to think, and that even though it may be more common in young people, yet that it is not confined to them. The patients I have just referred to were respectively of ages 37, 70, and 68 years. The cases have not been specially selected from a large series with a view to this point, but are taken from those I have seen in Guy's Hospital during the past five years. As a general rule the onset is gradual and insidious, extending over some weeks or more ; the symptoms are often indefinite, consisting of disturbances of digestion, pain in the stomach, and other symptoms commonly included by the patient under the term "dyspepsia."

The important fact in connection with the symptoms for us to remember is that any person past middle age, and especially at about 45 to 50 years, who develops symptoms of dyspepsia for the *first* time, with no adequate cause to account for it, should be looked upon with suspicion and as one who requires the most careful investigation of his case.

We will now turn our attention to certain signs and symptoms of carcinoma of the stomach, with special reference to some points upon which more observations have recently been made.

Pain.—Although one of the most frequent symptoms, yet it may be conspicuous by its absence. For instance, Fenwick (3) says that it is absent in about 13 to 14 per cent. of cases, and the degree of severity is also very variable, from quite slight attacks to those of a severe and persistent nature.

Dysphagia is a symptom which has attracted little notice. Perry and Shaw (5), in their most recent paper, specially refer to it. They point out that pain and discomfort felt immediately after taking food are often ascribed by the patient to a difficulty in swallowing, and so might easily have been put down by an inexperienced clinical clerk as "dysphagia." As a matter of fact, however, in eight out of the ten cases in which "dysphagia" was reported as present, actual obstruction was found to exist at the cardiac orifice.

In the case I have previously referred to (Specimen S. 05) of the patient who was under the care of Mr. Symonds, dysphagia was a prominent symptom, as also in the second case of Alice M— (*vide* p. 58), who was under me at the beginning of this year. In both of them there was obstruction at the cardiac orifice, and in one of these cases, and in four of those mentioned by Perry and Shaw, the difficulty in swallowing was so great that an operation had been carried out for its relief. Thus the conclusion may fairly be arrived at that if dysphagia be a prominent symptom it probably implies involvement of the cardiac orifice by growth. On the other hand, the cardiac orifice may be the seat of a growth, and yet it may give rise to no symptoms relating to the power of swallowing.

Vomiting, although a common symptom, is not so frequently present as pain. The characters of the vomit are well known to you—its faintly acid reaction, dirty brown colour, and unpleasant odour, and the great variations in amount that may occur in different cases.

In reference to the last of these characters, just as a large quantity vomited at long intervals may lead to a diagnosis of dilatation from pyloric obstruction, so, on the other hand, a small quantity vomited soon after the ingestion of food may imply a contracted organ. Such a case was that of John B— (*vide* p. 60), æt. 70 years, one of the patients to whom reference was made as having developed his symptoms suddenly. At the autopsy the stomach was found to be contracted and infiltrated throughout with growth.

Hæmatemesis is a symptom upon which comparatively little stress has been laid in connection with cancer of the stomach, and especially as the direct cause of death.

In many cases blood is present in small quantities in the vomit as one of the later manifestations of cancer. Fenwick (3) states that it is most frequent in association with growths of the pylorus or those of the lesser curvature. On the other hand, severe attacks of hæmorrhage in pyloric growths causing marked stenosis are rare.

An important point in connection with the bleeding that may take place is the very bad effect it may produce upon the health of the patient. The presence of the blood may not be recognised, as none is actually vomited, and so a slowly progressive anæmia develops, and the case may perhaps be mistaken for one of pernicious anæmia.

Attacks of bleeding such as occur in simple ulcer are, according to Fenwick (3), met with in about 10—12 per cent. of the cases, but hæmorrhage leading to death is certainly rare. Though this is the case yet it is not so uncommon as many of us believe. Most of us would, I think, say to ourselves, on meeting with a case of fatal or very severe hæmatemesis, that such an event almost puts a diagnosis of cancer of the stomach out of court. Our impressions, however, are not altogether in accord with the facts. Perry and Shaw (5), as the result of their analysis, pointed out that there had been hæmatemesis in 49 out of 306 cases and that in some of them the hæmorrhage was a very prominent factor in causing the death of the patient.

The following case will serve as a good example. It is not included in the paper referred to, as the patient was not admitted until 1901. The patient, æt. 35 years, was admitted on May 29th, 1901, under Dr. Perry, with a history as follows. For about six months he had noticed that he had been getting weaker, and he suffered from a feeling of faintness at intervals. After taking food he experienced sensations of sickness, with other symptoms of indigestion. For two months previous to admission the symptoms had been more pronounced and at times streaks of bright red blood had been present in the vomit. On June 6th, 1901, he vomited two "porringers" of dark blood. Melæna was present and he had a second attack of hæmatemesis the morning after the first one. From this date the pain became much more severe, and the patient gradually sank and died a fortnight later. At the autopsy a scirrhous growth of the pylorus was found.

Although such a sequence of events is rare, yet it is well to remember the fact that even in cancer fatal hæmatemesis does occasionally occur, and rather more frequently than is stated to be the case in text-books and monographs on the subject. *E. g.* Osler and McCrae (2) state that although hæmorrhage was profuse in some cases, yet that in no case that they had met with was it sufficient to cause death, although in some it hastened the fatal termination.

On the other hand, in six cases of Perry and Shaw's (5) series, hæmatemesis was the direct cause of death, and in five others fatal hæmorrhage into the stomach took place although no blood was vomited.

Appetite and digestion.—Although for some little time past the impression had been gaining upon me that loss of appetite and distaste for food were not symptoms so frequently present in the early stages of cancer of the stomach as I had thought, yet I was not prepared for the result which comes out from Perry and Shaw's (5) analysis. Some of us may have seen cases of cancer in which the appetite was good even beyond the digestive powers of the patient; and Osler and McCrae (2), to quote the words used by them, say that "in rather a surprising number the appetite was practically normal, though many of these complained that while the desire for food was present, the fear and knowledge of subsequent pain and distress restrained them."

The conclusion, then, that we may deduce from this is that the presence of even a good appetite

must not be laid too much stress upon as negativing a ·suspicion of cancer of the stomach, that
loss of appetite is present in a large number of
patients, but that it is variable in its time of
onset, and in some cases the appetite remains
good throughout, or is little impaired.

This loss of appetite may depend to some extent
upon the absence of HCl, which acid is, as you
all know, a powerful antiseptic; and when it is absent
fermentative changes become more marked and so
interfere greatly with the digestive processes.

Presence of free HCl.—It is not in relation to
the connection of HCl with the digestive processes that I wish to refer now, but to the value
of the determination of the presence of free HCl
in the diagnosis of cancer of the stomach. The
examination of the stomach contents in all doubtful cases is a procedure which must on no account
be omitted. Free HCl is absent much more
often in cancer of the stomach than in any other
disease : it is one of the few facts we know in
connection with the stomach and cancer. It is
true that free HCl is present in a small percentage
of these cases, while it is sometimes absent in
diseases of the stomach due to some other cause.
Notwithstanding this, the fact remains that in a
very large percentage of cases, 90 per cent. or
perhaps more, either no free HCl is found or only
a very small trace.

In some of the cases in which free HCl is
present it has been suggested that the amount of
destruction of the mucous membrane was not ·
very extensive and that the remainder was competent to secrete the acid. In connection with
this question I should like to draw your attention
to the conclusions arrived at as the result of
observations made by B. Moore (7), in collaboration with others, and reported in the ' Lancet' for
April 29, 1905.

These observers, being unable to satisfactorily
explain the absence of HCl in consequence of any
local condition in the stomach. surmised that it
might depend on a general condition. The conclusion they arrived at was that " the absence of free
HCl in cancer of the stomach is not due to local
action in that organ, for HCl is absent or reduced
in amount whatever may be the situation in the body
of the malignant growth." They made observations
upon seventeen cases, including growths from such
different parts as the stomach, the uterus, and the

mouth. This conclusion, if confirmed, will, although
lessening the value of the test in its direct relation
to the stomach, yet not affect its general importance
in association with cancer.

In testing for the acid the most satisfactory
reagent to use is phloroglucin and vanillin (Gunsberg's reagent). The vomit should be filtered
before the application of the test ; the evaporation
should be done on a water bath, only a drop or
two of each of the fluids being used.

Test meal. — Proteids and other nitrogenous
bodies combine with HCl, and therefore if these
substances be present in any large quantity
Gunsberg's reagent will not give a reaction. Carbohydrates and fat, on the other hand, do not
materially interfere with the secretion of HCl.
A very good test meal to employ is a pint of tea
with a little milk and sugar, and a round of toast
and butter. This meal should be given in the
morning before any other food is taken, and the
stomach contents siphoned off one to one and a
half hours later. It is of importance not to dilute
the stomach contents with water when they are
being drawn off.

Lactic acid.—Excessive formation of this acid
occurs in the stomach under certain conditions,
viz. : (1) Stagnation of food ; (2) deficiency of
free HCl ; (3) diminished power of digestion and
absorption of proteids. The general view is that
although absence of lactic acid cannot be taken
as evidence of absence of cancer, yet its presence
in association with other signs is much in favour
of the existence of carcinoma. For clinical purposes Uffelmann's test is the best   This reagent
is composed of a mixture of 3 grammes of carbolic
acid in 100 c.c. of distilled water. When applying
the test a drop or two of liq. .ferri perchloridi
is added. Free HCl renders the solution colourless, while lactic acid turns it a pale canary yellow
colour.

Microscopical examination.—This method also
may be most valuable in its results. Osler (2)
recommends that after washing out the organ any
solid matter present in the washings should be
placed between two glass plates and examined
against a dark background, and that any pieces
which it is desired to inspect should then be picked
out and examined under the microscope. He refers
to several cases in which malignant tissue was recognised in this way, and it is therefore clearly a method

of examination to which more attention should be paid than, I think, we for the most part are in the habit of doing.

Oppler-Boas bacilli should also be looked for, as they have been observed in a large number of cases. They give rise to lactic acid fermentation of carbohydrates. They are long, rod-shaped, non-mobile bacteria, often thicker at one end than another.

Some of the symptoms not so directly connected with the stomach will now be taken.

Pyrexia.—Many of you have seen cases in which in association with cancerous deposits in the liver, or elsewhere, there has been a rise of temperature. In cancer of the stomach the temperature is often raised a degree or two and sometimes more, but for the most part such a rise, even when it is above 100°, does not seem to be particularly related to any complications. All I wish you to remember is that pyrexia is often associated with cancer of the stomach, and that it has no special significance of its own.

Perforation, which is the next complication I shall refer to, is not one likely to supervene in the early stages of the disease as happens in gastric ulcer. As a rule it occurs quite late, and then very often with little or nothing in the way of clinical evidence to draw attention to its onset. In Perry and Shaw's (5) collection of cases there were twenty examples of perforation, and in only one of them was the patient in such a condition as to allow him to follow his occupation at the time when the rupture took place.

This patient is Case 138 of their series, J. G. C—, æt. 48 years, who for three months before admission had suffered from flatulence, vomiting, and epigastric pain. On the day of his admission he was at work, driving a tramcar, when he was suddenly seized with pain in the abdomen, so violent as to cause him to drop down.

On admission he presented symptoms of peritonitis ; his temperature was 100·5° and pulse 128. Death ensued five days later, and at the autopsy recent lymph and bile-stained fluid were found in the peritoneal cavity. A cancerous ulcer was present in the neighbourhood of the pylorus, the ulcer having perforated at the thinnest part on the anterior wall.

Thus, as a practical point in diagnosis, we may conclude that, unless there is definite evidence to the contrary, a sudden onset of symptoms indicative of peritonitis is not due to the perforation of a malignant ulcer.

When perforation does occur it may be either (1) into the general peritoneal cavity, or (2) into a space shut off by adhesions, so giving rise to a localised abscess. The onset may be associated with acute pain, or it may be so insidious as to be unrecognised.

To take examples of these two varieties I cannot do better than quote to you Cases 5 and 178 of the Guy's (5) collection.

CASE 5.—Henry C—, æt. 43 years, had been ill for twelve months. He was suddenly attacked at the end of this period by a severe lancinating pain in the hypochondria and scorbiculus cordis. He died some seventy-three days later, and at the autopsy an abscess cavity of considerable size was found between the liver and stomach and extending across to the spleen. There was a well-defined ulcer in the pyloric region of the stomach and about an inch from the pylorus a communication through the growth with the abscess cavity.

CASE 178.—William B—, æt. 39 years, was attacked with vomiting and severe pain in the stomach two days before he died. The pulse was 136. At the autopsy a general acute peritonitis was found. An aperture about as large as a pin's head was present in the anterior wall of the stomach near the pylorus, this part of the wall being the seat of a carcinomatous ulcer four inches in diameter.

Turning to cases in which there were no symptoms of peritonitis, or where such symptoms, if present, were not recognised, I will read to you abstracts of Cases 104 and 269 of the same series.

CASE 104.—Elizabeth C—, æt. 56 years, whilst carrying a tub of water, felt something snap on the left side, causing her pain and faintness. After this she vomited coffee-ground-like material for a week, and continued to do so at intervals of a fortnight up to the time of admission. She was in hospital for at least four months, and her history affords no evidence of any sudden attack of acute pain during that period. At the autopsy an abscess was found in the lesser sac of the peritoneum which communicated with a villous growth on the lesser curvature and posterior wall of the stomach.

CASE 269.—George H—, æt. 63 years, had suffered from vomiting after food, with pain in the epigastrium, for nine months previous to admission, and he died two months later. A tumour was felt which was thought to be connected with the liver. He gradually grew weaker and ascites supervened, but this was not apparently attended with any abdominal pain. At the autopsy a carcinoma of the lesser curvature was found. There was a perforation on the anterior surface of the stomach and a general suppurative peritonitis.

The absence of symptoms is, no doubt, in many cases due to the moribund condition of the patient, and consequent insensibility to pain and inability to react to stimuli which under a more lively condition would give rise to acute symptoms.

Perry and Shaw (5) also suggest that the fact that the peritoneum is in many cases the seat of cancerous deposits would render the serous membrane less sensitive to stimuli than would be the case when a perforation of an appendicular ulcer or a simple ulcer of the stomach occurred into a previously healthy serous cavity. The character of the gastric contents, especially in its freedom from HCl, might render it less irritating than usual.

When an abscess does develop, the chief symptom of its presence may be an intermittent pyrexia associated with a rapid increase of general debility. At the same time, you may remember that I mentioned to you before, that, in many of the cases with pyrexia, no special lesion was found to account for the rise of temperature, so that pyrexia alone cannot be accepted as evidence of the presence of an abscess.

REFERENCES.

(1) PERRY and SHAW.—'Guy's Hosp. Rep.,' vol. xlviii, 1891.

(2) OSLER and McCRAE.—'Cancer of the Stomach.'

(3) FENWICK.—'Cancer and other Tumours of the Stomach.'

(4) MOYNIHAN.—'Practitioner,' December, 1903.

(5) PERRY and SHAW.—'Guy's Hosp. Rep.,' vol. lviii, 1904.

(6) MAYO, W. J.—'Annals of Surgery,' July, 1903, and March, 1904.

(7) B. MOORE, ALEXANDER KELLY, and ROAF. —'Lancet,' April 29th, 1905.

(*To be concluded.*)

November 6th, 1905.

WE have received a copy of Sir James Crichton-Browne's address on 'The Prevention of Senility,' published by Messrs. Macmillan & Co. The author has succeeded in producing a most interesting little book, and his treatment of the subject is excellent. The following passages are taken from the work :

Metchnikoff believes very firmly in his slow-intoxication theory of old age, and, as I have said, contemplates the removal from all human beings of the whole of that large intestine which is the lair of these poison-breeding and old-age-inducing bacteria. He perceives, however, that we are not yet quite ripe for that heroic measure, and so has other and temporary expedients to suggest. These are directed against fermentation and putrefaction in the large intestine, and so we must use only sterilised milk ; we must drink 1½ litres of kephir or sour milk daily, which will furnish lactic acid that is antagonistic to the microbes of putrefaction, and we must exclude "wild microbes" from the alimentary tract by partaking only of food that has been thoroughly cooked or sterilised, and if we cannot in these ways eliminate all the harmful microbes from the flora of the intestines, we must resort to appropriate serums.

The prevention of putrefaction in the intestine is no doubt very desirable, not only for the prevention of old age, but for the maintenance of comfort throughout life, but I am not disposed to trust to sour milk or any serum as a specific. There is no short cut to longevity. To win it is the work of a lifetime, and the promotion of it is a branch of preventive medicine.

Believing that the impaired nutrition and degeneration which correspond with senility and end in death are due to a misdirection of that fermentation by which tissue construction and destruction are brought about, Dr. Allchin has been led to take a hopeful view of our power of controlling them. Founding on the experiments of Loeb, on what may be called the saline fertilisation of the ova of some of the lower forms of life, he argues that "if it be possible by the application of certain electro lytes to avert from the ovum what may be termed its natural death, similarly to avert the degeneration and death of the tissues of higher organisms may be looked upon as no longer a hopeless quest." It seems, therefore, that it is the abolition or indefinite postponement of systemic death that Dr. Allchin holds in view as a legitimate object of quest.

THE CLINICAL JOURNAL,

CLINICAL RECORD, CLINICAL NEWS, CLINICAL GAZETTE, CLINICAL REPORTER, CLINICAL CHRONICLE AND CLINICAL REVIEW.

EDITED BY L. ELIOT CREASY.

| No. 681. | WEDNESDAY, NOVEMBER 15, 1905. | Vol. XXVII. No. 5. |

CONTENTS.

NOTICE.

Editorial correspondence, books for review, &c., should be addressed to the Editor, 51, New Cavendish Street, W., Telephone No. 904, Paddington ; but all business communications should be addressed to the Publishers, 22½, Bartholomew Close, London, E.C. Telephone 927, Holborn.

All inquiries respecting Advertisements should be sent to MESSRS. ADLARD & SON, *Bartholomew Close, E.C. Telephone 927, Holborn.*

Terms of Subscription, including postage, payable by cheque, postal or banker's order (in advance) : for the United Kingdom, 15s. 6d. per annum ; Abroad 17s. 6d.

Cheques, &c., should be made payable to THE PROPRIETORS OF THE CLINICAL JOURNAL, *crossed " The London, City, and Midland Bank, Ltd., Newgate Street Branch, E.C. Account of the Medical Publishing Company, Ltd."*

Reading Cases to hold Twenty-six Numbers of THE CLINICAL JOURNAL *can be supplied at 2s. 3d. each, or will be forwarded post free on receipt of 2s. 6d. ; and also Cases for Binding Volumes at 1s. each, or post free on receipt of 1s. 3d., from the Publishers, 22½, Bartholomew Close, London, E.C.*

SURGICAL TREATMENT OF GALL-STONES.

Clinical Lecture delivered to the Advanced Surgery Class at the London Hospital.

By C. MANSELL MOULLIN, M.D., F.R.C.S.

Senior Surgeon and Lecturer on Surgery at the London Hospital.

GENTLEMEN,—The subject to which I wish to call your attention to-day is the surgical treatment of gall-stones, and particularly the conditions which render surgical treatment advisable, if not absolutely necessary. We have had a large number of cases in our wards of late. Many of them have been of great interest, and many of them have been in that stage in which, according to some, it is still an open question whether surgical measures should be advised or not. Many physicians apparently still think that gall-stones do not matter much, and should almost without exception be left alone. Patients, all but a few who are capable of taking a wider view, are usually of the same opinion. The risks of operating appear to be much graver than they really are because they are immediate. The danger of not operating is under-estimated because the consequences are insidious in their onset and remote.

Gall-stones, in fact, are usually regarded as harmless, unless they happen to be impacted. So long as they lie quietly in a gall-bladder, they are considered to be so inoffensive as not to require any special treatment. It is only when they cause mechanical obstruction, and give rise to recurrent attacks of colic, persistent jaundice, or distension of the gall-bladder, and when they cannot be dislodged by ordinary means, that the question of the advisability of operating is allowed to be raised. Gall-stones that do not give rise to any of these consequences are looked upon as of no importance, or at any rate as of so little importance that anything like operation is unjustifiable.

Now, a great deal of this is true. You must all of you have seen numbers of cases in the postmortem rooms in which the gall-bladder contained a quantity of gall-stones, and yet was to all appearance perfectly healthy and normal. The gall-stones had never done any harm. But it is not quite the whole truth. There are at least two other conditions besides continued impaction which must be excepted. One of these is when a gall-stone which has caused obstruction is simply dislodged without being passed. So long as it remains in the biliary passages there is always the possibility that it will cause obstruction again. The other is when gall-stones are associated with inflammation of the gall-bladder or the bile-ducts, cholecystitis or cholangitis. In neither of these cases is the presence of gall-stones unimportant, and in both operation may be required no less urgently than when a gall-stone is impacted in one of the chief ducts.

In order to avoid any possible misunderstanding I should like to say at once that I am in entire agreement with those who maintain that medical treatment, as distinct from operation, should be thoroughly tried first. If it succeeds and the calculi are passed, nothing could be better. It is all that is wanted. But I must point out to you that it is very necessary that we should be under no delusion as to what is meant by success in a case of this kind. Mere relief from symptoms is not success. Under the influence of Carlsbad salts, large doses of olive oil, massage and other remedies, gall-stones may be dislodged, pain may cease, the biliary passages may be able to empty themselves again, inflammation may subside, and the patient may congratulate himself that he has recovered. But unless the gall-stones, one and all of them, have been definitely cleared away the patient is not cured, although he may be discharged from the hospital as such. On this point it is as well that there should be no delusion. Relief from symptoms is not the same thing as cure.

Leaving the question of the treatment of persistent impaction upon one side, as a matter about which there can be no dispute, I am going to direct your attention to-day to the treatment of those two conditions which I have mentioned already, and first of all to that one in which it is clear that a stone has been impacted, and that the impaction has been relieved, but the stone has not

been passed. The patient has had an attack of biliary colic or of jaundice or of both. It is almost certain that the cause was a gall-stone, for the attack came on with great severity, and very suddenly, while the patient was apparently in perfect health. The stone has been dislodged, for all the symptoms have subsided, but it has not been passed. A most careful search—a matter which should never be neglected—has been made, and nothing has been found. There has been no inflammation. The difficulty throughout has been purely mechanical. The patient is comfortable once more, and naturally averse to any operation. What is to be done? Is an operation to be advised or not? If the stone cannot be dislodged, the case is clear. Nothing but misfortune, varying in degree according to the part involved, can follow unrelieved impaction. But if it has been dislodged, without having been passed, what then?

Well, gentlemen, the rule that we have hitherto followed, and one which I do not feel disposed to alter yet, is not to operate for a first attack, and not to hesitate about advising operation strongly if there has been a second, especially if the second attack occurs within a short space of time—such, for instance, as a year. I admit it is rather like that somewhat absurd law which allows every dog to have one bite and draws the line sharply at a second; but in practice there is a good deal to be said for one as for the other. If a stone has caused two genuine attacks of colic, or of jaundice, within a short space of time, and has not been passed or otherwise got rid of, in spite of a thorough course of medical treatment, it will almost certainly cause a third, and it is better to remove it at the earliest season that is convenient than to wait until an operation must be performed at a time when circumstances are very likely not nearly so favourable.

Each case has, of course, to be judged upon its merits. There is at present in our wards an old man who has had many attacks of colic, who certainly has a large number of gall-stones in his gall-bladder, for they can be felt, and upon whom I have declined to operate. Such cases are exceptions, and are to be treated as such. They do not invalidate our rule that in all ordinary cases we ought to aim at a permanent cure, not merely at giving relief. A patient who has twice had a serious attack of colic or of jaundice, caused by a gall-stone, cannot be considered to be cured, or to be safe from a third attack, so long as that gall-stone is there.

The other point which I wish to bring before your notice to-day is the treatment of those cases in which gall-stones are associated with inflammation of the gall-bladder or of the bile-ducts, cholecystitis or cholangitis. This is a condition which, it appears to me, deserves a great deal more consideration than it generally receives. The consequences that follow from it may be of the gravest possible character. In certain instances, fortunately not common, immediate operation may be required as imperatively as in the most acute abdominal disorder. Even in ordinary cases in which the attack is apparently not very severe the gall-bladder is often left so distorted and contracted as to cause more or less trouble for the rest of life. One attack, beyond all doubt, predisposes to another, and, what is graver still, it may be regarded now as proved that a succession of these attacks, even when they are slight, often ends in cancer.

Inflammation of the gall-bladder and bile-ducts is always septic, caused by septic organisms which, in the vast majority of instances, find their way into the biliary passages from the bowel. Gall-stones of themselves do not cause it. I have already reminded you of the frequency with which they are found after death in gall-bladders which show no sign of ever having suffered from them during life. They do not cause inflammation even when they are impacted. The cystic duct may be blocked and the gall-bladder distended to an enormous size, or the common duct may be closed and the patient intensely jaundiced, without there being a trace of inflammation. Gall-stones themselves, therefore, are certainly not the immediate cause; but though this is true, it is no less true that they are of the utmost importance as accessories and that without them, or without some similar assistance, septic organisms will rarely be able to effect much harm. As in the case of the urinary bladder, so it is with the gall-bladder. If it is healthy and uninjured, if the exit from it is free, and there are no foreign bodies or other agencies to act as accessory causes, septic organisms that find their way in are soon expelled. Unless they are exceptionally virulent, or there is something else there to help them, they are unable to maintain a permanent footing. They may affect the surface of the mucous membrane, and cause an attack of what is sometimes spoken of as catarrhal inflammation; and this, if it is severe, may cause so much swelling as to close the duodenal orifice. Then the tension rises, the mixture of bile and of pus secreted by the inflamed mucous surface collects behind the obstruction, the gall-bladder and bile-ducts are filled to their utmost, and jaundice and a certain amount of septic absorption naturally follow. But so long as there are no accessory causes there to lend their aid, the symptoms nearly always subside rapidly under the influence of careful dieting and drugs, the swelling disappears, the tension falls, the septic organisms are swept away. Gall-stones cannot cause inflammation by themselves, and septic organisms by themselves can only do so when they are exceptionally virulent. It is the combination of the two, the mutual action of the two, helping each other, that produces such grave results. The gall-bladder and the bile-ducts cannot get rid of the gall-stones. Nor can they, when gall-stones are present, especially when they are impacted, get rid of the septic organisms. Gall-stones and septic organisms both remain, assisting each other in causing inflammation; and the inflammation will continue as long as they both are there—varying, it is true, in severity, at one time perhaps almost subsiding and then breaking out again, but never entirely disappearing.

It is a fortunate thing that the bile is a fluid which is not very favourable to the growth of septic organisms—they can exist in it, but they do not thrive and multiply as they do, for example, in the contents of the bowel—and also that the walls of the gall-bladder and of the bile-ducts are very different in structure from, for instance, the walls of the appendix. Otherwise the consequences that would follow from the impaction of a gall-stone with a vigorous culture of septic organisms in the fluid dammed up behind it would be as frequent and as grave as they are in connection with the appendix. As it is, they are quite sufficiently serious. The worst form, acute phlegmonous cholecystitis, with sloughing or gangrene of the walls of the gall-bladder, is fortunately rare. When it does occur there can be no question as to the absolute necessity for immediate operation. It is not a matter that admits of discussion or of delay. The symptoms are those common to all acute infectious disorders of the viscera, partly toxæmic, partly due to shock, and vary according to the locality, according to the particular part of the biliary tract involved, and the extent to which the liver itself is affected. The constitutional symptoms are of the gravest possible character, delirium, with a rapid, feeble pulse, and often a subnormal temperature, being marked from the first. The local signs are of the same description as those that occur in cases of gangrenous appendicitis; and if this disease is complicated in its early stages by pylephlebitis, as it sometimes is, there may be considerable difficulty in diagnosis. In one case under my care the cutaneous hyperæsthesia, which is usually present in these affections in the short period that precedes the actual occurrence of gangrene, proved to be a most valuable distinguishing feature. When the gall-bladder is involved, the hyperæsthetic area lies above and to the right of the umbilicus. When it is the appendix, the most sensitive spot is always below, even in those cases in which the cæcum and appendix have failed to descend into the right iliac fossa. If gangrene has occurred already, before the case is seen, this sign may fail; but then the rest of the symptoms are more clear, and the difficulty is less.

Cases in which the severity of the inflammation is not so great as it is in phlegmonous cholecystitis are, however, of more interest, partly because they are so much more common, partly because there is not the same unanimity of opinion either as to the time when operation should be performed or as to the necessity for it. The effects vary in character and in degree according to the position of the gall-stones, whether they are impacted or not, and the virulence of the septic organisms. The gall-bladder may simply become distended more and more with a thin semi-purulent fluid until it forms a tumour that is visible on the front wall of the abdomen. I have known it so large that it filled the epigastric region, descended far below the umbilicus, and was mistaken for a hydatid cyst. Or, on the other hand, the gall-bladder may shrink up to a fraction of its former size, and its walls become so much thickened by inflammatory deposit that the cavity almost disappears. Localised peritonitis may occur around it, distorting it into all sorts of shapes and tying it down to the omentum, the pylorus, or any other neighbouring structure. A dense hard mass of inflammatory exudation may be formed around it, in which, except for the presence of gall-stones, it is almost impossible to recognise anything. The walls may ulcerate through, and if the patient is fortunate, the gall-stones may find their way in the bowel directly and be passed. In less fortunate cases general peritonitis or intestinal obstruction, due to the gall-stone becoming impacted in the narrower part of the bowel below, may follow; or suppuration may occur around, and the pus track for immense distances before it approaches the surface. Or, again, the bile-ducts may be invaded as well as the gall-bladder, with consequences that are even more serious. The inflammation now is no longer localised in the gall-bladder, which lies comparatively isolated: the liver is involved as well, and the bile, which normally is an aseptic fluid, now becomes mixed with pus and pyogenic organisms; jaundice and septic absorption follow; rigors are of common occurrence; the functions of the liver are seriously disordered; neither assimilation nor excretion is properly carried out; the patient becomes poisoned with the products of the pyogenic organisms and decomposing bile, until at last a form of cholæmia, associated with septic intoxication, follows. Whatever form the disease may take, whether it involves the gall-bladder only or the liver and the pancreas (for this becomes involved as well), whatever its severity, the essential point to bear in mind is that so long as the gall-stones are allowed to remain there, whether they are impacted or not, the gall-bladder and the bile-ducts cannot get rid of the septic organisms that have invaded them, and the inflammation will never quite disappear. It may be very slight, or it may be very severe. It may become chronic, so that the patient is never free from pain; or there may be recurring attacks at long intervals during which the patient is almost well; so long as the gall-stones are there the inflammation will continue, always progressing from bad to worse, each attack leading to the formation of more adhesions, or the accumulation of a greater amount of exudation, or a fresh attack of septic intoxication, until at last a stage is reached when mere removal of the gall-stones is no longer sufficient, and the whole gall-bladder must be excised, with, perhaps, part of the omentum and even of the liver.

These are the cases to which I wish to direct

your attention to-day, as especially in need of operation, and of early operation. It is recognised that phlegmonous cholecystitis admits of no delay. It is recognised, not so widely it is true, but still by most, that gall-stones should not be allowed to remain impacted, or to cause more than two attacks of colic or jaundice. In the same way it should be recognised that gall-stones should not be allowed to cause more than one or two attacks of inflammation. If there is definite evidence of inflammation around or in the gall-bladder, or if there are constitutional signs, such as rigors, associated with gall-stones, and the gall-stones cannot be got rid of in any other ·way, they should be removed by operation.

It may be said that such operations are attended with too much risk. This is a mistake. The risks of operation, so long as the parts around the gall-bladder and the walls of the gall-bladder itself are reasonably healthy, are very small. When the gall-bladder is shrunken up into an unrecognisable mass, the walls of which are too rotten to hold a suture, or, what is worse still, when the patient is poisoned by long-continued jaundice and septic absorption, the danger is, of course, infinitely greater. But that is the very reason for avoiding the danger, and by timely operation saving the patient from years of pain and suffering, and from the increase in the risk that must necessarily occur. The choice is a very simple one. It lies between curing the patient at once, with a very small amount of risk, or giving him partial relief and allowing him to continue more or less in pain, with health and strength steadily deteriorating, until at last a condition is reached when cure is either impossible or is attended with so much risk as to render the attempt scarcely justifiable.

There are at least two other reasons why early operation should be urged in these cases. One is the effect that gall-stones associated with inflammation of the bile-ducts have upon the pancreas. That terribly fatal disorder acute hæmorrhagic pancreatitis may, I admit, occur without the presence of gall-stones; but the two have been found together in so many instances, and under such peculiar conditions, that there can be no doubt as to the existence of some causal relation between them. And though chronic pancreatitis may be caused in other ways, there can be equally little doubt that the continuous presence of septic organisms in the common bile-duct is one of the agencies that lead to it. In the ordinary anatomical arrangement of the parts there is, of course, no difficulty in the germs finding their way from one duct to the other. So long as the pancreatic tissues are healthy, this may not be a very serious matter; they may be able to offer an effectual resistance. But it must not be forgotten that the persistence of such a condition will at last wear the strongest resistance; and there is good reason for thinking that chronic pancreatitis is a much more common and much more serious complication of gall-stones than is usually believed.

The other reason will appeal still more forcibly. There is now not the slightest doubt that in a large proportion of instances chronic inflammation of the gall-bladder, kept up by septic organisms in the presence of gall-stones, ends in cancer. What the exact proportion may be is unknown as yet, but it is certainly not a small one, nor one to be neglected. The results obtained by our late colleague Dr. Slade, whose untimely death is a very great loss, not only to the hospital but to the whole profession, have not, it is true, been entirely corroborated. As he himself pointed out, the numbers with which he was working were so small that the possibility of an accidental coincidence could not be eliminated; but they have been corroborated sufficiently to establish the main fact, and of that there can be no doubt. For many years past it has been known that a close connection existed between the presence of gall-stones and cancer. The frequency with which they occurred together was admitted, and even the possibility that there might be some more intimate relation between them. Now it may be regarded as proved that in every case of persistent or recurring inflammation of the gall-bladder, associated with the presence of gall-stones, there is very grave danger of the development of cancer, and the longer the inflammation lasts the greater the danger. It would be very difficult to find a stronger argument in favour of early operation.

November 13th, 1905.

JOCHMANN asserts that, as a rule, it is impossible to detect bacteria in the blood in progressing cases of pulmonary tuberculosis. When found post mortem, they are due to invasion, when the bactericidal properties of the blood have been lost.—*Journ. A. M. A.*, vol. xlv, No. 17.

WITH DR. FAWCETT AT GUY'S HOSPITAL.

CANCER OF THE STOMACH: ITS CLINICAL VARIETIES, DIAGNOSIS, AND TREATMENT.

(Concluded from p. 64.)

Tumour.—A tumour was noticed in 130 of the 306 cases from the Guy's (5) series, *i. e.* about 43 per cent. In Osler's (2) cases a tumour was felt in about 76 per cent. The greater proportion in the latter series is possibly to some extent due to improved methods of diagnosis, but we have also to remember that in the Guy's series the clinical histories of the cases are taken from the post-mortem abstracts, which are necessarily short and at times incomplete.

The position of the tumour varies with the position of the growth, but there are other conditions to which I shall refer which may cause it to alter its locality from time to time.

The mobility of a tumour of the pylorus is well known. A good example of it was that of Emily N— (*vide* p. 73), upon whom pylorectomy was performed. On admission the dilatation of the stomach was obvious to the naked eye, and a tumour, which could be readily moved about, was felt in the right hypochondrium. Another day no tumour was found on examination. This is a comparatively common occurrence in connection with tumours of the stomach, and in the case in question the disappearance of the tumour was due to the lavage, and consequent reduction in size, of the organ. In examining for a tumour it is important to have the patient you are examining in a good light, when the mass may not only be visible, but may be seen to move beneath the abdominal wall over a considerable area. The mobility of stomach tumours is remarkable in some cases. They may be as freely movable as a floating kidney, and it is hardly necessary to say that such tumours are usually situated in the pyloric region.

In relation to diagnosis inflation of the stomach is sometimes of value, as by its means a tumour previously not felt becomes palpable. Although tumours may be movable at first, yet they tend to become more and more fixed as time goes on. Both at operations and at autopsies we find, as a

rule, more or less matting to neighbouring parts. As a result the tumour may, for instance, become adherent to the liver and, moving up and down with it, give rise to a diagnosis of a growth of that organ, or of the gall-bladder.

Again, the implication of, and adhesion to, neighbouring structures may considerably increase the size of the mass which is felt, although the opposite condition is the more common one, viz. that a tumour appears to be smaller and more movable than it actually is. This fact should make us cautious in prognosis, cautious in saying that the tumour is one which from its apparent size can be excised. I have seen several cases in which before operation it was thought that the tumour could be removed, whereas directly the growth was exposed the impracticability of such an operation became obvious.

In the case of Elizabeth A— (*vide* p. 74), upon whom a gastro-jejunostomy was ultimately performed, the growth was only felt at times before the operation, and yet was found to invade an area of about four inches square in the pyloric region of the stomach.

In some of the cases of growth of the pylorus the tumour is so obvious as to render the diagnosis almost certain at sight. A patient, a man, who came to my "out-patients'" last year, and who was admitted later under Mr. Jacobson for operation, was an excellent example. The tumour, the dilated organ with its characteristic outline, and from time to time the regular peristaltic movements which you all know so well, were visible. On the other hand, regular peristaltic waves are not always present. Instead of these we may see irregular muscular contractions resulting in depressions or bulgings of a part of the dilated viscus, and these may lead to doubt as to the diagnosis, owing to the difficulty in deciding whether the movements originate in the stomach or the intestine.

This was what happened in the case of Emily N—(*vide* p. 73), to whose case I just now referred. I did not see her till the stomach had been washed out for some days, and consequently it had diminished in size, rendering the tumour less obvious, and so I was in considerable doubt at first as to the seat of origin of the peristaltic waves which were present.

Growths in portions of the stomach other than the

pylorus may also give rise to a palpable tumour. In the case of Alice M— (*vide* p. 58) a tumour could be felt projecting from beneath the margin of the cartilages bounding the epigastric angle on the left side. Another example is that of a patient, Alice B— (*vide* p. 73), æt. 37 years, who was in " Clinical " ward recently. A mass was easily felt in the epigastrium, which, on an exploratory operation being performed, was found to be a diffuse growth, causing general contraction of the stomach.

I now want to call attention to cases in which the tumour is thought to be connected with some organ, or structure, other than the stomach.

A good example is one reported by Dr. Cayley in the 'Path. Soc. Trans.,' and referred to by Fagge in his ' Text-Book of Medicine.' There was a firm, slightly movable tumour in the left hypochondrium, extending below the umbilicus. It was thought to be the spleen, but proved to be a stomach indurated by a carcinomatous growth. Another more or less common position in which such a tumour may be supposed to arise is the omentum, the organ in this case being contracted into a sausage-like shape, just as so frequently happens to the great omentum when infiltrated by secondary deposits.

A useful practical point to bear in mind in such cases is that the organ may be felt to contract, or, if inflation be performed, the gas heard, or felt, to fizzle through it.

In some cases of dilated stomach due to malignant disease no tumour is detected, and it is in these cases that the value of microscopical and chemical examination, as well as of the blood, is so great.

There is one, though somewhat rare, variety of case which may give rise to difficulty in diagnosis, even in the presence of a tumour, viz. where there is considerable induration and matting around an old duodenal or gastric ulcer.

A case in point was recently under the care of Dr. Pitt. Maria B—, æt. 44 years, was admitted in March, 1905, with a history of three months' pain after food, with vomiting. A tumour, 2 inches in diameter, was felt above and to the right of the umbilicus, which, when laparotomy was performed, proved to be a cicatrised simple ulcer.

"Latent" cancer.—We will now turn our attention to cases in which the symptoms are, so to speak, " latent," *i. e.* do not present any indication of the stomach being the organ primarily and chiefly affected.

This class of case is an important one, not because at the present time we can do much for them, but because the recollection of their existence may help us in the future to the recognition of their presence as methods of diagnosis become more exact. When this stage has been reached we shall have at any rate approached somewhat nearer to the possibility of doing something for their amelioration, or even for their " cure."

Perry and Shaw (5) include under this heading, not only the cases of patients who die from cancer of the stomach unrecognised during life, but also of those who have died of some other disease, and in whom cancer is found to be present at the autopsy. Of the twenty cases referred to by them, seven came under the latter category, death being due to such conditions as strangulated femoral hernia, pyelonephritis, heart-disease, and puerperal fever.

One of the points of greatest interest in this group is the extent of the disease, which is compatible with the absence of gastric symptoms. Of this I cannot give you a better example than Specimen No. 695, from our museum. The patient died as the result of a strangulated femoral hernia. There was no history of vomiting, nor any other symptoms of disease of the stomach, until the attack of intestinal obstruction commenced, four days before death.

In this specimen you can see a large ulcerated growth, which reaches from just within the pylorus along the lesser curvature for a distance of five inches. Both walls of the organ are involved, and the growth extends to and projects beneath the serous coat.

Having once obtained a mental picture of such a specimen as this, you will not be surprised in future when you meet with a patient obviously cachectic, perhaps presenting evidence of enlargement of the liver from secondary deposits, and yet who tells you that his illness only commenced a few weeks ago, or even less than that. You will remember that I referred to the apparent sudden onset of the disease in some cases, and that on examination of the patient it was often clear that the disease had existed for a much longer period than that from which the patient dated the commencement of his illness.

The second variety of case in which the cancer, though unrecognised, is the cause of death, may for clinical purposes be divided into two groups :

(1) Those in which the cachectic symptoms predominate.

(2) Those in which the symptoms are due to the secondary deposits.

In Group 1 the diseases with which the case is most likely to be confused are chronic renal disease, pernicious anæmia, and infective endocarditis.

A very good example of this group was that of a patient, J. B—, æt. 50, who was under my care in Clinical Ward in April 1900, and who died in June of the same year. He had been feeling weak since Christmas, 1899, and a little later he noticed swelling of his feet and then of the abdomen. On admission he was much emaciated, and œdema of the legs, and ascites, were present. The patient became gradually weaker, the ascites more marked, and there were signs of effusion in both pleuræ. No other physical signs of disease were detected in any organ. He was thought to be the subject of malignant disease somewhere in the abdomen, the pancreas being regarded as the most likely primary seat. At the autopsy a generally diffused carcinoma of the stomach was found, the organ itself being much contracted. There was some chronic peritonitis in the upper part of the abdominal cavity, with secondary deposits in some of the neighbouring lymphatic glands.

In Group 2 Perry's and Shaw's (5) collection of cases contain excellent examples, e. g. the symptoms presented during the course of the case being due to fractures of the bones, to ascites from peritoneal deposits, to paraplegia and hemiplegia from deposits in cord and brain, to enlargement of the liver, and jaundice from hepatic deposits.

In this class the secondary deposits which most often mask the primary disease are those in the liver or the peritoneum.

In Group 1 the difficulty of actually determining the presence of a growth of the stomach is greater than that of excluding diseases with more or less similar symptoms, and it is therefore by a process of exclusion that a probable diagnosis may be reached.

In pernicious anæmia it is common for gastro-intestinal symptoms to be present, and a lemon-yellow tint of skin may be misleading, as in some cases of cancer the complexion may have a more yellow colour, and less of the sallow appearance

than usual. If, however, by a blood examination a secondary anæmia is demonstrated—that is, the hæmoglobin bears a low percentage proportionately to the blood-corpuscles—then we can in most cases conclude that pernicious anæmia is not the cause of the condition.

In chronic renal disease the cardio-vascular and eye changes are the signs which, if the urinary condition is of doubtful significance, are the most likely to put us on the right track.

The examination of the blood in itself presents no special characters. Most cancerous patients are anæmic, and a blood-count shows that the type is that of a so-called secondary anæmia. In some cases the red corpuscular count is normal or higher than normal, this being usually due to persistent vomiting, or to a secretion of a large quantity of fluid into the stomach.

In connection with the diagnosis of pernicious anæmia from carcinoma of the stomach, there is a statement of T. P. Henry's, quoted by Osler (2) in his monograph, to the effect that he had never seen a case of cancer of the stomach in which the red blood corpuscles were below 1,500,000 per c.m., and never any case of pernicious anæmia coming to a fatal issue in which they were not below 1,000,000.

Henry also states that in cancer the diminution of the red blood cells does not keep pace with the cachexia, while in pernicious anæmia it out-distances it completely.

It is always advisable to make a careful blood examination before operation, because anæmic patients stand operation badly.

Glands.—The value of enlargement of glands as regards diagnosis is considerable, especially in cases of suspected or "latent" cancer of the stomach. The glands above the left clavicle, in the left axilla, and behind the left sterno-mastoid, are those most commonly felt. Glands of normal size may be felt above the clavicle in any condition of emaciation, and we must bear in mind the fact that the glands, though enlarged, may have been so for a long time as the result of old tubercular or other disease. The true significance of them is when they increase in size under observation.

One of the most important glands is that behind the lower end of the sterno-mastoid, and growth in it is stated to indicate primary disease in the stomach in more than half the cases, though such conditions as disease in the œsophagus, the mediastinum, and the pancreas may also cause its enlargement.

To take an example. A man, Henry G—, æt. 37 years, was admitted under Dr. Pitt on December 30th, 1901 ; throughout the course of his illness he exhibited no gastric signs. He was ill some eight months in all, the prominent features in his case being ascites and effusion into the pleural cavity. About the middle of his illness a gland was noticed in the left anterior axillary fold, and a few months later some small subcutaneous shot-like tumours were felt in the abdominal wall. The detection of these deposits led to a correct diagnosis of malignant disease of the stomach being made.

Treatment.—The situation of the disease renders treatment sufficiently difficult, and this difficulty is increased by that experienced in diagnosis in the early stages. Though this be true, yet we should not look upon treatment as hopeless, and certainly not as useless. The hopelessness of the treatment in some cases depends upon the fact that we do not recognise it early enough, the hopefulness of it that we may in the future learn to do so.

Surgical treatment in general is looked upon with approval by a large section of the public, as well as ourselves, nowadays—to such an extent, indeed, that an exploratory operation is regarded by some, whether patients or doctors, as of hardly more consequence, I have sometimes thought, than the taking or the ordering of a pill. There *are* circumstances under which an exploratory laparotomy is advisable, nay essential, to clear up a diagnosis, but such an operation should only be undertaken after thorough investigation of the case, both as regards the chemical and microscopical characters of the stomach contents, and in relation to other points that I have mentioned. Such investigations, if properly carried out, need not cause any loss of time to the patient, whilst their neglect will only end in discredit to the profession and to surgical operation in particular, and in the subjection of some people, however pleased they themselves or their friends may be at the idea, to needless surgical interference.

In the surgical treatment of these cases, just as in cancer of the breast or elsewhere, lies for the present our best hope, and therefore is it all the more necessary to advise it, without needless delay it is true, but only after due consideration of all the facts obtainable in any particular case.

We should remember too that many patients with carcinoma of the stomach stand operation badly. Their general condition may previously appear satisfactory and yet directly after, apparently as a result of, operation, they, in some cases, rapidly become weaker and die. To give you an example : Emily N—, æt. 67 years, was admitted under Dr. Pitt on December 30th, 1904, and came under my care two days later. There was considerable dilatation of the stomach, with a tumour in the right hypochondriac region. At the operation a movable and limited growth was found in the pyloric region. It was easily resected and a gastro-jejunostomy was performed, but the patient, for no obvious reason, never rallied after the operation, and died in about thirty-six hours.

Though operation has a depressing effect upon some patients, yet in others the reverse is produced, the beneficial effect upon their mental condition being most striking. The patient Alice B—, who, when I saw her on April 1st, was little more than "skin and bone," had undergone an exploratory operation in March, 1905, when a diffuse carcinoma of the stomach was found present. Nothing could be done and the wound was closed again. After the operation she showed considerable improvement, both mentally and bodily ; and five weeks later she had not lost weight, her pain had diminished, the vomiting was lessened, and her appetite and digestion better than before the operation.

To produce this result, however, an operation is not necessary. Osler (2) refers to the visit of an "optimistic consultant" to a patient with malignant disease of the stomach, and how, as the result of the doctor telling the patient that he was the subject of chronic gastric catarrh, a remarkable improvement commenced, and continued for nearly three months, despite any particular change in the treatment, which had consisted of lavage and careful feeding.

Unfortunately, or perhaps fortunately, exploratory laparotomy does not always produce this beneficial effect, so that no reliance can be placed on a development in this direction by one who has recommended such an operation lightly or inadvisedly.

I have already referred to the importance of examining the blood in patients about to be operated upon, pointing out that anæmic patients are not favourable subjects.

Concise rules for operation. — The conditions under which an exploratory operation may be advised may be generally laid down as follows :

A middle-aged patient who, having previously been healthy, becomes the subject of progressive and intractable stomach disorder should be subjected to most careful examination.

If the facts obtained from the chemical and microscopical examination of the stomach contents, if the condition of general nutrition and the result of the examination of the blood are consonant with those usually met with in cancer of the stomach, then an exploratory operation should be advised, the patient having had explained to him the danger of further delay. As regards the operation to be performed a partial

the two papers to which references are given at the end of this lecture.

Moynihan (4) in a paper in the 'Practitioner' for December, 1903, after analysing a large number of cases (more than 700) recorded by Kronlein and Mikulicz, comes to the conclusion that gastrectomy is, where possible, a better operation than gastro-enterostomy. It gives the patient some ten months longer to live, and, during that time, in greater comfort; there is also the possibility that the disease may be removed in some cases.

As regards gastro-enterostomy Moynihan points out that Kronlein and Mikulicz and others recommend that gastro-enterostomy should only be performed where there is a stenosis at or near the pylorus, or where stasis of the stomach contents is

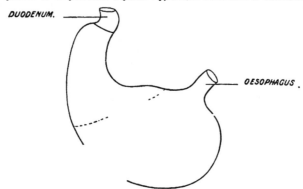

DUODENUM.

OESOPHAGUS.

gastrectomy with an independent gastro-jejunostomy would appear to be the best where possible. Mayo (6) states that one of the main reasons that only 5 to 8 per cent. of gastric cancer cases have been cured by extirpation lies in the fact that a part of the organ has been retained in which the vascular and lymphatic connections with the diseased area are close and direct. He recommends removal of the pyloric portion, and of the main lymphatic connections, but omitting what he calls the "dome." In the "dome" the lymph current is feeble and in the opposite direction to that elsewhere. The incision is made along a line in the direction shown in the diagram from the region of the cardia to that of the greater curvature in the pyloric region.

You will find full particulars of the operation in

certain. In such cases there is no doubt that although the duration of life may be only prolonged for some three to four months on the average, yet that the well-being and comfort of such patients are materially increased.

I may refer you to an excellent example of this in a patient who was under my care in February, 1905.

Elizabeth A—, æt. 39 years, was admitted on February 4th, 1905. The patient first noticed that she had some discomfort, not amounting to actual pain, after meals, in August, 1904. Her weight at that time was 14½ stone. At the end of August she began to suffer from pain after food and to lose flesh. In September vomiting commenced. She also had anorexia. Pain usually supervened immediately on taking food, and was followed by vomiting at intervals of two to four hours; when she was given a fluid diet sickness only took place at intervals of two to three days.

On admission the patient was thin, having lost about three stone in weight. A hard, irregular tumour could be felt in the epigastrium just to right of middle line: a succussion splash was present. No free HCl in stomach contents, but lactic acid was present. The presence of obstruction was shown by the fact that when the stomach was washed out at 11 a.m. (February 6th) a meal consisting of bread, some meat, and an egg having been given at 10 p.m. the previous evening, there was a large quantity of the meal in the washings.

February 10th.—Sir A. Fripp performed gastro-jejunostomy.

After the operation the patient was only sick once or twice, and the pain was relieved; her weight while in hospital increased 5 lbs.

Another case, under the care of Sir C. Perry, in 1901, is a very good instance of the relief that may be afforded by the same operation. The patient, Henry T—, æt. 42 years, first began to be sick after taking food about eight months before admission. This symptom increased in severity for the six weeks previous to admission to such an extent that it lasted sometimes for most of the day. For two months after the operation he was altogether free from pain and sickness, but at the end of three months he was again admitted to hospital, the anorexia and sickness having returned, and he ultimately died in October, about fourteen months from the commencement of symptoms.

In cases, however, in which there is no stenosis and no stasis a gastro-enterostomy is of little value; it will probably not prolong life; it will bring little, if any, increased comfort.

Medical treatment.—It is, of course, clear that the general nutrition of the patient should be maintained as far as possible, in addition to surgical treatment; or where the latter is impossible, medical treatment may be of much use in maintaining or improving the comfort of our patients. Food should, as a rule, be given in small quantities and in a readily assimilable form, and, as owing to the absence of free HCl, fermentative changes readily occur, the amount of carbohydrate and fat should be limited.

Alcohol is often useful, and of all the routine methods of treatment Osler (2) considers that lavage is probably the most valuable. He points out that a history of hæmorrhages and the presence of ulceration is no contra-indication if a soft tube be used with ordinary care. He recommends that this procedure should be carried out at bedtime and about four hours after the last meal.

With regard to other treatment, apart from that of those cases which require morphia or other narcotic, antiseptics are at times of use in controlling fermentation, and for the treatment of the constipation cascara, or glycerine suppositories, may be recommended.

REFERENCES.

(1) PERRY and SHAW.—'Guy's Hosp. Rep.,' vol. xlviii, 1891.

(2) OSLER and McCRAE.—'Cancer of the Stomach.'

(3) FENWICK.—'Cancer and other Tumours of the Stomach.'

(4) MOYNIHAN.—'Practitioner,' December, 1903.

(5) PERRY and SHAW.—'Guy's Hosp. Rep.,' vol. lviii, 1904.

(6) MAYO, W. J.—'Annals of Surgery,' July, 1903, and March, 1904.

(7) B. MOORE, ALEXANDER KELLY, and ROAF. —'Lancet,' April 29th, 1905.

November 13th, 1905.

Resection of Ovary.—Menge has succeeded in maintaining menstruation in three women on whom he operated for removal of bilateral ovarian cysts that had substituted the normal ovary. He accomplished this by making an oval incision around the base of the tumour, which he then shells out with his fingers, leaving an oval plate of ovarian tissue not more than 1 or 2 mm. thick at any point. The edges of this plate are then turned in until the raw surface is entirely covered and the tissue is sutured, the resulting roll being shaped something like a sausage, in the place of the normal ovary. This little roll contains the germinal epithelium of the albuginea and a strip of connective tissue. The three patients exhibited a few symptoms of the artificial menopause immediately after the operation, but they rapidly subsided, and menstruation has been apparently entirely normal since. The patients were from 25 to 34 years of age.—*Journ. A. M. A.,* vol. xlv, No. 17.

A LECTURE

ON

PRURITUS AND ALLIED CONDITIONS AFFECTING THE VULVA.

Delivered at the Medical Graduates' College and Polyclinic.

By FREDERICK J. McCANN, M.D.Ed., F.R.C.S.Eng., M.R.C.P.Lond.,

Physician to In-patients, Samaritan Free Hospital for Women.

LADIES AND GENTLEMEN,—I have been tempted to lecture on this subject because I have noticed that in the medical journals from time to time questions are asked about the treatment of pruritus. It is a condition which causes a good deal of trouble in treatment, and as you know it occasions considerable distress to the patient. I have stated in the short syllabus which has been handed round the various causes of pruritus, and after considering them we shall speak of the local changes produced, and then the treatment.

Now, with regard to the causation of pruritus, you know that there are many conditions which cause it, and that it is not a disease, but a symptom of many diseases. One of the most important causes is eczema. And although eczema may in many cases be the cause, it is also frequently the result of the pruritus, because patients continue scratching and rubbing the vulva until they produce the condition of eczema. Without going into the causes in the order in which they are in the syllabus, I would first direct attention to one or two actual cases of pruritus of a kind which are commonly seen in practice. And first of all, a very common cause of pruritus is smegma. You frequently see patients who have been suffering a long time from pruritus, and when you make a local examination you find that there is an accumulation of secretion around the clitoris and the labia minora, and that that is causing a great deal of irritation—in fact, producing a condition analogous to balanitis in the male. It is curious that people who may be very cleanly in their habits are not at all cleanly with regard to the genital organs. This condition is readily curable. The treatment is to get rid of the smegma by cleanliness, followed by the application of lanoline or other simple ointment.

The presence of pediculi is another common cause of pruritus, carbolic oil or mercurial ointment being the best treatment for this condition. There is another very common condition associated with pruritus, and that is the presence of tender spots. Examples are met with both in single and in married women. When you make a local examination you will frequently find on one or other side of the vulva one or more tender spots, and unless these tender spots are treated you will not be successful in combating the cause of the pruritus. It is best to search for these spots by using a probe, and when you touch the affected parts the patient will tell you that that is the cause of the pruritus. The best treatment is the application of pure carbolic acid or tincture of iodine to the tender spot. These tender spots also occur at another period in life, namely, at the menopause, and they are associated with a peculiar change in the mucous membrane characterised by the loss of epithelium and the presence of clumps of vessels, so that you see a number of bright red spots and patches, and often in addition a vascular urethral caruncle. These spots at the menopause are also a frequent cause of dyspareunia. The treatment of these spots is to touch them with the cautery or with pure carbolic acid, or with tincture of iodine, and having done that, you will get a complete cure. After using the caustic, whether it be carbolic acid or the actual cautery, you should employ regularly some simple ointment. Such cases are very common, and as a rule they are not successfully treated simply because these local patches are not dealt with systematically.

We have grouped here together acne, boils, and herpes. It is not uncommon to find patients suffering from a crop of boils on the vulva, and sometimes the infection passes from one sex to the other. These boils are situated on the mons veneris or on the labium, and there is much pruritus accompanying them and a good deal of pain. They are sometimes very troublesome to treat. The chief reason that they are troublesome to treat is because of the vulvar hairs. The hairs about the vulva are most important factors in spreading infection, and these boils are in reality abscesses of the hair-follicles. When the abscess bursts, the hairs become matted together and reinfection takes place, and you cannot get these cases well until the hairs are clipped short. To treat the abscesses properly you should open them and apply pure carbolic acid to the base. In these cases, as I say, you frequently see a crop of boils, but you find that if you treat them in that way, by cutting the hairs short and applying pure carbolic to the boils, the patients get perfectly well. These are some of the common examples which are associated with pruritus.

Now as to the other morbid states associated with pruritus, there is the great group of cases where the condition of the urine is at fault, either the presence of sugar in it, or, what is very much more common, hyperacidity of the urine. For one case which you meet with of pruritus vulvæ associated with glycosuria you will probably see thirty or forty due to hyperacidity. In those cases where there is excessive acidity of the urine the urine acts as an irritant and causes pruritus for some time after micturition. But first with regard to the cases of glycosuria associated with pruritus. Whenever you have a patient coming to you with severe pruritus, you should never omit to examine the urine. These cases of glycosuria are interesting in this, that they frequently occur at the meno-pause. They are not instances of true diabetes, and the glycosuria may disappear without any treatment. Many patients condemned to lifelong diabetes have completely recovered. I have had under my own care three or four patients who were so condemned but who got quite well. This climacteric glycosuria is a very curious disease. It frequently occurs in fat women, and often in those of the Jewish race. There may be a very high percentage of sugar in the urine, and there is very troublesome pruritus, the sugar being the irritant and the local manifestations being aggra-vated by scratching and rubbing. There may actually be crusts forming on the labia, which when removed expose a raw bleeding surface. These cases are best treated by the administra-tion of opium, and the opium is best given in the form of a pill, one grain three times a day, and three grains at bed-time—that is to say, six grains in the twenty-four hours. This should be kept up, increasing or diminishing the quantity according to circumstances, for a month or two. After that period you can reduce the dose to half, and even-tually discontinue the opium. Such cases are not much influenced by dietetic treatment, although it is well to give the dietetic treatment at the same

time. I doubt, however, if the pruritus is much benefited by the dietetic treatment. Locally I know of nothing better than sulphuret of potas-sium, ten grains to the ounce of a simple ointment. If that treatment is persevered in, it will cure these cases. You know you cannot always cure diabetes—some people go so far as to say you never cure it—but you can cure this climacteric glycosuria with its accompanying pruritus by the treatment I have just outlined. For hyperacidity of the urine the best treatment is the administration of alkalies and the use locally of an ointment. The best ointment to use is one containing carbonate of bismuth, ten grains to the ounce. The carbonate of bismuth is a good preparation to use to prevent irritation of the vulva, or to diminish it when it occurs. There is nothing which acts so well in protecting the vulva from irritation by urine, even in the case of a fistula, and you use it either as an ointment or as a paste, made with glycerine or with castor oil, rubbing up as much bismuth as the castor oil will take. A good alkaline mixture to give is bicarbonate of potash combined with acetate of potash and camphor-water. In addition you will remember to diminish the amount of meat taken by the patient in her diet, and to enjoin the other dietetic rules applicable in the treatment of hyperacid urine.

With regard to other causes, there are vaginal and uterine discharges, congestion during and after menstruation and during pregnancy. It is very common just when menstruation commences, but more especially after it has ceased. I should think probably there is nothing more common in practice for which doctors are consulted than cases of pruritus just at the end of menstruation, and, if any of you take the trouble to study that question, you will find that the pruritus is caused by an irritating discharge which supervenes on the top of the ordinary menstrual loss. If that discharge be examined, it will be found to teem with micro-organisms, and evidently they produce some acid products which are exceedingly irritating to the vulvar mucous membrane. The best treatment for these cases is this bismuth ointment ; you require to protect the mucous membrane against the irri-tating discharge and to use an injection of some bland fluid, such as a solution of permanganate of potash in water, five or ten grains to the pint. The important point is to protect the mucous membrane against this irritating discharge, which stops the pruritus, and you use the permanganate of potash to lessen the amount of discharge.

Some very troublesome cases of pruritus occur during pregnancy. When you get this kind of case the best treatment is to make the patient rest in bed. If a woman suffers badly from pruritus in pregnancy, you will not cure her—indeed you may not even relieve her—if you allow her to go about. But you will certainly relieve her and you may cure her if you put her to rest. Rest in bed in cases of pruritus associated with pregnancy is essential, combined with treatment by laxatives. These two together are most beneficial in that condition.

I have not said much about the local treatment, because .I desire to speak of that in connection with all the conditions together, and to do so will save repetition. But I wish to mention one or two other points with regard to the local condition. When you get bad pruritus in women after the climacteric, you should always be suspicious of the presence of epithelioma. If an epithelioma is not present under such circumstances, it may soon appear, as it is a very curious observation that people literally scratch themselves into epithelioma. If you go over the history of a group of cases of epithelioma affecting the labium, you will find that first of all the patients had pruritus for two years, or probably longer, and that then an epithelioma formed, and the patients have had that peculiar parchment-like condition of the skin which is exactly comparable to the skin of the hands of a washerwoman who has had them almost constantly immersed in soda ; that is to say, there is a peculiar sodden aspect, with cracks intermixed, and that condition, as the irritation goes on, will frequently have supervening on top of it the development of epithelioma of the labium. That is one of the local changes. But sometimes, instead of that, you may find well-marked redness of the whole of the ano-vulvar region, and extending down the thighs, redness and congestion also extending into the vaginal canal. That is another type of local change.

Lastly, there are cases where you examine the patient but fail to find anything wrong at all. These cases are those which occur in neurotic women especially. They will tell you there is a great deal of local irritation. You make an examination but can find no cause for it ; there is no marked change in the skin and mucous membrane, except perhaps traces of scratching. These cases are a little difficult to treat, as we shall see presently.

We will now speak of the symptoms caused, and I have put them in the paper before you. The usual complaint is of periodic irritation, or irritation which only occurs after walking or getting warm in bed, and all this is of course increased by scratching or rubbing. In the treatment of these cases the patient can help you a great deal if she has enough resolution to refrain from scratching, because, as you know, continual rubbing and scratch- will baffle the effects of any treatment you may employ. This irritation may vary in intensity from being very trivial to a degree in which it almost drives the patient mad. Moreover, under any circumstances it is associated with nerve-depression, because there is nothing so depressing as continual irritation. These cases sometimes result from masturbation, and sometimes they cause masturbation. It is a common experience for those who do asylum work to come across many of these bad cases of pruritus in which there is masturbation or in which probably it has originated it. I have seen one or two feeble-minded patients who have been exceedingly bad instances of pruritus, in whom the whole vulva was injected and torn with scratching, and the same trouble extended up the vaginal canal. It has been said that you cannot cure masturbation, but I doubt that statement. I think you can cure it in some cases due to local causes, and certainly you can alleviate it considerably in the way we shall mention later on. Remember, then, the relationship of masturbation to this trouble. In making a diagnosis in these cases what you have to pay attention to is your method of examination. You should examine the vulva to see if you can ascertain any local cause, because unless you can make out a local cause your treatment will not be so successful. You should also examine the vagina and the cervix, the rectum and the urine. Having done that, you are in a position to proceed to the intelligent treatment of the condition. Frequently the presence of threadworms in the rectum is a cause of very marked pruritus. I have myself seen threadworms pass into the vagina from the rectum.

Now, coming to the local treatment, I am quite convinced that practitioners fail in the treatment of pruritus through not getting properly at the disease ; and the reason is that they have followed the advice of the books as to the application of the different remedies ; that is to say, you are usually told in the books to apply the lotion or ointment, or whatever it be, on a piece of lint or cotton-wool and place it between the labia. It is curious that pruritus of the vulva has a close relationship with pruritus ani, and it is now beginning to be understood that the cause lies within the entrance to the bowel, that there is there a crack or ulcer, and unless you get at that cause you can paint all the preparations of the pharmacopœia on the anal region without curing the disease. I have gone through the experience myself ; I have tried—and I hope intelligently—to carry out the directions in the books, but I have failed to cure the patient. And the reason is that the most sensitive area in the vulva is just at that part where it joins the vagina, in that ring of tissue, and if you examine carefully you will find cracks and fissures and tender spots right round that ring, and a degree of inflammation extending into the vaginal canal. That being so, no treatment is of any avail unless it is also applied to the lower part of the vagina ; that is the secret of the treatment of these cases. I have had many cases of pruritus under my care, and I have not had a failure since I have been working on these lines. Undoubtedly the best material to use in the treatment of pruritus is carbolic acid. Carbolic acid must cure the pruritus ; it is only a question of strength. It is, as you know, a local anæsthetic, and you also know it is a strong antiseptic. You begin with a solution of 1 in 40, if that is not strong enough, use 1 in 20, and if that is not strong enough use 1 in 10. A bad case of pruritus you will never cure if you allow the patient to go about. The usual treat-ment is to allow the patient to walk about, to put a little wool between the labia, and to give her a lotion or ointment for application to the part. That may alleviate her, but it certainly will not cure the condition. If you get a bad case you have to put the patient to bed ; the relief obtained by the horizontal posture diminishes the local con-gestion, and she gets very much better. The way to apply the carbolic acid is to cut strips of lint and steep them into 1 in 20 carbolic. They should be about three inches in length. One inch of the strip is introduced into the vagina, and the

remainder, which is spread into the form of a fan, is allowed to lie between the labia. If two or three such pieces are put into the vagina and left there over night, you will find the pruritus is quite stopped, and the patient will probably have had the first night of relief for some time. That is the important point, that all applications, whether they be lotions or ointments, must be used so that, according to a common phrase, they "touch the spot." That spot is just inside and around the vulvar orifice and inside the vagina. Any of you who care to investigate this matter for yourselves and examine cases of pruritus should pass a specu-lum, and you will be astonished to find that the congestion is perhaps half way up the vagina. Now, is it likely that treatment directed to the vulva alone will ever cure it? It may perhaps alleviate it, but the pruritus will recur. So you must get at the lower part of the vagina and treat that, with the tender spots and cracks around the vulvar orifice.

You should then apply a large pad of boracic wool. Boracic wool readily gives off the boracic acid, and a fine powder is left on the vulva. And if you put a large pad of boracic wool and fix it with a T-bandage, you have not only the action of a powder and the drying action of the wool, but it is a very effectual method of preventing the patient from scratching herself. After you have used the carbolic once or twice and got the local conditions improved, you will find the use of carbonate of bismuth ointment of great benefit. I prefer to make this carbonate of bismuth ointment with lanoline. It is true that you may make a rather thick ointment, but you can diminish the thickness of it by adding glycerine. But that it should be fairly thick is most important, because it forms an effectual coating to the mucous membrane and the skin in that region. These are the important points with regard to the use of carbolic acid in this condition. There are various other remedies which are used. Supposing you should see a case which the carbolic acid has not cured, though I think it is very unlikely you will have such a one, the next best application, in my experience, is chloroform and olive oil (Chloroform 3j, Ol. amygdalæ 3j). This should be applied on a camel-hair brush, or you can apply it on a piece of wool or lint, and in applying it you must also put some inside the vagina. A very useful ointment is Ung. conii (hemlock ointment) either alone or with 30ℳ. of purified creosote. This is a very good ointment for allaying the local irritation. But if you use the hemlock ointment you must get some of it into the vagina, otherwise you do not cure the disease. In addition to that, it is very useful to advise hot Sitz baths, simply because in many cases of this kind where there is a lot of discharge it aids cleanliness. These Sitz baths ought to be tepid, and ought to contain bicarbonate of soda. You know that baths with bicarbonate of soda are useful in cases of general pruritus of the skin—half a pound of bicarbonate of soda to the usual size of bath. For a Sitz bath you diminish the quantity of soda in proportion to the amount of water employed. After a patient has had a Sitz bath she should dry the vulva carefully, and then introduce the plugs of carbolic, and put on the boracic wool with a T-bandage. After removing the plugs and pad in the morning, she should use one of the ointments which I have mentioned, such as the hemlock ointment, with or without creosote, or the carbonate of bismuth. There are several lotions recommended. One of the best to use is :

   ℞. Sodii Biborat . . ʒj
       Olei Menth. Pip. . . ℳv
       Aq. ad. . . Oj

Another good lotion is Liquor carbonis detergens. Sometimes this acts like a charm in these cases. These lotions are especially useful when you find the irritation has been alleviated by the carbolic, and you want a preparation which the patient can continue using to keep the pruritus from returning.

   ℞. Liquor carbonis detergens ℳx
       Plumbi subacetatis . . ℳx
       Aq. ad. . . . ʒj

This lotion should be diluted with an equal quantity of warm water. If you prefer to give it as an ointment, a very good combination is :

   ℞. Liquor carbonis detergens ʒj
       Hydrarg. ammon. chlor . gr. x
       Lanoline . . ʒj

There is no doubt that lanoline is very much better than vaseline in cases of local irritation in the vulvar region. It is, however, more expensive. Ointments act much better than lotions, and this is one of the best.

Additional formulæ.—Lotions.

   ℞. Zinci oxidi . . . ʒj
       Calamini . . ʒj
       Mucilaginis tragacanthe ʒj
       Aquæ calcis . . ʒiv
       Aquam ad. . . . ʒj

Strong infusion of tobacco with addition of eau de Cologne to mask the odour.

Lotio nigra, Corrosive sublimate lotion.

Dilute hydrocyanic acid (ʒj–ʒxv).

Ointments.

   ℞. Lanoline . . . ʒij
       Vaseline . . . ʒij
       Oxide of zinc . . ʒij
       Starch . . . ʒij

You may add ten grains of resorcin or fifteen grains of salicylic acid.

   ℞. Ung. zinci . . . ʒij
       Pulv. calamini . . ʒij
       Pulv. amyli . . ʒiv

   ℞. Ung. plumbi iodidi . ʒj to the oz.

   ℞. Acidi hydrocyanici dil ʒj
       Ung. Bismuthi . . ʒj

Other local applications may be mentioned : silver nitrate, 10–20 per cent.; solid menthol, compound tincture of benzoin; cocaine, 4 per cent. solution. A weak continuous current is useful in the so-called neurotic cases.

For the general treatment of these cases rest and diet are important ; and another most important precaution is to prevent the patients taking alcohol, because the pruritus is so depressing that as a rule when they take alcohol they imbibe too freely. One of the best drugs to give as a local sedative is bromide of sodium, 20-grain doses three times a day.

And lastly, a word or two with regard to surgical treatment. If you get a bad case which nothing, not even carbolic, can cure, there is always the possibility of affording relief by excising the whole ring of mucous membrane at this sensitive area, including the ring of the urethra, and bringing mucous membrane and skin together. But another condition which is frequently associated with pruritus is gaping of the vulva, and in this condition fæcal matter may pass into the vagina and considerable local irritation results. An operation undertaken to diminish the size of the vulva will also cure the pruritus.

November 13th, 1905.

THE CLINICAL JOURNAL,

CLINICAL RECORD, CLINICAL NEWS, CLINICAL GAZETTE, CLINICAL REPORTER,
CLINICAL CHRONICLE AND CLINICAL REVIEW.

EDITED BY L. ELIOT CREASY.

No. 682.   WEDNESDAY, NOVEMBER 22, 1905.   Vol. XXVII.   No. 6.

CONTENTS.

*Specially reported for the Clinical Journal. Revised by the Author.

NOTICE.

Editorial correspondence, books for review, &c., should be addressed to the Editor, 51, New Cavendish Street, W., Telephone No. 904, Paddington ; but all business communications should be addressed to the Publishers, 22½, Bartholomew Close, London, E.C. Telephone 927, Holborn.

All inquiries respecting Advertisements should be sent to MESSRS. ADLARD & SON, Bartholomew Close, E.C. Telephone 927, Holborn.

Terms of Subscription, including postage, payable by cheque, postal or banker's order (in advance) : for the United Kingdom, 15s. 6d. per annum ; Abroad, 17s. 6d.

Cheques, &c., should be made payable to THE PROPRIETORS OF THE CLINICAL JOURNAL, crossed " The London, City, and Midland Bank, Ltd., Newgate Street Branch, E.C. Account of the Medical Publishing Company, Limited."

Reading Cases to hold Twenty-six numbers of THE CLINICAL JOURNAL can be supplied at 2s. 3d. each, or will be forwarded post free on receipt of 2s. 6d. ; and also Cases for binding Volumes at 1s. each, or post free on receipt of 1s. 3d., from the Publishers, 22½ Bartholomew Close, London, E.C.

ECHINOCOCCUS COLONIES (HYDATIDS) IN THE HEART, WITH ESPECIAL REFERENCE TO THE PREFERENCE OF THE PARASITE FOR AREOLAR TISSUE.

By J. BLAND - SUTTON, F.R.C.S.,

Surgeon to the Middlesex Hospital and to the Chelsea Hospital for Women.

IT has become customary in describing the vegetable and animal parasites infesting man to speak of the Flora and Fauna of the human body. This application of a natural history expression is useful, perhaps even picturesque, and it is certainly an improvement on many of the dry and commonplace terms used in medical writings ; moreover the expression is true.

As the living things in a brook thrive best in certain haunts, so the vegetable and animal forms which infest animal bodies exhibit a marked preference for certain organs and tissues in which to live and grow. For example, the *Demodex* prefers the hair-follicles, whilst *Ankylostomum* selects the mucous membrane of the duodenum ; the malaria parasite finds its way into an erythrocyte ; filariæ swim freely in the liquor sanguinis ; *Coccidium oviforme* finds its way into the epithelium cells of the biliary passages, and the embryo of *Tænia echinococcus* prefers subserous areolar tissue ; whilst the adult form of this tapeworm chooses the mucous membrane of the dog's intestine, where it " occurs in considerable numbers, sometimes in many thousands between the villi, so that only the milk-white proglottides project " (Leuckart).

It is to this peculiar preference of the embryo of *T. echinococcus* for subserous areolar tissue that I wish to draw attention. In writings on Echinococcus disease (hydatids) the topographical distribution of the colonies and cysts so characteristic of this infection is based on the organs affected, and from the clinical point of view this is sufficient ;

but a more critical examination of infected organs from the pathologist's standpoint demonstrates that even in solid organs like the liver and spleen the primary seat of the parasite is in nearly all instances in the connective tissue immediately beneath the peritoneal investment or in the fissures. Occasionally a cyst or colony will be found deep in the iver substance without any connection with the tissues in the portal or hepatic fissures, and in very exceptional instances a liver will be thickly and unformly infested with cysts. One of the best examples of this is a liver described by Peacock ('Path. Soc. Trans.,' vol. xv, p. 247), which was obtained from a sailor who died in St. Thomas's Hospital in 1864. This liver weighed twenty-five pounds, and is occupied by hundreds of cysts apparently uniformly distributed in the organ. A portion of the liver is preserved in the Museum of the Royal College of Surgeons, and is the source of Fig. 1. The sailor had cysts in his lungs, spleen, kidney, omentum, and on the right ventricle of the heart. I carefully re-read Leuckart's account of his feeding experiments for the purpose of ascertaining if they would throw any light on this particular specimen. I think they do. Leuckart's greatest success occurred with the pig, which he says "may be very readily infected by the eggs of *Tænia echinococcus*," and he points out that "it is remarkable that the cysts were all thickly distributed under the serous covering of the liver, and that upon both the concave and convex surfaces." Leuckart also distinctly notices the relation of this parasite to the connective tissue of the liver, for he distinctly states in more than one place in his book that these early cysts were " everywhere in direct continuity with the connective-tissue trabecular network of the liver." And he writes : " In all cases, moreover, it was the interlobular tissue that contained the parasites." This supports the teaching of Naunyn, that the embryos are distributed through the vascular system.

In the liver of the sailor we have an example of infection exceptionally severe, in which the interlobular connective tissue of the organ lodged the parasites, as well as the subserous tissue.

My first serious study into this question was made in regard to the occurrence of echinococcus disease of the female pelvic organs, and I was soon satisfied that many examples loosely recorded as hydatids of the uterus and ovaries were part of a general echinococcus infection of the subperitoneal tissue of which the mesometria (broad ligaments) form part. As a matter of fact, in the British Isles the occurrence of an isolated echinococcus colony in connection with the uterus, ovary, or Fallopian tube is exceedingly rare. In the few known examples connected with the uterus the colony grew beneath the subserous covering of the fundus, and simulated a pedunculated fibroid (Altormyan, Martin). Those supposed to have arisen in the ovary are remarkable examples of the credulity of

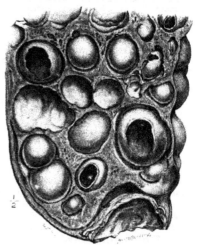

Fig. 1.—Portion of a liver which weighed 25 lb., in which the interlobular tissue throughout the organ was infested with echinococcus cysts. (*Museum Royal College of Surgeons.*)

compilers and the carelessness of recorders. Some years ago I hunted up the original descriptions of primary hydatids in the ovary referred to by Neisser in his oft-quoted paper " Die Echinococcen Krankheit," 1877, and in none of the records that I had access to was the description satisfactory, and one proved to be an ordinary multilocular ovarian cyst. The cases recorded since that date are equally unconvincing. Dr. Eden has since made a literary search ; and though he is credulous enough to accept a case imperfectly recorded by Pean, and which to my mind is unconvincing (for Pean merely states his impression but gives no description of the specimen), agrees with me in the absence of proof that primary echinococcus disease occurs in the ovary. In 1901 I found a solitary colony in the mesosalpinx in the course of an abdominal operation which, so far as the mere needs of practical surgery are concerned, could be regarded as a "hydatid" cyst of the ovary, but a careful dissection of the parts revealed clearly enough that the colony arose in the loose tissue of the mesosalpinx, and as it grew flattened the ovary over a part of its circumference (CLINICAL JOURNAL, October 23rd, 1901). This is true also of a specimen recently reported by Cullingworth, but in this case the pelvic colonies were associated with general echinococcus disease of the subperitoneal tissue generally.

Indeed, the cases recently reported support the view expressed by me, that the ovaries and testes are immune from primary echinococcus infection.

In order to test the reality of this affection of the echinococcus embryo for loose areolar tissue I have made a critical study of echinococcus cysts (hydatids) in relation to the heart. In most descriptions of "hydatids of the heart" attention is in the main directed to the relation of the cysts and colonies to the chambers of this organ, but a critical examination of the reports and specimens serves to show that the parasite exhibits the same fondness to abide in loose areolar tissue in this organ as in others.

The heart contains in the auriculo-ventricular groove a large amount of loose adipose tissue which is strictly subserous. This loose tissue, which serves as a bed for the coronary vessels, penetrates deeply between the adjacent walls of the auricles and indicates on the ventricular surface of the heart the line of the interventricular septum.

A critical examination of some of the available specimens makes it clear that in the majority of instances the parasite lodges in the loose tissue of the auriculo-ventricular septum.

The Museum of the Middlesex Hospital contains a specimen which illustrates this (Fig. 2). The heart was obtained from a man, æt. 19 years, who died in Guy's Hospital, with extreme suffering and the ordinary symptoms of mitral imperfection. On examining the heart, Moxon ('Path. Soc. Trans.,' vol. xxi, p. 99) found a projection the size of an apple on the back of the auricles, "off their septum near where it joins the septum of the ventricles; from its extent it implicated all those parts men-

tioned." The cyst had completely blocked the coronary sinus. The cyst which contains daughter vesicles was unbroken.

A careful study of this specimen is interesting, and shows that the colony arose in the loose tissue of the auriculo-ventricular groove and came into close relation with the four cardiac cavities. It is a noteworthy fact that the cyst is in very intimate relation with the interventriculum septum, and I have come across several records in which the cyst is described as occupying this septum, and, on examining the specimen described by Peacock ('Path. Soc. Trans.,' vol. xxiv, p. 37), which is

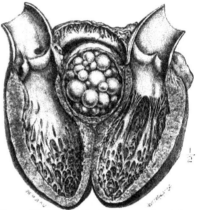

FIG. 2.—The left ventricle of a heart opened vertically to expose an echinococcus colony growing in the loose tissue of the auriculo-ventricular septum on the posterior aspect of the heart. (*Museum of the Middlesex Hospital.*)

preserved in the Museum of the Royal College of Surgeons, the cyst will be seen to occupy the upper end of the septum.

The effects of echinococcus colonies on the heart and circulation are important. A cyst may exist for a long time and give no indication of its presence, and then death occurs suddenly and the cause is manifest at the post-mortem examination (Peacock's case). In others the cyst, or colony, embarrasses the action of the heart and produces serious symptoms of valvular lesion (Moxon's case). More often the cyst bursts into one of the cavities of the heart, the vesicles and membrane being deported as emboli. When the cavities on the left side of the heart are invaded the vesicles are distributed by the systemic vessels. Oesterlin (Virchow's 'Archiv.,' bd. xlii, p. 404) recorded a case in which a girl, æt. 23 years, developed gangrene of the right leg ; this was amputated, and she died of pyæmia. An echinococcus colony the size of a pigeon's egg, situated in the wall of the left auricle, had burst into the cavity of the auricle, a piece of the cyst wall was discovered in a thrombus in the right common iliac artery, and an entire vesicle had lodged in the deep femoral artery.

Altmann ('Inter-Colonial Medical Journal,' 1902, p. 573, of Australia) has recorded a case which illustrates the tragic way in which an echinococcus colony of the heart may destroy life. A servant-girl was gathering chips at a wood-heap ; she fell down as if in a fit, and died within ten minutes. On post-mortem examination an echinococcus colony as big as an orange was found on the posterior aspect of the left auricle, and had ruptured into the auricular cavity. A daughter-cyst had been conveyed into the left internal carotid artery and blocked it at its entrance into the cranium. A complete examination was not permitted.

When a "colony" bursts into one or other cavity on the dextral side of the heart the vesicles and fragments of membrane are carried as emboli into the lungs. Budd described a good example of this ('Path. Soc. Trans.,' vol. x, p. 80).

Echinococcus cysts seated in the tissues of the heart are said to be primary, but the vesicles and membrane of a colony may find their way into the heart as emboli. This, however, is a very rare phenomenon, and after a careful search I can only refer to one—the classical observation reported by Luschke to Professor Leuckart. A woman, æt. 45 years, died suddenly. In the posterior border of the liver there was an echinococcus cyst about the size of a child's head, which had burst through the walls and discharged some of its contents into the inferior vena cava. The daughter-cysts had reached the right chamber of the heart and had been driven thence into the pulmonary arteries and caused rapid death.

In writing this article I have no intention of dealing with echinococcus disease of the heart exhaustively (although it provides ample material for an interesting monograph), but to illustrate the preference of the six-hooked embryo for areolar tissue. In the course of the inquiry I was surprised to find so many hearts affected with this disease in the London museums. The most impressive feature connected with the clinical side of this study is the dramatic suddenness with which an echinococcus colony will often cause death, although this is no novelty in connection with grave cardiac disease of all kinds.

November 20th, 1905.

OPERATIVE TREATMENT OF SIMPLE FRACTURES.

By W. ARBUTHNOT LANE, M.S., F.R.C.S., Surgeon to Guy's Hospital, and Senior Surgeon to the Hospital for Sick Children, Great Ormond Street.

HAVING decided that it is advisable to operate rather than to attempt to obtain a moderately good result by the use of splints and similar apparatus, the surgeon should proceed to render the patient's skin as clean as possible. The surgeon should not be satisfied with cleaning the skin in the immediate vicinity of the fracture, but in the case of a fracture of a long bone he should render the skin of the entire extremity as free from organisms as he can.

In order to render the operation as simple as possible, and also for the safety of the surgeon, radiograms should be taken in planes crossing one another at 90°.

Having in this manner determined the situation and character of the fracture, the surgeon must next consider from which aspect of the limb the fracture can be best approached so that the patient suffers a minimum of damage from the procedure.

The surgeon should not hesitate to make a free incision ; the only disadvantage which accrues from increasing the length of the incision is the greater hæmorrhage which may result from it. Such hæmorrhage is readily controlled by the use of specially constructed compression forceps fitted with terminal teeth, having a spring sufficiently strong to obliterate the lumen of the vessel if left on for a sufficient length of time, thus obviating the necessity of applying a ligature.

The advantages of the long incision are that any vessels which are cut through are readily exposed and seized by compression forceps, and the fragments of the fractured bone can be cleared from the surrounding soft parts and can be handled by means of special forceps.

As soon as the incision is made through the skin sterilised cloths are attached to its margins in their whole length by means of forceps made for that purpose. In this manner the skin of the patient is excluded from contact with the wound or with the bone which can be extruded from between the edges of the wound during the processes of manipulation. On no account whatever should the skin of the surgeon's hand be allowed to come in contact with the surfaces of the wound, and similarly no portion of an instrument that has been grasped by the hand should be permitted to touch the raw surfaces of the wound. Also any sterile swab or cloth introduced into the wound for the purpose of soaking up blood must be held in forceps and must not be touched by the hand.

Having done this, the surgeon must next consider the best mechanism at his disposal by means of which he can retain the fragments in apposition. The most effective means by which such accurate apposition may be obtained is by the screw, and if this instrument is suitable it should always be employed.

Fig. 1 illustrates the result of an operation for fracture of the tibia and fibula. The patient was treated in a large London hospital for simple frac-

FIG. 1.

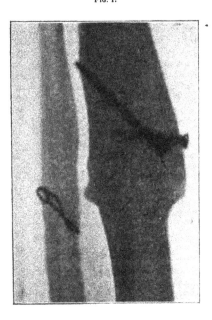

FIG. 2

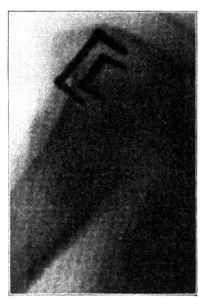

To avoid accidental infection by instruments it is preferable to employ elevators and retractors in which one extremity alone is intended for the wound, the other extremity having special handles for the purpose of grasping, so avoiding any chance of indiscriminate introduction. By the employment of forcible traction, approximation, and leverage the surgeon should, in ordinary circumstances, be able to establish accurate apposition of the fractured surfaces and so restore the bone to its original form.

ture of the tibia and fibula, but when the case came under my care, nine months afterwards, he could not bear his weight upon the limb because of pain in the seat of the fracture and in the ankle-joint. The fractures of the tibia and fibula were freely exposed, and the situation of the fragments and the alterations in axes were carefully gauged. The bones were sawn through in different planes to admit of the fragments being brought together, so that their axes returned to the normal relationship with one another. The tibial surfaces were then secured by two screws, and silver wire was used for the fibula. The result of the operation was excellent.

The use of the staple is well illustrated in Fig. 2, which represents the result of operative treatment of a fracture of the upper end of the humerus. In this case apposition was effected with extreme difficulty since the upper extremity had rotated round an antero-posterior axis in such a manner that the fractured surface looked outwards, while the upper extremity of the lower fragment was displaced inwards and forwards. In these circumstances neither the screw nor wire would have been of much use, since a screw could not be introduced in such a direction as to obtain an effective grip on the upper extremity, while a wire could not have been employed efficiently, partly because of the mobility of the upper fragment and partly because of the depth at which the fragments lay at the bottom of a bruised and swollen wound. The result of the operation was excellent, the patient obtaining a perfectly useful arm.

In the case of comminution of fragments the pieces of bone are better connected together by wire than by staples, since it is usually impossible to drive one limb of the staple into a mobile fragment.

Should there be much hæmorrhage it is well to employ drainage for a period of time varying from twenty-four to forty-eight hours, but in the majority of cases it is unnecessary. The risk involved by operative interference in skilled hands is very small, but one can readily recognise that infection of such a wound due to any want of care on the part of the surgeon is certain to be followed by serious, if not disastrous, consequences.

November 20th, 1905.

New Dressing for a Suprapubic or Biliary Fistula.

—The dressing is described in a paper by G. H. Colt, M.B., B.C., in the ' Lancet ' of November 4th, 1905. It consists of a glass vessel applied over the fistula, from which the urine is led away by a side tube. The glass vessel is attached in a watertight manner to the skin of the patient by a rubber flange and an aseptic solution of pure rubber in naphtha. This arrangement is efficient and a boon to the patient ; it also effects a saving of time in treatment. The makers are Messrs. Down Bros., Ltd., St. Thomas's Street, S.E.

ALCOHOL AS A THERAPEUTIC AGENT.*

By ROBERT HUTCHISON, M.D., F.R.C.P., Assistant Physician to the London Hospital.

MR. PRESIDENT AND GENTLEMEN,—It is a good thing for us, I think, to review our position from time to time with regard to the remedies which we most commonly employ, and to ask ourselves what we really expect them to do for us, and whether we are using them in the right way and in the right sort of case. Especially is this true of such a therapeutic agent as alcohol, in the use of which we can hardly expect to escape being biassed, partly by tradition and partly by predilections derived from a study of its effects as exerted in our own persons. Accordingly, when you were kind enough to invite me to address you here to-night, I thought that we might profitably occupy our time by considering together the uses of alcohol as a remedy in disease. I have purposely restricted the scope of the remarks which I shall have to make to the use of alcohol as a *remedy*. Of the advantages or otherwise of the habitual use of alcoholic beverages I shall have little to say, for I believe that in the last resort that is a question which every man must decide for himself—indeed, whatever we as doctors may lay down the average man is pretty sure to do so. But of the remedial uses of alcohol it is for us, and us alone, to judge, and it is of the first importance that we should try to arrive at some degree of unanimity on the subject. That such unanimity is at present pretty far to seek I think every unprejudiced observer of medical practice will admit. I remember a friend of mine telling me that he went some years ago, when suffering from some slight disorder or other, to consult a distinguished physician, since dead. At the close of the interview he asked this eminent man if a glass of port at dinner would be of any benefit to him, and was assured that he might with positive benefit allow himself this indulgence. My friend then did what, of course, you and I cannot at all approve of; he crossed the street and consulted another distinguished physician for the same symptoms. He again put his question about port wine, but on this occasion was solemnly assured that he must on no

* An address delivered before the Ealing Branch of the British Medical Association.

account touch it, for it was little better than poison to him. Need I say that his faith in the infallibility of our profession received a severe shock!

Now, gentlemen, such occurrences are not creditable to us. About the advisability or otherwise of ordering such a potent agent as alcohol as a medicine there ought to be no two opinions amongst us any more than there is with regard to the use of such drugs as strychnine, quinine, or digitalis; yet if anyone studies the practice of different physicians regarding the administration of alcohol in such conditions as fevers, heart failure, stomachic disorders, or gout, he will find, I think, that the greatest diversity prevails. Now, what I should like to do to-night is to lay down some rules which in my judgment should guide us in ordering or withholding alcohol, and then to hear how far you agree with me and what opinions you have yourselves formed as the result of your daily experience at the bedside.

Now, at the outset we are met with this difficulty, that the conclusions arrived at by pharmacologists, who study the action of alcohol in laboratories, and those formed by physicians, who observe its effects on patients, do not by any means always coincide. This applies, of course, in greater or less degree to every agent in the Pharmacopœia, but it is more striking in the case of alcohol, I think, than in that of any other drug. Nor is the reason for this far to seek. Most of our patients are habituated ·more or less to the action of alcohol from its daily consumption in small doses, but the animals on which the pharmacologist makes his experiments are not accustomed to the action of alcohol, for the liquor problem is unknown in a community of rabbits and frogs. Hence it is that man may be expected to react differently to alcohol from the lower animals; hence it is also that, valuable though such pharmacological experiments may be, we as clinicians must not allow ourselves to be too much influenced by them.

In the last resort the question at issue can only be settled empirically, and the results of observation at the bedside must outweigh the teachings of any number of experiments, no matter with what ingenuity they are planned or how carefully they are carried out.

In order that we may proceed along the easiest and plainest way in our study of the subject, it will be best to follow alcohol through the body, and to concentrate our attention upon the effects which we believe it to be capable of producing at each point of its passage.

Use of Alcohol in Gastric Disorders.

On the mucous membrane of the stomach alcohol acts as an irritant. This is most marked in the case of the stronger alcoholic liquids, such as whisky and brandy—hence the chronic gastritis of spirit-drinkers—but one sees it even in such a weak alcoholic liquid as beer, if taken in large amounts and on an empty stomach. For this reason alcohol should be avoided in cases of chronic gastric catarrh. In virtue of its slightly irritating effects, however, and in part also it would seem from direct chemical action, alcohol increases the secretion of the gastric juice and also stimulates the movements of the stomach wall. Physiological experiment has clearly shown that, unless in large quantities, it has, in virtue of these actions, an effect upon digestion which is favourable rather than otherwise. It is in the atonic forms of dyspepsia, such as are so common in overworked men of sedentary pursuits, or in ₵onvalescence after severe illness, that the beneficial action of alcohol is most apparent. To such patients the admonition "Take a little wine for thy stomach's sake" is still sound advice. In those cases it is not a matter of indifference what form of alcoholic beverage is selected. What we may describe as the mental effect of different articles of food and drink upon digestion is so marked that it is important that the beverage employed should be pleasing both to the eye and to the palate, or in other words that it should possess some æsthetic properties in addition to containing a certain proportion of alcohol. Now, no one I think really *likes* a mixture of whisky and water, and it cannot be said to be particularly pleasing either to the eye or to the palate. For that reason it is better to select some sound wine with a certain amount of bouquet. Burgundy is very suitable, and possesses an alcoholic strength which, while not so great as that of the fortified wines, is greater than that found in natural wines such as claret and hock, and it has rightly gained a high reputation as a digestive. Some patients, however, prefer a glass of well-matured port, though others, probably those who have a tendency to gastritis, complain that port makes them " bilious," whilst if there be an inclination to acidity, a good Rhine wine may suit best of all. Beer, in spite of its low alcoholic strength, has many advantages as an aid to digestion, for it is a bitter, and the carbonic acid which it contains helps to stimulate the stomach movements, but it is rather too bulky for general use in the atonic cases in which the quantity of fluid consumed should be kept within narrow limits. The effervescing wines have a definite place in gastric disorders; alcohol is a much better solvent of carbonic acid than water is, and carbonic acid is a powerful anæsthetic to the nerves of the stomach. For this reason an effervescing wine, of which champagne is by far the best, is a very useful aid in the treatment of many cases of vomiting, particularly if of nervous origin.

The stimulating effect which alcohol exerts on gastric secretion contra-indicates its use in cases in which there is already a tendency to the formation of an excess of acid. Such a tendency exists in the acid dyspepsia so often met with in healthy young subjects and in patients who suffer from gastric ulcer, and in all such cases alcohol is best avoided. The same is true, I believe, of carcinoma, in which there is so often, perhaps always, some accompanying gastritis.

The use of alcohol in dilatation of the stomach calls for special remark. It has been shown by physiological experiment that alcohol is rapidly absorbed from the gastric mucous membrane, but that as it passes into the blood-vessels it causes a considerable osmosis in the opposite direction to take its place. The result is that the amount of fluid in the stomach is really increased in spite of the absorption of the alcohol and as one wishes to prevent a dilated stomach from becoming filled with fluid, alcoholic beverages are best avoided when that condition is present.

Alcohol in Disorders of the Circulation.

It has been pointed out above that alcohol is rapidly absorbed through the wall of the stomach. Entering the blood, it is able to exert its effect upon the circulation and it is here that the results of clinical observation and of physiological experiment begin to be in conflict. It is generally agreed amongst pharmacologists that alcohol produces some dilatation of the peripheral blood-vessels, and in this view all clinical observers will readily acquiesce. Indeed, it is popularly recognised

when we speak of a man as being "flushed with wine." We can turn this property of alcohol to therapeutic account when there is a mal-distribution of blood in the body with a tendency for it to stagnate in the internal organs, as in some stages of fever and when the skin is blanched and the internal organs congested after exposure to severe cold. On the other hand, in febrile conditions accompanied by a "bounding" pulse and an already dilated system of peripheral vessels alcohol is obviously contra-indicated. So far we are on fairly sure ground. It is when one comes to study the effects of alcohol upon the heart itself that confusion creeps in. We are all accustomed to believe, and to act on the belief, that alcohol is a cardiac stimulant—i. e. that it spurs the heart on to more frequent and more powerful contraction; and even although we may not suppose that it is capable of supplying the organ with a real amount of potential energy, at all events we habitually act as though alcohol were capable of enabling the heart to draw upon its resources. But many prominent physiologists deny that alcohol stimulates the heart at all. How are we to reconcile these conflicting views? Is the practice of using alcohol as a cardiac stimulant based upon a fallacy, or is there some error in the physiological experiments? To some extent perhaps the contradiction may depend upon the way in which alcohol is given. When taken by the mouth there seems to be no doubt—and as regards this even the physiologists are mostly agreed—that it increases for at least a short time the force and frequency of the heart-beats. This effect is probably a reflex one, exerted through the mucous membrane of the œsophagus and stomach, for it takes place too rapidly to permit one to believe that the alcohol has had time to be absorbed. Now, for clinical purposes of course alcohol is usually given by the mouth, but in the laboratory it is perhaps oftener injected straight into the circulation or even applied directly to the isolated heart, the reflex effect being in either case eliminated. But if this be the explanation what becomes of our attempts to stimulate the heart by the administration of alcohol by the bowel? Is everyone here, indeed, convinced that such a method of administration is efficacious? In any case, the reflex stimulating effect of alcohol is purely transitory, useful it is true in cases of sudden syncope, but of little value when one is dealing with a slow failure. But it is just in the latter class of case that alcohol is so often given as a stimulant, and I am bound to say that I can find in physiological writings but little justification for such a use. I must confess, too, that for my own part I am not thoroughly convinced that alcohol is of much use in cases of chronic heart failure from valvular disease or myocardial degeneration. On this point I should be very glad indeed to hear what your experience has been. If the muscle failure is the result of overwork from the attempt to overcome the resistance offered by contracted peripheral arterioles, then I can understand that alcohol may be of service—not by directly stimulating the heart, but by unlocking the closed gates of the circulation and so lessening the work of the left ventricle ; for we must never forget the aphorism of a distinguished French physician, that "pour fortifier le cœur il faut diminuer son travail." Is it only in such cases, then, that alcohol is of service, or does it really, despite the physiologists, enable a failing heart to pull itself together, so to speak, no matter how impotent it may be to affect the healthy organ ? For we must always remember, in considering this subject, that the clinician deals with abnormal hearts and not, as the physiologist does, with healthy conditions.

Uses of Alcohol in Diseases of Metabolism.

From the blood alcohol reaches the cells and exerts an influence upon metabolism. The often discussed question whether alcohol is to be regarded as a food or as a poison to the cells may be regarded as settled in the sense that it is both. It is a food inasmuch as it is capable of being oxidised and yielding energy in the body in the shape of heat, whilst it incidentally spares fats from combustion and to some extent proteids also ; but it is also a poison of the narcotic class which leads ultimately to a paralysis of protoplasm ; and which of these effects predominate depends, it would seem, mainly upon the quantity consumed. It is the properties of alcohol as a food which chiefly interest us as clinicians. It is true that we do not often consciously use it for this purpose—perhaps not as often as we should. The constituents of the food which alcohol is best calculated to supplement or replace are the carbohydrates. There seems, indeed, to be a certain complementary action between alcohol and these substances which is to some

extent perceived even by the laity. I have been told, for instance, by men who served in the South African War, that so long as an abundant supply of sweets in the shape of jam and other preserves was forthcoming the want of alcohol was not felt, but that so soon as such supply failed the craving for alcoholic stimulants reasserted itself. There may, therefore, be a physiological reason for the popular belief that abundant meat-eating and an inclination to indulge in alcohol go together. The chief use wé can make of the power of alcohol to replace carbohydrate is found in the treatment of diabetes. In that disease I believe it to be of great value, both as an aid to the digestion of a sufficiency of fat and as a means of helping to replace sugars and starch. The form of alcohol selected is to a large extent a matter of indifference, provided always that the beverage chosen be free from carbohydrate. All malt liquors are naturally contra-indicated, and the same is true of the sweeter wines, but any sound natural wine is admissible as well as all forms of spirits, the small traces of sugar which these may contain being quite unimportant. In the treatment of incipient diabetic coma the stimulating properties of alcohol are also of value.

The power of alcohol to interfere with the combustion of fat renders its use deleterious in obesity, especially, of course, if the beverage habitually taken contains carbohydrates, as the malt liquors do. As regards the use of alcohol in gout it is difficult to lay down general rules, for it depends so much upon the condition of the patient's digestion and circulation, but on the whole there can be little doubt that the less it is indulged in the better.

Use of Alcohol in Fevers.

I suppose that alcohol is more largely used in the treatment of fevers than in that of any other disease. The fashion in this respect was set by Todd, who often employed it in heroic doses, and since his day it has become the custom to prescribe it in cases of fever of any prolongation almost as a matter of routine. That the physiological properties of alcohol entitle one to expect that it will prove useful in febrile conditions there can be no doubt. Its power of dilating the surface blood-vessels, to which reference has already been made, causes it to be, to some extent at least, an antipyretic, whilst its capability of lessening the destruction of body-fat renders it a means of restraining tissue waste. I fancy, however, that most of us, when we order alcohol in a case of fever, have little thought in our minds of such modes of action as these. It is, without doubt, for its supposed stimulating properties that alcohol is usually prescribed for febrile patients, and the organ which we mostly wish to stimulate is the heart. Now, I do not wish to call in question the wisdom of the elders in our profession nor to pose as an iconoclastic upsetter of established practice, but I merely wish to ask, Are we sure that alcohol is capable of stimulating the heart in fever? I have already pointed out that many physiologists deny that alcohol has any power of directly stimulating the heart at all and I would only add that recent and careful observations (Cabot in America) showed a surprising inertness of alcohol as regards the circulatory system generally. But yet I think it must often have fallen to the lot of every one here to see a rapid, feeble, and irregular pulse in a febrile patient become slower, steadier, and more regular in its beat under the judicious administration of alcoholic stimulants. How, then, are we to explain this apparent contradiction? I would suggest that the explanation may be found in the action of alcohol on the nervous system. It may well be that the beneficial influence of alcohol on the heart in fever is exerted through the medium of its nervous apparatus and not upon the heart directly. By slightly narcotising the nervous mechanism which presides over the movements of the heart it may render the latter insusceptible to the influence of high temperature and the toxins of fever and so enable it to maintain the even tenor of its way unaffected by disturbing influences. Be this as it may, I think no good clinical observer will deny that in many cases of fever with failing circulation alcohol *is* useful, and may even indeed be the only means of saving life. But its use should be reserved for such cases. Fever alone is no imperative indication for its administration and its routine use is to be deprecated on all grounds.

I think I am right in saying that it is in the septic fevers that alcohol seems to exert its happiest effects. Here again we are in disagreement with the experimentalists ; for all bacteriological observations unite in showing tha alcohol tends to lessen rather than to increase the power of the organism to resist infection, whilst the liability of chronic alcoholics to suffer severely from septic processes

is notorious. In reply to this I can only repeat that we are not compelled to accept the results of experiments on the lower animals in such a subject as this as being directly applicable to man, whilst the fact that chronic alcoholism lowers tissue resistance and damages the kidneys is no argument against a possibly beneficial action of the drug in otherwise healthy persons. So long as we believe, as I think we do believe, that patients suffering from erysipelas, septicæmia, puerperal fever, and the like derive benefit from alcohol, so long we are justified in continuing to use it.

As regards the mode in which alcohol is to be administered in fever, there is perhaps too great a tendency to give it always in the form of spirits. In acute cases and where large doses have to be given that form is convenient, but in the more chronic cases, *e. g.* in typhoid, I think there is something to be said for the more nutritive forms, such as the malt liquors. If spirits are used, a good whisky is certainly preferable to an inferior brandy ; though if the effects of the ethers are desired good brandy is best of all, but to this point I shall return in the discussion of delirium. In deciding at what intervals the dose is to be repeated we should avoid routine instructions and take the pulse as our guide, any signs of flagging of the heart being an indication for repetition.

Use of Alcohol in Nervous Disturbances.

Alcohol is popularly regarded as a brain stimulant, but I need not remind such an audience as this that all physiological evidence is opposed to such a view. There is, on the contrary, good reason to believe that the action of alcohol on the brain is essentially that of a narcotic. It gradually paralyses the brain-cells, beginning, it would seem, with those in the highest centres which are connected with the psychical processes and passing down finally to the basal centres which preside over the functions of organic life. It is doubtful even whether the initial feeling of exhilaration which alcohol produces is not due rather to a paralysis of inhibition, a slackening of the rein over some centres, than to any truly stimulant effect. Consciously or unconsciously, it is probably for its anæsthetic effects that the ordinary man flies to alcohol, regarding it with Omar Khayyam as—

" The subtle Alchemist that in a trice
 Life's leaden metal into gold transmutes,"

which by slightly numbing the brain renders it less sensitive to the thousand frets and jars of existence.

It is to its anæsthetic effects too, I believe, that alcohol owes its utility in disorders of the nervous system. When the brain is excited by fever, so that the patient is tremulous, sleepless, and delirious, alcohol calms down the cortex and renders it less responsive to the heat of the blood and to the poisons which it contains. Its action is comparable to that of a dose of bromide but more rapid and evanescent, whilst by its effects upon the heart it at the same time increases and steadies the circulation through the cortex. To some extent too, it seems to restore a sick man's nerve, giving him courage again—even if it be but Dutch courage —with which to fight down his malady.· And this is one of the chief services which alcohol can render us in fevers.

Of the best form in which to give alcohol in order to produce these effects it is difficult to speak dogmatically. Anstie believed that those alcoholic beverages which contain the largest proportion of volatile ethers are the most potent and of these there is none better than genuine Cognac brandy. There is something to be said, too, for bottled stout, especially if sleeplessness be a prominent symptom for stout is possessed of great soporific virtues— probably by reason of some of the ingredients of the hops which it contains—and I have known it render yeoman service in cases of delirium tremens. In regulating the dose we must be guided by the effect produced and that in turn seems to depend greatly upon the previous habits of the patient as regards alcohol, for if the brain has been habituated to its presence large doses may be required to pro- duce the desired effect.

Remote Effects of Alcohol.

The oxidation of alcohol in the body, in non-in- toxicating doses, is very complete even in conditions of health. In febrile states the power of the cells to destroy it seems to be increased, and enormous quantities may then be consumed without intoxica- tion resulting. It is well to remember, however, that unoxidised alcohol acts as an irritant, especially to the liver and kidneys, and for this reason it should only be given to patients who suffer from hepatic cirrhosis or chronic nephritis when imperatively indicated, and there is reason to believe, I think, that such patients stand it badly even in medicinal doses. That alcohol is sometimes given with the best intentions in doses that are toxic there can, I think, be little doubt and one has sometimes seen patients who have been rendered drunk by it. Certainly when unoxidised alcohol can be smelt in the breath one can feel pretty sure that too much is being given.

To sum up, gentlemen, the points to which I would specially wish to direct attention are these : that in chronic disease alcohol is chiefly of use to us from its action on the stomach, and that its effects upon appetite and digestion are the guides to its usefulness, whilst in acute disease it is of service both from its action upon the circulation and upon the brain, and that so long as it is render- ing the pulse slower and steadier and the brain calmer so long, and so long only, is it doing the patient good.

November 20th, 1905.

THE RATIONAL USE OF "INFANTS' FOODS."

By G. A. SUTHERLAND, M.D., F.R.C.P.,
Physician to Paddington Green Children's Hospital and to the North-West London Hospital.

IT may be regarded as one of the signs of the times that when we speak of "infants' foods" we are understood to refer to the different patent and proprietary foods which are thrown so profusely on the market by enterprising manufacturers. Within recent years there would appear to have been a failure in the maternal supply of milk, and, in addition, so many dangers have been credited to cow's milk that mothers have fallen back on some tinned or bottled food as the best nourishment for their infants. This evil has been largely aggravated by the ingenious but misleading statements of the advertising manufacturer, who describes the mar- vellous life-saving properties of his own preparation and illustrates his statements with pictures of fat rachitic babies, each of whom appears to the young mother to be an infant Hercules.

The force of circumstances and the responsibility of our position as medical advisers have compelled us to take up a position which may appear as extreme to outsiders. The circumstances are that the maternal mind is so saturated with the belief that patent foods are fattening, strengthening, bone-producing, brain-producing, and teeth-pro- ducing ; that the foods are easily procured, easily preserved, and easily prepared ; and that they "stay down" in a manner which proves that all must be well. Has the mother not learned these facts from every paper, magazine, and poster she has read ? Consequently she will welcome any suggestion as to a patent food by her medical adviser, and she will attribute every satisfactory symptom in her child to that food, and she will feed all her other babies on that food also. Hence we have to proceed cautiously.

At the Paddington Green Children's Hospital printed instructions on the feeding of infants are issued to the mothers attending the Out-Patient Department. The only reference to "infants' foods" in these instructions is as follows : "On no account give any infants' food, condensed milk, bread, biscuits, or tops and bottoms until the child is nine months old—except by doctor's orders." It must not be concluded from this notice that all "infants' foods" are disapproved of, but the regulation of their use amongst out-patients is so difficult, and their abuse is so frequent and so disastrous, that it seems better to omit any mention of them. In the wards, on the other hand, there is always a supply of various proprietary foods, and these are used should the case seem suitable for such treatment. To put the matter briefly, it may be said as regards the use of "infants' foods" that the tendency of the mother is exactly the opposite of that of the physician. When the child is well the mother longs to employ a patent food, but when the child is really ill she usually returns to milk and water. The physician considers milk and water the best food for an infant, but in diseased conditions he may employ a proprietary food as one of his means of treatment. The young practitioner must remember how authoritative his words may be considered—at times. "May I give the baby a little of Rickett's Food?" says the young mother. "Oh, certainly," says the young doctor. Six months or a year afterwards she takes her child, who has been steadily fed on increasing amounts of this food, and is now a fine specimen of fully-developed rickets, to another doctor, who at once declares the child to be suffering from the effects of improper food. "But the doctor ordered it!" exclaims the mother. As during these months she has been telling all her friends of this "doctor's order," it is impossible to say how many other babies have been put on "Rickett's Food," and how many little tombstones have been erected in consequence.

With regard to the feeding of infants it must be remembered that the feeding during the first nine months, if physiologically carried out, differs greatly from that after the same period. A similar distinction must be drawn as regards the use of "infants' foods" during these periods.

During the first nine months the following dietetic principles have been endorsed by the highest medical authorities, and may therefore be taken for granted: (1) That breast milk is the best food for an infant; (2) that, failing this, fresh cows' milk and cream, suitably diluted, is a complete diet. It follows, therefore, that the rule of the nursery should be that no "infants' food" is to be given to any baby under nine months, except by the doctor's order.

Many monthly nurses and mothers start the babies very early on patent foods, without any reason save that they were handy or that some other baby had thrived on them. Such a course of procedure must be severely condemned, and the employment of a milk diet should be advised.

Advice may have been sought for some infantile ailment, and the doctor, finding tinned foods entering largely into the diet, suggests a trial of fresh milk only. The reply often is, "My baby cannot take cow's milk." The only attitude to adopt in the face of such a statement is one of complete scepticism. Lay statistics, drawn from the experience of mothers, would lead one to believe that about 99 per cent. of babies cannot take fresh cow's milk, while medical experience would put the number at about 1 per cent. If we eliminate from the crowd of infants who are stated to be congenitally unable to digest cows' milk all those who have been over-fed, or too frequently fed, or fed on milk improperly prepared, we shall find only a very small residue who possess this undesirable quality. We have, therefore, firmly, but politely, to waive aside this sweeping assertion, and advise a trial of a milk diet under proper rules.

Another difficulty may present itself when a mother asserts that the infant is thriving on the patent food, and is an extremely healthy baby. A cursory examination may tend to confirm this statement, for one of the dangers connected with the use of patent foods is that they are insidious poisons, and do not necessarily manifest their evil effects for some time. Scurvy, rickets, and anæmia may not show any obvious signs for months after the adoption of such a diet, although the constitution is being steadily undermined all the time. It is difficult to convince the mother of these prospective dangers, or to explain to her the etiology of an affection which develops so long after the diet has been begun. Further, as long as the food has been "staying down" satisfactorily she will trace all acute disturbances, such as diarrhœa or convulsions, to teething, or nervousness, or something which runs in the father's family, and never dream of the food poison the infant has been absorbing. These points must, however, be explained to her as clearly as possible.

So far we have been discussing the use of "infants' foods" when the infant is under lay control, and the conclusion drawn is that their employment is in most cases injurious to the child. Under medical control, circumstances may arise in which the use of an " infants' food " may be advisable.

The various foods on the market may be classified as : (1) Peptonising powders, with or without starchy matter; (2) dried milk; (3) condensed milk ; and (4) starchy foods, non-converted, partially converted, or wholly converted. Of these the starchy foods from their composition cannot be regarded as in any way resembling breast-milk, or suitable for the physiological feeding of infants under the age of nine months. If used by medical advice, they are only employed as adjuncts to the proper food. Some infants appear to have the digestion of an ostrich, and will thrive on any food, but the rules of infant feeding cannot be drawn up from such exceptional cases.

The chief indications for the use of an "infants' food " are three in number : (1) vomiting, (2) diarrhœa, and (3) wasting.

(1) *Vomiting.*—After the preceding remarks the writer will not probably be understood as suggesting that in cases of vomiting an "infants' food " is to be tried. The physician will, of course, try to find out what is the cause of the vomiting, and more especially what is the error in the feeding which has produced this result. But failing to effect a cure after careful examination and treatment, one may with advantage try predigested milk. The nutritive value of peptonised milk is probably less than that of fresh milk, but its " staying down " power in a much harassed stomach is greater. Similarly, dried milk, either the whole milk or the remainder, after all the cream has been removed, may sometimes be tolerated and digested, especially if it is very well diluted. In other cases condensed milk may be successful. These are methods of resting the stomach by giving it less work to do than is required by the tough curds of fresh cow's milk, and in the digestion of fat. No added cream should be used under these circumstances, and the dilution should be carried far beyond the printed instructions on the tins, the object being not to fatten the infant but to rest the stomach.

(2) *Diarrhœa.*—An acute attack of diarrhœa in an infant frequently necessitates the temporary disuse of fresh cow's milk. As the cause of this trouble is often traceable to impure milk, and the active poison flourishes in that medium, the usual practice is to discontinue milk entirely during the acute stage. When convalescence has set in the irritable stomach and intestines must be treated very gently at first, and so a return to milk food is best made with predigested, dried, or condensed milk. In addition we may add in small quantities one of the starchy foods, if fully converted, as they are not specially favourable to the growth of the diarrhœa-producing organism.

(3) *Wasting.*—With all the advances made in the treatment of infantile disorders, marasmus still holds its own as a fatal and puzzling malady. Probably many cases are due to a complete breakdown of the digestive organs, which have been sorely tried by " infants' foods " during the first few months of life. At any rate, one frequently meets with infants who, with or without vomiting and diarrhœa, continue to waste in spite of every attempt to feed them on a pure milk diet. Here, again, we are led to try some of the peptonising powders or foods or preserved milk. My own experience is that the best results are obtained by the use of a peptonising powder, and that if progress is made with full predigestion we should then reduce the peptonising period to the shortest time possible. In other words, if we secure improvement by peptonising for half an hour, we should then gradually reduce the period to fifteen or ten minutes, or even less, until we have found the limit that is tolerated. By this means we can educate the stomach to do a certain amount of its proper work, and allow time for the atrophied cells to recover their function. In such cases also the predigested foods, or the converted starchy foods, advertised for infants may serve to increase the nutrition. The latter class may be used along with cow's milk, first, because they mechanically aid the digestion of the milk, and, secondly, because they add certain food elements which the disordered stomach can retain and digest. In some infants, as in many adults, the drinking of plain cow's milk produces indigestion, but if the milk is mixed with some solid material the difficulty in the digestion is removed. In the case of young infants, however, we must not push this too far, or else the relief of one trouble will be followed by the supervention of others. Whenever dried milk or condensed milk or a starchy food is being used the degree of dilution must be explicitly stated.

Apart from actual illness there are times when

fresh cows' milk is not obtainable, as on board ship or on a long railway journey. Again, fresh milk may be obtainable, but there may be an epidemic in the neighbourhood, and the milk supply may have fallen under suspicion. In such cases the physician will be called on to advise, and condensed milk of a good brand is probably the best temporary substitute for a healthy infant.

In all cases in which these more or less unnatural foods are being used certain rules of procedure ought to be followed as safeguards both of the infant's health and the doctor's reputation.

(1) In acute illness a return to natural feeding should be made before the patient is discharged.

(2) In chronic illness no "infants' food" should be continued longer than is absoluely necessary. If the infant is apparently thriving well on the food, it will in all probability actually thrive better on a fresh milk diet.

(3) In all cases where a predigested or preserved food has been used for more than two weeks, orange or grape juice (half an ounce) in water should be given daily to avoid the risk of scurvy.

(4) Under similar circumstances the addition of fresh cream or cod-liver oil to the diet should be made as soon as possible, because the fatty element is usually deficient in all "infants' foods" (as prepared for use), and is specially essential.

After the age of nine months the question of "infants' foods" is not of so much importance, because the risks attached to their use are not so great. Personally I do not see that, in the case of healthy children, there is any necessity for them. They have no advantages over freshly-prepared milk foods, porridge, bread and milk, puddings, etc. They have the disadvantages that they do not encourage to the same extent the use of the teeth or the development of the gastric functions. At the same time, the presence in the cupboard of a starchy food which can be quickly mixed with fresh milk is much appreciated, and as long as fresh milk and other natural foods are also employed there is no reason to object. The curious point in this connection is the very great respect with which the mother regards any such food. If the infant is consuming a pint and a half of milk daily, with bread and pudding, and an ounce of " Rickett's food," whenever we ask the mother what she is feeding the infant on, she will at once reply " Rickett's food." And every virtue—mental, moral, or physical—which the child develops will also be unhesitatingly traced to " Rickett's food."

November 20th, 1905.

ANTISEPTICS IN OBSTETRICS.

By THOS. G. STEVENS, M.D.Lond., F.R.C.S.Eng., M.R.C.P.Lond.

Obstetric Tutor, St. Mary's Hospital ; Assistant Physician, Hospital for Women, Soho Square.

ALTHOUGH it is an established principle that antiseptic measures are absolutely essential in the practice of obstetrics, it is common to see letters in the medical press denying this, and advocating mere cleanliness as the one desideratum for the successful conduct of a normal labour. The writers of these letters rarely specify exactly what they mean by cleanliness, but one gathers that it means washing the hands in soap and water, adopting the same as a means of cleansing the patient's genitals, and probably paying attention to the question of clean clothing for doctor and patient. Æsthetic cleanliness of this nature is pleasing to the eye, makes a considerable show of carefulness, and must be as balm to the conscience of those who can look back to, or have heard of, the times, not so many years ago, when the washing of hands even was not universally practised before attending a labour. How far short of the real surgical cleanliness necessary for the safety of the lying-in woman this method is can not only be imagined but has actually been demonstrated during the last few years. Bacteriologists in all countries have demonstrated the utter impossibility of rendering the hands surgically aseptic, or even diminishing to any degree the number of bacteria upon them, by any methods short of the most stringent antisepsis. Soap and water alone has very little effect in diminishing the numbers of bacteria upon the skin of the hands. Even if a prolonged immersion in a strong antiseptic is made use of after the preliminary scrubbing, it depends largely on the kind of antiseptic whether few or many bacteria can afterwards be cultivated from the skin. Of course it is true that most people's hands contain no truly pathogenic bacteria, *i. e.* pus-producing organisms : but, nevertheless, those which are present are capable of setting up putrefactive changes if they are deposited upon a suitable food material, and so must always be regarded as of the greatest danger to the lying-in woman. There can be no doubt that the lying-in woman owes her comparative safety to this fact, that there is no suitable food material upon which bacteria can be deposited in the majority of cases. The constant outflow of lochia and the efficient contraction and retraction of the uterus conspire to prevent the retention of a suitable culture medium, whilst the absence of any intra-uterine manipulation in the majority of cases insures the absence of bacteria from the uterine cavity. This cannot, however, be made an excuse for the slightest neglect of careful hand preparation before conducting even a normal labour.

Danger to the patient does not, however, only arise from the hands of others : the bacteria present upon the vulva and in the lower third of the vagina are sometimes a source of infection. The exact amount of danger from this source has been a bone of contention since the bacterial origin of sepsis was first demonstrated, and the question cannot be said to be even on a fair way towards settlement. The normal protective powers of the vaginal secretions in a non-pregnant woman, demonstrated first by Döderlein, and dependent upon the bacillus vaginæ and its product lactic acid for its powers, are not present in the parturient woman to anything like the same degree. The vagina during the puerperium has been shown by many observers to contain various kinds of bacteria, and these can only flourish if the normal protective mechanism is in abeyance. The reason for this seems to lie in the alkaline reaction caused by the neutralisation of the lactic acid by the copious lochial discharge, and the large quantity of food material thus provided for other organisms which may gain entrance. If these organisms should happen to be pathogenic, then we cannot doubt but that they would be a considerable source of danger to the patient. For-tunately, however, they are most frequently only harmless saprophytes, and, unless there is some retention of placenta membranes or clots in the uterus, they find no food material there, and so do not gain entrance to the uterine cavity.

That much can be done towards eliminating this source of danger is admitted on all sides, and the cleansing of the vulva and vaginal entrance must take a place almost as important as that of the hands in the midwifery technique. The same argument, however, applies equally here as in the case of the hands : no mere perfunctory wash over with soap and water will do the least good, and a single vaginal douche, even of a strong antiseptic, is more likely to be an actual source of danger than a safeguard. To give a vaginal douche to a parturient woman so that no danger from the carrying upwards of organisms of the vulva shall result, is almost as difficult a task as to perform an aseptic operation elsewhere. We must agree, how-ever, that the vulva and vaginal entrance must be rendered as surgically clean as possible before delivery, and we cannot but believe that simple douching is *not* the way to do it. After delivery the same argument prevails that douching can do no good. and may be a source of much harm if carelessly performed. Leopold showed that a large series of cases treated by vaginal douching after delivery actually had, if anything, a rather higher morbidity percentage than a similar number of cases treated without douching. Looked at from a common-sense point of view, what g$_{oo}$d can a vaginal antiseptic douche do to a parturient woman? The application is but momentary ; no appreciable quantity of antiseptic can remain in the vagina for a sufficient time to kill organisms, and any that does remain is quickly diluted with the secretions from the uterus. If, however, it is known that an infective discharge is present before delivery, such as would be set up by a gonorrhœa, the douche can do some good, if only by washing away the dis-charge, and so limiting the growth of bacteria by doing away with their food material.

What, then, are we to regard as the absolute essentials of the antiseptic technique in obstetric practice?

The desired technique must be simple and easy to carry out in the poorest house, nothing being required of the patient but two basins and hot water. It must be effective—that is, able to render the skin as nearl aseptic as possible, and it must be carried out in a routine manner, each procedure being timed by the watch. Whatever the method used, the same may be employed for hands. vulva, and vaginal entrance, so as to avoid multiplicity of antiseptics. On all sides it is agreed that alcoholic solutions of antiseptics produce the best results in rendering the skin poor in bacteria, and for practical use a 1 in 1000 solution of corrosive sublimate in 80 per cent. alcohol (pure methylated spirit will serve) has been found to give good results. Although this is agreed to be the best yet attained antiseptic solution, still there are drawbacks to its general use in obstetrics. There can be no doubt that it is not convenient to carry about a pint bottle of spirit, and although it is ignominious to admit as much, it is none the less true that an inconvenient technique will never be carried out by the majority of the profession. The most convenient form of antiseptic to be carried, of course, is some chemical in the compressed form which can be readily dissolved in hot water. If corrosive sublimate is chosen for this purpose, it must be used in not less than 1 in 1000 strength. With, perhaps, the ex-ception of lysol (1 in 150 of water), no other anti-septic can be accepted as giving any good result or as being so convenient for routine use. Let it be clearly established as an axiom to which no exception will be accepted from anybody, that 1 in 1000 corrosive sublimate is the very least in the way of an antiseptic that must be used for the hands in all obstetric practice.

All that must be carried by the medical man or midwife is a sterilisable nail-brush, soap, and the antiseptic. The hands must be scrubbed for five minutes with two changes of water preferably, and then scrubbed for another five minutes in the antiseptic solution. Merely holding the hands in the solution is not sufficient, and the amount of time used in the process must be taken by the watch.

The accusation may be brought that there is nothing new in this technique; undoubtedly this is true, but will even a nail-brush be found in every person's bag who practises midwifery? If there are only a few such brushless bags, it is an excuse for repeating again and again so time-worn a principle. If it be suggested that undue prominence is given to the sterilisation of the hands, let it be remembered that whatever any individual opinion may be, it is the opinion of the masters of obstetrics throughout the world that the hands are still the most dangerous source of puerperal sepsis.

The most efficient way to cleanse the vulva and vaginal entrance before delivery is not by douching but by scrubbing the parts lightly with pledgets of absorbent wool, first impregnated with hot soap and water and then with a strong antiseptic. Lysol in the strength of 1 in 150 to 1 in 200 seems to fulfil the requirements here best, chiefly because it is non-poisonous. Corrosive sublimate 1 in 1000 is decidedly dangerous to use in this way, as the writer has seen a mild mercurial poisoning set up by a single application. If used in strengths much less than 1 in 1000, corrosive sublimate ceases to be a really effectual antiseptic. It must be remembered that only the vulva and vaginal entrance need be treated in this way; the vagina in most cases requires no treatment. It is only where an infective discharge is present that the same procedure must be applied to the vaginal walls. If the objection is raised that it is not the custom to prepare the patient thus, it can only be said that it *ought to be*, and that no intelligent woman would object to it if it was explained that her safety partly depended on it.

Rubber gloves have been recommended and are largely used on the Continent in midwifery practice. Very little can be said against this practice and everything for it. The only objections are the inconvenience of sterilising the gloves by boiling and the slight limitations of touch (easily overcome by practice) which they impose. To those who can disregard these objections the rubber gloves will be the greatest boon that has been invented in modern times. When sterilised by boiling and carefully put on (so as to avoid infection) the gloves render the hands absolutely sterile, a height

to which no known method of chemical sterilisation can attain. Nevertheless, it has been recently shown in a continental clinic that the results of a large series of cases in which gloves were used were no better than those of a similar series in which the hands conscientiously chemically sterilised were employed. There is, however, one great use for rubber gloves : they can and should be used by anyone who has to deal with a case—midwifery, surgical, or otherwise —which is already septic. The hands can in this way be protected from infection, and a "clean" case may be attended afterwards without fear of infection from the former. If the hands have presumably become infected from a septic case of any kind, the opposite procedure may be adopted if a "clean" case arises. After chemically sterilising the hands and then putting on a pair of freshly boiled rubber gloves, there is no scientific reason why a midwifery case should not be attended although the hands may have been infected. The gloves alone, however, cannot be accepted as an excuse for not chemically sterilising the hands in such a predicament.

In the after-treatment of a labour case it is a safe rule that the external genitals should be washed with an efficient non-poisonous antiseptic every time the urine is voided or the bowels act. The most convenient way to do this is to syringe the parts, not to dab them with cotton-wool pledgets : in this way the hands do not come into contact with the genitals, and if there are any lacerations no pain is given. It need hardly be said that at all times the nurse must chemically disinfect her hands in the manner already described, when helping in any way before labour or dealing with the after-treatment. With regard to instruments and appliances used it goes without saying that sterilisation by heat must be adopted for all things which can be so treated, while the rest must be chemically sterilised before use.

The above technique embodies the principles carried out in lying-in hospitals throughout the world : and apart from general hygiene it cannot be doubted by any thinking men that it is just this adoption of stringent antiseptic principles which has caused the mortality in lying-in hospitals to drop to almost *nil*

November 20th, 1905.

WE have received from Jeyes' Sanitary Compounds Company a sample of the new disinfectant "Cyllin," a germicide prepared from a new series of oxydised hydrocarbons existing in coal-tar. By a system of standardisation of disinfectants (carbolic acid being taken as a unit) "Cyllin" is shown to be much more effective and also cheaper than other preparations made for a similar purpose. The system is known as the Rideal-Walker method of standardisation and accurately gauges the germicidal value of disinfectants.

THE CLINICAL JOURNAL,

CLINICAL RECORD, CLINICAL NEWS, CLINICAL GAZETTE, CLINICAL REPORTER,
CLINICAL CHRONICLE AND CLINICAL REVIEW.

EDITED BY L. ELIOT CREASY.

| No. 683. | WEDNESDAY, NOVEMBER 29, 1905. | Vol. XXVII. No. 7. |

CONTENTS.

* *Specially reported for the Clinical Journal. Revised
by the Author.*

ALL RIGHTS RESERVED.

NOTICE.

*Editorial correspondence, books for review, &c.,
should be addressed to the Editor, 51, New Cavendish
Street, W., Telephone No. 904, Paddington ; but
all business communications should be addressed to
the Publishers, 22½, Bartholomew Close, London,
E.C. Telephone 927, Holborn.*

*All inquiries respecting Advertisements should be
sent to* MESSRS. ADLARD & SON, *Bartholomew
Close, E.C. Telephone 927, Holborn.*

*Terms of Subscription, including postage, payable
by cheque, postal or banker's order (in advance) : for
the United Kingdom, 15s. 6d. per annum ; Abroad,
17s. 6d.*

Cheques, &c., should be made payable to THE
PROPRIETORS OF THE CLINICAL JOURNAL, *crossed
" The London, City, and Midland Bank, Ltd., New-
gate Street Branch, E.C. Account of the Medical
Publishing Company, Limited."*

Reading Cases to hold Twenty-six numbers of
THE CLINICAL JOURNAL *can be supplied at 2s. 3d.
each, or will be forwarded post free on receipt of
2s. 6d. ; and also Cases for binding Volumes at 1s.
each, or post free on receipt of 1s. 3d., from the
Publishers, 22½ Bartholomew Close, London, E.C.*

THE PROGNOSIS AND TREATMENT OF ALCOHOLIC CIRRHOSIS OF THE LIVER.*

By H. CAMPBELL THOMSON, M.D., F.R.C.P.,

Assistant Physician to the Middlesex Hospital ;
Physician to the Hospital for Epilepsy
and Paralysis, Maida Vale.

MR. PRESIDENT AND GENTLEMEN,—I think you
will probably agree that cirrhosis of the liver, as
ordinarily met with in this country, might to a
large extent be spoken of as a preventable disease,
for although our knowledge of the different stages
of its production is by no means complete, the
majority of instances are undeniably associated
with the habitual use of considerable quantities of
alcohol.

The precise way in which alcoholic drinks bring
about the characteristic changes in the liver is
doubtful ; for experiments tend to show that alcohol
itself is unable to produce cirrhosis, and it therefore
seems likely that its effects in this direction are
largely due to the formation and absorption of
poisons from the alimentary canal which arise
through the disordered digestion that always
accompanies chronic alcoholism.

The varying nature and potency of such secondary poisons would afford an explanation of the
unequal effects which drinking has upon the livers
of different persons ; for they suffer very dispro-
portionally to the quantity they take, though it is
possible that quality may have some influence,
since it is generally considered that cirrhosis is less
frequently met with in the upper than in the
lower classes. While the drunkard may escape,
there can, however, be no safety guaranteed to him
who exceeds the strictest moderation ; for "excess"
here, as elsewhere, is a relative term and must be
considered individually and not collectively.

These interesting but debatable points need not
detain us this evening, for, speaking generally, the

---

* Read before the South-West London Medical Society.

broad fact remains that intemperance is the chief cause of cirrhosis of the liver.

From what has already been said it will be seen how impossible it is to predict with any degree of certainty the course, or even the onset, of cirrhosis in any individual instance of chronic alcoholism; and it is only by dealing with averages that it is possible to indicate the order in which symptoms may be expected to arise, and to suggest the different methods of dealing with them; for although nothing can be done to remove the connective tissue in the liver after it has once been formed, its further progress may, fortunately, often be retarded and the resulting symptoms greatly ameliorated. As the newly-formed connective tissue contracts, the freedom of the circulation through the portal capillaries becomes hampered, and the mucous membrane of the stomach and intestines, the functions of which have already been impaired by the alcohol, becomes still more congested and the digestion and nutrition of the patient suffer in proportion. Loss of appetite, morning sickness, irregularity of the bowels, and general weakness are now among the principal symptoms complained of.

At the same time, the blood, finding its flow through the portal veins obstructed, endeavours to make its way through the channels that unite the portal to the general circulation, and so what is generally known as a compensatory circulation is established. These connecting vessels become enlarged, and if too much strain is put upon them they break, and so hæmatemesis, or bleeding from the bowel, is liable to occur. Hæmatemesis is an important event in the course of cirrhosis; for, although it may take place any time after the disease is fairly established, it is most often met with at what may be termed the mid-period of the disease—that is, some time after the digestive disturbances have been felt, but yet some time before the time at which ascites usually sets in. Hæmatemesis in this respect has an important significance; for while it indicates that the liver changes have advanced far enough to strain the collateral circulation to the breaking point, experience shows that it is still often possible, even at this stage, to arrest the general symptoms, provided the patient can be persuaded to make a radical change in his habits. Like hæmoptysis in the early stages of pulmonary tuberculosis, an hæmatemesis may sometimes be a useful warning.

A patient illustrating this is at present attending my Out-Patient Department at the Middlesex Hospital. Seven years ago he had a severe attack of hæmorrhage, with other signs of commencing cirrhosis; but with a complete change of work, which up to that time had been that of a potman in a public house, his health has been sufficiently preserved to enable him to lead a useful life.

Unfortunately, however, one cannot depend upon the hæmorrhage taking place at the right time, for it may be absent throughout, or it may only arise during the last weeks of life, when the fatal signs of general toxæmia have already become manifest.

As the inflammatory changes progress they do not remain confined to the interior of the liver, but gradually spread on to the surface and invade the capsule, which becomes thickened and adherent.

From inflammation of the capsule of the liver it is but a short step to the general peritoneal surface, the resistance of which has already been lowered by the congestion to which it has been subjected, and so chronic perihepatitis merges into chronic peritonitis. Chronic peritonitis is often accompanied by exudation of fluid and so the next stage—that of ascites—is ushered in.

Ascites is undoubtedly the symptom that stands out among all others in cirrhosis of the liver. It is of grave omen to the doctor, and in the mind of the patient the onset of dropsy dispels any lingering doubts which may previously have been cherished as to the seriousness of his complaint.

Later on another factor has to be taken into account in the production of ascites, namely, the toxæmia which occurs towards the end, and which is closely analogous to the uræmia of chronic kidney disease.

It is the omission to take into account the different underlying causes of ascites (some of which predominate at one time and some at another) that has given rise to differences of opinion regarding the gravity of this symptom. Variation of cause also explains the different ways in which cases behave; for in some the appearance of the fluid is the precursor of early death, while others, after perhaps being tapped a number of times, improve in health and are able to get about for a long time.

An accurate prognosis in these cases depends upon the possibility of analysing the various factors in each case, and this is naturally often a matter of considerable difficulty. The ascites, that depends upon chronic congestion and chronic peritonitis, is a local condition, which may be described as being associated with the cirrhotic liver, rather than directly depending upon it, and as such it is capable of being relieved for so long a time as the liver keeps sufficiently healthy to carry on its functions. There is nothing particularly dangerous about the ascites itself; it is the cause which underlies it with which we are specially concerned, and where this is a combination of chronic peritonitis and congestion there is usually no immediate cause for fear. So it happens that these cases are tapped time after time as occasion requires, while their general health is not necessarily greatly affected by the local condition which causes the fluid to collect.

Quite otherwise is it at a later stage, when the ascites depends upon the general toxæmia, which is the forerunner of coma and death. Here the underlying cause is the toxæmia, and the exudation of fluid is associated with it in much the same way as it is liable to accompany a condition of uræmia. The ascites may now be said to depend directly upon the condition of the liver, and is but one of the signs that these functions of the liver have fallen below a point which is compatible with life. Drawing off the fluid at this stage, beyond relieving pressure upon neighbouring organs, does no good, and, indeed, it is an open question as to whether it does not sometimes do harm.

Recognition of these underlying causes of the effusion is a great help towards forming an opinion as to the probable results of treatment; but, of course, it is often difficult to decide at exactly what stage the patient is in, especially if there is the disadvantage of not having seen the case in the earlier part of the illness. Moreover, clinically, cases do not necessarily pass through one stage before they reach another, for a patient may evade many of the early symptoms only to find himself more or less suddenly entering upon the terminal toxæmia.

Again, the several conditions underlying the production of the ascites may be mixed up together and so defy any accurate analysis; for the effusion associated with chronic peritonitis may merge imperceptibly into that depending on toxæmia, or the earlier form may never appear at all, and the first sign of ascites may be coincident with the onset of final toxæmia.

Considerable difficulty will often be found in judging these underlying factors with any degree of accuracy, but the general state of the patient is a great guide, for when the effusion depends upon a local cause the general health is not necessarily very much lowered. Rapid wasting, slight signs of jaundice, and œdema of the legs are all signs of bad omen, and early œdema of the legs is of great importance; for, where the ascites is merely a local manifestation, the swelling of the legs, when it occurs, will come after the enlargement of the abdomen and chiefly as a direct result of the increased abdominal pressure, but when a general toxæmia is threatening it has been shown by Dr. Hale White that swelling of the ankles is very likely to appear before the onset of ascites, and is then but one manifestation of the impending general disturbance.

This was well illustrated by a patient whom I had been in the habit of seeing occasionally, and whom I knew to have a large liver which was evidently cirrhotic in nature. He came one day complaining of swelling of the legs, and on examination some considerable puffiness was found around the ankles. Investigation failed to reveal any definite physical signs to account for this, and the liver being, as far as one could tell, in the same condition as usual, I did not feel that I had satisfactorily explained the cause of this new symptom. Its true significance, however, became apparent only too soon, for it persisted in spite of rest, and in a few weeks was followed by ascites, toxæmia, and death.

The prognosis of the ascitic stage depends, then, upon our judgment as to the exact nature of the changes which underlie the collection of fluid, and when those are clear it will not be difficult to predict the effects of treatment.

The cases which do well by tapping are those in which the presence of fluid depends upon chronic peritonitis and congestion, and these are often relieved time after time, and occasionally the fluid ceases to recur.

Tapping in such cases is a rational form of treatment, just as it is in an ordinary pleural effusion, but quite otherwise is it with the toxæmic class. Here the fluid effusion is but a small part of a severe general condition, and it is as hopeless to think you are going to cure the patient by drawing it off as it would be to suggest that a uræmia could be cured by tapping a pleural effusion which was associated with it.

Dr. Hale White has shown conclusively how badly these cases do, and how they seldom live long enough to require more than one tapping. Withdrawal of the fluid at this period is only of use inasmuch as it relieves the pressure on neighbouring organs, and so contributes to the comfort of the patient.

But not only is tapping of no permanent value at this stage of the disease, but the question has been asked as to whether it may not even be injurious, for it undoubtedly happens that patients often appear to go downhill very rapidly after it has been done. It is generally considered that such cases are coincidences, and that death, already so near at hand, is not in any way accelerated by the operation, but personally I cannot feel sure of this, and it does not seem difficult to believe that the withdrawal of a very large quantity of fluid, which is rapidly followed by the secretion of more, must have a distinct and probably an adverse influence upon a patient who is in a severe state of general toxæmia.

Now, if it be granted that tapping in these terminal cases is undertaken to relieve pressure and not with any view to permanent relief, any doubt on this point can be got over by only partially emptying the abdomen and stopping the flow when the desired comfort has been obtained, and I feel sure that this is a better plan in many cases than attempting to drain off every possible drop. Here, again, there is the analogy of the pleura, where removal of a moderate quantity is usually considered sufficient.

Last, there is the question of operative treatment to be considered. The plan (which was introduced to the notice of the medical profession in this country by Drummond and Morison and which is also associated with the name of Talma) is to produce adhesions between the peritoneum, omentum, and liver, and the idea was conceived on the supposition that the congested portal circulation would be relieved by the development of new veins in the adhesions and a consequent increase of the collateral circulation.

This explanation is, however, open to doubt, and it is certainly difficult to believe that new veins

are formed with such rapidity and of such calibre as to be almost immediately capable of draining off the recurring fluid, which is often poured out at a great rate, and moreover, physiologically, it does not appear to be beneficial to make a very free communication between the portal and general circulation, for if the contents of the portal vein are made to empty themselves directly into the vena cava without first passing through the liver the animal becomes poisoned and dies.

Dr. H. D. Rolleston has suggested that the presence of vascular adhesions over the surface of the liver would relieve venous engorgement and so allow a freer supply of arterial blood to the liver and a consequent improvement in the nutrition of the liver-cells. In a previous paper * on this subject I suggested that the obliteration of the peritoneal cavity by adhesions would in itself be sufficient to account for the non-recurrence of the fluid, just as it is in the case of the pleura and pericardium.

The results of this operation as shown by statistics cannot be considered to be very satisfactory, and Dr. Rolleston in his recent work on diseases of the liver considers that on the whole the results are somewhat disappointing, though of course this may be partly due, as has been suggested, to cases being left too late before being operated upon.† It will be quite clear that it is useless to operate upon patients who are in the last stages of the disease ; for then ascites is very apt to be only one of the symptoms of a general collapse, and, generally speaking, the cases which are most likely to benefit are those which have already survived several tappings. It must not, moreover, be overlooked that patients sometimes make a satisfactory recovery after tapping alone, and numerous illustrations of this fact were brought forward by Dr Cheadle in his Lumleian lectures on

---

* ' Med.-Chir. Trans ,' 1902, vol lxxxiv.

† Rolleston quotes Greenough, who collected 122 cases in which the operation had been performed. After deducting 17 in which the disease was not cirrhosis and one case in which the result was not given, there are 104 cases of cirrhosis in which the operation had been performed. Of these, 31 died within 30 days of the operation, and 29 were in no way improved, so that 60, or 57 per cent., not only received no real benefit from the treatment, but possibly had their lives shortened, 44 or 42 per cent. were improved, and of these 9 were living and in improved health two years after the operation

"Some Cirrhoses of the Liver." If, however, as certainly seems the case, the formation of extensive peritoneal adhesions is beneficial to the patient at certain stages of the disease, it is still open to question whether such adhesions could not be produced by some simpler means than those of opening the abdomen ; for the patients cannot, as a rule, be considered to be in a favourable condition to undergo an operation, and in my former contribution to this subject I referred to a case recorded by Dr. W. Cayley * in which the patient, a cabman, after the fourteenth tapping for recurrent ascites, developed symptoms of peritonitis and the fluid did not collect again. He was discharged convalescent and was seen by Dr. Cayley to be well and driving his cab two years after. In commenting on this case Dr. Cayley suggests the possibility of relieving ascites by exciting adhesive peritonitis, as often happens in the cases of peritoneal tuberculosis.

A further contribution to this subject has been made recently by Dr. H. W. Plant and Dr. Patrick Steele, † who have treated cases of serous effusion by the injection of adrenalin chloride after the manner suggested by Dr. Barr in 1903, and from their reports this method seems to be a promising one for the treatment of selected cases of ascites in hepatic cirrhosis.

November 27th, 1905.

* 'The Middlesex Hospital Journal,' March, 1897.

† 'Brit. Med. Journ.,' July 15th, 1905. The following was the method adopted: As much as possible of the fluid was withdrawn by a two-way trocar cannula, and through the cannula, still *in situ*, 1 drachm of adrenalin chloride (1 in 1000) diluted to ½ oz. with sterile water, was introduced by means of an exploring syringe.

WE regret to learn from Messrs. John Wright & Co., the Bristol medical publishers and printers, that by the fire arising in a neighbouring warehouse on November 4th the whole of their offices, factory, and stock were entirely destroyed. There are, however, a few copies of most of their publications at their London agents, Messrs. Simpkin & Co., Ltd. These can be supplied so long as any remain. In the meantime a re-start has been made in a temporary factory, and most of the volumes are reprinting by themselves and by other firms throughout the country. In a few weeks they hope to re-issue the most urgent volumes, and confidently trust to the forbearance of their friends for any temporary inconvenience thus unavoidably caused.

A CLINICAL LECTURE

ON

HÆMATURIA.*

By J. W. THOMSON WALKER, M.B., F.R.C.S.,

Assistant Surgeon to the North-West London Hospital and to St. Peter's Hospital for Stone and other Urinary Diseases.

GENTLEMEN,—Hæmaturia is a significant symptom of urinary disease and one which may afford you much trouble and anxiety in trying to reach a diagnosis of its source and cause.

The urinary system presents a long and complex surface from which bleeding may take place, and you will often find that the accompanying symptoms tend rather to confuse than to throw light upon the diagnosis.

The loss of blood in itself may not be serious ; the quantity removed from the circulation is seldom so great as to constitute a surgical emergency, although the constant leakage may render the patient profoundly anæmic.

The importance of accurately localising the source of the hæmaturia lies in the fact that this symptom leads in many cases to surgical intervention. Even if the operation is restricted to an exploration to discover the cause of the bleeding it is essential that the situation of the bleeding point be accurately known. We have it in our power, by the help of symptoms or of special methods of diagnosis, to localise the source of the bleeding in every case of hæmaturia, and this should be done before any question of operation arises. Exploratory operations for the purpose of discovering the source of the hæmorrhage sometimes fail, and when successful they frequently necessitate a second operation upon the real seat of hæmorrhage. They are unnecessary since equally accurate information may be obtained without an operation.

In discussing hæmaturia it is usual to complicate matters by including such forms as occur in scurvy and many other extra-urinary diseases. I shall presume, however, that you are able to exclude such diseases where the hæmaturia is, after all, a matter of very secondary importance, and shall discuss with you only the hæmaturia of urinary disease.

* Delivered at the Medical Graduates' College and Polyclinic.

The difficulties of your task will be less formidable if you go to work systematically, and in the first place carefully localise the source of the hæmorrhage, and only then try to estimate the significance of the symptom. Unless you do so your diagnosis will be little more than guesswork, based upon what you believe are the most common causes of hæmaturia.

The diagnosis of hæmaturia should therefore be considered under these headings :

(1) The localisation of hæmaturia.

(2) The significance of hæmaturia.

I shall only have time to discuss the first of these headings with you to-day and must leave the consideration of the second for some future occasion.

I. THE LOCALISATION OF HÆMATURIA.

The presence of blood in the urine may of itself give rise to marked and even severe symptoms quite apart from the pathological changes which lead to the hæmorrhage. Thus, you may meet with renal colic from the passage of clots along the ureter, frequent and urgent micturition from the irritation of the blood, and temporary blockage of the urethra, or even complete retention of urine from distension of the bladder with masses of blood-clot. The latter complication is the most formidable that can occur to a patient suffering from hæmaturia. The distress of the patient, the difficulty of removing the clot, and the imminent danger of infecting this mass of clot in your attempts to do so all combine to render this occurrence a disaster.

Hæmaturia may, however, be accompanied by symptoms of urinary disorder which give you the clue to the source of the hæmorrhage. These are the simpler cases and we shall consider them first.

(1) Hæmaturia with other Symptoms.

(a) Hæmaturia with pain.—In a lecture before you in October last I considered the localising value of pain in urinary disease at some length.* I shall not, therefore, do more than touch briefly upon pain at present, and I must ask you to accept without further explanation the term "posterior renal pain" as signifying an area at the angle of the twelfth rib and the erector spinæ muscle into which the patient tucks his thumb to demonstrate kidney pain and "anterior renal pain" as a spot

* CLINICAL JOURNAL, February 8th, 1905.

above the level of the umbilicus near the costal margin as representing pain from disease of the renal pelvis. Further, ureteral pain may be "renal colic" or fixed dull pain at some spot along the line of the ureter or nearer the groin, bladder pain is usually supra-pubic, prostatic pain may be across the base of the sacrum or in the perineum or rectum, while pain at the end of the penis may be caused by irritation at the bladder base or prostatic urethra. These are the principal pain areas, and the only ones likely to be of service to you in localising the source of hæmaturia.

In a case, therefore, in which you find hæmaturia with posterior renal pain on one side, you will say that the source of the bleeding is that kidney, and will then look for other symptoms or signs which will give you a hint as to the cause of the unilateral renal hæmaturia ; or, where the renal pain is bilateral you will judge that disease of both kidneys is present.

You must not, however, forget that certain fallacies in regard to renal pain exist, and these fallacies may, if you are not careful to corroborate your diagnosis by other means, lead you astray.

Referred pain from a diseased kidney to its sound neighbour may lead you to believe that the latter is diseased ; a papilloma or a malignant growth at the vesical orifice of one ureter may give rise to hæmaturia and pain in the corresponding kidney, and give you the impression that this kidney is the source of hæmorrhage. These cases are not common, but they occur in sufficient numbers to lead now and then to grave blunders. In making your diagnosis you must therefore reckon with them, the more so, that hæmaturia frequently demands surgical interference, and a mistake in diagnosis will lead to a useless operation.

Bladder pain, I have said, is supra-pubic. This pain is little likely to help you in localising a hæmaturia to the bladder. A bladder full of clot will give this pain, but the source of the bleeding is not of necessity vesical. Urethral obstruction, whether from prostatic or true urethral disease, will also cause it. Pain at the end of the penis will lead you to look for some source of bleeding at the bladder base or prostatic urethra, but make certain before you commit yourself to this that the pain is not merely a sign of blockage due to a clot. Prostatic pain at the base of the sacrum, in the rectum, or at the perineum, is more reliable as a guide, and you will here have other symptoms of prostatic disease to help you, and, moreover, the gland is readily examined from the rectum. Renal pain from back-pressure is often present in such cases, and may be unilateral ; but it is slight and of a dull, aching character, and you are more likely to overlook it than to over-estimate its significance.

(*b*) *Hæmaturia with frequent micturition.*—In frequent micturition you have a symptom which so evidently points to bladder irritation that you will at once conclude that the bleeding point is in the bladder. In the majority of cases this is true, but not in all. The presence of blood in quantity in a healthy bladder may of itself cause frequency of micturition just as the swallowing of a quantity of blood may cause vomiting in a healthy stomach. If the blood is clotted it is the more likely to stimulate vesical contraction, and if a clot become engaged in the orifice of the internal meatus, temporary obstruction will follow and the bladder contraction may amount to strangury. This fallacy must ever be present in your mind when you find the combination of hæmaturia with frequent micturition. It is often possible to discount the irritation caused by the blood by a few questions. Did the frequency of micturition commence simultaneously with the bleeding ? And if the bleeding be intermittent, as it not infrequently is, does the frequency diminish or cease when the water clears? If such be the case, you will be inclined to look upon the frequent micturition as resulting from the irritation of the blood and will lay more weight upon other localising symptoms ; or you will a least withhold your diagnosis of bladder disease until you gain some further information.

An even more difficult problem may confront you where known kidney disease is present, and frequent micturition is so marked and persistent as to point to the bladder being involved. A severe hæmorrhage in such a case will tax your powers of diagnosis as to its source. And the question may become urgent from the necessity of operating to staunch the bleeding.

Hæmaturia combined with frequent micturition may have a prostatic source, as you will recognise when you remember the relation of the act of micturition to the prostatic urethra and the symptoms which accompany prostatic disease. You will not, however, have much difficulty in distinguishing

such cases, for the prostatic symptoms will have been clearly marked and the hæmorrhage is merely an incident in the course of the disease.

(*c*) *Hæmaturia with frequent micturition and pain.*—You may have this combination, and where both localising symptoms coincide your diagnosis of the source of the bleeding will, of course, be strengthened.

A hæmorrhage occurring with pain at the end of the penis and frequency of micturition will point to prostatic or bladder disease, and, when other prostatic symptoms are absent and you can exclude prostatic disease with the finger, the inference will be that the blood has come from the bladder. Or, on the other hand, the remaining symptoms may point to prostatic disease and a rectal examination corroborates this diagnosis. The sources of fallacy referred to above must be as carefully considered here as they would be with a single localising symptom.

When the localising symptoms do not coincide you will find yourself in difficulties once more.

With bladder disease causing bleeding and frequent micturition you may, as I have already pointed out, have pain in one kidney from blockage. With kidney disease causing pain and bleeding you may have frequent micturition from irritation of the blood. You will usually find, however, that one or other symptom predominates. The aching renal pain in the first case is less marked than the frequent micturition, or the frequent micturition in the second case is evidently dependent upon the blood, and the renal pain may amount to colic. You will sometimes, however, be left in doubt and will have to settle the diagnosis by other means than symptoms.

In any case you will be wise to use every means of examination which may throw fresh light on the case, however certain you may be of your symptomatic diagnosis.

(*d*) *Hæmaturia with obstruction to micturition.*— I have already told you that clotted blood may completely block the urethra and distend the bladder so that no urine can escape.

Usually, however, when a patient complains of difficulty in emptying his bladder and is passing blood in his urine, you will suspect urethral disease.

It is unusual to find a stricture causing hæmaturia of a pronounced type apart from the passage of instruments. In the following case, however, the hæmaturia was profuse, and the obstruction so slight that a stricture was only discovered on attempting to pass the cystoscope.

C. D—, æt. 53 years, was sent to me at St. Peter's Hospital by Major H. N. Dunn, R.A.M.C., complaining of hæmaturia. Blood had first appeared in his urine fourteen months before, and lasted four weeks on that occasion. The hæmaturia was accompanied by marked frequency of micturition during the day and at night. These symptoms disappeared until six days before I saw him, when they re-commenced. The urine usually commenced quite clear, and at the finish pure blood was passed. There was a burning sensation along the urethra when the blood was passing, but no real pain. The patient had served in India and Afghanistan, but had not been in Egypt or South Africa. The prostate was small on rectal examination, and the bladder base apparently free from disease.

A tentative diagnosis of papilloma of the bladder was made, and I thought it probable that a portion of the growth was engaging in the urethral opening. To my surprise on attempting to pass the cystoscope, I met with obstruction in the bulbous urethra, and found a readily bleeding stricture which gripped a $\frac{4}{}$ steel sound. After gradual dilatation extending over five weeks, I introduced the cystoscope into his bladder, still expecting to find some vesical disease. I was again mistaken, for the bladder, except for some slight trabeculation, was perfectly healthy and the ureteral openings natural and pumping clear urine.

The bleeding had apparently come from the stricture or from the congested mucous membrane behind it. The urine cleared when the stricture was dilated, and the hæmaturia has not since recurred.

You must be careful to dissociate hæmaturia after the passage of an instrument from spontaneous hæmaturia; and it is not sufficient that you should inquire whether the patient has noticed blood in his water—you must expressly ask him whether the blood followed instrumentation, or he may unwittingly mislead you on this point.

When hæmorrhage recurs repeatedly after the passage of instruments through a stricture you will watch for malignant disease of the urethra, and more especially is this the case where the blood appears spontaneously in the urine. But although hæmaturia with obstruction is always present in

the later stage of malignant growths of the urethra, this rare disease may first attract attention by the appearance of a copious discharge which becomes bloody. The following case was sent to me by Dr. Oliver Kerr, and I watched its progress with him for over two years, until the patient died.

A. B. D—, a thin, rather nervous man, æt. 57 years, had suffered from a urethral discharge for five months. The discharge had appeared four weeks after an illicit connection. Thirty years previously he had contracted gonorrhœa and a phagedænic ulcer had destroyed a part of the glans penis. There was a history of a blow upon the penis eighteen months before I saw him. After the discharge had continued three months he noticed that there was blood in it. At this time there was no difficulty in micturition and no straining.

Hæmaturia had been observed on four or five occasions and each time the blood was dark and appeared at the end of micturition. He had lost weight during four months. The whole penis was swollen and the skin rather reddened. A long prepuce hid the glans and meatus and could not be retracted. The whole of the penile and bulbous urethra was thick and indurated, and in the penis this induration passed round on each side almost to the middle line on the dorsum. The penis was curved downwards by the traction of the indurated mass.

Under astringent injections the discharge ceased and it was found on examination with the urethroscope that the urethra was considerably narrowed about $1\frac{1}{2}$ inches from the meatus. Behind this stricture there were numerous papillomatous nodules and some of these projected through the lumen of the stricture.

Under iodides the induration steadily improved, and I began to doubt my original diagnosis, when he suddenly developed a secondary mass in the liver and began to emaciate rapidly.

Ultimately nodules appeared on the ribs and in the left side of the chest, and repeated attacks of hæmatemesis hastened the end.

In this case there was never severe obstruction, and the discharge and induration led one surgeon who saw the case to make a diagnosis of gonorrheal urethritis.

Hæmaturia with obstruction has most often a prostatic source. Sometimes the cause of the symptoms is inflammatory and you may find a patient suffering from tuberculous disease of the prostate complain of obstruction for a few days, and this is followed by a little hæmaturia and some "matter" appears in the urine from the rupture of a tuberculous collection into the urethra.

The obstruction in such a case is, however, transient and the prostatic cause for hæmaturia with obstruction is more often simple enlargement of the gland. Here the symptoms are persistent and increasing.

The hæmorrhage in these cases is really vesical, for it comes from the surface veins on the nodules which project into the bladder.

Malignant growths of the prostate rarely give rise to bleeding.

You are not usually taught that obstruction may be one of the prominent symptoms of a papilloma of the bladder, yet such may be the case.

Where a papilloma is anchored to the base of the bladder by a long pedicle it may be swept into the urethral opening as the bladder empties and cause blocking of the flow. The same may be observed in the case of a papilloma which abuts upon the urethral opening, and there need not be a long or well-defined pedicle in such a case.

This patient suffered from complete retention of urine, requiring catheterisation on several occasions.

F. L. M—, æt. 53 years, was sent to me at St. Peter's Hospital by Mr. Canny Ryall. Two years previously he had been seized with continued desire to micturate, and after straining for some time, he passed a quantity of blood. After this he suffered from increased frequency of micturition, urgency and straining. There was always some blood in the urine after the first onset, but it varied a good deal in quantity. During this time he had complete retention of urine on five occasions and was relieved each time by catheterisation.

On cystoscopy two large masses of growth could be seen close to the opening of the urethra.

I afterwards opened the bladder and removed two papillomatous masses from the lips of the urethral opening.

II. HÆMATURIA WITHOUT LOCALISING SYMPTOMS.

You will meet with cases in which hæmaturia occurs as a solitary symptom of disease. In such cases the bleeding is usually considerable, often it is copious. You will have difficulty in tracking the blood to its source, and you may have to call special means of diagnosis to your aid.

In your text-books you will find certain rules laid down for your guidance by which you may find the source of the bleeding. I shall deal with these in considering the first means of diagnosis.

1. Inferences to be drawn from the Examination of the Urine.

(a) The amount of the blood.—You will gain little knowledge as to the source of the hæmorrhage by noting the amount of the blood in the urine. Chronic inflammatory changes in the kidney so slight as to require the microscope for their detection may be the cause of hæmorrhage as severe and prolonged as a bladder growth. Severe hæmorrhage may arise from any part of the urinary tract. The renal diseases which most frequently give rise to copious hæmaturia are some forms of nephritis and renal growths. In the bladder severe hæmorrhage most often arises in papillomatous growths and the intra-vesical projection of enlarged prostates.

(b) The colour of the bloody urine.—This may give you a hint as to the source, but it is little more than a hint, and you must not look upon the colour as of great diagnostic value.

The urine may be brown (coffee-coloured), brownish (smoky), purple, red, bright red, or delicate pink. These colours depend upon many factors. Recently shed blood from an arterial source will, according to its quantity, cause the urine to assume a pink tinge to a bright red colour. It is said that "the brighter the blood the nearer is the source to the external meatus," and this is in some sense true. The nearer the source to the meatus the more likely is it to be passed quickly, and the more likely is there to be bleeding at the time of micturition. When we have to deal with bladder ulceration or with inflammation of the prostatic urethra, we will almost certainly have frequent micturition. The blood is therefore passed out quickly and some degree of vesical spasm is nearly certain to be present, so that a drop or two of blood is squeezed out at the end of the act and added to the last of the urine as it passes.

Deep purple urines derive their colour from venous blood being added in quantity to the urine. In the bladder you have the most favourable conditions for such bleeding, and you will frequently get this dark purple colour in blood derived from the intra-vesical projection of an enlarged prostate or from a papilloma. When you meet with such a bloody urine, therefore, you will be influenced to some degree by the colour, and look for a vesical source, but do not be led into a snap diagnosis based upon this, for you may find the same colour in copious renal hæmaturia. The longer the blood remains in contact with the urine the more likely it is to be discoloured. We look, therefore, for a renal source in smoky or coffee-coloured urine. With the former you will probably, but not certainly, be right ; with the latter you will frequently go astray. Any cause of urinary stasis, such as an enlarged prostate, may prolong the contact of the blood and urine, and a decomposing urine will very quickly change the colour of the blood and throw your calculations completely out. Again, you are told that " blood well mixed with the urine is derived from a renal source." The significance of a well-mixed blood and a poorly-mixed blood, if you take it apart from the type of hæmaturia which I shall presently discuss, has, I think, received rather more than its due value.

Blood poured out from the kidney must be well churned up with the urine by the vermicular contractions that propel it down the ureter, and it is projected into the bladder urine with considerable force, so that it is to some extent diffused in it. On the other hand, bleeding from a bladder source is more likely to form a layer which is only disturbed by the act of micturition. We look, therefore, for well-mixed blood from renal disease, and blood in layers from bladder disease. At the same time, too much weight must not be placed upon the fact that the blood is well mixed with the urine, and where the blood is present in quantity it will be well mixed, whatever its source. I think you would be less likely to be led astray if these rules read as follows :

If the quantity of blood in the urine be small and well mixed and of a brownish or smoky tint, it is probably derived from the kidney. If, on the other hand, the colour is a delicate rose-pink, the bleeding probably took place in the bladder. But if the bleeding is copious, no inference may be drawn from the colour.

(*c*) *The type of hæmaturia.*—You will recognise several types of hæmaturia, and may infer with

tolerable accuracy the source of some bleedings from the type they present.

For convenience of description I shall divide them into partial hæmaturias and total hæmaturias, meaning by these terms that the blood may appear only at some part of the flow, or may be present from the beginning to the end of the act.

Partial hæmaturia.—A patient may commence micturition with clear urine, or at least with urine free from blood, and at the end of the act the urine becomes red, and he finishes with a drop or so of pure blood. You will best demonstrate this by directing the patient to pass urine in two or three glasses—in these cases you will almost invariably find that frequent micturition and some spasm is a factor in the case, and these will give you a valuable clue as to the source of the blood. Apart from this, however, this terminal type of hæmorrhage will point to some pathological condition of the prostatic urethra or the bladder, and you can rely upon the symptom as a valuable means of localising the source of bleeding.

Where frequent micturition accompanies terminal hæmaturia the patient will usually tell you that the frequent micturition commenced first, and after a time a drop or two of blood appeared at the end of micturition. Such a history usually means some ulceration or inflammation in the bladder or the prostatic urethra. You will sometimes meet with it in malignant growths of the bladder, very rarely in papilloma.

I do not think you will often come across blood at the commencement of micturition and find the urine finish clear.

This form of hæmaturia is urethral in its origin, and is seldom seen apart from instrumentation. Sometimes the blood clots and is projected from the urethra as a worm-like mass with the first urine, but clotted blood with the first of the urine may have a vesical source.

The blood in partial hæmaturia is usually small in amount and bright red in colour.

In total hæmaturia there is blood throughout the whole flow of urine. It may be small in amount or copious, bright or dark. It may be continuous over a long period or it may last for a week or a month and suddenly cease, and recur again later on. This will not, however, give you a clue as to its source. A bladder growth may bleed copiously for a time and suddenly cease, but the same may be observed in hæmorrhagic nephritis.

The presence of clots.—A good deal of importance has been given to the presence and form of blood-clots in the urine.

It is said that blood from the kidney does not often clot, and again, that long worm-like clots are casts of the ureter and mean renal hæmorrhage. The clotting depends a good deal upon the proportion of blood in the urine. Blood rapidly poured out from a renal source or from the renal pelvis or ureter will clot as readily as blood from other parts. Worm-like clots if present may help you to localise the hæmorrhage to the kidney, renal pelvis, or ureter, but you will not very frequently find such clots.

Large flat or irregular clots are formed in the bladder, but they do not necessarily arise from bladder hæmorrhage, for renal hæmorrhage may fill the bladder with blood-clot.

Urethral clots have already been referred to. They resemble ureteral clots in their worm-like form. You will not gain much reliable information in regard to the origin of the bleeding from the presence of blood-clots in the urine.

Extraneous substances in the urine apart from blood.—In urine that is deeply tinged with blood you will have little chance of discovering tube casts, for they may be hidden by the blood present in the specimen. With less blood you may be more fortunate, and if you do find casts you have a very important hint as to the origin of the bleeding.

I have examined the urine in a number of cases of hæmaturia that after operation proved to be cases of slight chronic nephritis, and have submitted these bloody urines to expert analysts without gaining any hint by the discovery of tube-casts. If, however, these casts should be found, their significance is undoubted. If you have the opportunity of examining the urine at a time when the bleeding has ceased, you are much more likely to gain important information than when it is teeming with blood-discs. The presence of crystals in the urine gives you no help as to the source of the bleeding.

Newman, of Glasgow, points out that by estimating the amount of hæmoglobin and of albumen and comparing these an excess of albumen over the proportion of 1·6 to 1 hæmoglobin points "not only to an independent albuminuria, but also to a renal affection as the cause of the hæmaturia."

The patient suffering from hæmaturia will sometimes tell you that he has passed pieces of growth. You must, however, receive such statements with caution, for you will often find it difficult to make up your own mind as to whether a shred of tissue is a piece of decolorised blood-clot or growth or merely necrotic shreds from an ulcer or masses of pus and mucus with particles of granular phosphate. If you have a difficulty in this matter, resort at once to the microscope. Should the tissue prove to be growth, you may presume that the hæmorrhage is vesical, since the great majority of papillomata are situated in the bladder. You will remember, however, that similar growths have been found in the renal pelvis and ureter.

In addition various forms of epithelial cells may be found in the urine. It is not always easy to give these cells their proper place in localisation and diagnosis. V. Jaksch says: "It is very difficult to distinguish between the epithelial cells which are derived respectively from the bladder, ureters and renal pelvis." "It follows that a particular affection in one of these situations can hardly be localised by the characters of the urinary epithelium." This authority believes, however, that certain inferences may be drawn from their number "Given a disease of one of these parts, it may be assumed to involve the ureter alone when the epithelial forms are very few. When in greater quantity and superimposed upon one another like the tiles of a roof, they probably come from the pelvis, and when in very great abundance they indicate cystitis. These points must not be strongly insisted upon, but taken in conjunction with other symptoms, they should carry some weight in a differential diagnosis." Do not place too much confidence on the discovery of a few tailed cells. They are said to come from the renal pelvis, but you may find them in an ordinary gonorrhœal urethritis.

The ova of the *Bilharzia hæmatobia* in the urine would indicate a vesical source for the bleeding, but you would have already concluded that the bleeding comes from the bladder from the presence of increased frequency of micturition, which is an important symptom of all these cases.

I cannot leave this subject without giving you a word of warning against placing the microscopic and chemical examination of the urine on too high a plane in the diagnosis of these cases. Independent reports are of extreme value when taken in conjunction with the clinical facts of the case, but I can see a tendency to go too far and to place too much reliance upon urine analyses considered apart from the clinical examination of a case. Diagnoses based solely upon the examination of the urine and advice in regard to treatment, which, I regret to say, is sometimes issued with these reports, must both be accepted with reserve.

(2) *Examination of the Patient.*

In a case of hæmaturia without localising symptoms you may be able to ascertain the source of the bleeding by examining the patient and without employing any special methods of diagnosis. ⁴In any case even if you have been able to point to the source of the bleeding from the symptoms alone you will do well to neglect no means by which you may corroborate your diagnosis or amplify it.

The following case illustrates the fallacy of a diagnosis which depends upon symptoms alone.

B. C—, a carpenter, æt. 41 years, came under my care at St. Peter's Hospital in February, 1905. He had first noticed pain in passing water in August, 1904. He thinks that he had a slight touch of the same pain each summer for two years before this and passed one or two clots of blood each time, but he took no notice of it. In August, 1904, he "caught a cold" and had pain and frequent micturition. The pain radiated along the urethra and he also had some pain across the pubes. The pain was most marked at the end of micturition.

The frequency of micturition was at first hourly and increased to half-hourly, and later he made water every ten minutes, and rose three or four times at night. He was seen by a surgeon, who made a diagnosis of "cystitis." Nine weeks before he came under my notice he began to pass a little blood. This ceased for about a week and then he had a severe attack and passed some clots. Another severe attack of hæmorrhage, lasting two days, came on three weeks ago. When I examined him there was a trace of blood in the urine and the frequency of micturition was one hour during the day and two hours at night. He had a little pain along the urethra on passing urine, but no lumbar or abdominal pain. He had lost a stone in

weight in two months. There was a tubercular taint on the maternal side of his family and one sister had died of phthisis. Cystoscopy showed a rigid distorted right ureteral opening with the surrounding mucous membrane heaped up and infiltrated and covered with flakes of muco-pus. Above and behind this was a patch of inflammation and there was a similar area near the apex of the bladder. The base was spongy and the left ureter was normal. On palpation of the right kidney a large, hard, slightly tender mass was felt. I afterwards removed a large pyonephrotic kidney with numerous cavities and pockets surrounded by tough sclerosed kidney-tissue. There was a small calculus in one of the pockets. After the operation the cystitis gradually subsided.

(*a*) *Testicles and epididymes.*—You should commence the physical examination of all male cases of hæmaturia by palpating the testicles and epididymes. Tubercular nodules in the epididymes or thickening of the vasa deferentia are the points you will most frequently come across in such cases, and will at once give you the hint for which you were searching.

Do not forget that the sudden development of a varicocele in a middle-aged man, especially if it be on the right side, is a point of importance in the diagnosis of renal growths (Morris).

(*b*) *Rectal examination* will follow as a routine practice, and you will gain information which is of positive value in many bladder hæmaturias, and if nothing is found the fact has a certain negative value. The prostate first claims attention. You are not likely to find much there in hæmaturia without other symptoms. An enlarged prostate will give signs of obstruction and frequent micturition along with the hæmaturia. In a man over fifty you will palpate the prostate to ascertain whether you are dealing with a case of this sort. Do not be too certain that the prostate is not the source of hæmorrhage if you cannot feel an enlargement from the rectum. Some prostates project into the bladder without showing much change in their extra-vesical portion. Do not neglect to make a bimanual examination in these cases.

A malignant growth of the prostate may be present, but hæmaturia is rarely an early or a prominent symptom in such cases.

A buried nodule in the prostate, especially if the patient be a young or middle-aged man, when combined with hæmaturia coming at the end of micturition, and marked frequency of micturition, may give you a valuable point in the diagnosis of bladder tubercle. In such a case you may find the seminal vesicles hard and nodular. The trigone of the bladder lying above the prostate is readily palpated, and sometimes gives the clue to diagnosis. In tubercle of the bladder the examination of this region is usually negative. I have, however, felt the trigone clearly mapped out and thickened in a case of tubercular disease of the bladder.

I saw the case, of which the following are the particulars, at first with my colleague, Mr. Swinford Edwards, and later he came under my care.

M. W. I—, a golf-club maker, æt. 30 years, was seized with pains across the lower part of his abdomen in April, 1903, and for about six weeks had repeated attacks of shivering. He had pain during micturition at the base of the glans on the dorsum penis, and there was increased frequency of micturition to three hours during the day and from two to three hours at night, with a good deal of urgency. He had been losing flesh for about a year. His urine was pale and cloudy and contained many fine dots and flakes.

On rectal examination the prostate was rather small and there was a pea-sized nodule in the left vas deferens. The trigone was distinctly mapped out as an indurated thickened area. To the right of this, near its base, was a small and hard nodule, which was probably a nodule in the right vas deferens.

On cystoscopy the bladder base was covered with tubercular granulations. The rest of the bladder mucous membrane was healthy.

A calculus in the bladder, even when of large size, is seldom palpable from the rectum, for it is separated from the finger by a thick contracted bladder wall. You may feel the thick ridges of hypertrophied bladder muscle, but this condition meets the finger in other forms of obstruction. I have, however, felt a hard mass in the region of the bladder base in a case of enlarged prostate, and, on performing prostatectomy, removed two large calculi which were lying in the post-prostatic pouch.

A simple papilloma of the bladder base cannot be felt from the rectum. A malignant growth may give merely a slight loss of elasticity in the earlier stage of its infiltration. Later you will feel a hard, tough area, and when the growth has spread widely you will feel a hard, resisting mass with a smooth rectal face. Do not neglect to search for enlarged lymphatic glands. The lymphatics of the bladder and prostate are within reach of the finger as they pass out to the side wall of the pelvis. A hard lymph-gland in a case of hæmaturia may be suffi- cient evidence on which to base a diagnosis of malignant growth of the bladder.

The following is a case in point :

M .J—, æt. 59 years, came under my observa- tion at St. Peter's Hospital in January, 1904. For six months he had been losing vigour and had felt languid and heavy ; for a month he had lost weight. Four and a half months before I saw him he had a sudden burst of thick black blood before the urine, and since that time had occasionally noticed blood in his water. There had been some dull sacral-base pain since the hæmorrhage com- menced. On rectal examination the prostate was normal, and no induration or loss of elasticity could be detected at the bladder base. Above and to the right of the right lobe of the prostate, but quite separate from it, was a hard, flattened, smooth nodule about the size of the thumb-nail, which was evidently a lymph-gland. A diagnosis of malignant growth of the bladder was made. A subsequent cystoscopy showed an irregular epitheliomatous mass at the bladder base, and bimanual examina- tion under an anæsthetic showed strings of enlarged hard glands along the course of the internal iliac vessels.

Before finishing the rectal examination you will palpate the lower end of the ureters. A thick ureter combined with hæmaturia is most likely due to tuberculous disease. A single nodule in the ureter is probably a stone, and an impacted cal- culus in this position may give rise to bursts of hæmaturia from time to time.

(c) *Examination of the kidneys.*—If, in examining a case of hæmaturia, the patient has told you of pain in the loin, you will feel yourself bound to palpate this region, and you are more likely to neglect the rectal examination than that of the kidneys. If, however, the localising symptoms point to a bladder complaint, you are more likely to overlook the palpation of the kidneys. Do not fall into this mistake, for in either case you may be led astray by symptoms and miss some condition which merely awaits your palpating finger to give you the clue to the source and cause of the bleeding. In illustration of this I would refer you to the case I have detailed at the beginning of my remarks on the examination of the patient.

In many cases of hæmaturia your examination of the loins will reveal nothing. The kidney cannot be felt on either side, and there is no tenderness in this region. This negative result is not to be taken as a final test that there is no renal disease. Some of the most severe and prolonged renal hæmorrhages may reveal nothing abnormal on palpating the loin. But you will sometimes gain positive information of extreme value. Tenderness in this region if well marked will indicate the presence of some inflammatory condition. It may be the tender kidney of an ascending pyelonephritis, or the pressure of your hand may rub the jagged surface of a stone against the inflamed mucous membrane of the renal pelvis. A pricking sensation may be produced by a renal or pelvic stone by your handling or by plunging with the finger-tips (Jordan Lloyd).

A movable kidney may be discovered and it may be tender from the addition of inflammatory changes.

In the following case a movable kidney was the source of almost continuous bleeding over a considerable period of time.

S. F—, a thin, anxious-looking woman, æt. 39 years, was sent to me at the North-West London Hospital by Dr. C. O. Hawthorne in September, 1904.

She gave a history of continuous hæmaturia like dark coffee, which had lasted for two months. There had been some gastric trouble for twelve months. In winter she could not hold her water, and it sometimes dribbled at night. There was fixed anterior renal pain. All her symptoms were increased on walking or when she worked about the house, and she was much improved by rest. On palpation of the right loin the kidney was felt low down and somewhat large. The range of mobility was not great, but the fingers could be pushed above the kidney.

On cystoscopy the right ureter was a tiny pin-hole which did not show any change for many seconds and then gaped once or twice without emitting any urine. On squeezing the right kidney a jet of dark brown much diluted blood was shot out with a sudden jerk.

The urine of each kidney was collected separately with Luy's separator. The left urine was normal, the right urine was hazy and pink and contained flakes ; there was a small amount of albumen present, and with the microscope there were red blood-corpuscles and pus-cells. There were a few granular casts and some flat round clumped cells and a single tailed cell in one of several specimens.

The right kidney was explored and fixed in position, and the symptoms had completely disappeared before she left hospital.

An enlarged tender kidney may be calculous, pyonephritic, tubercular, or merely inflamed. An enlarged kidney which is not tender is most probably hydronephrotic or the seat of a growth. Any of these conditions may lead to hæmaturia. A renal growth may bleed for many months before any change can be detected in the size of the kidney.

But these are merely suggestions. It is difficult to lay down exact rules for your guidance that will cover all cases.

(*d*) *Instrumental examination.*—You may be tempted to use one of the two common instruments which are certain to be at your hand. Let me, therefore, say a word to you in reference to the value of the sound and the catheter in the diagnosis of hæmaturia.

In a case of hæmaturia in which you have no symptoms to guide you as to the source of the bleeding, sounding the bladder will suggest itself to your mind as a possible way out of your difficulty. You will hope by this means to feel the grating or metallic ring of a calculus or to appreciate the uneven surface of a tumour if one is present. And if your examination reveals neither of these sensations, you may feel satisfied that the stone or growth is absent or that the bleeding is renal and not vesical.

If you have the opportunity of following a number of cases in which your sounding was negative to a final diagnosis, you will become dissatisfied with the conclusions you have drawn, and the more so if you have taken the trouble at each stage of your examination to note your diagnosis. In the first place, the number of cases in which a vesical stone is accompanied by copious or even moderate hæmorrhage without giving rise to other well-marked symptoms of its presence is very small. You may exclude vesical stone in such cases by symptoms alone, and the sound gives you no additional informàtion of a reliable nature.

Severe hæmorrhage may occur, indeed, in cases in which an enlarged prostate is complicated by calculous formation, and it is notorious that in such cases the irritant symptoms of stone are absent, or very slight. But the hæmorrhage here is prostatic and has no relation to the presence of the stone. In these cases you are little likely to touch the stone with a sound, for it lies' deeply behind the projecting prostate, well out of reach. If you base any statements upon a negative sounding in such a case, you may get an unpleasant surprise when the bladder is opened. Difficulties also beset you when you set out to feel the unevenness of a simple or malignant growth with the sound.

A papilloma is too soft to give any impression to the finger and thumb holding the sound. Papillomata not infrequently become incrusted with phosphatic deposit, and may give a soft grating sensation that may lead you to infer the presence of a phosphatic stone, and the same conclusion may result from the phosphatic coating on a malignant ulcer, or even on an inflamed mucous membrane. You will sometimes feel an indefinite fulness at one or other side of the bladder, and if you have acquired a delicate touch you may estimate some differences on the two sides or some irregularity or unusual toughness that may guide you in your diagnosis of a malignant growth. Or, again, if your experience is sufficient, you may detect a crumbling sensation in entering the bladder when such a papilloma or malignant growth lies near the neck of the viscus.

On the whole, you are little likely to gain any addition to your knowledge in regard to a case of symptomless hæmaturia by the use of the sound, and you may be led astray in the manner I have indicated. I should therefore advise you to lay aside your sound when you approach such a case.

The use of the catheter in these cases may give some definite information. I say *may give*, for it will only do so in a small number of cases, and in the others the negative result of the operation is of no value either in regard to localisation or diagnosis. You have been taught to fish for a piece of growth with a catheter, and when the instrument is removed with a small plug of papillomatous material in its eye you will have gained very certain and

important evidence. It is not always an easy matter to distinguish with the naked eye between a fragment of old blood-clot and a scrap of a papilloma, especially if they are powdered with phosphatic material. If any doubt remains, float the tissue in water and finally settle the point by having a microscopical section made.

But you will meet with many cases of hæmaturia in which you cannot fish out a piece of growth in the eye of a catheter, and some of these will afterwards turn out to be villous growths of the bladder.

You will frequently find in washing out the bladder or in draining off the urine that the flow stops with a sudden thud. This may be so sudden and sharp that you almost believe that a stone is present, or you may think that the softer thud is a portion of growth. I do not say that a growth could not produce this sensation, or that a very small stone might not be swept into the eye of a catheter, but this sensation is usually due to blocking of the eye of the catheter with soft swollen mucous membrane.

If in a case of hæmaturia which is copious and continuous you wash out the bladder and find that after the first bladderful the fluid returns quite clear, you may take it as likely that the cause of the bleeding does not lie in the bladder, and that you are probably dealing with a renal hæmaturia. On the other hand, if you find that the fluid constantly returns tinged with blood, and especially if the blood is bright pink, you will be pretty certain that the blood comes from the bladder. If on further washing the bleeding increases, you may accept the hæmaturia as vesical.

This test applies with even greater certainty to cases of pyuria, and although we are not considering this symptom to-day, I should like you to note the value of this means of separating bladder from renal pyuria.

3. *The Use of the Cystoscope.*

The means by which hæmaturia can be localised with absolute certainty is by the use of the cystoscope.

In the washing preparatory to the cystoscopic examination you will often get the hint that I have just mentioned to you in regard to the persistence or increase of the blood ; but it is only when you obtain a view of the bladder mucous membrane and the openings of the ureters that you can state with certainty the origin of the bleeding in those cases where hæmaturia is the solitary symptom.'

I could quote many cases to you where, in order to test the value of this means of diagnosis I have used every other method of examination and then committed an opinion to paper before cystoscopy, only to find my statement wide of the mark.

There are, of course, difficulties to be overcome in cystoscoping such a case. In renal hæmaturia everything is simple and straightforward ; a rapid survey is sufficient to assure you that the bladder itself is healthy, and your attention is then concentrated upon the ureteral openings. Often without any actual disease being present a pink blush may be observed at the edges of the ureteral opening on the bleeding side, whether from irritation or from mere staining I am unable to say. This is a useful hint where the bleeding has ceased at the time of examination.

When the bleeding is still going on you will see a jet of blood issue from the ureter and slowly fade away, much like the puff of smoke which bursts out from the mouth of a gun when it is fired. There is no need for undue haste in getting the ureter into view, for the amount of blood projected at each contraction of the ureter amounts only to a few drops and you have plenty of time to observe it. Sometimes, on examining the ureteral orifice, it remains passive for quite a considerable time. It may help you if an assistant squeezes the loin on this side while you keep your eye on the ureteral opening. Usually, however, the jets of bloody urine are projected more rapidly and with greater force than in the normal condition.

In vesical hæmaturia the examination may not be so simple if the bleeding is still in progress, for there may be difficulty in obtaining a clear medium by washing.

A large mass of papilloma may envelop the beak of the cystoscope and obscure the view, but unless the growth is very large and near the urethral orifice this is not likely to happen. As a rule a papilloma is easily seen and forms a beautiful cystoscopic picture.

Malignant growths of the bladder are often difficult to examine thoroughly, for a bladder which is the seat of a malignant growth appears to have a remarkable tendency to cystitis quite apart from the passage of instruments. The presence and nature of these growths is, however, readily recognised by means of the cystoscope.

Stone, tuberculous ulceration, and bilharzia cystitis rarely cause bleeding without other symptoms, and the same holds good in bleeding from prostatic enlargement. I must, however, except from this statement a few cases of tuberculosis of the bladder. In these frequent micturition is not a marked symptom and the bladder permits of a normal distension with fluid.

The following case illustrates a difficulty that arose in regard to cystoscopic diagnosis :

N. W—, a schoolmaster, æt. 43 years, came under my observation at St. Peter's Hospital, complaining of pain at the base of the frenum penis. The pain came on at the end of micturition and was increased by exercise. There was increased frequency of micturition, especially in the evening.

These symptoms had lasted for fourteen months ; occasional hæmaturia commenced ten months before I saw him. It was slight at first and always accompanied by other symptoms. The blood appeared only at the end of micturition, was bright in colour, and at no time was it copious. While under observation he passed a small phosphatic shell. On cystoscopy there was a rounded brilliantly white body rather larger than a pea lying above and behind the right ureteral opening. He passed some pieces of phosphatic *débris* and was relieved of his symptoms. A month later he returned with a recurrence of his symptoms. On cystoscoping him the same pea-sized white body was lying outside and behind the right ureteral opening, but now a small fleshy ridge could be seen peeping out behind it. I admitted him to the hospital and after careful washing was successful in clearing the surface of a small papilloma of the coating of phosphates which had hidden it. I afterwards removed the little growth through a suprapubic wound.

I have elsewhere discussed the relation of the separator to the localisation of hæmaturia and stated my opinion that for this purpose the instrument is unreliable. I shall not, therefore, go over this ground again.

The X rays may give you some help in localising the source of hæmaturia ; a shadow of a renal or a ureteral calculus will not only show you the source but also demonstrate the cause of the hæmaturia.

November 27th, 1905.

THE CLINICAL JOURNAL,

CLINICAL RECORD, CLINICAL NEWS, CLINICAL GAZETTE, CLINICAL REPORTER, CLINICAL CHRONICLE AND CLINICAL REVIEW.

EDITED BY L. ELIOT CREASY.

No. 684.   WEDNESDAY, DECEMBER 6, 1905.   Vol. XXVII. No. 8.

CONTENTS.

* *Specially reported for the Clinical Journal. Revised by the Author.*
ALL RIGHTS RESERVED.

NOTICE.

Editorial correspondence, books for review, &c., should be addressed to the Editor, 51, New Cavendish Street, W., Telephone No. 904, Paddington; but all business communications should be addressed to the Publishers, 22½, Bartholomew Close, London, E.C. Telephone 927, Holborn.

All inquiries respecting Advertisements should be sent to MESSRS. ADLARD & SON, *Bartholomew Close, E.C. Telephone 927, Holborn.*

Terms of Subscription, including postage, payable by cheque, postal or banker's order (in advance) : for the United Kingdom, 15s. 6d. per annum; Abroad 17s. 6d.

Cheques, &c., should be made payable to THE PROPRIETORS OF THE CLINICAL JOURNAL, *crossed* "*The London, City, and Midland Bank, Ltd., Newgate Street Branch, E.C. Account of the Medical Publishing Company, Ltd.*"

Reading Cases to hold Twenty-six Numbers of THE CLINICAL JOURNAL *can be supplied at 2s. 3d. each, or will be forwarded post free on receipt of 2s. 6d.; and also Cases for Binding Volumes at 1s. each, or post free on receipt of 1s. 3d., from the Publishers, 22½, Bartholomew Close, London, E.C.*

A LECTURE

ON

THE PROGNOSIS OF CHRONIC GRANULAR KIDNEY.

Delivered at Guy's Hospital,

By W. HALE WHITE, M.D., F.R.C.P.,
Physician to the Hospital.

I THINK, gentlemen, many of you have seen, when they were alive, the two patients whose cases I thought we might discuss this afternoon. The first is a man who for a long while lay in No. 6 bed in Addison Ward. He was 37 years of age, and he came in, you will remember, because of bleeding from the bowel and shortness of breath ; he told us that three months ago he noticed that he passed some blood from the rectum. He also said he passed a great deal of water. He then went on to tell us that the blood from the rectum was very large in amount. He felt very weak, and his eyelids were puffy in the morning. He had a high-tension pulse, his arteries were thick and tortuous, and also we found that the urine had a specific gravity of 1007, it contained a fair amount of albumen, and there were granular casts in it. On looking at his eyes we found that he had albuminuric retinitis, and the subsequent history of the case can be summed up by saying that he often bled from his rectum, he was very anæmic, very weak, and suffered a great deal from headache. You will remember that he was often so short of breath that he could not get up, although we told him to get up whenever he liked, and it was remarkable that he had no cyanosis. He was very drowsy, he coughed up blood, and no treatment which we prescribed for him, unfortunately, did him any good. He gradually sank and died, and here are his kidneys ; you can see perfectly well that they are typical granular kidneys. And that assemblage of symptoms made such diagnosis quite certain.

The other man I propose to talk about was in No. 17 bed in the same ward. He was 48 years of age, and he was sent up because he was passing a quantity of blood in his urine; so much blood was passed and there was so much pain with the passing of it that it had been suggested by more than one person who had seen him that he had a tumour of the bladder. When he came in he also complained of loss of eyesight, pain in the head, and sleeplessness. He told us that he had had headache and had slept badly for eighteen months. Six weeks ago, he said, his eyesight suddenly became blurred and misty. Three days after that he noticed blood in his urine. When he came in he had had hardly any sleep for seventeen days. He vomited a good deal; he had had no œdema. The urine was of a specific gravity of 1007, and it contained blood and albumen, and under the microscope there was seen to be a little pus and blood, bladder epithelium and epithelial and granular casts. His pulse was a very high tension,' and his arteries were thick. We could not estimate the size of his heart because of his emphysema. He had well-marked albuminuric retinitis and, of course, with that granular kidney was easily diagnosed. On the day after his admission there is a note that he slept very badly and had severe headache. Two days after he came in he was passing blood in his motions, he had been sick, and next day he vomited and the vomit contained blood. On the next day he was very restless and had much headache. Two days later he had twitchings and was again very restless and suffering from great headache; you may remember that we were going round at the time and saw him restless and excited, so that he hardly knew what he was doing. He was tossing about the bed, and we gave him chloroform, which did what we hoped it would do, namely sent him to sleep. He fell into a deep sleep, and there is a note on the next day that he was better, no doubt as the result of the sleep. Three days later, however, he became comatose, the urine secreted sank almost to nothing, and he died on the next day. Here I show you the kidneys from the case, presenting the appearances which we knew that they would. By looking at the kidneys our diagnosis is confirmed. Here is one typical granular kidney, and the other is also in a granular condition but larger, because there is a good deal of superadded tubal

nephritis. Here is the hypertrophied heart, which is so characteristic of the disease. There is also present, in the intestines which I show you, what you saw so admirably in the post-mortem room, an extreme degree of enteritis.

I propose now to tell you something chiefly about the prognosis of these two cases, both of which are obviously typical cases of chronic Bright's disease.

The first thing about which some of you were in doubt is where these patients ought to be placed among the varieties of Bright's disease; not long ago I gave you a clinical lecture on the relationship of the varieties to one another, and that lecture was published in the CLINICAL JOURNAL, June 15th, 1904, and the diagrams I put upon the blackboard were repeated there, so I will not spend more than a minute or two to remind you what the diagram, which I again show you, means, because you can look up the lecture for yourselves. A certain number of patients with acute Bright's disease recover, like the boy in No. 9 bed in John Ward, who is getting well; some die during the acute stage; some become chronic, and get a large white kidney. All people with a large white kidney sooner or later die from their disease. Sometimes, as I have just said, large white kidneys follow upon acute Bright's disease. Sometimes they are a chronic condition throughout the whole illness. So much for acute Bright's disease. Next we consider what our two patients are examples of, granular kidney. All cases of granular kidney are irrecoverable; no man with granular kidneys ever got well. Many of them live a number of years, but they never recover. Supposing a man has granular kidneys, two things can happen to the kidneys: the new fibrous tissue in them can contract more and more, so that at last they become small granular kidneys, often called red kidneys, but I think it is a pity to introduce the word "red" because redness only depends on the amount of blood in the organ. That is the kind of kidney you see before you, and that is the last stage of granular kidney. With other cases of granular kidney some tubal nephritis occurs subsequent to the fibrosis. These are cases of mixed nephritis, partly tubal but chiefly interstitial. A few cases of acute Bright's disease—much fewer than many text-books give you to understand—arrive at the same condition, because although the tubal disease of such patients improves, a good deal of interstitial change occurs, and then later an extra attack of tubal disease supervenes and so you get the same condition as you arrive at from the granular kidney—that is to say, a contracted kidney with added tubal change. Such kidneys are generally called mixed contracted white kidney, and many would restrict the term "chronic Bright's disease" to them whether they originated in granular kidney or acute Bright's disease. I show you such a kidney here. I hope by the aid of this diagram that you understand the relation of the various kinds of Bright's disease to one another. But as I say you can look for the full details in the lecture itself, so we will not spend any more time on this to-day. Nor will we spend much on the symptoms, except a few which these cases illustrate particularly well.

You will have noticed that the first man bled from the rectum. Large clots were passed, and you observed while he was in hospital that he also coughed up blood. He was very sick and on one occasion he vomited some blood. The next man, you will remember, had so much blood in his urine, and there were such large clots, that pain was caused by passing them, and because of the pain and the blood a fairly confident diagnosis of tumour of his bladder had been made. You noticed that he also vomited blood, and passed blood from the rectum. So both these patients bled a good deal from various places ; and a fact which you cannot too importantly remember is that a person with Bright's disease may bleed from anywhere ; there is no point from which such a patient may not bleed. You get into your minds very readily that sufferers from this disease bleed into their brains, because that kills them, you also remember that they bleed into the retina, because you see the hæmorrhages with the ophthalmoscope, but you are inclined to forget that they may bleed from anywhere else. The most dramatic instance of that which I remember to have come across was that of a young man, æt. 30 years, who casually asked me one day what was the matter with the lobe of his ear. He had a hæmatoma, and I found albumen in his urine, and it was clear that he had chronic Bright's disease. He had been bleeding into the lobule of his ear ; he died of uræmia a month afterwards. And I often tell you the tale of a doctor who first knew that he had chronic Bright's disease because he had some hæmoptysis.

One of our patients here had hæmoptysis. These patients illustrate the fact that the subjects of granular kidney may have blood pass from the bowel, but often the most difficult variety of hæmorrhage to interpret is that from the urinary tract, like that of the second case. At the post mortem his bladder showed what we expected to find : under its mucous membrane there were hundreds of hæmorrhages. Hence his Bright's disease admirably explained why he should have such profuse hæmaturia and pain on passing his urine. If you forget that people with Bright's disease may bleed from anywhere, you make bad mistakes, as has been done over and over again, chiefly with regard to bleeding into the urinary tract.

Another symptom which the books do not sufficiently emphasize, and which these patients illustrate, is that most sufferers from severe chronic Bright's disease become weak, so much so, that I think you may often successfully save yourself a mistake by looking at the urine of a patient who only complains of general weakness. A person with chronic Bright's disease often presents himself first to his doctor as a man who is pale, weak, feeble, and who says that he cannot get about as much as he should. I saw only a day or two ago a woman who went to her doctor because she felt weak and out of sorts. There was no œdema, no high-tension pulse, none of the classical signs of Bright's disease. On examining the urine it was 1005, with plenty of granular casts and a ring of albumen. There was not the slightest doubt that she had granular kidney. So whenever anybody comes before you for general weakness, wasting, and pallor which you cannot quite explain, please let it pass through your minds whether the patient may not be an example of granular kidney and examine for it.

Another group of symptoms which these patients illustrate, and which I want to direct your attention to because they illustrate them so well, are some symptoms of uræmia. You will have noticed in regard to the second patient about whom I read to you how bitterly he complained of headache and insomnia. Both are striking symptoms in many cases of uræmia. And you will remember that one day when we were going round the wards he was restless and hardly in his right mind, and he was throwing himself about. That, again, if you saw him for the first time, might not have caused you to think of uræmia. Coma is more generally remembered. Both our patients, towards the end, became comatose. You will remember also that our first patient had much shortness of breath, and that will serve to recall to your minds that you must never overlook uræmia as a cause of dyspnœa.

The last symptom to which I think I need direct your attention now, as it is illustrated so well by our patients, is diarrhœa. There is much difficulty about the diarrhœa of Bright's disease. In the first place, it is often artificially induced, because the fact that the patient has uræmia necessitates giving him jalap or some similar aperient, and that induces diarrhœa. Again, diarrhœa itself is a symptom of uræmia. Probably it is caused by the attempt to get rid of the poison. But apart from that, there is actual enteritis, which is associated with Bright's disease, as has been taught here for many years. Our museum contains plenty of examples of it, and I have had brought some in for you to look at afterwards. Here is one in which the inflammation begins at the top of the alimentary canal, for it is an example of membranous gastritis associated with Bright's disease. This patient was under Dr. Pavy in 1870. His kidneys were small and granular, and his colon was ulcerated, showing that he had enteritis as well as gastritis. Here is a very interesting little specimen, which also helps us very much ; it is from a woman who was admitted here in 1855, and you can see there is a blood-clot attached to the mucous membrane of the stomach. She bled on account of Bright's disease and so illustrates what I have been teaching you. Here is another good specimen, from a woman who was under Dr. Fagge. It shows very well the entero-colitis which is associated with Bright's disease, and if you look at it afterwards you will be able to see plenty of ulcerations. She had interstitial nephritis, and the account says there are many ulcers at the lower end of the ileum, and also upon the colon. Here is another, a magnificent specimen, in which you can see the extensive ulceration of the mucous membrane, illustrating this most important complication of Bright's disease. That man was in here as long ago as 1828. At death his kidneys were found to be diseased. Here is another one in which you can see the change in the colon, and that is from a man who had advanced Bright's

disease. You will see that the colon is in a condition of acute inflammation. Here is another one, showing ulcerative colitis associated with Bright's disease. So you have actually before you now one recent specimen of inflammation of the intestine from our own case, and six museum specimens of severe enteritis associated with chronic Bright's disease. The enteritis is mostly in the colon. It may be so extensive as to be in the small intestine also. There is a case which Dr. Goodhart showed at the Pathological Society some time ago illustrating that. It was a woman, æt. 54 years. The lower twenty-six inches of the ileum were claret-coloured and so much honeycombed by ulceration as to produce a sloughy aspect of the intestine. The cæcum and colon had large sloughy ulcers and the kidneys were granular and cystic. In one place the ulceration had perforated, and the woman died from perforative peritonitis. So enteritis is a very serious condition. It may kill by its diarrhœa ; it may even, as in Dr. Goodhart's case, kill by perforative peritonitis. Perhaps I ought to go back to this specimen for a moment, the one where there is a blood-clot on the stomach, to explain to you that it has been said by some people that the cause of all this intestinal ulceration is the fact that there are hæmorrhages under the mucous membrane of the gastro-intestinal tract, and as the hæmorrhage gets washed away so there is an ulcer left. That such hæmorrhage may occur is undoubted, but hæmorrhage cannot be the explanation for such extensive ulceration as you see in these specimens.

Now I pass on to what I wanted to tell you about chiefly in this lecture, namely, the prognosis of this disease, chronic granular kidney. I have tried, very roughly, to arrange the symptoms according to their prognostic value. And please do not go away with the impression that the prognosis does not matter, because, as a matter of fact, in a sense it is the most important thing in medicine. Usually you can find out what is the matter with your patient, and having found out, usually your text-book will tell you what to do for him. Your greatest skill will be shown in trying to estimate whether the patient will get well, and that is what the friends, naturally, always want to know. The mother, whose child is ill, does not care very much what is the matter with the child or what you do for it so long as you can promise her you can get it well. And you have not finished your proper mental estimate of a case if you have merely made a diagnosis and ordered the treatment; you have not completed your work until you have in your mind tried to foretell what will be the result of the case. Do not, for goodness' sake, mention what you consider will be the result unless you are asked, because, unfortunately, we are so often wrong in estimating the result; but sometimes you will have to give an estimate because you will be asked straight out what the result is going to be.

To go back to Bright's disease, everyone is agreed, without a doubt, that the most valuable prognostic feature is the presence of albuminuric retinitis. But in saying that we have to distinguish. There are two broad varieties of retinal changes in association with Bright's disease. One is largely inflammatory, and is best shown by optic neuritis when present. This may occur with acute Bright's disease, and may get well as the patient gets well. Putting that aside, the second variety of trouble in the eye is mainly degenerative. Both our patients showed the most beautiful shiny, bright, white patches, almost like mother-of-pearl, let into the retina. Those are degenerative changes. The nerve-fibre layer undergoes fatty degeneration and so changes chemically that it becomes a brilliant shiny white. This change has a very bad prognostic value, and it is doubtful whether patients showing it ever recover. Only twice in my life have I ever come across patients who showed degenerative changes indistinguishable from albuminuric retinitis and who had not, as far as could be made out, any disease of the kidney. In one set of cases 85 per cent. of the patients were dead within the first year after the discovery of the degenerative retinitis, and 9 per cent. were dead in the second year; that is to say, 94 per cent. were dead within two years of the discovery of the trouble. So there can be no doubt whatever that the most valuable prognostic sign, and the most certain which you can have, is the occurrence of the degenerative form of albuminuric retinitis. If you want actual cases, I may mention that Dr. Sutton, who was house-physician here, published a number of cases in our 'Guy's Hospital Reports' for 1895.

I should think that perhaps the next most important thing in prognosis is the age of the patient. Young subjects with chronic granular kidney rarely, if ever, do well. Fortunately it is a rare disease in young subjects, and by that I mean anybody under forty years of age. You will have noticed that the age of our first patient was thirty-seven, and we diagnosed that he had granular kidneys. He illustrated this point very well, poor man, because he died within a few weeks of his admission to the hospital. You do occasionally see recorded in the papers the cases of young people who improve and live a long while, but such are very rare, and I hardly think you ought to hold out any hope to anyone under the age of thirty who has granular kidney. I am not at all sure that these cases in the first half of middle life are not a different disease, possibly, from the cases in later middle life, for while people in later middle life may die from cerebral hæmorrhage, or pneumonia, or various conditions which are associated with granular kidney, those in the first half of life who have granular kidney almost invariably die of uræmia, and it was so in this man.

Then I should have put high up in the list of things which are bad for prognosis the general weakness. That I have mentioned already, and I need not now go any further into it. Both our patients were very weak, both were wasted, and I think the pale, wasted, thin type of patient with chronic Bright's disease as a rule does badly. You may say, speaking broadly, that when anybody with granular kidney voluntarily takes to his bed he will probably die before long.

Another point which is rare, and which neither of our patients illustrates, is that, apart from that red blush, or erythema, which often occurs on any œdematous part readily, people with Bright's disease are liable to a severe form of dermatitis. As a rule when a patient with Bright's disease has the dermatitis which is associated with it he dies. And even if the dermatitis improves, the granular kidney remains, and the patient having had dermatitis will not live very long. Another point is the enteritis. You have only to look at these specimens to see how enteritis may be associated with Bright's disease. If diarrhœa is slight, it may be due to purgatives or to slight chronic uræmia; but severe, long-continued diarrhœa in Bright's disease, inasmuch as it points to some colitis or entero-colitis, is of very dangerous prognosis.

Another thing of prognostic value is uræmia. There is no doubt, as Fagge says, that sometimes most remarkable recoveries occur. Patients who are so comatose that the friends of the patient and the doctor are hopeless occasionally get well enough to go out of the hospital. But they are exceptions. As a rule, when uræmia is as severe as it was in our second patient, who was restless and had twitchings, and insomnia lasting a fort-night, with intense headache, so that he was scarcely in his right mind, I do not think you often find the patient recover. At any rate, you will be justified in taking a very grave view when talking to the patient's friends. Certainly, as you will remember, our patient did not recover. And I cannot help reminding you here, because it is so important, that in such a condition the best thing is what we did here, give chloroform. The patient will then go off to sleep for a long while, and you can, if necessary, repeat it after he wakes.

Talking of such symptoms reminds us of cere-bral hæmorrhage, and that, of course, is of bad prognosis, but it is not of nearly such bad prognosis as most of the symptoms which we have already mentioned. In fact, there is a saying that the third cerebral hæmorrhage kills, which shows that many people at any rate have two. It is nearly always associated with granular kidney, so it does strictly come into this lecture. When you are at the bedside of the patient who has cerebral hæmor-rhage, and his friends are saying " Will he get better ? " the points for you to bear in mind are, if his coma is not less at the end of twenty-four hours, he will almost certainly die ; if he has Cheyne-Stokes' breathing as a result of cerebral hæmorrhage, he will almost certainly die ; if there is much mucus in the lungs, he will probably die ; if his paralysis is bilateral, he will probably die, and so he will if his temperature is very low, because that shows there is a considerable loss of blood, or if the temperature is very high because this shows that his thermotaxic mechanism has been thoroughly upset. Then, putting epistaxis aside, I think as a rule these patients are doing badly when they bleed elsewhere than from the brain. I mentioned earlier in the lecture the man who bled into his ear, and the doctor who bled into his lung. Both of our patients of whom we are speaking to-day bled extensively, and I do not like the outlook in a case of granular kidney if the man has the variety which is asso-ciated with repeated hæmorrhages from various parts of the body.

You know that pneumonia and pleurisy are both of them complications of Bright's disease, and peri-tonitis and pericarditis too, for the matter of that. When any of these supervene upon granular kidney they usually kill the patient.

Now we pass on to consider the urine. By far the most important point in connection with it is whether or not it is suppressed. Remember the case of the second of these two patients. Towards the end he had suppression. The outlook is always grave in granular kidney if the patient gets suppression of urine. If the specific gravity is very low and the urine is pale, that, as a rule, is of bad prognosis, because it means that the kidney is not getting rid of much solid matter. You should always look for casts in a case of granular kidney. The value of blood-casts in estimating the prognosis is great, because they may mean that the patient has an acute attack supervening upon his chronic trouble, or he may be bleeding from his kidney simply because he is a patient with chronic Bright's disease. So that blood-casts in the urine of a patient with chronic granular kidney, whatever their cause may be, are of bad prognosis. Then, although they are not so important, granular casts, being chiefly degenerate epithelial casts, or degene-rate blood-casts, show that the epithelium is being shed, or that the kidney is bleeding, therefore they are of bad prognosis. And so are epithelial casts. Hyaline casts we do not know much about ; we do not understand their significance. They are often passed by people who are apparently perfectly healthy, and so I do not want you to attach any particular importance to them in trying to estimate the prognosis of Bright's disease. Of course if there are epithelial or blood cells adherent to the hyaline casts, then they become important. You might think that the amount of urea passed was of importance in prognosis. Theoretically that is so, and von Jaksch has published observations which show that the prognosis is bad in proportion as the amount of urea passed is low. But for ordinary clinical purposes it is almost valueless, because, as you know, the amount of urea depends on the intake of nitrogen, and your conclusions would not be correct unless you compared the output of nitrogen in the urine and fæces with the intake of nitrogen in the food. Let us turn now to the chlorides. A healthy man, as you know, excretes 10 to 15 grammes of chlorides every twenty-four hours, and it has been shown that in severe chronic Bright's disease the diminution of the chlorides in the urine is very considerable, and it has been suggested that the cause of the œdema in Bright's disease is that the chlorides are retained in the tissues, and that they attract water and hence œdema. But much work will have to be done before we know whether that is true. It would be an admirable subject for some of you who want a thesis if you would systematically work at the subject and see whether the cases with œdema excrete less chlorides than those without œdema. Those who uphold that theory maintain that if they withhold chlorides from the food they can reduce the amount of the œdema, and further that the prognosis is bad in proportion as the amount of chlorides in the urine is small. But I do not know that this is of much practical value, because a man in ordinary practice has not time to estimate quantitatively day by day the amount of chlorides excreted, nor is it any good his doing so unless he knows the amount of chlorides taken in the food. But for hospital work, anybody who is inclined to work at it scientifically would find it a good subject to take up.

Another mode of investigation which has been used in prognosis is that which is called cryoscopy, and that, too, is a subject upon which some of you might do original work. The freezing point of any fluid depends on the amount of solid in it, and the freezing point is lower the greater the amount of solid and its molecular weight—*i.e.* upon the molecular concentration (osmotic pressure). It is found that the urine in health freezes between 1° and 2° C. below zero. And in granular kidney, owing to the fact that not much solid is excreted in the urine, the freezing point of the urine is raised—it may be as high as —0·56° C.; and at the same time, owing to the failure of the kidney to excrete solids, the freezing point of the blood, which in health is —0·55° C. to —0·57° C., is lower—it may be to —0·77° C. The best results would be obtained by comparing the raised freezing point of the urine with the lower freezing point of the blood; and such results, it is said, are of considerable value in estimating the prognosis of Bright's disease, but it is quite possible that results of considerable value would be got by noting the freezing point of the urine only, and the patient might object to having his blood frequently examined. Cryoscopy will probably be of especial

use in determining whether the other kidney is sound in cases in which we know one to be diseased. For example, if a surgeon wishing to operate on a diseased kidney finds that the freezing point of the blood is normal he has evidence that the other kidney is working as in health; or, if we obtain, by means of a separator, the urine from each kidney and then compare the freezing points of the two specimens, we shall have a guide to determining which kidney is diseased.

Methylene blue has been given to patients with chronic Bright's disease, and the interval between its appearance in the urine has been compared with the interval in a healthy man; it usually takes longer to appear in the urine if the kidney is diseased. But this proceeding is not of much prognostic value, for the kidney might well be unable to excrete the poisons which cause uræmia and yet be able to excrete methylene blue, and it is obvious that this method, cryoscopy, the estimation of chloride and of urea, are hardly applicable to every-day practice.

The next point we need consider to-day is the value of albuminuria for purposes of prognosis. You must remember that albumen in the urine does not of itself matter much, for many who pass it have not Bright's disease; they may be suffering from a specific fever, from heart-disease, renal calculus, cystitis, and other maladies. Again, the amount of albumen lost in the urine is often so small that it cannot affect the general health of the patient. Sometimes patients seriously ill with chronic Bright's disease pass hardly any. The amount of albumen in the urine is of very little value in prognosis; its presence may be invaluable for purposes of diagnosis; a steady increase in its quantity indicates that tubal nephritis is supervening, and if tubal nephritis is already present a lessening of the albumen indicates that the tubal change is receding.

Much may be learnt about the prognosis by a careful examination of the cardio-vascular system. If the artery is thick or the tension of the pulse high, the patient is, ás you know, liable to cerebral hæmorrhage. Let me beg of you not to depend solely on your finger for estimating the blood-pressure, for you cannot then accurately compare the pressure on different occasions. For a small sum you can now buy the instrument recently described by Dr. C. J. Martin ('Brit. Med. Journ.,' 1905, vol. i, p. 865). Here is one and I will now show you how to apply it. [The lecturer then gave a demonstration of how to use the instrument.] The time allotted to this lecture has now elapsed, so I cannot go into the question of the value of an examination of the heart in prognosis, nor is this necessary, for much of this properly falls in a lecture on heart-disease.

December 4th, 1905.

A CLINICAL LECTURE

ON

ACUTE INTESTINAL OBSTRUCTION.

Delivered at Westminster Hospital.

By CHARLES STONHAM, C.M.G., F.R.C.S.,
Senior Surgeon to the Hospital.

GENTLEMEN,—There is a very important subject which I want to say a few words to you about, namely, acute intestinal obstruction. A knowledge of this condition, of its symptoms, and of the proper way to examine and treat a case when it comes before you is so easily acquired that it is astonishing to me how many cases one sees in which obstruction has been allowed to persist for five or six or even more days, before further advice is sought, when practically the last hope for the patient has gone. I am sure those of you who have been about the wards for the last year or so must remember cases of acute intestinal obstruction which were sent in too late. If you can do nothing more, at least make a correct and early diagnosis, and then you can call in a surgeon if need be to effect such treatment as the case demands. To-day I shall only discuss the general facts of acute intestinal obstruction ; I shall not go into its various causes.

The diagnosis of the condition has to be made from three standpoints. First of all you have to diagnose the *fact* of obstruction. Having established this, you must then determine (as near as may be) the *seat* of the obstruction, and lastly you have to diagnose the *nature* of the obstruction. To diagnose the fact is simple ; to diagnose the approximate seat of the obstruction is usually easy ; to diagnose the cause of the obstruction may be very easy or very difficult, and it may be only actually discoverable after the abdomen has been opened. Bear in mind another point with regard to acute obstruction, and this is that the history may perhaps point to dyspeptic trouble extending over some period of time, and very likely associated with alternating attacks of constipation and diarrhœa, with a feeling of fulness and distension after food, and general ill-health. Acute intestinal obstruction following on such a history is probably due to some cause, *e. g.* a growth, which has led to gradual obstruction of the lumen of the bowel. It is a by no means uncommon thing for a patient who has a growth in the colon to suddenly get acute obstruction, due, in the vast bulk of instances, in my experience, to the sudden blocking of the narrow lumen by some indigestible material or hardened mass of fæces.

Now, with regard to the symptoms pointing to the *fact* of obstruction. First of all the mode of onset. The onset is sudden. The patient feels perfectly well perhaps (except under the circumstances before mentioned) until he is suddenly seized with acute pain in the abdomen, pain which is sometimes of great severity, and may induce a condition of extreme collapse. The pain is usually felt in the neighbourhood of the umbilicus, and it is referred to that situation no matter where the obstruction itself is, although there may be local pain and tenderness in addition. You must not take the situation to which the pain is referred as an indication of the situation of the cause of the pain—that is to say, of the obstruction. The pain is usually felt round the umbilicus owing to the fact that it is reflected through the solar plexus, which is situated on a level with and just to the right of the umbilicus. The pain is fairly characteristic in its nature. As a rule it is paroxysmal. The patient may have a severe attack of colicky griping pain, which lasts perhaps five or ten minutes, or even longer, and then gradually subsides, and the patient becomes easy again. Probably in a very short time he will have another attack. Such attacks may be determined by palpation of the abdomen, or again, may be brought on by giving him an enema or food by the mouth. Occasionally you will find that the pain becomes constant, but when so it is always liable to paroxysmal exacerbations. When the pain becomes constant it tends to show that the obstruction is more or less complete. The cause of this pain is of course the strong peristaltic action of the intestine attempting to push its contents past the obstructed point. The rest or comparative freedom from pain comes when the intestine has, as it were, given up the task for the time, the peristalsis stops, and there is a period of ease. You will find, further, that as the case progresses the pain often becomes more diffuse ; there is not only the paroxysmal colicky pain, but a general pain, associated very likely with superficial tenderness, all over the abdomen. Such a condition tends to show that acute peritonitis is being set up at the point of the obstruction, and is gradually spreading over the whole abdomen ; and I need hardly say that if you meet with this general condition of tenderness, the prognosis of the case is proportionately more grave, naturally enough, since acute peritonitis is, apart from intestinal obstruction, a very serious condition.

There is one point in connection with pain which it is important to remember, and that is, do not be taken in by the fact that a patient after receiving some drug, the nature of which he may not know, feels better. He can only tell you that he has had some drug and since then the pain has been much less severe. Always, under such circumstances, examine his pupils carefully and try to form an opinion as to whether he has been given morphia or not. Of course morphia is very largely used in intestinal obstruction. Its use is right and proper provided you do not allow it to deceive you. If you allow the amelioration of the symptoms due to morphia to persuade you that it is evidence of the obstruction being overcome, so much the worse for the patient.

The next symptom of importance which I want to speak of—and perhaps I ought to have put it first because it is the most important—is vomiting. The vomiting in intestinal obstruction is characteristic. It comes on tumultuously ; the vomited matter is brought up without any retching, and without any effort on the part of the patient ; it comes out with a gush, and very likely the patient may bring up pints of vomit, which is a remarkable fact in view of the circumstances that he has probably not taken any food or any liquid for some time. The vomiting is associated with intense nausea, which, unlike the nausea accompanying other conditions, is not relieved by the vomiting. The vomit varies somewhat in its profuseness and in its nature with the position of the obstruction. It tends, sooner or later, in nine tenths of the cases, to become stercoraceous. The contents of the stomach are very likely mixed with bile, and then there is a feculent-smelling fluid, and after that fæces only. You never get true feculent vomiting if the intestinal obstruction is high up in the abdomen, you will see fœtid vomiting under these circumstances, but not feculent. If the obstruction is very low down—say it is an obstruction due to a carcinoma situated in the cæcum or in the rectum, or somewhere about there—the vomiting is not so intense and the feculent character is not so marked. This feculent vomiting is not, as was previously supposed, dependent upon inverted peristalsis, but it is due to a central return wave from the point of obstruction.

Another important symptom is constipation, but this, again, may vary a good deal. If the obstruction is in the ileum, it may be that the colon is full of fæces at the time the obstruction takes place, and the colon may empty itself, and is especially likely to do so if the patient be given an enema. At the same time, very often the colon will not empty itself; the fact of an obstruction existing in the middle part of the intestine paralyses the intestine to a certain degree, and the lower end remains inactive. Even if you have a history of a certain amount of diarrhœa associated with vomiting, and associated with pain, there still may be intestinal obstruction, so do not place too much reliance on statements bearing on the action of the bowels. Diarrhœa is sometimes an evidence of constipation, just as so-called incontinence of urine is evidence of retention. Further, the patient does not pass any flatus by the rectum. Here again, however, there is a source of fallacy which you must guard against, for if the patient has had enemata, a quantity of air may have been introduced, and this being passed may lead the attendants to think that the patient is passing flatus. He frequently brings up a lot of flatus by his mouth, and fœtid eructations are very characteristic indeed of intestinal obstruction situated anywhere in the small intestine. These eructations become, of course, proportionately rare as the obstruction is lower down. Another symptom which is met with is diminution in the quantity of urine. It used to be said that the diminution in the quantity of urine was proportionate to the height at which the obstruction took place. That is really not quite true. Diminution in the urine may occur in connection with obstruction situated anywhere, and the probability is that it is dependent upon a reflex inhibition of the kidneys through the nerves of the solar plexus. Another reason possibly that urine is diminished is that a patient is taking but little fluid, and at the same time is bringing up large quantities of fluid in his vomit, and as you know, if you get rid of fluid from the body in one way you will not do so in another.

The general condition of the patient is fairly characteristic. As a rule he is in a state of extreme collapse, that collapse being more marked if the obstruction is in the small intestine than if it is in the large intestine. It is more marked if the obstruction is very high up, and it is more marked if a large piece of bowel is involved than if a small piece is involved. The expression of the patient's face is generally more or less characteristic. It is drawn, and he has an anxious look about him, one of intense pain, with his brows contracted. If you look at a man who has an obstruction in his small intestine, I think you will after a little experience be able to make a shrewd guess at the diagnosis before asking him any questions.

As a rule the temperature is diminished. If the case is associated with profound shock, the temperature may fall to 95° or 96° F.; but it rarely falls below 97° F. Sometimes in the course of intestinal obstruction the temperature begins to rise, and this is a symptom of rather ominous import, since it tends to show that there is peritonitis extending from the point of obstruction. The pulse, again, is generally diminished in frequency, and is small and wiry; but it may increase in rate if acute peritonitis supervenes.

There are one or two other general symptoms. One is the condition of the patient's respiration. You will find that these patients in great measure cease breathing with their abdominal muscles, the respiration becoming more costal in character; it is often shallow, and increased in rapidity. Sometimes the embarrassment of respiration is very great indeed, and this is especially the case when the obstruction is situated low down in the colon. In such a case the colon itself becomes enormously distended, presses upon the diaphragm, and thus hampers respiration and the heart's action. Such cases become markedly cyanotic, the pulse fails, and the patient generally dies of acute cardiac failure unless the obstruction be speedily relieved.

Now, the symptoms that I have discussed are those which will lead you to diagnose the fact of obstruction quite apart from any examination of the abdomen. Bear in mind that the symptom which is the most urgent and prominent one, and which should never be neglected, is vomiting. Directly the patient brings up vomited matter

which smells fæcal you ought to promptly seek for and relieve the obstruction. It is not the least use—indeed, it is most deplorable—to temporise any longer. Prompt operation usually means recovery; delay spells death.

Having arrived at the diagnosis of obstruction, you have next to try and find out what is the situation of its cause, and this you will do by examining the patient and by bearing in mind the facts ascertained as to the history of the case. The history should inform you whether the patient has ever had any such attacks before, whether he has suffered from chronic dyspepsia, if his bowels have been acting regularly, if he has had alternating attacks of constipation and diarrhœa, and, in fact, anything pointing to some gradual involvement of the bowel, as by a growth, either inside or outside the colon. Again, inquire carefully whether he has had attacks of gall-stone colic, whether he has ever had jaundice, and whether subsequent to the jaundice he has had chronic intestinal trouble, pointing, of course, to the fact of intestinal obstruction being occasionally caused by a large gall-stone impacted in the lower end of the ileum. Again, inquire particularly, especially in the case of women, for any evidence pointing to mischief in the pelvis, such as pelvic peritonitis or pelvic cellulitis, by which bands of adhesions may have been formed under which a coil of bowel may slip. Also try and find out if there is any history of appendicitis, because the appendix may be tied down and form an arcade under which the patient's bowel slips, giving rise to obstruction, of which I have seen several cases.

Having got the history, you should next examine the abdomen. The first thing you would examine for is all the usual and unusual places for hernia—the inguinal, femoral, umbilical, obturator, and sciatic regions. If you find hernia, ascertain exactly what its condition is. Find out if it is very tense—if it is very painful, whether it is reducible or irreducible. If you find a tense and more or less painful hernia, you must cut down upon it forthwith; but you must constantly bear in mind that the mere fact of a hernia being irreducible and being associated with evidence of intestinal obstruction does not prove that the hernia is strangulated and responsible for the condition, for there may be some other cause. I have seen the abdomen opened on more than one occasion for intestinal obstruction when it was found to be dependent upon hernia which had not even been looked for. In examining the abdomen, it is important, when possible, to make the examination during a paroxysm of pain, and also during an interval. During a paroxysm you may be able to see the coils of intestine gradually contracting and the gas passing along them, but suddenly stopping at some particular spot, indicating thereby more or less accurately the situation of the obstruction. In the early stages of intestinal obstruction the abdomen is more or less tense, and very soon it becomes very tense and hard; in many cases the serrations of the recti will show up plainly, and if you put your hand on the abdomen at this time it will feel board-like. This depends upon the irritation of the lower costal nerves, causing contraction of the muscles to protect the damaged parts beneath. Not very long after the obstruction has become manifest the patient suffers from meteorism; the abdomen becomes distended with gas, the distension depending in some measure upon the position of the obstruction, but in the main it is due to the interference with the blood-supply of the mesentery. It has been shown experimentally in animals that if you produce artificial intestinal obstruction by tying a ligature round the intestine, meteorism is not developed to any great extent, but that if you interfere with the vascular supply, especially with the venous supply in the intestine, by ligaturing the large veins, leaving the lumen of the bowel unaffected, meteorism is extreme. Therefore you would expect to find that, if a large portion of bowel and consequently a large portion of mesentery were affected, the meteorism would be proportionately great: And so it is. In very thin people it sometimes happens that you can see the coils of intestine moving about under the abdominal wall, the so-called borborygmi. In fat people of course you will not see this. By inspection you may very likely be able, except in fat patients, to form a very good opinion as to whether the obstruction is situated in the great or in the small intestine. When it is situated in the small intestine the chief swelling occupies the centre of the abdomen round the umbilicus, and in this area the tympanites is most marked. There will, of course, be resonance in the flanks and iliac fossae; but it will not be absolutely tympanitic there as it would be over the distended coils. If, on the other hand, the obstruction is situated low down in the colon, then you will find that the centre part of the abdomen is more or less flattened—comparatively; but there is a huge coil of distended intestine extending right the way round and down to the right iliac fossa, and associated with this there will be evidence of impairment of respiration, and feeble action of the heart due to the distended colon pressing on the diaphragm, as I have already mentioned.

Having examined the abdomen by inspection, the next thing is palpation. Palpation will, of course, confirm much of what you have learnt by inspection, but it may also reveal the presence of increased resistance at some part of the abdomen, or in some cases, as for example in intussusception, you may detect the presence of a very definite tumour. But too often, unfortunately, it does not reveal anything, and after palpation you are about as wise as you were before. Finally, you should examine the rectum, and, in the case of married women, the vagina.

Now, gentlemen, supposing that an exhaustive examination reveals nothing definite, yet the fact of obstruction is manifest from the symptoms, and you are still in ignorance as to where the obstruction is, whether it is in the great intestine or whether it is in the small, and you are equally ignorant as to the nature of it, what is your next duty? It is immediate laparotomy. Do not temporise; to do so is not only useless but is positively harmful, and too frequently robs the patient of such chances as may be his. Open the abdomen between the umbilicus and the pubes, and having opened it you should promptly introduce your hand and find the caecum. Having found the caecum, pick up the lowest coil of the ileum and examine it; if this be quite normal in appearance, is empty and not distended with flatus, you may be certain that the obstruction is in some part of the intestine higher up. Therefore under these conditions you next proceed to pass the coils through your fingers until you come to the cause of the obstruction, which is then treated according to its nature. Then go further up in the same way, to make sure that there is not another cause for obstruction higher up still; by neglecting this rule many patients have been relieved of only one source of obstruction. And this is a fatal mistake which you must guard against in every case. I remember once seeing a case in which a coil of intestine was found strangled by a band ; this was freed, and the bowel put back again. But the symptoms were not relieved, and eventually the patient died. At the post mortem it was found that two other bands existed higher up. Supposing, however, that you find the lower coils of the ileum to be distended, and that the cæcum is distended too, then work right the way round the great intestine until you discover the obstruction, which will in all probability be in the sigmoid flexure or high up in the rectum. If you proceed on this plan of examining the intestine, you will cut your operation shorter than you otherwise would, you will inflict less injury on the patient, and produce much less shock, and naturally enough the results of your operation will be far more satisfactory in every way.

I do not know whether it is advisable or even wise to tell you anything about the treatment of intestinal obstruction other than the operative. My view is that any man who waits when he has once made up his mind that the case is one of intestinal obstruction is violating surgical common sense and courting disaster. At the same time, there are cases, I suppose, in which one may justly have a doubt as to whether one is dealing with acute obstruction or not ; and if so it may be necessary to treat your patient temporarily until either the diagnosis becomes perfectly clear to you or until somebody has given you help to clear the matter up.

In the first place, I would like to say a few words about morphia. Do not give a patient with intestinal obstruction morphia unless he is suffering great pain, and when you do give it only give a sufficiency to give him ease. And further, remember always that he has had morphia and that he will improve under it. He improves in every way. Morphia tends to diminish shock, to stop or at least diminish vomiting, to relieve pain, and encourage sleep. But do not allow yourselves to be taken in by this improvement.

Another question is that of feeding. Speaking generally, you are not to give these patients any food whatever by the stomach. The first reason is that they will probably bring it up if you do ; secondly, if it is not brought up, the stomach will not digest it. Very likely the stomach has already got a lot of feculent material in it, and so long as that is there the stomach is not likely to digest the food which you put into it. And even if it did digest it the small intestine will not absorb it, and, therefore, it is useless. In feeding these patients, with very few exceptions you should do so by the rectum. Feed them with small nutrient enemata and meat suppositories. If the obstruction is low down, say in the sigmoid flexure or in that neighbourhood, it is obvious that you cannot feed your patient by the rectum, but these are the very cases in which you can feed the patient by the mouth, because in such the stomach is not in a very disturbed state nor is the upper part of the small intestine. Probably such a patient has not vomited very much, and he will keep his food down if it is given to him in suitable form and in small quantities which he will be able to digest and absorb.

Another point is with regard to the use of enemata in these cases. It is the customary thing in acute intestinal obstruction to give an enema to see what fæces there may be in the lower bowel ; sometimes large enemata are given with the idea of overcoming the obstruction. Personally, I do not see the use of giving an enema unless there is reason to believe that the colon is loaded. In any case the enema has the disadvantage that it very often excites a paroxysm of pain, it adds to the patient's discomfort and increases his collapse, and as regards the employment of large enemata with the view of overcoming the obstruction I regard it as the pernicious treatment of a bygone age, except in cases due to fæcal impaction.

Finally, I beg of you to learn at any rate the common signs of intestinal obstruction, so that you may recognise its existence without delay. Whether you can ascertain the cause of it or not is of much less importance. Having diagnosed the condition, act immediately, and never let a patient die in default of operation, as too many have done in the past. Remember that every hour counts.

December 4th, 1905.

WE have received from the publishers, Messrs. Heinemann, London, a copy of Dr. S. Squire Sprigge's book on 'Medicine and the Public.' We hope before long to find space for an adequate review of this most interesting and fascinating volume, and therefore for the present content ourselves with complimenting the author on the practical and useful book he has written.

A CLINICAL LECTURE

ON

A CASE OF CARCINOMA WITH VENOUS THROMBOSIS AND ENDOCARDITIS.

By ARTHUR HALL, M.A., M.D.Cantab., F.R.C.P.,

Physician to the Sheffield Royal Hospital ; Consulting Physician Mexborough Montagu Hospital ; Joint Lecturer on Clinical Medicine, University of Sheffield.

GENTLEMEN,—The case which forms the subject of my lecture to-day presented so many features of interest in connection with diagnosis that, although any form of successful treatment was out of the question, yet it is worth careful consideration and study. It may seem at first sight that in a case where nothing can be done to cure the patient the labour of making a diagnosis is largely wasted effort, but that is not so. The study of medicine is something more than the immediate case with which you are dealing at any one time ; and whilst deploring your helplessness in saving the individual life or alleviating the individual suffering, you should endeavour to acquire all the information that can possibly be obtained from as full and complete a study of the case as if you hoped thereby to save a life.

One can never say from what seemingly unimportant or hopeless—it may be rare or it may be common—disease a careful and thorough observer may not gather, if not some hitherto unknown fact, at least some new item of information which may prove of future use in dealing with other cases.

The patient whose case I propose to discuss was a labourer, æt. 39 years.

His family history was good, and his habits had been temperate in every way.

He said he had always enjoyed good health in every way until two or three months ago, when he began to suffer from loss of flesh and pains in his legs. This gradually prevented him from walking and he took to bed four weeks ago. He had "pains flying about" him up to a week ago, but they had now all "settled" in his legs.

You will see from this brief statement that the history limited itself almost entirely to the lower extremities, with one or two important exceptions.

He said that the first thing he noticed was pain and weakness in the left leg, so that he gradually had to give up work and could not get about, that the left leg swelled and was painful, that later the right leg became painful, so that he had difficulty in moving it.

These were the chief symptoms to him. Taken with the signs which were present on admission and which developed later, there was no difficulty in diagnosing all these as due to thrombosis of the veins of the legs causing obstruction. This might have been due to a simple phlebitis, extending into the iliac veins and the inferior vena cava, had it not been that he told us he had lost three stone in weight in three months, a statement which his emaciated appearance fully supported. This at once removed the possibility of the case being a simple phlebitis and nothing more ; for, as you know, such an affection, though it may be serious, and though it may lead to grave and even fatal complications, either by extension to other veins, or by producing an embolism of sufficient size to block the pulmonary artery, yet it would never lead to such a serious loss of flesh as three stone in three months. For that one must look to some such condition as malignant disease, tuberculosis, diabetes, an acute fever such as typhoid, or possibly a nervous condition such as anorexia nervosa.

Of none of these did he offer any evident history, his only statement being, as I have already told you, that a week or two ago he had pains "flying about" his body for some days, which eventually seemed to "settle" in his legs. There was no cough or expectoration ; there were no physical signs of disease in the lungs. The urine was normal, and although his temperature was raised, there was no evidence of any acute febrile disease nor of any nervous affection.

As regards malignant disease, there was, however, some evidence on examination, namely, an enlarged liver, with a hard, smooth portion of surface in the region of the gall-bladder. Taken with the history of loss of flesh, this hardness over the liver surface became very suggestive of malignant disease. and it seemed probable, therefore, that the primary or chief disease was not the thrombosis to which his symptoms had chiefly attracted attention, but some form of cancer.

Two questions then arose. First, Where had the cancer begun ? and secondly, Had the phlebitis any relationship to it at all, or was it merely, so to speak, a coincidence, a purely chance complication?

Let us take these two points in order.

Where had the cancer started? As you know, "cancer" is a term used by the public to signify a new growth or malignant tumour, and of these there are at least two varieties, the carcinomata or epithelial cancers and the sarcomata or connective-tissue cancers. Between those two varieties there are many differences, which you will learn more about in the proper place. But there are also certain similarities between the two varieties, and one of these, the most important, the chief character of malignancy common to both, is, that whilst each begins as a single primary tumour in some single site, it sooner or later develops multiple secondary tumours at distant sites. Moreover there are both for carcinoma and sarcoma certain sites where primary tumours are commonly found and other sites where it is quite unusual to find them, these being different for each variety.

To return, then, to our first question. Where is the primary tumour in this case? You will remember that the only demonstrable evidence of a tumour was on the anterior surface of the enlarged liver. Now, in either form of cancer the liver substance is a rare position for a primary tumour, whilst, owing to its large and varied vascular supply, it is a very common situation for secondary growths. Therefore, whenever you find what appears to be an enlarged liver, containing a malignant deposit, the probability is that it is merely secondary to some primary malignant tumour elsewhere. Cancer of the liver is a very common diagnosis, but it is usually an incomplete one. In this man there was no history to suggest where that primary tumour was. It was certainly not on any part of the body surface, it was not in the rectum, there was no evidence of any other swelling in the abdomen except that of the liver or of any distension of the bowels such as is commonly produced by a cancerous stricture of the bowel; in fact, there was nothing to point to any disease of the bowels.

Similarly with regard to the stomach, there had been no pain after food, no vomiting, no distension.

Another common site of cancer is the head of the pancreas, and in such cases the emaciation is usually rapid, but jaundice is generally present sooner or later from obstruction to the adjoining bile-duct, which was not so in his case. Moreover, although the abdominal wall was quite relaxed and palpable, no tumour could be felt over the pancreatic region.

So you see that to locate the site of a primary growth was not perfectly simple and straightforward.

Before further considering this question, let us consider the second, viz. Had the thrombosis anything to do with the growth? Now, there are two ways in which venous thrombosis may occur in malignant disease. In the first place, the tumour may press upon or surround or even invade the walls of a vein and so obstruct it, leading to thrombosis in the part obstructed, or in the second place so-called "marantic thrombosis" may occur in cancer, as in other diseases, accompanied by much wasting and exhaustion, such as typhoid fever, tuberculosis, influenza, or even chlorosis.

In the excellent article on "Thrombosis" in Allbutt's 'System of Medicine,' vol. vi, by Professor Welch, which, together with that on "Embolism," I should advise you to read for yourselves, reference is made to cases in which peripheral venous thrombosis was the first symptom to attract attention, in cases of latent cancer of the stomach, as it was in the case of Trousseau himself, the famous French physician. Such cases are not common, but they do occur.

It was thus impossible to lay too much stress on the thrombosis of the inferior vena cava as a possible localiser for the primary growth. Still, it was open to argument that the primary growth had started in, or in front of, the bodies of the lumbar vertebræ and surrounded and obstructed the inferior vena cava and so caused the symptoms due to thrombosis in the legs.

Nothing could be seen or felt in the abdomen in support of this, but as you know, any vigorous palpation of the neighbourhood of a venous thrombosis is not permissible for fear of loosening some clot and causing a fatal pulmonary embolism.

The diagnosis therefore made on the patient's admission to hospital was "thrombosis of iliac veins, probably secondary to malignant growth of which the primary seat was unknown; secondary deposits in liver."

So far the case, though interesting, seemed fairly straightforward. One week after admission, however, he was suddenly seized in the early morning with paralysis of the right side and complete aphasia, without any loss of consciousness, and this continued up to the time of death, three days later, this being preceded for some hours by coma.

This hemiplegia offered many interesting patho-logical points for consideration, and it is to these I want particularly to call your attention.

Briefly we may say that there were four possible causes of the hemiplegia :

(1) An ordinary cerebral hæmorrhage, due to a ruptured cerebral artery or aneurysm.

(2) Thrombosis of a cerebral artery.

(3) Embolism.

(4) Secondary malignant deposit in brain.

(1) *Cerebral hæmorrhage.*—Against this was the absence of loss of consciousness, the sudden com-pleteness of the paralysis, and the absence of any evidence of arterial disease elsewhere. This, taken with his age, 39 years, and the general low tension of the vascular system in such an emaciated condi-tion, made such a diagnosis unlikely.

(2) *Thrombosis.*—Similar considerations as to arterial disease elsewhere and age would again hold good, and although such a diagnosis was not to be absolutely negatived, yet it was not probable. You might naturally think that the presence of throm-bosis in one part of the body would suggest thrombosis in another part, and that is not un-reasonable ; but in this case it would be throm-bosed *veins* in the leg and a thrombosed *artery* in the brain. No cerebral *venous* thrombosis would account for a sudden complete hemiplegia such as this, although it might produce a certain one-sided weakness. As a matter of fact venous and arterial thromboses are usually due to distinct and separate conditions and do not run coincidently in different parts of the body.

(3) *Embolism.*—The history of sudden onset without loss of consciousness suggests embolism, but if so, where did the embolic plug arise ? As you know, an embolism is often formed by the loosening of a piece from the free end of a venous thrombus, but such a plug carried along the veins in the direction of the blood-stream must reach the right side of the heart, and from there can only be driven into the lungs, where it will be arrested as soon as it reaches a branch of the pulmonary artery too small for it to pass through. It cannot reach the left heart *via* the lungs unless it is small enough to get through the lung capillaries. If it is small

enough to do this, it is too small to block any cere-bral artery larger than the minutest arteriole, which could not produce a hemiplegia ; for, as you know, the amount of brain-tissue involved in the motor function of one side is considerable, and to cut off its blood supply requires something more than a clot which can get through the lung capillaries.

There is, however, one way by which a good-sized venous thrombus might get from the right heart into the left and so to the systemic arteries, without traversing the lungs, and that is by being pushed through a patent foramen ovale in the interauricular septum from the right to the left auricle. This is spoken of as "paradoxical em-bolism " and the condition, though rare, is by no means unknown. It offered at least a working hypothesis.

A careful examination of the heart gave no evidence of disease of the valves of the left side of the heart to suggest any endocardial vegetations, the usual cause of arterial emboli.

(4) *Secondary malignant growth in the brain, or tumour embolism.*—Although the brain is not a common site for secondary deposits of carcinoma such a complication is not unknown and it seemed a possibility, although a complete sudden hemi-plegia is not a common way for such a deposit to first show its presence.

Putting together the pros and cons, it seemed probable that we had in this hemiplegia either a "paradoxical embolism " or a secondary intra-cranial growth. How far the diagnosis was correct and how far incorrect the autopsy showed.

Autopsy.—September 17th, 1905 : Emaciation. Right leg œdematous and foot blue.

On opening the abdomen the liver was found to be much enlarged (7½ lb.) and infiltrated with large masses of secondary carcinoma, one of which had been felt in the region of the gall-bladder. The peritoneum was normal. The pleuræ and inner chest walls studded with small deposits of new growth, and secondary pleurisy with adhesions. These were more marked at the bases and chiefly on the right side, and had probably been directly infected through the diaphragmatic lymphatics. The mediastinal glands were infected.

There was a small primary new growth in the large intestine at the splenic flexure, not causing a stricture. The intestines were collapsed, small, and showed no distension.

The prevertebral lumbar glands were consider-ably infected and surrounded the inferior vena cava behind and towards the middle line. The latter contained a thrombus reaching as high as the level of the renal veins and extending from there downwards. Along the left iliac and its con-tinuations this was pale and more or less completely organised, whilst along the right it was more recent, red, and unorganised. The heart was of normal size, musculature flabby, nothing abnormal except at the mitral valve, where there was a complete ring of recent vegetations, projecting freely from the auricular surface, indistinguishable to the naked eye from ordinary rheumatic endocarditis. The kidneys and spleen each contained fairly recent simple infarcts. An embolus was found in the left middle cerebral artery at its first large division, causing complete obstruction.

In every respect the original diagnosis on admission was confirmed ; the unknown site of the primary growth proved to be quite a small tumour of the splenic flexure which had caused little or no obstruction and consequently no symptoms; it was tucked away under the spleen and so escaped palpation.

The prevertebral glands in the lumbar region were enlarged and closely surrounded the inferior vena cava, but probably the thrombosis was merely a so-called "marantic thrombosis." Our speculations as to the hemiplegia were quite wrong ; there was no "paradoxical embolism," there was no need to assume anything unusual, for the man had a well-marked ring of endocarditis at the mitral valve, which had been throwing off simple emboli, freely, to the kidneys and spleen and finally to the left brain, causing hemiplegia.

One naturally looks back to see if there was anything to call attention to this unexpected endocarditis. There was no history of rheumatic fever, and no murmur was heard in the heart at any time.

It is worth noting that he volunteered a state-ment as to pains flying about him a few weeks before, also that he was always sweating profusely, but seeing his general condition, no stress can be laid upon these. Probably the feeble, emaciated musculature of the heart had not sufficient force to cause a murmur during his last few days. What, then, is the relationship of these three factors, carcinoma of the bowel with secondary deposits in glands, liver, and pleuræ, thrombosis of inferior vena cava and its lower branches, and endocarditis? That the carcinoma was primary there can be no doubt.

Venous thrombosis does occasionally occur in cases of cancer, and that it is in some way connected with the wasting and diminished power of resistance of the tissues seems probable, as I mentioned above. Endocarditis also occasionally occurs as a terminal infection in cases of wasting disease such as cancer, probably due to the diminished bactericidal power of the tissues and fluids of the body. The combination, however, of these three processes, cancer, thrombosis, and endocarditis sufficient to produce embolism, is unusual and interesting.

December 4th, 1905.

MESSRS. ALLEN AND HANBURYS have sent us a specimen of the "Allenburys" feeder, and draw attention to a considerable improvement they have recently effected in the shape of the teat. They point out, quite rightly, that a frequent cause of complaint in all feeders in which the teat is placed on the neck of the bottle is that the child pulls the teat off. This trouble is effectually overcome by the new patent "Allenburys" teat, which possesses the great advantage of automatically holding on to the neck of the bottle, and does not involve the necessity of an independent fastening. There is but little fear that the child will pull the teat off, as it requires a very strong pull to do so. To put the teat on to the bottle it is well to follow the advice given in the instructions, to wet the neck, when the teat is easily stretched into its place on the bottle. This change in construction is an improvement of considerable value which will be much appreciated by the mother and nurse, and is well worth the attention of medical practitioners. To preserve and keep these pure rubber teats sweet and clean they should be washed in clean water both inside and out immediately after use. This may be done by rubbing the teat between the finger and thumb or by turning it inside out, taking care to re-turn the teat as soon as clean. The teats are perforated in four different ways—for milk, thin food, food of medium thickness, and for use with thickest food. It is well to remember that in hot climates these teats are best kept in cool water to which a pinch of bicarbonate of soda has been added.

THE CLINICAL JOURNAL,

CLINICAL RECORD, CLINICAL NEWS, CLINICAL GAZETTE, CLINICAL REPORTER,
CLINICAL CHRONICLE AND CLINICAL REVIEW.

EDITED BY L. ELIOT CREASY.

No. 685.   WEDNESDAY, DECEMBER 13, 1905.   Vol. XXVII.   No. 9.

CONTENTS.

*Specially reported for the Clinical Journal.   Revised
by the Author.

ALL RIGHTS RESERVED.

NOTICE.

*Editorial correspondence, books for review, &c.,
should be addressed to the Editor,* 51, *New Cavendish
Street, W., Telephone No.* 904, *Paddington ; but
all business communications should be addressed to
the Publishers,* 22½, *Bartholomew Close, London,
E.C. Telephone* 927, *Holborn.*

*All inquiries respecting Advertisements should be
sent to* MESSRS. ADLARD & SON, *Bartholomew
Close, E.C. Telephone* 927, *Holborn.*

*Terms of Subscription, including postage, payable
by cheque, postal or banker's order (in advance) : for
the United Kingdom,* 15s. 6d. *per annum ; Abroad,*
17s. 6d.

Cheques, &c., should be made payable to THE
PROPRIETORS OF THE CLINICAL JOURNAL, *crossed
"The London, City, and Midland Bank, Ltd., New-
gate Street Branch, E.C. Account of the Medical
Publishing Company, Limited."*

Reading Cases to hold Twenty-six numbers of
THE CLINICAL JOURNAL *can be supplied at* 2s. 3d.
each, or will be forwarded post free on receipt of
2s. 6d.; *and also Cases for binding Volumes at* 1s.
each, or post free on receipt of 1s. 3d., *from the
Publishers,* 22½ *Bartholomew Close, London, E.C.*

WITH DR. SAMUEL WEST IN THE WARDS OF ST. BARTHOLOMEW'S HOSPITAL.

GENTLEMEN,—This man came into the hospital, with a history of a few weeks' illness, at the beginning of September. He had the signs of very dense consolidation of the right upper lobe, which looked like pneumonia, only the history did not quite agree with this. The dulness was so extreme as to suggest fluid, but I had never seen an empyema at the apex. The consolidation of the lung continued, and the evening temperature usually reached 103° F. A patch of dulness then developed in the lower part of the chest and this I explored with a needle, withdrawing some blood-stained fluid. Excluding empyema, the diagnosis seemed to lie between new growth and tuberculous consolidation, though with new growth there ought not to have been a high temperature. Next day we put in an aspirating needle, with the intention of drawing off what fluid we could. I do not like aspirators for drawing off pleuritic effusions, but as I knew we had a difficult case to deal with we did not use much suction. Six ounces of blood-stained fluid were all we could obtain. This proved to be sterile, and showed no evidence of new growth. Next day the whole side was found resonant and it was obvious that pneumothorax had developed. The pneumothorax was only discovered by physical examination. This patient has had no symptoms whatever to suggest it, and said he felt better. As he has had no urgent symptoms, we have not interfered and the air has been spontaneously absorbed, but his temperature has continued as high as before. I do not know that the aspirator was responsible for the pneumothorax, though I have seen the lung burst many times by its injudicious use and personally I never use it if I can help it.

The aspirator is going out of use for the tapping of serous effusions altogether, and rightly. If I want to tap the pleura, I do it by syphonage, which gives eighteen to twenty-four inches of negative pressure. This is ample, and if the pleura cannot be evacuated with this the aspirator will not succeed better. The case is an illustration of the fact that pneumothorax may develop without any urgent symptoms at all and be discovered by physical signs alone.

The indications for operation in pneumothorax are urgent dyspnœa and distress ; it is better to leave the patient alone for a time if you possibly can. This case had no urgent symptoms ; therefore he was left alone. The pneumothorax does not affect the question of diagnosis, but it is an interesting complication. I think it most likely that the case will prove to be one of acute tuberculosis, of what used to be called acute caseating pneumonia, or the acute pneumonic form of phthisis. He has no cough and no expectoration. If this be a case of caseating pneumonia, I remember a case of a similar kind, in a young lady, æt. 16 years. It was a very acute case and lasted 3 months. She never coughed until the last week of her life, and she never expectorated at all.

This boy is suffering from tubercular meningitis. You will notice that he has Cheyne-Stokes' breathing. There is the well-marked crescendo and diminuendo, the up and down followed by a pause, and then the cycle commences again. It is a very acute case, and the boy has been ill only a few days. When he came in he was practically as unconscious as he is now.

There are two types of tubercular meningitis, the one in which the various stages are run slowly through, and the other in which the patients become unconscious almost at once and die in a few days or hours. That type is connected with very large effusions—that is to say, with acute hydrocephalus or the rapid effusion of fluid—into the ventricles. I put the lad yesterday on full doses of perchloride of mercury, for it is the only drug which seems to be of any use.

A few cases of tubercular meningitis are recorded as having recovered, but it is fair to say that most of them were recorded before the distinction was drawn between the posterior basic form, which sometimes recovers, and the tubercular, which practically never recovers. I have seen one case of recovery myself from what I believed to be

tubercular meningitis. But of course in the cases which recover there is no absolute proof that they were tubercular. The child I am referring to had a sister at the same time in the hospital, also with meningitis, and this was found post mortem to be tubercular.

Cheyne-Stokes' breathing is met with in two groups of cases ; in the one it is of great clinical importance, while in the other it is not.

In morbus cordis, though there may be no other sign to give anxiety, Cheyne-Stokes' breathing is of fatal omen before long. Such cases practically never recover. This is a good clinical point, but I do not like to put it absolutely, because there will be always exceptions quoted. You will find cases recorded of Cheyne-Stokes' breathing which is said to have lasted for years or even for the whole of life. But these are not cases of Cheyne-Stokes' breathing in the ordinary clinical sense of the term. In nervous diseases Cheyne-Stokes' breathing may occur, and if the patient recover from the nervous disease the Cheyne-Stokes' breathing may also pass off ; but if the patient is moribund at the time it occurs, however interesting it may be, it is of no clinical importance. There is another kind of periodic respiration, which has not been distinguished as sharply as it should be from Cheyne-Stokes' breathing. In true Cheyne-Stokes' breathing, though the rate of breathing per minute is perhaps forty, the breathing may only last for twenty seconds and the rest may be a pause, so that the actual breathing rate while it lasts is 120 per minute. In the other form of periodic respiration there are groups of two, three, or four slow, sighing respirations of equal depth, with no crescendo or diminuendo, so that the number of respirations in a minute may not be more than eight or ten. The only condition in which this form occurs so far as I know is in meningitis, generally in the posterior basic form, and some of these cases recover.

Here is a man of middle age who spits up a pint of thick muco-purulent fluid in twenty-four hours. He came into the hospital, with difficulty in swallowing. He cannot swallow liquids, and if his food is not in a more or less solid form he gets distress and cough from it. There is no doubt that he has got some mischief in his mediastinum. There is some difference in the breathing on his right side, into which air does not enter so freely as into the left, and he has an area of dulness in his right interscapular space, where the vocal vibrations and vocal resonance are increased. In the diagnosis we have to choose, it seems, between new growth and aneurysm. He has lost flesh, but the difficulty with his food may account for that. His colour does not suggest malignant disease, but I have never seen aneurysm cause the symptoms of which he complains. Unless he happens to have an abscess, or something of that kind, I think the diagnosis must be malignant disease. The secretion is not pure pus, and does not look like that from an abscess, and the temperature is normal.

In this bed there is a woman who was operated upon yesterday for empyema. About five weeks ago she was said to have had pneumonia, and the result of the pneumonia was that she aborted, having a seven months' child. After these two events she developed shortness of breath and apparently had an empyema. Her doctor sent her in with that diagnosis. The questions arose, Was it a pneumococcal infection, or due to staphylococcal or streptococcal infection following parturition? In the pneumococcal form the prognosis is good, but not so good in the streptococcal. I think it is pneumococcal, but investigation will clear that up. [It proved to be pneumococcal.] We put in a needle, but at first we did not succeed in getting pus. We then put it in in another direction and struck pus. The needle was then used as a director and the side opened. It is a rule which should never be departed from that a needle should be inserted first to find where the pus is before the knife is used. We had a case a little while ago in the ward where a needle was inserted and pus extracted. Being sure that pus was there when the operation was done, the needle was not put in again, and when the incision was made no pus was found. The man got quite well, but as a piece of his rib had been removed, it might have been awkward. In the present case my housephysician who performed the operation told me that he did not get pus where he expected, nor in the amount which was anticipated. It was a fairly big empyema, and could be felt to be loculated when the finger was inserted through the incision ; there were bands which divided it into compartments. After the operation a great deal more escaped no

doubt because the adhesions gave way. This is a good instance of the necessity for the rule to use the exploring needle immediately before operating. I could give a long lecture on that subject, supported by a number of illustrative cases. I have departed from this rule myself and have regretted it, but I never depart from it now. Trousseau laid down that rule years ago and he was right. I remember a case some years ago in which what was apparently a large empyema was opened, but not very much pus was obtained from it. It was a septic case and the patient ultimately died. Oddly enough, the child had suppurative pericarditis also, which was evacuated by incision through the pleural opening. The child died a week later, but the pericardium had got completely well, except for general adhesions. On post-mortem examination three compartments were discovered in the pleura ; one had been opened, the other two not ; each contained a different fluid.

The question of washing out the pleura has been raised. If it is necessary to wash it out, there is no reason why it should not be done. If the pus is curdy, the pleura ought to be washed out to get it clean. I do not know where the statement originated that washing the pleura out is attended with serious risk. I have washed out the pleura very many times and have never seen any harm come of it, so that I never have any hesitation in doing so, either at the time of the operation or afterwards if necessary.

Here is a female baby with congenital hydrocephalus. The head has been tapped. It is three months old, and the condition developed three weeks after birth ; that is to say, it was then that the head was noticed to be enlarging. We took away twelve ounces of fluid from it in about twenty minutes, and there was no apparent harm. The temperature has been raised since and there is retraction of the head. I asked my surgical colleague, Mr. Bowlby, if he would like to do anything more in the way of establishing a drain, but he did not recommend any operation. The chief interest in the case is the quantity of fluid removed, and that its withdrawal caused no fits or disturbances of any kind, the child seeming neither worse for the procedure nor better.

Some of you saw this next little patient last time

we met. It was shown to you as a case of impetigo facialis, corporis et capitis, a general vesicular eruption, which had been most obstinate. It has been nearly well once or twice, but has regularly relapsed. The other day the child got a cold, which travelled down its pharynx and trachea, and developed into broncho-pneumonia. At the time I mentioned that perhaps the fever would cure the skin disease, and that is what has happened. This skin affection vanished as by a charm. The skin is now comparatively healthy and smooth. Previously it was a sad spectacle. The same thing is observed sometimes in connection with pemphigus. If some fever—*e. g.* pneumonia, or scarlet fever, or measles—intervene, up goes the temperature and away goes the rash. But when the illness vanishes the skin trouble often returns. I am afraid that may be the case here ; we shall see.

December 11th, 1905.

. FROM CLOUD TO SUNSHINE. By ALFRED S. GUBB, M.D.Paris, M.R.C.S.E., etc. Pp. 50.

THE title is one which is sure to command attention at this season when we, in England, are better able to judge of the quality of fog than of sunshine. It is positively aggravating to reflect that within some fifty or sixty hours of London there exists a spot "where the glad ocean dances in the sun," and "milder moons emparadise the night." Decidedly such a region must possess unsurmountable attractions for those who are not compelled by professional, social, or political exigencies to remain in the gloomy north. Dr. Gubb, however, deals with the climate from the therapeutical rather than the æsthetic point of view, and our readers will find in this little volume a summary of the morbid conditions that are likely to be benefited by a sojourn in the mild, equable climate of Algiers, together with much useful information concerning the choice of a dwelling, clothing, and habits. His description of Algiers corresponds to the sort of place said to be so healthy that a doctor could neither live nor die there. A climate free from sudden oscillations, and in general mild both by night and by day, cannot but be beneficial to those whose powers of resistance have been reduced by age, overwork, or disease, so that the contra-indications are few. Incidentally details are given of other health resorts in Algeria—Biskra, Hammam R'Irha, etc.—and full information is afforded as to the various modes of transport, with their cost.

A
RATIONAL BASIS FOR ORGANO-THERAPY.*

By W. LANGDON BROWN, M.D., M.R.C.P.,
Senior Assistant Physician, Metropolitan Hospital ;
Demonstrator of Physiology and Junior Demonstrator of Practical Medicine, St. Bartholomew's Hospital.

THOUGH the use of organic extracts has enormously increased during the last decade, yet it is but the revival of a very ancient method. Homer relates that the wise physician Cheiron trained Achilles on marrow to give him strength. Celsus and Galen also testify to the antiquity of organo-therapy.†

The first ·Pharmacopœia, published in 1618 by the College of Physicians, contains several preparations of animal extracts. In 1677 preparations of a man's heart in powder were given for epilepsy : the horn of the unicorn was prescribed, but whence obtained I know not.

There were also several preparations from a man's skull and even from the mummy.

Macaulay tells us that in the last illness of King Charles II "the patient was largely bled, a hot iron applied to his head, a loathsome salt extracted from human skulls was forced into his mouth." Really after all this one can understand why the king apologised for being "an unconscionable time a-dying." He might well have mistaken the intentions of his physicians.

But amused though we may be at the efforts of these old-world organo-therapists, we must sometimes have an uncomfortable suspicion that the physicians of the future may smile contemptuously at tablets of brain-extract in the treatment of insanity and nervous disease, or extracts of bronchial glands for phthisis. If the older physicians used powdered heart-muscle, we squeeze it into a tablet and call it cardin. Wherein is the difference ?

"Advance in organo-therapeutics is not to be expected from the indiscriminate use of the gland extracts in every sort of disease, such as is too popular at present. Such progress as has been made hitherto in this field has been due to careful

---

* The substances of papers read before the Abernethian Society October 12th, 1905, and the Æsculapian Society October 20th, 1905.

† See A. T. Davies, 'Hunterian Society's Oration on Organo-Therapy,' 1902, for a history of the whole subject.

observation and experiment and not to haphazard use of the hypodermic syringe." (Cushny.)

The basis of rational organo-therapy is an intelligent study of the active chemical substance—how it acts, when it acts, and (an important point) the order in which it acts. Starling in his recent generalisation concerning hormones * has pointed the line along which advance lies, and it behoves us to put our own house in order and see how far we are applying and how much further we can apply organo-therapy rationally.

As Starling says, "the practice of using drugs rests on the supposition that the functions of the body can be influenced in a normal direction by chemical means. . . . If the mutual control . . . of the body be largely determined by the production of definite chemical substances in the blood, the discovery of the nature of these substances will enable us to interpose at any desired phase in these functions and so to acquire an absolute control over the workings of the human body. Such a control is the goal of medical science."

The development of a nervous system is a comparatively late event in evolution. The stimuli to which the most primitive forms of animal life respond are chemical, as the facts of chemiotaxis show. The nervous system enables very rapid reactions to occur, but where less sudden responses are needed the primitive method is retained.

For instance, in the digestive system the secretion of saliva may occur even before the food is taken. The first part of gastric secretion is started by the taste of the food in the mouth, whereas the second occurs only after absorption has begun. In the case of pancreatic secretion all attempts to prove the existence of nervous stimuli have failed.

Now, it is not too much to say that the old view was that all the organs are directly under the control of the central nervous system, but act practically independently of each other. The modern conception is one of close interdependence of the different organs. Though the central nervous system might start a series of events, the subsequent chapters are due to chemical interactions, one organ producing a chemical substance necessary as a stimulant to the rest in series.

For these substances Starling suggests the name

* Starling, 'Croonian Lectures,' Royal College of Physicians, 1905.

"hormones" (ὅρμαω—I excite). At present only the following are known :

TABLE OF HORMONES.   (Starling.)

(a) Katabolic Reactions.

Origin.	Hormone.	Reacting organ.
Muscles.	CO_2.	Respiratory centre.
Suprarenals.	Adrenalin.	Sympathetic nervous system.
Stomach (pylorus).	Gastric secretin.	Stomach (fundus).
Duodenum.	Pancreatic } secretin.	Pancreas.
	Hepatic	Liver.
Pancreas.	Pancreatic juice.	Intestine.

(b) Anabolic Reactions.

Thyroid.	Iodothyrin.	Nervous system, skin, etc.
Ovaries.	.	Uterine mucous membrane.
Fœtus.		Mammary gland.

The distinction between anabolic and katabolic reactions is merely one of convenience, for increased anabolism results in increased katabolism and vice versâ. Thus we see that "internal secretions" are simply examples of the more widely distributed hormones.

Ehrlich classified the substances which produce physiological or pharmacological effects into two main divisions :

(1) The substances closely allied in their chemical character to the proteids, which are designated as toxins; all are produced by the agency of living organisms. As a result of their introduction, the body reacts by development of an antibody.

(2) Includes all the common drugs, which probably act on the protoplasmic molecule by reason of their molecular configuration, and act without any incubation period as soon as they reach the cells they chiefly affect. Although repeated doses can set up a certain degree of tolerance, they never give rise to the production of an antibody.

We should expect hormones to belong to the second class, because if they excited the production of an antibody, larger and larger doses of them would be required to produce their physiological effect and thus defeat their own object.

The general features of a hormone, based chiefly on adrenalin and secretin are :

(1) They are bodies of comparatively small

molecular weight; for instance, adrenalin which was prepared in a pure state by Takamine and has been synthesised from pyrocatechin by Dakin, possesses the formula :

$$OH\langle\rangle CH(OH)CH_2NH,CH_3.$$

(2) They are not destroyed by simple heating, but rapidly lose power by prolonged boiling.

(3) They are rapidly destroyed by oxidising agents.

(4) They are destroyed in the tissues which they excite and do not escape in any of the secretions.

(5) They are not, as a rule, absorbed unaltered from the alimentary canal.

It is clear that CO_2 and iodothyrin present exceptions to these rules. From the practical point of view we may note especially :

(1) That, so far, we can usually employ a typical hormone only by local application or injection.

(2) That as they can be added to boiling water without loss of strength, the question of sterilisation for purposes of injection is much simplified.

(3) That as they disappear rapidly, probably from oxidation in the tissues they excite, they are more useful in producing sudden than prolonged effects.

Our list of hormones will probably become much larger; I would suggest that the opsonins will be found to fall into this class, for they are chemical excitants to the phagocytic activity of the phagocytes and I understand that they do not give rise to any antibody. Rhodopsin in the retinal rods may be another.

Carbon dioxide as a hormone.—Not much need be said of this. Haldane and Priestley * have shown that while the respiratory centre is very tolerant of alterations of the oxygen in the blood, it is remarkably sensitive to variations in the amount of CO_2. In fact, the movements of respiration are exactly regulated so as to keep the tension of CO_2 in the lungs constant. The clinical application of this is very limited, but Pembrey has shown that Cheyne-Stokes' respiration can be abolished by increasing the percentage of CO_2 in the respired air.

Adrenalin as a hormone.—We know that adrenalin is found in the medullary portion of the suprarenal capsules which is developed as a direct out-

* ' Journal of Physiology,' May, 1905.

growth from the sympathetic system ; and it is of great interest to note that this substance is also found in the sympathetic paraganglia and structures such as the carotid body. Prof. Langley has laid down the important generalisation that the action of adrenalin or any tissue is the same as stimulation of the sympathetic nerves to that part. It will not act on a muscle that at no time in its history has been innervated by the sympathetic. Elliott in extending these observations has brought forward some facts which suggest that after excision of the suprarenals the muscles innervated by the sympathetic cannot be thrown into activity even by electrical stimulation of the nerves. Adrenalin appears then to be a chemical body whose presence is essential to the activity of the sympathetic. If this be so, it should be impossible in Addison's disease to cause reflex dilatation of the pupil by pinching the skin of the neck. Cocaine, which stimulates the long ciliary nerves, ought not to cause dilatation of the pupil in this disease. This would provide us with two simple tests, but they would probably only be operative in advanced cases, where the diagnosis would scarcely be in doubt.

We are on safer ground in stating that in applying adrenalin therapeutically we have to consider what would be the effect of stimulating the sympathetic nerves to the part in question.

I shall omit its applications to surgery because the blanching effect of this drug is so well known. It may be noted in passing that larger doses of local anæsthetics can be used if adrenalin is simultaneously injected, as the resulting vaso-constriction diminishes the absorption of the anæsthetic into the general circulation.

Alimentary canal.—Since Grünbaum suggested the use of adrenalin in hæmatemesis several instances of its successful use have been reported. But we know now an additional reason for its use in this condition is that it stops the peristalsis of the stomach. For a similar reason it has been found useful for vomiting, in doses of ten minims of the 1 in 1000 solution diluted with water.

I have found it of service in typhoid hæmorrhage when administered by mouth in doses of half a drachm of the solution in half an ounce of water. Like the sympathetic, it not only constricts the bleeding point, but keeps the intestine quiescent. Herein lies its advantage over ergotin and the like.

It is always an anxious time when the bowels are being opened by enema after an intestinal hæmorrhage ; and as a precautionary measure I am accustomed to give a similar dose about a quarter of an hour before the enema, to take advantage of this action and of the closure of the ileocæcal sphincter which accompanies it. This affords the ideal condition for emptying the large intestine by enema, keeping the blood-vessels of the small intestine constricted, the walls flaccid, and the door of communication with the large bowel closed.

Exner found that intra-peritoneal injection of adrenalin delays the absorption of poison introduced into the stomach or peritoneal cavity. For instance, strychnine requires twenty times as long to produce its toxic effect. This gain of time is most valuable, and suggests the administration of a full dose of adrenalin pending the employment of other remedies.

Heart and blood-vessels.—Adrenalin augments and accelerates the heart's action like the sympathetic, but by raising the blood-pressure so much it stimulates the cardio-inhibitory centre in the medulla so that slowing might occur in this way. This could be avoided by the simultaneous injection of atropin, but it seems to me there is a simpler method at hand, and one which has an additional advantage. The chief objection to injection of adrenalin for failing heart is that by suddenly constricting the peripheral blood-vessels the work of the heart is greatly increased, and failing to meet this increase, dilatation of the cavities may occur. Dilatation combined with vagal inhibition is a danger that would outweigh any advantage to be derived from the stimulating effect of the adrenalin. But if we give amyl nitrite at the same time, we flush the peripheral vessels, thus avoiding both extra work and stimulation of the cardio-inhibitory centre. The effect of both drugs is about equally sudden and transitory. I propose to try this plan in cases of cardiac failure in future ; at present, I have only employed intravenous injections of fifteen minims, and in spite of the possible dangers I have pointed out, the effect seemed to be good. Recently in a case of failing heart in a child, apparently on the point of death, this treatment caused a distinct rally which lasted about six hours. Fortunately, it has been shown experimentally that adrenalin does not constrict

the coronary arteries, for if it did, it would almost certainly produce anginal attacks. In cases of shock where the blood-pressure is lowered from dilatation of the splanchnic blood-vessels, adrenalin is free from the risks I have mentioned.

In accordance with the general law that adrenalin only acts on structures which have a sympathetic innervation it is interesting to note that Baum finds it has no effect in bleaching nævi, and only a very transitory effect on unsound flesh.

On this law too we should expect to find that adrenalin has no constricting effect on the pulmonary vessels, which have no sympathetic vasoconstrictors. In fact, so far as any result will be obtained it will be an injurious one. The blood which is being squeezed out of the rest of the blood-vessels will be forced into the pulmonary vessels, which are unable to protect themselves by vaso-constriction, and hæmorrhage will be aggravated. The only reason that serious harm has not been done more frequently is that the drug has been administered by mouth, so that it has had no effect. But if injected into the circulation it would have a most injurious effect in hæmoptysis because of the pulmonary engorgement which results.

Serous membranes.—Injection of adrenalin to prevent recurrence of ascites or pleural effusion was first advocated by Barr, of Liverpool, in 1903. A drachm of the adrenalin chloride solution in two drachms or half an ounce of sterilised water is injected through the trocar when the serous exudation has been withdrawn. In view of the transitory effect of adrenalin, it is difficult to see why this should be effective. But it apparently is. Plant and Steele [*] suggest that as adrenalin added to serous exudation causes some coagulum it glues together the layers and thereby promotes adhesions. They noted pain and a rise in temperature in some of their cases as a result of the injection, but I have not seen any bad effects in the cases where I have used it, with chloretone. It seems free from risk and well worth employing.

Bladder.—Like the sympathetic, adrenalin inhibits the movements of the body of the bladder, while contracting the muscles at the base of the urethra ; perhaps this could be applied to some cases of incontinence of urine. Its use in vesical and uterine bleeding I need not refer to.

In Addison's disease its use must be pronounced

[*] ' Brit. Med. Journ.,' July 15th, 1903, p. 125.

a failure up to the present. For this I would suggest three reasons :

(1) The cortex of the suprarenal capsules must have some function, and as we have seen, it does not secrete the adrenalin.

(2) The gland probably contains other active principles.

(3) Above all, as adrenalin is not absorbed from the alimentary canal it is useless to administer it by mouth.

We may conclude that at present the therapeutic applications of adrenalin are limited to cases where either by topical application or by hypodermic injection we can produce a local effect, while for a general effect intravenous injections must be used. If necessary, the danger of a sudden rise in blood-pressure must be avoided by simultaneous use of amyl nitrite. In all cases the drug will imitate the effect of sympathetic stimulation.

Some observations of Dakin's on the synthesis of bodies allied to adrenalin give hope for wider application in the future. Some of these bodies produced less sudden and more prolonged effects. The presence of a catechol nucleus with unsubstituted hydroxyl groups is essential to them all. From analogy with other substitution compounds we may expect that some of these bodies may be more stable, and even, resisting digestion, may be absorbed from the alimentary canal.

Deleterious effects.—Like all powerful drugs, adrenalin has its dangers. Elliott has summarised these under three heads :

(1) The mechanical effects of high blood-pressure.

(2) Direct toxic action on the tissues, leading to necrosis, especially of the kidneys and liver.*

(3) It may cause glycosuria.

The hormones of digestion.—I have already said that the secretion of gastric juice occurs in two stages, the first depending on the stimulation of the sense of taste, while the food is yet in the mouth, the second occurring when absorption has begun. The mechanism of this second secretion has been shown by Edkins to depend on a chemical factor. The pyloric glands differ widely in structure from the glands in the fundus of the stomach. They

are non-granular, they form no hydrochloric acid, and only $\frac{1}{15}$ of the amount of pepsin supplied by the fundus glands. This suggests that they have some additional function. Edkins finds that an extract of pyloric glands made with products of salivary digestion, such as dextrin or maltose, if injected into the circulation of a fasting animal, provokes a flow of gastric juice containing both hydrochloric acid and pepsin. A similar extract of fundus glands produced no effect.

Bayliss and Starling had previously shown that the contact of hydrochloric acid with the epithelial cells of the duodenum (and to a less extent of the jejunum) causes the production of a substance they called *secretin*, which is absorbed from the cells by the blood-stream and carried to the pancreas, where it acts as a specific stimulant to secretion. Thus for pancreatic secretion to occur normally hydrochloric acid must descend from the stomach, which will only happen in the presence of food. And undue acidity of the duodenal contents with consequent excessive secretion of pancreatic juice is prevented, for von Mering has shown that injection of acid into the duodenum leads to closure of the pyloric sphincter. Not until this undue acidity has been neutralised by the pancreatic juice it has produced will the sphincter relax and more of the acid contents of the stomach pass into the duodenum. In this way pancreatic secretion is exactly regulated to the amount of food to be digested.

Moreover fresh pancreatic juice contains inactive trypsinogen. Before this can become active trypsin it must be acted upon by another ferment, *enterokinase*, which appears to be present only in the succus entericus. The best way to produce a flow of active succus entericus is to place some pancreatic juice in a loop of intestine. Indeed, the intestinal mucosa of the fasting animal will not yield enterokinase. By this "double locking" it is insured that under normal conditions active trypsin can only be liberated in the presence of food. We see also that although the secretions of digestion are initiated by nervous stimuli, they are continued by chemical stimuli, each stage in digestion being necessary to the production of the appropriate excitant to the next stage.

We shall not find in these secretins the panacea for digestive disturbances. The organs must be excited in their correct order. If secretin be

---

* In one case I found these areas of necrosis after intravenous injection of fifteen minims, followed four hours later by ten minims. (I am describing the case fully in the forthcoming volume of the ' St. Bartholomew's Hospital Reports.')

injected into a fasting animal, active pancreatic juice is set free and the animal dies from extensive digestion of the intestinal walls.

But note the importance of hydrochloric acid throughout the process.

(1) It is necessary in gastric digestion to activate the pepsin.   .

(2) It is necessary to stimulate pancreatic digestion. Therefore without a due secretion of acid, not only gastric, but pancreatic digestion is interfered with.

(3) It regulates the pyloric sphincter.

(4) It is antiseptic, preventing fermentation.

Elaborate classifications of functional dyspepsia have been made, but Leonard Williams * points out that they really fall under two heads—(a) the *sthenic type*, in which there is excess of hydrochloric acid; (b) the *asthenic type*, in which there is diminution or absence of hydrochloric acid. As he forcibly puts it, "all else is chaff and dust, which let the wind blow whither it listeth."

The *asthenic type* is much the commonest. To treat this with alkalies after meals may temporarily relieve symptoms by neutralising any acids of fermentation, but the hydrochloric acid of the gastric juice, already deficient, will also be neutralised and without it pepsin is powerless. As this acid is also antiseptic, fermentation will proceed apace in its absence, while digestion is arrested. The use of alkalies should be restricted to the period before meals, when its solvent action on mucin will help the stomach hampered by catarrhal exudation. After meals acids should be given freely, combined with nux vomica.

I have tried various methods to induce the stomach itself to form the acid, but with indifferent success. Meat extracts are perhaps the best stimulant to a secretion of acid—and here we are really employing organic extracts again.

The *sthenic type* is usually met with in patients otherwise robust, though sometimes they may be gouty. The pain comes quite at the end of digestion, the appetite is often voracious, and the pain is relieved by taking food, especially indigestible substances, such as fat. The explanation is clear : the hydrochloric acid is given some work to do ; it can attack the food instead of irritating the mucous membrane of the stomach, while fat inhibits the secretion of gastric juice. The result of hyper-

* CLINICAL JOURNAL, May 10th, 1905, p 55.

chlorhydria is not only pain but pyloric spasm—for the reasons stated above. In both types the food is retained too long in the stomach and pancreatic digestion cannot begin, but the cause and, therefore, the treatment is different.

In the sthenic type the administration of hydrochloric acid will only aggravate the patient's sufferings. Here alkalies after food are clearly called for. Perhaps the best method of administering them is by means of the bismuth lozenges (B.P.), which should be slowly sucked, as recommended by Sir William Roberts. In this way not only is a sedative and an antacid taken but a large quantity of alkaline saliva is swallowed. Leonard Williams advocates bismuth subnitrate, gr. xv, with cerium oxalate, gr. x, in a cachet after food. The pain is relieved, the pyloric sphincter relaxes, and pancreatic digestion can proceed.

Thus, though we must not influence pancreatic activity directly by means of secretin injections, we can do so indirectly by regulating the hydrochloric acid in the stomach.

Secretin and diabetes.—Dale has shown that after repeated injections of secretin the intertubular clumps in the pancreas are greatly increased in number. It is strongly maintained by some observers that these clumps are the seat of disease in pancreatic diabetes. It is reasonable, then, to try secretin in diabetes, but Spriggs found no benefit from this treatment. The easiest way of giving secretin by mouth would, of course, be by feeding the patient on tripe—and no doubt we shall yet hear of the "tripe cure" of diabetes. But this would hardly be "rational organo-therapy," for we have no reason to believe that secretin is absorbed from the alimentary canal.

Iodothyrine as a hormone.—Thyroid preparations are absorbed readily from the alimentary canal, probably because the gland used formerly to discharge its secretion into this canal through the thyroglossal duct. This simplifies the therapeutic application of iodothyrin, which we may regard as a hormone having a specific action on the central nervous system and on the skin and subcutaneous tissues. Its success in the treatment of cretinism, myxœdema, and various skin affections confirms this view. I do not propose to dwell on these points, which are familiar to all.

The effect of iodothyrine on metabolism is that it reduces weight, one sixth of the loss being due to increased nitrogenous waste, the remainder being due simply to the marked diuresis it causes. It may produce glycosuria. It is, therefore, not very effective in the treatment of obesity, and its use is not free from danger, as a fatty heart may not be able to maintain the accelerated rhythm.

I wish, however, to call attention to its effect on the metabolism of the liver and a practical application thereof.

Apart from the discoloration, the chief sufferings of a jaundiced patient are due to the bile-salts circulating in the blood, for they cause:

(1) The intense itching which is so troublesome.

(2) The slow pulse and depression.

(3) Headache.

(4) Small subcutaneous hæmorrhages.

Now it has been found that after ligature of the bile-duct there is an increase of colloid in the follicles and lymphatics of the thyroid gland. It appeared possible that this was a defensive step against intoxication by bile-salts, and accordingly Gilbert and Herscher * administered thyroid extract to seven cases of jaundice ; in six the pruritus was benefited.

The only reliable qualitative test for bile-salts in urine is, of course, Hay's test—*i. e.* their presence lowers the surface tension so much that flowers of sulphur sink through the fluid. The urine must be cold. Under thyroid treatment this reaction gradually diminished and then disappeared. After cessation of treatment the reaction returned until thyroid extract was again administered. They concluded that thyroid extract must modify or destroy the bile salts. Outside the body they did not find that thyroid has any effect on bile salts.

This point seemed to me worthy of further investigation. At the outset it was necessary to have some method of estimating bile-salts in urine, and for this purpose I have employed Grünbaum's method of counting the number of drops discharged from a 2-c.c. pipette fitted with a rock quartz nozzle. With urines diluted to a uniform specific gravity of 1010, the number of drops discharged will be proportional to the surface tension, which will depend on the percentage of bile-salts.

For the details of calibration I must refer you to Grünbaum's paper.† I can confirm Gilbert and Herscher's statement that the administration of

* ' Compt. Rend. Soc. de Biol.,' Paris, 1902, liv, p. 1087.
† ' Path. Soc. Trans.,' 1904.

thyroid extract diminished the amount of bile-salts in the urine with great relief of pruritus.

I found that on keeping urine with a known amount of bile-salts at the body temperature and comparing it with a similar mixture to which I had added iodothyrin that the iodothyrin did not destroy a perceptible amount of bile-salts, though a small amount did disappear on prolonged heating in a water-bath. Similarly, iodothyrin had no destructive effect on bile-salts ad ed to blood even after incubation for twenty-four hours.

Evidently one must look to the liver itself for an explanation ; is it possible that iodothyrin inhibits the formation of bile-salts by the liver ? To test this I gave a cat weighing 7 lb. iodothyrin and sometimes elixir of thyroid with its food for a week : under chloroform and ether a cannula was introduced into the gall-bladder, the common bile-duct clamped, and the bile collected for an hour, during which time seven injections of bile-free secretin were given to stimulate the flow of bile. The bile-salts were then estimated and found to amount to ·026 grams. In a control cat weighing 6 lb. 2 oz., which had had a similar diet without iodothyrin, ·067 grams were secreted under similar conditions in an hour. This strongly suggests that iodothyrin positively diminishes the formation of bile-salts and provides us with a rational method of diminishing the disagreeable symptoms in jaundice due to their presence in the circulation.

Of the last two instances of hormones I shall speak very briefly, for I have no first-hand knowledge of them, and for further particulars I must refer you to Professor Starling's ' Croonian Lectures.'

Ovary.—Marshall and Jolly believe that the changes in the uterus which determine menstruation are due, not to ovulation, but to an internal secretion arising from the ovary, probably from its interstitial cells. Extirpation of the ovaries in early pregnancy prevents the fixation of the ovum, and Fraenkel states that the destruction of the corpora lutea by the galvano-cautery is as efficacious as total removal of the ovaries in bringing pregnancy to an end. Now, the corpora lutea are also derived from the interstitial cells of the ovary. It would appear that these provide a secretion which is essential to the activity of the uterine mucosa. In animals where the ovaries have been removed the phenomena of heat may be reinduced by the injection of ovarian extracts.

It is highly probable that such extracts or extracts of corpora lutea might be useful in those cases where abortion occurs repeatedly in the early months of pregnancy.

Mammary gland.—Why should the mammary gland undergo hypertrophy in pregnancy and become functionally active as soon as pregnancy terminates? No nervous connection has been made out between the uterus and other glands, and a chemical stimulant appeared to several observers the most probable agent. Professor Starling and Miss Lane-Claypon have apparently found this in the fœtus. Extracts of the fœtus injected into virgin rabbits led to distinct hypertrophy of the mammary glands ; in multiparous but not pregnant animals the injection caused a distinct secretion of milk.

The active principle is contained in all parts of the fœtus, apparently resists boiling, and can be passed through a Berkefeld filter. To the possible practical applications of these observations I need not refer here ; they are entirely for the future.

In this hurried survey I have not attempted to consider exhaustively all the conditions in which organic extracts have been applied and with what measure of success—it is sufficient if I have been able to indicate the lines on which we must proceed towards a rational system of organo-therapeutics. Much of the work is quite new and many points await confirmation, so that my remarks must aim at being suggestive rather than conclusive.

But I believe that the hormones offer a profitable field for pharmacological research. It is only by an exact knowledge of the bodily processes in health that we can learn to intervene effectively in disease. And what can be more rational than to use those very drugs in disease by which the body is enabled to do its own work in health ?

December 11th, 1905.

In cases of congenital dislocation of the hip, Klapp (*Centralblatt für Chirurgie*, No. 37, Sept. 16th, 1905) applies a flat piece of board over the hip and leaves the central part of it uncovered by plaster bandage, in order to take an X-ray picture of the joint after reposition, to make sure of the presence of the head of the femur in the acetabulum. The method has no disadvantages as far as the patient is concerned.—*Therapeutic Gazette*, 3rd series, vol. xxi, No. 11.

THE TREATMENT OF CONGENITAL TALIPES.*

By H. A. T. FAIRBANK, M.S.Lond., F.R.C.S.Eng.

Surgical Registrar, Charing Cross Hospital, and Surgical Clinical Assistant, Hospital for Sick Children, Great Ormond Street, W.C.

MR PRESIDENT AND GENTLEMEN,—Before proceeding to the subject proper of this paper, perhaps I may be allowed to refer briefly to the occurrence, varieties, and anatomy of this class of deformity. Congenital talipes is by no means rare ; it forms about 18 per cent. of all congenital deformities ; it is met with at least once in every thousand births. The deformity occurs nearly twice as frequently in boys as in girls. In nearly half the cases both feet are affected, and in over 90 per cent. of these the deformity is the same on the two sides. When only one foot is at fault, the right foot is rather more commonly the seat of the trouble. In a few cases (4 per cent. Waller, quoted by Whitman [1]) some other deformity is present, such as hare-lip, spina bifida, etc. I will not trouble you with any of the theories that have been advanced as to the cause of the deformity, but in this connection I should like to mention two deformities which occasionally accompany talipes. The first is the absence of one of the bones of the leg. The fibula is more frequently absent than the tibia. Absence of the former naturally leads to severe valgus, while suppression of the latter is associated with varus. When the tibia is at fault the chance of making a useful limb is extremely small. The other deformity is spina bifida. Paralysis of the legs may or may not be present. The association of the two deformities seems to be a mere coincidence ; paralysis, if present, has nothing to do with the formation of the talipes, though deformity may result from it later. The feet should be treated according to the principles set forth below.

As to the varieties of talipes most commonly met with at birth, three fourths of the cases belong to the group equino-varus. Next in order of frequency we find cases of calcaneo-valgus—the exact opposite of the previous deformity—calcaneus alone, and valgus alone. A pure equinus is the rarest of all.

---

* A paper read before the Southend on-Sea and District Medical Society.

Speaking generally, the cases of equino-varus are more severe, are more difficult to treat, and are more prone to relapse than are any of the other varieties. The following anatomical points may be briefly recalled, as bearing on the treatment of these cases:

(1) The deformity is a distortion capable of complete cure if treated early.

(2) There is no paralysis of muscles. Certain muscles are shortened, others are stretched. The shortened muscles are irritable, and have a tendency to spasmodic contraction. The opposing muscles are somewhat weak, and tend to become weaker from disuse.

(3) At first the limb is well nourished, but if the case is neglected the muscles waste from disuse.

(4) The bones are more or less deformed even at birth in all but the mildest cases; but the bones, being largely cartilaginous in infancy, are readily moulded to their normal shape, if over-correction of the deformity be maintained sufficiently long.

(5) Certain ligaments are shortened.

Apart from the distortion of the foot there is one deformity which deserves mention, and that is inward rotation of the leg occurring with talipes equino-varus. This rotation of the leg often persists after the deformity of the foot has been corrected, and it calls for special treatment, for not only is it unsightly, but it also predisposes to relapse. If a man with normal feet turns his toes in, his feet tend to assume a position of slight varus, while, at the same time, the arch of the foot is increased. The rotation may take place anywhere between the hip and ankle-joints. It usually takes place between the knee and ankle, the tibia and fibula being twisted in a spiral manner. Whitman (2) says the rotation takes place, in the majority of cases, in the knee-joint. In some cases laxity of the ligaments of the knee-joint accounts for most of the rotation. Genu valgum may co-exist with talipes at birth, but more especially is it acquired later, if the case be untreated.

With these introductory remarks I now pass to the treatment of the various forms of talipes.

All authorites agree that in all but the mildest cases treatment must be continued for several years. For long after the deformity has been corrected the child requires careful supervision, so that the slightest sign of relapse may be recognised and dealt with at once.

In every case we have to do three things:

(1) To correct, and to overcorrect, the deformity.

(2) To retain the foot in the corrected position till the muscles have regained their balance and the bones have acquired their normal shape.

(3) To correct any accompanying deformity, such as rotation of the leg, genu valgum, etc.

Two factors in the treatment cannot be overestimated; these are—(a) commencing treatment early, and (b) continuing the treatment and supervision of the cases for years.

I will not trouble you with the outlines of the many methods of treatment which are adopted by various surgeons, but I will rather describe in detail one of these methods. I venture to think that success is more easily achieved by this method, more especially in the hands of those whose experience of orthopædic surgery is necessarily limited, than by any other method. The method is essentially one of gradual correction of the deformity; the apparatus used is of the simplest, and is readily removed and re-applied. The contracted tissues, if not divided with the knife, are stretched rather than torn, with the result that little scar-tissue is formed. The more scar-tissue there is formed the greater the tendency to relapse of the deformity by contraction of that scar-tissue, and the greater the difficulty experienced in dealing with a relapse, should such occur (Tubby [3]).

Plaster of Paris is used by many with success, but it has been my experience that this method of fixation of the foot requires much greater skill than does any other method.

It is no easy matter to apply a plaster-of-Paris bandage to a baby's foot sufficiently tight to control the foot without causing undue pressure on one or more points of the skin.

The advantage of using a splint which the mother can remove with ease is obvious when we remember that it is impossible to keep any apparatus applied to an infant's legs from being soiled by excreta.

I would suggest that plaster of Paris be reserved for cases in which the parents are unusually ignorant or careless. Another advantage of the use of removable splints is that massage and manipulation can be carried out daily. The principles of this treatment I learnt from Mr. A. H. Tubby, for whose kindness in demonstrating his methods to me I cannot be sufficiently grateful. Talipes equino-varus forms the bulk of the cases, so this may with advantage be considered first. The treatment of this deformity will serve to indicate the line of treatment to be adopted in all.

It is convenient to divide the cases into groups according to the severity of the deformity in each. We may, therefore, divide the cases into the four following groups :

(1) The mild cases, which respond readily to treatment.

(2) The severe cases, which require tenotomies, etc.

(3) Relapsed cases, and cases that have been neglected.

(4) Inveterate cases in adolescents and adults.

In this deformity, equino-varus, the foot is, of course, adducted and inverted, and at the same time the foot is extended, or plantar-flexed.

Many infants normally hold .their feet inverted, but in these there is no limitation of evertion—*i. e.* there is no shortening of tendons or ligaments. In the mildest cases of varus the foot can be brought into line with the leg or even slightly everted, but the moment the foot is released it springs back to its faulty position. The equinus is also slight—*i. e.* dorsiflexion is but slightly limited. These cases may be treated successfully by manipulation and fixation on a simple straight malleable iron splint. This splint is easily bent to fit the leg, and its shape is altered as the deformity improves.

It is fixed in the antero-external aspect of the leg and foot by a calico bandage, which should take a couple of turns round the leg before the splint is applied. The mother or nurse is taught to manipulate the foot in two definite directions. For the first manipulation the heel and ankle are grasped firmly with the fingers and thumb of one hand, while the other grasps the fore part of the foot ; the latter is then gently but firmly turned outwards, and at the same time everted, as far as possible, and held in the corrected position for some moments, and then let go. This movement is repeated again and again, the utmost possible correction being obtained each time : The second manipulation is then performed as follows : The malleoli are grasped in one hand, while the other seizes the foot and dorsiflexes it as far as possible, holds it in the corrected position, and then lets go. This movement is also repeated many times. The

leg and foot are then carefully massaged, special attention being paid to the muscles on the outer side of the leg. In manipulating the foot the pressure must be steady, and as much as possible of the hand should be employed in grasping the foot so as to avoid hurting the child. If the manipulations are roughly performed, or are too violent, the shortened muscles contract reflexly and make further manipulation at the time useless. The child should not be made to cry.

The manipulation and massage being finished, the malleable iron splint is bent to the required angle and applied to the antero-external aspect of the limb, the foot being held in as good a position as possible. When the varus is fully corrected the splint may be bent to a right angle and applied to the back of the leg ; the equinus is controlled better in this way. Two or three times a day the splint is removed, and the manipulations and massage repeated. On each occasion the mother should spend at least a quarter of an hour manipulating one foot. Day by day the foot is further corrected, till full over-correction is obtained. The treatment must be continued till all tendency for the foot to return to its faulty position has disappeared. In the mildest cases the child may be completely cured before he learns to walk. In others the foot may still need watching after walking has commenced. In such cases it is well to manipulate the foot every night, and let the child wear a splint during sleep. In a few cases it may be found that the equinus cannot be completely corrected by this method, though the varus gives way without difficulty. Tenotomy of the tendo-Achillis will then be required. The tin shoe, to be mentioned later, may be used for the mild cases, especially when the equinus is obstinate, though I prefer the straight splint for the correction of the varus. A few of these mild cases may require a boot with irons for walking, but the majority will not require this. We now pass to the ordinary case of some severity, in which the deformity is marked. This class includes all those seen in early infancy, and which cannot be cured without division of some at least of the resistant structures. No hard and fast line can be drawn between mild and severe cases ; every surgeon has his own views on the subject. My practice is to make use of tenotomy in any case in which the foot cannot be brought into line with the leg by ordinary pressure with the fingers. The varus should be corrected first, the equinus left till later.

By leaving the tendo-Achillis undivided in the first stage of the treatment, we have a *point d'appui* for correction of the varus. Moreover the mother or nurse has to learn only one manipulation to begin with. During the first week or two of life simple manipulations may be employed. In the third week, if the child be in good condition, tenotomy may be performed. Mr. Tubby (4) says tenotomy is a justifiable operation in the first week of life. What structures are to be divided? I always divide the tibialis anticus tendon and the inner band of the plantar fascia, and very often the anterior part of the internal lateral ligament of the ankle. These may all be divided through the same puncture of the skin, to the inner side of the tibial tendon. Most writers on orthopædics divide the tibialis posticus in almost all these cases. Judging from my experience, I do not think it is necessary to divide this tendon so often. The tendon is best divided above the internal malleolus, through an open incision. Other structures which may require division are the extensor proprius hallucis, the abductor hallucis, and the flexor longus digitorum. The tenotomies having been done, a pad of gauze is placed over the puncture and a rather firm bandage applied ; the foot is then fixed in its *faulty* position by means of the malleable iron splint, bent to a suitable angle. The splint is removed after four days, and bent in the opposite direction before being re-applied and the daily manipulations commenced.

The mother is directed to remove the splint every morning and evening, and manipulate the foot outwards in the manner already indicated, and thoroughly massage the leg. The case should be seen at least twice a week at first, to make sure the mother understands her part of the treatment. When the foot can be fully abducted and everted without undue force being used, the second stage, or correction of the equinus, may be commenced. The first stage usually lasts about four weeks. It may last three months if the case is a severe one or the mother rather stupid or careless. The tendo-Achillis is now divided subcutaneously ; the foot is put up with the varus corrected, but with the equinus still present, for four days. In some cases the posterior ligament of the ankle also requires division. Then the foot is gradually brought up by manipulations and the use of some simple fixation apparatus. I use one of two splints. The better is Adams' varus splint, which is quite simple, and yet it absolutely controls the foot. The other is a tin shoe, with a quadrant, so that the degree of flexion of the ankle may be altered. This is very useful for the milder cases and is particularly useful in hospital practice, as it is by far the cheaper of the two instruments. But for severe cases Adams' apparatus is the better. Although more complicated, it can be removed, replaced, and even adjusted by the mother or nurse. It has also some control over the internal rotation of the leg if such be present. The strap passing over the front of the ankle is fixed first, so that the heel is " well down." It is also useful to have the sole-plate extended and to screw it up after the heel is fixed, especially in the early stages of treatment. The control obtained by this instrument over the adduction of the foot is excellent. The tin shoe is fixed to the limb by a bandage. Whatever apparatus be used, it is removed two or three times a day, and massage and manipulation performed as before. This treatment is continued till the child is allowed to walk—*i. e.* till about the end of the second year, though the equinus is usually corrected in from four to six weeks. If the case proves obstinate, or if the deformity be allowed to relapse, owing perhaps to interruption of treatment during illness, the foot may need wrenching under an anæsthetic. The padded wedge used by Lorenz for these cases and for the reduction of congenital dislocation of the hip will be found useful. The foot is laid on its outer side on the wedge, and the force applied with the hands to the fore and back part of the foot. Damage is more likely to be done while overcoming the equinus. In nearly all cases it is advisable to order a surgical boot and iron for walking purposes. In cases without any internal rotation of the leg the irons need not be extended beyond the knee. A varus T-strap is always used. In the worst cases a light toe-elevating spring may be added, with a stop to prevent over-dorsiflexion, while in the milder cases a back-stop to prevent plantar-flexion may be sufficient. In the majority of the cases it is well to continue the inner iron to the upper part of the thigh, while the outer iron is continued to a pelvic band. A ring catch at the knee-joint with double knee-caps is also useful.

By means of this large apparatus the internal rotation of the limb, wherever this rotation may have taken place, is controlled, and as the child grows gradually corrected. Laxity of the ligaments at the knee and hyperextension at this joint are also dealt with by this apparatus, which, by means of the knee-caps, restricts the movements of the knee-joint.

This apparatus must be worn for a year at least and often for three or more years. At night a simple rectangular tin shoe, without a quadrant, must be used, and it is well to manipulate the foot as of old every night. The cause of relapse is leaving off treatment too early : the more severe the case the longer must the case be watched.

One more word with regard to the rotation of the bones of the leg. If this be present—and it usually is present—something may be done to correct it before the walking apparatus is employed. The upper and lower ends of the tibia and fibula are seized by the two hands, and an attempt made to twist the lower ends outwards (R. Jones [5]). This manipulation may be included in the daily routine of massage, etc. Osteotomy of the tibia and fibula has been performed for this deformity (Tubby [6] and Swan [7]).

We now pass to the cases in which treatment has been neglected till after walking has commenced, or in which relapse of the deformity has occurred. Rigidity of the foot is a feature of these cases, particularly those that have relapsed. Spasm of the shortened muscles has been induced by walking, and in the relapsed cases the resisting structures are more or less welded together. Perhaps no bands of plantar fascia stand out, inviting division of the tenotome.

Some of these feet can be successfuly treated by the method already detailed. Forcible wrenching under anæsthesia on more than one occasion will probably be necessary. Thomas's wrench may be used with advantage, though it is not absolutely necessary. A more powerful appliance than those mentioned above — e.g. some form of Scarpa's shoe—may be necessary. In spite of all we can do by these methods some cases will still remain imperfectly corrected. The deformity of the bones is is too much for us. The operations that have been devised for these cases are numerous. I believe that—with no method can it be said that relapse is impossible—Phelps' opera-

tion, which involves division of all the resisting tissues on the inner side of the foot down to the bones, does not seem to have found much favour in this country, though Mr. Muirhead Little (8) speaks well of it in selected cases. The formation of a large wound, which heals by granulation, and is necessarily followed by the formation of a large amount of scar-tissue which has a strong tendency to contract, seems to me to invite relapse. Covering the wound with a skin flap or grafts does not appear to do away with this tendency. Mr. Arbuthnot Lane's (9) operation of subcutaneous division of everything on the inner side of the foot together with all the structures behind the internal malleolus, is considered unnecessarily severe by many orthopædic surgeons. Division of the chief resisting structures, tendons, fasciæ, and ligaments will form part of the treatment in all cases. Beyond this two operations appear to offer the best prospect of restoring the foot to its proper shape without interfering with its functions. These are (a) removal of the astragalus, (Lund's [10] operation), and (b) Ogston's (11) operation.

Astragalectomy would seem to be called for in cases in which equinus forms the chief part of the remaining deformity. In these cases the shape of the superior articular surface of the astragalus plays a part in the prevention of dorsiflexion to the normal extent. The anterior part of this surface is too wide to pass between the malleoli. Astragalectomy removes this difficulty at once, and at the same time allows the varus to be further corrected. The operation which Professor Ogston described in 1902 depends on the fact that for the first few years of life the tarsal bones consist of a shell of cartilage surrounding a bony nucleus. The operation consists in incising the cartilaginous envelope and scooping out the contained bone. The foot is then forcibly corrected, the cartilaginous shells being crushed. The advantage of this operation over cuneiform tarsectomy lies in the fact that the small joints of the tarsus are not interfered with, so the elasticity of the foot remains unimpaired. The astragalus, cuboid, and anterior part of the os calcis are treated in this way. I have some skiagrams here showing the condition of the tarsal bones at various ages.

Professor Ogston says this operation may be performed up to six years of age or even later.

Every case must, of course, be treated on its own

merits. Some surgeons never operate upon the bones before about twelve years of age.

Of the treatment of inveterate cases I need say little. The use of Scarpa's shoe, with frequent wrenching, combined with or followed by tarsotomy or tarsectomy, may eventually render the foot fairly useful.

Now let me say a few words with regard to the treatment of the less common varieties of congenital talipes. The calcaneo-valgus and calcaneus cases are, as a rule, of a mild type, and rarely call for tenotomies. In these cases the tendency to relapse is small. Manipulations in the direction of inversion and plantar flexion, with or without the use of a malleable iron splint, will generally suffice to cure the deformity before the child is old enough to walk. In cases of pure valgus the peronei may require division, if the deformity is severe, and when the child begins to walk a boot and iron will be necessary. The sole of the boot should be thickened slightly along the inner side, with the inner part of the heel carried forwards. A valgus pad and a valgus T-strap buckling round the outside iron complete the apparatus. In milder cases thickening the sole along the inner side and carrying the heel forwards will often be sufficient.

Pure varus is rare ; its treatment has already been considered.

In cases of absence of the fibula the valgus should be corrected, and later a boot with an outside iron and valgus T-strap ordered. The leg will be considerably shorter than the other. In conclusion, I venture to state that the secret of success in the treatment of all these, often troublesome, deformities is perseverance.

REFERENCES.

(1) 'Orthopædic Surgery,' 1904, p. 743.

(2) Op. cit., p. 745.

(3) 'Deformities,' 1896, p. 397.

(4) Op. cit., p. 400.

(5) Quoted by Tubby, op. cit., p. 425.

(6) Op. cit., p. 426.

(7) 'British Medical Journal,' June 15th, 1895.

(8) Ibid., 1903, p. 977.

(9) 'Lancet,' 1893, p. 432.

(10) 'British Medical Journal,' 1872.

(11) Ibid., 1902, p. 1524.

December 11th, 1905.

THE PRINCIPLES OF CLINICAL PATHOLOGY. By LUDOLF KREHL. Translated from the third German edition by ALBION WALTER HEWLETT, M.D., with an Introduction by WM. OSLER, M.D. 1904. Philadelphia and London : J. B. Lippincott Company. 21s. net.

THIS is a book which it is a genuine pleasure to read, for all throughout it makes the reader consider what the phenomena of disease really mean. We can strongly recommend it to anyone who takes a genuine interest in his profession. There is much matter in a small space, but the condensation does not make it too hard to understand for everyone who reads it seriously and is already familiar with the subjects of which it treats. The chapters on the heart, the blood, and fever are perhaps the best, but all the abnormal manifestations of the body are considered. The main fault of the book should be to English readers an attraction, for Prof. Krehl has almost entirely neglected all American and English work, and therefore we in this country derive a good bird's-eye-view summary of German opinion. As an example of it may be mentioned that when discussing variations in the volume of the blood Prof. Krehl does not allude to Lorrain Smith's work. An instance of similar kind is the failure to refer to the French work on the relations of chloride of sodium to œdema, but the editor has inserted a short account of this. A glance at the references at the bottom of the pages show that they are almost entirely German. This may wound our pride, but it is good for our education, especially when, as is the case with some of the teaching in the book, we feel that a view different to that of the author may be true, or, on the other hand, we recognise that our accustomed explanation is not as good as his. This translation will, indeed, as Prof. Osler says, " be most helpful to all students and teachers who wish to know the scientific basis of our art," and it raises the science of medicine to a higher plane than most of the books which are written.

THE CLINICAL JOURNAL,

CLINICAL RECORD, CLINICAL NEWS, CLINICAL GAZETTE, CLINICAL REPORTER, CLINICAL CHRONICLE AND CLINICAL REVIEW.

EDITED BY L. ELIOT CREASY.

No. 686. WEDNESDAY, DECEMBER 20, 1905. Vol. XXVII. No. 10.

CONTENTS.

* *Specially reported for the Clinical Journal. Revised by the Author.*

ALL RIGHTS RESERVED.

NOTICE.

Editorial correspondence, books for review, &c., should be addressed to the Editor, 51, New Cavendish Street, W., Telephone No. 904, Paddington; but all business communications should be addressed to the Publishers, 22½, Bartholomew Close, London, E.C. Telephone 927, Holborn.

All inquiries respecting Advertisements should be sent to MESSRS. ADLARD & SON, *Bartholomew Close, E.C. Telephone 927, Holborn.*

Terms of Subscription, including postage, payable by cheque, postal or banker's order (in advance) : for the United Kingdom, 15s. 6d. per annum : Abroad 17s. 6d.

Cheques, &c., should be made payable to THE PROPRIETORS OF THE CLINICAL JOURNAL, *crossed "The London, City, and Midland Bank, Ltd., Newgate Street Branch, E.C. Account of the Medical Publishing Company, Ltd."*

Reading Cases to hold Twenty-six Numbers of THE CLINICAL JOURNAL *can be supplied at 2s. 3d. each, or will be forwarded post free on receipt of 2s. 6d. ; and also Cases for Binding Volumes at 1s. each, or post free on receipt of 1s. 3d., from the Publishers, 22½, Bartholomew Close, London, E.C.*

A CLINICAL LECTURE

ON

THE DIAGNOSIS OF PNEUMONIA.

By W. P. HERRINGHAM, M.D., F.R.C.P., Physician to the Hospital.

GENTLEMEN,—In a clinical lecture which I gave you recently I tried to impress upon you the fact that although we were perfectly right to be exceedingly careful in testing and observing the physical signs of heart disease, yet when all was said and done, the most important symptoms for prognosis and for treatment were not those usually called physical signs, which rather point to the actual disease of the valves, but those more general symptoms that show us the condition of the cardiac wall, affections of the myocardium as distinct from the conditions of the valves. And in this lecture I want to take up a similar subject, and to tell you that although in most cases the diagnosis between pneumonia and other somewhat similar diseases of the lungs is comparatively easy to those who are careful over their physical signs, yet you will find a considerable number of cases in which physical signs alone will not be sufficient for you to form your diagnosis upon.

I suppose that all of you here know quite well the typical presentment of a medical case of acute or lobar pneumonia. You know that a man will come to you saying that at such and such a time in the day he was perfectly well, or that he went to bed perfectly well one night, when he was suddenly taken with a shivering attack, possibly accompanied by an attack of vomiting, and that he had sudden pain in the side and that from that time onward he has felt very ill, that he has probably been obliged to be in bed, that he has had a cough which has hurt him and given him a pain in his side, that he has been very feverish, and perhaps that within a day or two of his first attack he noticed an eruption upon his face. If you ask him, he will probably tell you that he has been bringing up some blood when he coughed. When you come to examine him you find a remarkably high temperature, and if you watch it for a few days you find the tempera- ture does not vary ; it keeps at 103° or 104°. You will find that his pulse is very quick, and that his respiration is even quicker than it should be in ratio to his pulse. In no other disease do you get the ratio of respiration for pulse so high. Then you will find that he has probably spat up a certain amount of bloody sputum, that his complexion is very dusky, and that his skin is burning hot. All these things are familiar to you in any ordinary case of acute pneumonia.

And when you come to examine him physically you find, as a rule, first of all that his affected side is perhaps larger than the other side, and that it is not moving so well. Secondly you will notice when you put your hand on the chest that the vocal vibrations on the affected side are increased, that the percussion note is diminished, that the breath sounds are loud and roaring, that there is bronchial breathing and bronchophony and that the vocal resonance is increased. When you get a case like that it is perfectly true, as is constantly said in text-books, that there is no disease so easy to diagnose as acute pneumonia.

But I want you to remember that in a great many cases—more than many of you would believe —these signs do not fall into their regular place, and that if you rely upon the physical signs alone you will be misled. That is perhaps not so difficult to understand if you come to analyse what the meaning of the different physical signs is. Of course the enlargement of the chest is nothing peculiar to pneumonia. It may happen that it is due to pneumonic enlargement of the lung itself in consequence of the stuffing up of the tubes and cells by inflammatory products. But it may equally happen that it is due to enlargement as a result of malignant disease, a thing which is easily separated by the absence of fever, or, which is a more common difficulty, that it is due to a pleural effusion between the lung and the chest wall. In either case the intercostal spaces will be flattened, and in some cases will even, perhaps, bulge. The absence of movement of the chest wall is equally common to various diseases. It is due to the inability of the lung to be filled with air and to expand. That may be caused either by the

stuffing up of the lung itself by inflammatory products or it may be due to its complete collapse under the pressure of fluid. So on the inspection of the chest the signs are common to two quite different diseases.

When we come to palpation of the chest we are constantly impressing upon you that vocal vibrations are increased in pneumonia and diminished in pleural effusion. But in many cases it is not so. What is the meaning of vocal vibrations being increased ? Vocal vibrations are the vibrations which you make in your larynx, conducted down through your pipes and damped on their way to the chest wall by the vesicular structure of the lung, and therefore vocal vibrations are less palpable lower down than in the throat. If you put your fingers on the larynx, you will feel a thrill much more plainly there than if you put them on the chest wall. The fact that it is damped down on its way to the chest wall proves that the vesicular structure of the lung is a bad conductor to these vibrations. We know as a matter of experience—and one would not have known it except as a matter of experience, because there is no a priori reason why it should be so—that lung consolidated by inflammation is a better conductor of these vibrations than natural lung, and as a matter of common rule it is perfectly true that a pneumonic lung conducts vocal vibrations better than a natural one. But we do not know why it is so. And when we come to look at the excep- tions we are very much puzzled. We suppose naturally that pneumonic lung is a better con- ductor because it is solid, just as a bit of wood is a better conductor than pneumonic lung. But there are two exceptions, or rather, two exceptions com- monly acknowledged. One is when the tubes of the lungs are filled with a sort of fibrinous coagulum. That I have seen several times in the post-mortem room in a lung which in life was a bad conductor. There were bad vocal vibrations in the chest, and the bronchi were found to be filled with fibri- nous coagula at their entrance. Another exception which is acknowledged is what is called a massive coagulation of the lung, by which I suppose is meant a very large or a very close inflammatory exudation. That is, again, a bad conductor. But why should that be ? If a pneumonic lung con- ducts better because it is solid, why should a more solid pneumonic lung conduct worse ? Moreover, there are other cases. For instance, in the early stage of pneumonia one frequently finds that the lung does not conduct vibrations well. Neither of those explanations, if they are explanations, can apply to that. So, just as I do not believe we know why a pneumonic lung conducts better than an ordinary lung, so I do not think we know why these exceptions conduct worse. I only wish to bring them before you because I want you to remember that there are a certain number of cases in which this sign of increased vocal vibration is absent in pneumonia.

The next sign is that of the percussion note. Of course the resonant percussion note over ordinary lung is due to the lung itself. You can test that in the post-mortem room by percussing a patient's lung cut out on the table, and you will find that natural lung is resonant and a pneumonic lung is dull. That is exactly the same on the chest wall. The percussion note is impaired, whether you get the dull lung against the chest wall as in a case of pneumonia, or whether you get dull, collapsed lung cut off from the chest wall by fluid. But when you are percussing fluid and dull lung, as in pleural effusion, the percussion note is very much more stony than the percussion note over pneumonia. And you are constantly being told in the wards that the amount of dulness is a considerable help in forming a diagnosis between pneumonia and pleural effusion. That, I think, is because a pneumonic lung contains more air than a collapsed lung due to pleural effusion.

A second thing which you find in percussion, but which you cannot hear with your ears, though you can feel it with your fingers, is a sense of resistance. There is a great difference between pleural effusion and pneumonia in this respect. In pneumonia the chest wall is still resilient and elastic, and it gives under your finger as you percuss. But when you percuss a chest-wall over effusion it is not so; it is more like percussing a brick wall because it is so resistant. The reason for that is not at all difficult to understand. There is nothing so incompressible as fluids; and if you get fluid under a chest-wall it simply cannot go in or out, it is an inert wall; it cannot possibly vibrate and give you any sense of resiliency and elasticity, which it can perfectly well do so long as it has only got solid lung beneath it.

Then we come to the signs of auscultation.

You are always told—and it is perfectly true as a general rule—that in pleural effusion the sounds are very weak, but that in pneumonia there is loud bronchial breathing. But there are exceptions on both sides of the line. I have heard some pleural effusions over which there was loud bronchial breathing, and I am familiar with a large number of cases of pneumonia in which there is hardly any breathing to be heard at all. Therefore the signs may be reversed: you may get a pneumonia with the auscultatory signs of pleural effusion, and you may get a pleural effusion with the auscultatory signs of pneumonia. What the meaning of that is we do not certainly know. I suppose it is that whereas as a rule in pleural effusion no air reaches the collapsed lung, and therefore no breathing is heard over it, yet there may be certain exceptions in which the lung is partially collapsed and breathing is heard over it to a certain extent. The meaning of pneumonia with weak breathing we do not know, unless it be that the tubes are plugged by fibrinous coagula such as I mentioned in connection with vocal vibration.

The mixture of these different signs therefore makes you sometimes have exceedingly difficult cases to diagnose. During the last year I have had at least eight or ten cases in which we were in considerable doubt. The first, which I remember very well, was that of a young woman who was in for appendicitis, was operated upon, got suppuration in the wound, subsequently had parotitis, and then an attack in her lungs, for which I was called to see her. She had a temperature which was not typical of pneumonia, it was a temperature of about 102°; she was very ill and with considerable dyspnœa, was very blue—for she had bad heart disease as well—and when I came to examine her lungs I found an immovable chest, entirely absent vocal vibrations on the right side, a perfectly stony dulness, a dulness as stony as any I have ever heard in my life, and an entire absence of breath-sounds. I thought, without the slightest hesitation, that she had pleural effusion, and very possibly empyema, seeing that she had had a good deal of suppuration in other places and was a septic subject. We sought it carefully with tears—the tears of the patient—and explored in several directions. But we found no fluid, and she never had any fluid in her chest, as far as I know. The whole thing was a pneumonic consolidation of the lung, showing no such high state of fever as is usual in pneumococcal cases, because it was a septic case. Her case lasted a long time and she recovered. When the case is surgical and is due to septic absorption it is not, I think, as a rule an empyema or a pleural effusion, but is usually one of pneumonia. That is what I should suspect first.

The next case was that of an elderly woman, æt. 51 years, who was admitted during September last year. She came in with a history of acute onset and "stitch" in her side four days before. Her temperature was perfectly normal, and she had a perfectly slow pulse, not a febrile one. She was comfortable, slept well, and so forth, and when we came to examine her chest we found just the same condition of affairs as in the last case, that of the girl ; that is to say there was dulness, almost stony, and absence of breath sounds We explored her also, and in vain, but in her case there was another symptom, which tended to make the diagnosis of pneumonia easier, and that was green sputum. The sputum of pneumonia is different in different cases. The most common form of pneumonic sputum is coloured rusty. It is exactly the colour of rust. That is the typical sputum of the disease, and when you see that you may not need any other sign. But the sputum in this particular case, as I say, was green, and sometimes what these patients bring up looks like greengage jam. We have had a case in the wards lately in which the sputum was bright yellow, like apricot jam. Both these forms of pneumonic sputum are due to the colouring matter in the blood, but are a variation of the ordinary rusty sputum. And in bad cases, where it is a very congestive form of inflammation, you get that which is known as prune-juice sputum—that is, very darkly coloured hæmorrhagic sputum. In this woman, as I say, we found greengage sputum, which is a fairly diagnostic sign of pneumonia. Her physical signs were indistinguishable from those of pleural effusion.

The next case was that of a man, a drunken meat porter, who came in a little while ago ; and his history was—and it is the case which made me think of giving you this lecture—that he was taken on May 25th with vomiting and shivering and sweating, followed by a cough and pain in his left side. He also had, afterwards, herpes in the face. When we examined his lungs four days later we found he had a diminished percussion note, that the vocal vibrations were entirely absent, and that he had faint bronchial breathing and a crepitant friction sound at his left base. So in that case again, as far as physical signs went, they were confusing as between pneumonia and pleural effusion.

When physical signs are like that, confusing, what have you to go upon ? In the first place you have the general symptoms, and those are always of great importance in a case of pneumonia. Pneumonia is a fever, and if you have acute and general fever in a case of doubtful lung disease, it is far more probable that it will be a case of pneumonia than that it will be anything else. The high temperature, the dusky face, and the very rapid respiration compared with the pulse are typical of cases of pneumonia.

Then you have the further evidence, in cases of large pleural effusion, of displacement of other organs, and that is evidence which is irrefutable. No pneumonia ever displaces the heart or ever pushes down the spleen or the liver. If you get those facts in any case in which you are doubtful whether there is pneumonia or pleural effusion, be sure there is an effusion in the chest. The displacement of other organs is one of the most certain signs of pleural effusion. But, of course, it may be due to something else ; it may be due to a tumour, and continually happens in aneurysm or mediastinal tumour. So do not think every case of displacement is necessarily one of pleural effusion. But if you have no reason to diagnose thoracic tumour, and there is displacement of viscera, you may safely put it down to pleural effusion. Unluckily, it is only the large effusions which displace. Small effusions, just the cases which most resemble pneumonia, cause no displacement.

And, lastly, comes the evidence which you get from paracentesis—that is to say, exploratory puncture of the chest, and that of course is the best test of all. One does not want to do that in every case, but when you are in doubt it is the course to pursue. But even there, how often does one puncture a chest and not find the fluid which is there ! It happened to us the other day. We had a little child whose signs were very doubtful, as they very often are in children, far oftener than in adults, and for several days we were in doubt. We punctured it two or three times, and at last, by poking about—that really is the correct word for it—we did eventually hit upon the purulent pleural effusion, and find the empyema which was at the bottom of the symptoms.

Therefore, I want you to remember that however exact and however true it is as a general rule that the signs of pneumonia are quite distinct from those of pleural effusion, yet there are many cases in which the best of us may be deceived, because the signs are not regular ; and in those cases you have to rely, not upon physical signs only, but also upon general symptoms, and eventually upon Paracentesis thoracis.

December 18th, 1905.

WITH DR. WALDO AT THE BRISTOL ROYAL INFIRMARY.

TWO CASES OF AORTIC ANEURYSM.

GENTLEMEN,—I propose to direct your attention to the important points in connection with two cases of aortic aneurysm which have been under my care in the infirmary during the last few weeks. The subjects are both males in about middle life; one is 54 years of age and the other 51 years. You must have observed that aneurysm seldom occurs in women, and that it is chiefly found in hard-working men. The patient I now show you has been occupied in carrying railway iron on his shoulder. He states that in lifting the rails he has to make a great effort, with his breath held and his chest fixed. It is generally assumed that for an artery to give way under a severe strain there must be some disease in the arterial coats, and the recognised causes of this are thought to be either the abuse of alcohol, or the presence of syphilis, or Bright's disease. I can assure you that neither of these conditions has existed in this case. With the exception of the sacculated aneurysm of the aorta there is no evidence of disease, with the exception of some emphysema of the lungs, and the man has been a total abstainer for many years. His superficial arteries do not show any signs of thickening or degeneration, and it seems impossible to take any other view but that overwork is the only likely cause of his chest trouble. Most probably an arteritis of the aorta was first of all set up, followed by degeneration, but the initial factor was the nature of his work.

In the other case the recognised causes in addition to strain cannot be so surely excluded.

The symptom for which these patients seek admission to hospitals is usually severe pain in the chest, and it was present in this first case to a marked degree, and always increased upon the least exertion. It was located at the site of maximum pulsation, namely under the left clavicle and shot through to the left scapula in the back and down the left arm, accompanied with numbness of fingers. It was of a throbbing character and was always much relieved by the recumbent position. Although this patient has been confined to bed for some time, the pulsation is quite perceptible and the percussion note over it is decidedly dull. There is no diastolic shock to be felt, nor with the stethoscope do you perceive a very accentuated second sound, which is often described in these cases as ringing or clanging. The heart sounds are audible over the tumour as well as a systolic murmur. This aortic systolic murmur is also heard at the second right interspace, where there is some visible pulsation just beside the sternum. In the second case the normal pulsation is in much the same situation, and with the dull note limited to the upper part of the sternum and under the left clavicle, the aneurysmal tumour in both cases springing from the transverse part of the arch or perhaps a little to the left of it. You must not think that the presence or absence of a murmur is of much consequence in diagnosing these conditions. In the second case you may observe there is no murmur present. The pain, as well as all the other symptoms, depends upon pressure exerted by the aneurysmal sac on important structures. If you see one of these cases cured, you will notice how remarkably the sac shrinks and so relieves the contiguous parts from the pressure. Dyspnœa is another pressure symptom which has caused much discomfort and anxiety. This man describes the attacks of short breath as occurring at times only, and chiefly upon exertion. His voice is not clear, and he says that it has changed very much during the last few months. These two symptoms would lead you to examine the larynx, and you would observe the left vocal cord to be quite motionless. You know that the left recurrent laryngeal nerve, a branch of the vagus, winds round the aortic arch, and pressure upon this accounts for the difficult breathing and the husky voice. Dyspnœa may arise from the trachea or one of the bronchi being pressed upon. In the second case there is very feeble breathing all over the left lung, depending, no doubt, upon the left bronchus being involved. When the difficult breathing comes in paroxysms and resembles an asthmatic attack, it mostly means that a vocal cord is paralysed, as in this case. But the trachea is accounting for some of it, as upon one occasion (August 20th last) he coughed up some blood-stained sputum. I asked him if his cough was anything like a child with croup and he said it resembled whooping-cough. This kind of cough is what you would expect with a vocal cord fixed.

This patient has complained of difficulty in

swallowing solids for some long while, and one is justified in coming to the conclusion that this is owing to direct compression from the aneurysmal sac, or indirectly from its setting up spasm. It may be that the left vagus is pressed on in this case, which would account for the motionless vocal cord and the difficulty of swallowing. It is a somewhat rare symptom and is mostly seen when the third part of the aortic arch is the seat of the bulging. If a man consults you for dysphagia, do not attempt to pass a bougie until you have satisfied yourself that aneurysm can be excluded. The pupil of the left eye is slightly contracted and is to be explained by the sympathetic nerve in the neck being irritated, and so causing paresis of the ciliary muscle. It is said to produce pallor, or sweating on one side of the face exceptionally. The flow of blood in the left subclavian artery may be interrupted by the sac from without, or its mouth may be blocked by a piece of fibrin. In some cases the intermittent is converted into a continuous stream and the pulse at the wrist is almost imperceptible. The explanation of this is that the distended aorta acts as a reservoir and so the heart's impulse is lost in this space. Osler reports a case of obliteration of pulse in abdominal aorta and lower limbs. In one of these cases the pulses are equal, in the other the left is the weakest—the sphygmograph shows the difference more accurately than the finger. Retardation of one pulse may also occur. The veins are more or less pressed on in one of these cases, and the patient's hands become œdematous and blue sometimes. Tracheal tugging is only slightly present, but pulsation is transmitted to some extent through the trachea to the hand. This is probably pathognomonic of an aneurysm of the aortic arch.

A radiograph photograph of the thorax gives no distinct shadow. All these means of forming a diagnosis which I have mentioned should be carefully sought for in the case of any male patient in middle life who complains of a constant fixed pain in his chest. Even if you discover a motionless vocal cord you may rightly conclude that the large majority of cases with this condition are primarily owing to an aortic aneurysm.

To give a reliable prognosis in any diseased condition is one of the most difficult problems in he practice of medicine. I must tell you that ie probability of curing an aortic aneurysm is very unlikely, and one is almost always obliged, from former experience, to be a prophet of woe. But I am inclined to prognosticate a favourable termination for this case (the man who was engaged in carrying railway iron), my reasons being that his arterial system appears to be healthy, that he is a total abstainer, and that he is likely to carry out the very trying instructions which it is so necessary to lay down in these cases. In the treatment your object is to induce blood-clotting and consolidation in the aneurysmal sac, which is more likely to occur if you can insure quiet of mind and body. Absolute rest in bed is the most important curative agent, and almost as important is a minimum amount of nourishment provided the patient does not lose much weight. Liquids must be taken in very small quantities, as your wish is to keep down the pressure within the arteries. Many drugs are advocated and I suppose that iodide of potassium has a first place. It certainly appears to relieve pain in these cases, as it does in angina pectoris ; it has been called the opium of the heart, but I am inclined to think it has been much overrated and that it is to the rest that the relief should be chiefly attributed. There is no reason to suppose that the blood clots more readily from any inherent virtue contained in iodides ; on the contrary, I should imagine it would be otherwise. It may assist clotting indirectly by lessening arterial tension, but this is at the expense of causing much depression of spirits, and sometimes even more unpleasant symptoms. There are other drugs which lessen arterial tension better and more effectually than iodides. It has been shown by Wooldridge, who experimented on animals, that a fatty diet is best adapted to produce the formation of clot in an aneurysmal sac, and for this and other reasons I should be inclined to prescribe cod-liver oil twice daily for these patients. But after all the chief thing to enforce is rest, which must be absolute.

It is an important matter to avoid constipation and consequent straining at stool ; and it, therefore, may be good treatment to administer a laxative occasionally, always obliging the patient to use the bed-pan ; but the less of other drugs the better, unless pain persists in spite of the prolonged rest, in which case it may be necessary to give morphia hypodermically. If the veins are pressed on to the extent of producing alarming cyanosis and swelling, the condition may be best relieved by venesection in the arm to a moderate amount. The diet should consist of plain, ordinary food, of which milk may form a part. It has been thought that one reason why patients convalescing from enteric fever so often suffer from thrombosis may be owing to the milk diet they consume, although personally I think it is more likely to arise from toxines circulating in their weak blood-flow.

[Since giving this lecture I have read Professor A. E. Wright's paper in the ' Lancet,' in which he shows that calcium and magnesium salts undoubtedly increase the coagulability of the blood. The man in whose case I have ventured to give a favourable prognosis has now left the infirmary and is under the care of Dr. J. J. S. Lucas, of Bristol, who diagnosed the presence of aneurysm and sent the patient to the infirmary. He intends to carry out Professor Wright's views, and I hope he may be successful in bringing about a cure of this oft incurable condition.]

December 18th, 1905.

A CONSIDERATION OF MEDIAN HERNIA AND ITS OPERATIVE TREATMENT.

By LAWRIE McGAVIN, F.R.C.S.Eng.,
Surgeon to the Seamen's Hospital Society ; Assistant Surgeon to the Hospital for Women, Soho Square.

To those who are in the habit of dealing with the many unfortunate conditions to which the female sex is liable, and especially to those of its members who are reaching or have already entered the fourth decennial period of their lives, the various forms of median hernia, if I may use the term, appear to me to present a ceaseless appeal, and one which has always, I fear, fallen on somewhat barren ground.

For if one considers the wealth of literature which has been lavished upon the question of inguinal and femoral hernia, and the ingenuity of the methods adopted for the treatment of sacs and the closure of canals, one cannot but be struck by the comparative poverty which has attended the efforts, both literary and operative, of our profession in dealing with a condition quite as distressing to its victims as those on which so much time and ingenuity have been expended. It is possibly due to the fact that man not having been condemned to suffer to the same extent from the

condition to which these remarks refer, his companion of the weaker sex has had to await, in this as in many other matters, the awakening of the interest which her condition most justly demands. Those of us who happen to be attached to hospitals reserved exclusively for women perhaps see more of abdominal hernia and the results of its neglect than do others ; and I feel sure that many will agree with me that much more might be done in these cases than is at present attempted, both by practitioners and by surgeons, whereby comfort and increase of years might be secured to many.

The following remarks are suggested to me by an appreciation of these facts, and by many cases which have come under my care, and by many to which I have had access while under the care of other surgeons, during the last six or seven years.

The Classification of Median Herniæ.

I have chosen the term "median" as applied to hernia to include all protrusions of the abdominal viscera in the middle line of the body ; it is therefore made up of two varieties, viz. umbilical and ventral hernia. Now, in casual conversation, and indeed in many text-books, it is commonly the custom to confound these two conditions, no proper distinction being made between them ; but not only are the terms etymologically different, but the conditions to which they refer are, in their anatomy, topography, etiology, prognosis, and to some extent in their treatment, things quite separate.

First, umbilical hernia is that which appears through, and within the limits of the umbilical ring, once patent, subsequently closed or partially so, and now expanded and its coverings stretched and bulged forwards. Of this there is only one variety topographically. Secondly, ventral hernia is that which presents through any portion of the abdominal wall bounded by the costal margin and epigastric angles above, and Poupart's ligament and the crest of the pubes below, and a vertical line drawn through the anterior superior spine of the ileum on either side. It is rarely seen away from the median line of the body, except as the result of wounds, when it differs essentially from the form under consideration. Occurring in the median line, it may be termed complete, when it involves the whole length of the abdomen (complete separation of the recti) or partial, when it may be above the umbilicus (median epigastric hernia), or below it (median hypogastric hernia). The former is comparatively rare, the latter is very common.

Consideration of the essential anatomical differences between umbilical and ventral hernia will at once reveal several points which may be here noted.

Anatomical Differences in Umbilical and Ventral Hernia.

(a) Umbilical hernia appears through a patch of preformed scar-tissue, which it expands almost indefinitely. The healing of the umbilicus in the young child causes a puckering of the deeper tissues, just as it does in the skin, and at some points of the patch the puckered material is stronger than at others ; consequently the stretching is irregular and as the weaker portions give way first, one sees the commencement of that sacculation of the peritoneum which is so characteristic of this form of hernia. Ventral hernia (excluding that which results from wounds) is not preceded by any formation of scar-tissue, and is not therefore thus complicated ; it is rather the outcome of a gradual stretching of the non-cicatricial intermusclar septum between the recti muscles, and a bulging forwards of the abdominal contents.

(b) The umbilicus represents the site of a potential canal, still occupied by the withered remains of the cord ; as such it is still capable of reopening before sufficiently persistent pressure from within. This canal has a very definite ring-like boundary, which can be easily detected in those cases in which the hernia is yet early and reducible, if the finger be passed through the umbilicus, the skin being invaginated by it. This ring-like structure is not the result of irritative thickening, although in the later stages it may be thus augmented ; it is not found in cases of ventral hernia even when of long standing, since no canal has ever existed here along which pressure might be directed.

(c) The thickness of the abdominal wall at the umbilicus is represented by one thin layer of fascia, exclusive of the feeble peritoneum, fat, and skin ; above this point, and below it for about two inches the two stout layers of the sheath of the rectus muscle, becoming conjoined, form a strong barrier ; below the semilunar fold the absence of the posterior layer is well compensated for by the close approximation of the bellies of the powerful rectus abdominis muscle. Consequently, hernia at the umbilicus is much commoner than at any other point of the median line.

(d) An essential factor in the determination of hernia at the umbilicus is to be found in the fact that at this point is the chief linea transversa, which, although serving several useful purposes, is yet, being a fibrous structure, liable to stretch, and therefore a weak spot in the abdominal wall. Below the umbilicus it is unusual to find a linea transversa (although such occurs at times), and this may render hernia less prone to occur at this spot. The rarity of hernia above the umbilicus, where there are commonly two of these lineæ, may be accounted for by three factors, viz. the support of the ribs and the narrowness of the epigastric angle, the presence of the left lobe of the liver, and the slighter influence of gravity here as compared with the lower part of the abdomen, especially when filled with pelvic tumours or ascitic fluid.

(e) The last point of difference between these two forms of hernia anatomically is to be found in the character of the skin covering the tumour. In the case of umbilical hernia at least some portion of this is composed of that which originally formed the cicatrix of the umbilicus ; it is therefore thin, ill-nourished, since there is little underlying fat to carry its vessels, and extremely prone to ulceration. A ventral hernia, on the other hand, is protected by skin of good texture and fair blood supply ; unless, therefore, the hernia becomes exceedingly pendulous, with a constricted base and the development of eczema intertrigo (a condition common enough in the subjects of extreme obesity), ulceration is unusual ; nor do we see as the result of this ulceration when it does occur adhesion of the skin to the hernial contents so commonly in this as in umbilical hernia.

From the above points it will be seen that there are well-defined differences between these two forms of hernia. Now, as a consequence of these, certain results naturally follow which have a very important bearing upon the prognosis and treatment. Thus, in umbilical hernia ulceration, suppuration in the sac, and strangulation are common and often early, while the prognosis as to cure is often good, whereas in ventral hernia, although these evils are rare, the prognosis (at least in this respect) is frequently doubtful. The reason for this difference is not far to seek. The neck of an umbilical sac, as already pointed out, lies within a more or less circumscribed area, bounded by a firm fibrous ring ; outside this is the margin of the rectus muscle on either side ; being thus circumscribed, the hernia does not tend to the same extent as elsewhere to encroach upon, push aside, and attenuate the muscles ; nor do these, being here reinforced by the lineæ transversæ, undergo the adaptive narrowing which is seen so markedly below the umbilicus. Consequently, in the performance of a radical operation the abdomen will usually be more easily closed in dealing with umbilical hernia than with the median hypogastric variety, where wide separation, narrowing, and atrophy are the rule. Further, the bulging sac of a ventral hernia can always contain a much larger mass of abdominal contents than can the narrownecked and somewhat restricted pouch of an umbilical rupture, and occasionally to such an extent does this occur, that by no means in our power could the viscera, so long divorced from their proper domain, be returned to it.

Etiological Considerations.

It has usually been the custom to accord to these two conditions, viz. umbilical and ventral hernia, the same etiology, that of increased intraabdominal tension due to pregnancy, tumours, ascites, etc.; and although in such tension may be found the essential element of all herniæ, there are other particulars in which the cause of umbilical hernia differs from that of ventral. Were it not so, the two forms of hernia should be frequently met with in the same patient ; but this is, at least in my experience, not by any means common. Two facts here seem to me to stand out, viz. that the former condition is almost exclusively met with in women who are excessively obese, some of whom have never borne children, whereas the latter frequently occurs in thin subjects, most of whom have borne many children. Taking these facts with the anatomical points already discussed, one may conclude that umbilical hernia is the result of gradual increase of intra-abdominal pressure resulting from obesity especially, and induced by the presence of the peritoneal dimple or depression which exists in most of us at the umbilicus ; while ventral hernia (median hypogastric) occurs most commonly as the result of the great weight and pressure, often repeated, of the gravid uterus upon

the lower portion of the abdominal wall, the predisposing element being present in the form of a congenital, though often slight, separation of the recti muscles, this separation being easily increased by the stretching which takes place during pregnancy. That this explanation fails to account for the epigastric form of hernia is, of course, true ; but, as I have already mentioned, this form is rare, and as when it is present it is only seen either as a complication of umbilical hernia or as part of the bulging through the whole extent of a congenitally wide linea alba, accompanied by general gastroenteroptosis, its etiology is probably, unlike that of the hypogastric form, that of general pressure of obesity.

That the burden of patients afflicted with median herniæ is a severe one is undeniable and yet how little is done to relieve their condition ! Noting the obesity of the patient and the evidences of slight pulmonary trouble, and giving undue weight to the possibility of recurrence, surgeons have, I think, been too ready to regard the condition as one best left alone, and a truss, that curse of progressive surgery, applied, and this at times even to herniæ which have not been reducible for years.

Meanwhile, what is occurring as the result of this inaction ?

The nausea, which was at first but slight, now gives way to retching, due to dragging on the omentum, which has gradually become adherent to the sac ; little by little more of this omentum becomes involved owing to the frequent straining and coughing of the patient ; standing up causes pain, the contents of the sac becoming congested, while lying down is often worse owing to the dragging of the stomach and colon upon the imprisoned omentum, and so upon the sympathetic plexuses ; thus quiet rest and sleep become impossible. Arising out of this dragging, a very important condition results ; the stomach, gradually drawn down, becomes inactive, restricted in its movements, atonic and dilated, fermentation takes place, and one of the most constant complications of median hernia—viz. flatulent dyspepsia—is established. Similarly the colon, whose normal position in the abdomen is that of a festoon having its lowest point just above the umbilicus, becomes unduly kinked, with the result that flatus accumulates, giving rise to tympanitic distension, and, the fæces being retarded, their fluids are reabsorbed.

In these two points one can trace the origin of the obstinate constipation so characteristic of these cases, and, provided the transverse colon itself is in the sac, the explanation of the frequency of incarceration in a portion of the alimentary canal, in which the contents are normally only semi-solid.

But this constipation is favoured in other ways ; the patient, noticing the great increase in the size of the hernia which takes place on going to stool, is under an ever-present apprehension that the " belly may burst," * and consequently avoids opening her bowels. How far such a fear is justified is difficult to say, but the accident must be very rare ; it is, however, very alarming to the patient. The pain and backache too, which result from dragging upon the omentum and irritation of the splanchnic area, act as powerful deterrents and both of these causes, when combined with the coincident loss of power in the recti muscles owing to their separation, tend to favour a plethoric and slothful state, in which, exercise being studiously avoided, obesity is allowed to take its course and something of the nature of a " vicious circle " is the result.

But many median herniæ, although they are not so marked as this, are, perhaps, the more dangerous; for there are certain cases, usually early ones, and only seen in very obese patients, in which the symptoms may be present without the appearance of any protuberance at the navel. On several occasions I have seen patients whose trouble did not go beyond a slight nausea (especially on lying down), backache, and umbilical tenderness, and in whom no hernia could be felt, and yet in whom such was demonstrated by operation. To such herniæ the term " blind " may be aptly applied ; they are the result of a very small opening at the navel, which allows little to escape, covered by a very large amount of abdominal fat, which completely masks the presence of the protrusion. These cases are especially dangerous in that strangulation may occur before their presence is even suspected by the patient or her medical man. In this fact, and in the fact that these strangulations are commonly extremely tight, and at times of the variety known as Richter's hernia, is to be found one explanation of the higher mortality of kelotomy here than in the case of inguinal or of femoral hernia. A further cause is undoubtedly the serious

* A case was reported by Davies of Liverpool, ' Lancet,' 1898.

impression which must be made upon the sympathetic system of the upper abdominal region by the strangulation of organs so intimately connected with the semilunar ganglia as are those which are commonly involved at the umbilicus. The shock thus originated is greatly increased by the vomiting, which is more forcible and frequent, and by the pain, which is more griping and exhausting, than in other forms of hernia ; consequently the post-operative condition is one in which pulmonary hypostasis, broncho- and lobar pneumonia, and bronchitis are among the commoner causes of death.

Some Reasons for Unsatisfactory Results of Treatment.

That the treatment of these cases has been, and to some extent still is, most disappointing is, I believe, due to a number of causes, most of which are within our control, but many of which we neglect. First, a tendency on the part of the patient to fancy the condition one of no great moment, especially when the hernia is small and not causing pain. Secondly, a failure on the part of the practitioner to recognise the serious and inevitably progressive nature of these cases. Thirdly, the unfortunate and ill-advised belief in the time-honoured truss or belt, the use of which puts off till too late an operation otherwise of promise. Fourthly, the supposition (often quite erroneous) that the patient is too stout to undergo any operation. Fifthly, the undoubted lack of interest shown by our profession in the study and treatment of obesity, a lack of interest which equally overshadows the study of alopecia and other common ailments, which have become most unwarrantably the Utopia of the quack and the charlatan. Sixthly, the lack of sound technique ; and lastly, that curse of so many abdominal operations, too short convalescence in the recumbent position.

Now, there is little doubt that if these cases are to go untreated to the end the patient has at least one of three conditions to face, and at times all three ; for chronic discomfort and ill health will attend him or her always, incarceration may repeatedly threaten life, and strangulation may end it in a few hours.

What is to be said of the truss and the belt ? Although both are of use in their proper place, it is to be feared that by many their purpose has been misunderstood, and that they have been permitted to take the place of more modern surgical methods.

I have said that the condition is progressive, and the almost constant increase of obesity and the repetition of pregnancy in women are the chief factors in this ; therefore, it is easy to see that the simplest form of median hernia, small and easily reducible when at first a truss is applied to it, becomes quite uncontrollable when in the course of a few years the interposition of two or even more inches of mobile fat has raised the truss from the site of its original utility, and when pressure has thinned out the skin and irritation sealed down the hernial contents to the umbilical margin. Again, the belt, affording relief to the discomforts of the early stages of an enteroptosis between separated recti, has constantly lulled the patient to a false sense of security, only to prove a broken reed when later years have brought atrophy and fibrosis to muscles which were once succulent and elastic, and the time for action has been lost.

As an alternative to operation, trusses and belts may at times present the only means of treatment at our disposal, but it is not too much to say that the number of unfortunate sufferers which we see crowding the out-patient room (and indeed in private practice), condemned in later life to the thraldom of these instruments, is a standing witness to our professional inertia in the earlier days of their affliction.

The question of obesity has, I think, been given too prominent a place in the consideration of operative interference, since it is not the fact of obesity *per se* so much as the conditions which commonly give rise to it and those which complicate it which is of importance. There is a great difference between general and abdominal obesity; few patients are too stout to undergo an operation for the cure of median hernia, provided their obesity is uncomplicated by the plethora of cardiac and pulmonary disease or by albuminuria—and this is especially the case when their obesity is confined or chiefly limited to the abdominal walls. In most of these cases it is the rule to find the recti muscles, at least in the earlier period of the trouble, of good development, and stout enough to lend themselves to firm suturing ; for it is only in the later years that narrowing and attenuation take place. The chief effect of obesity upon

operations is to compel the making of a larger and a deeper wound ; to necessitate very careful drainage, in view of the exudation of oil or blood from so large a mass of fat, and the proneness of such tissue to undergo disintegration ; and to render the accurate suturing of the skin rather more difficult than in other cases.

That many patients who are plethoric are refused operation on the score of the dangers to which a general anæsthetic might expose them is a misfortune which it is at least possible to a great extent to combat, the gradual perfection of local anæsthesia having placed within the surgeon's grasp many conditions which were hitherto regarded as of little promise ; but although several British surgeons have done much to strengthen its position in this country, its general adoption in suitable cases still falls short of being an accomplished fact. It is very far from my intention to advocate the adoption of local anæsthesia to the almost complete exclusion of the older method—a practice which has, unfortunately I think, become almost a fashionable craze in some countries; but in the case of plethoric and obese subjects, the victims of median hernia and many other surgical affections complicated by cardiac and pulmonary troubles, it is a method of first importance.

How many of us ever consider for a moment the prospects of a young woman with an early umbilical or ventral hernia and commencing obesity, or our duty towards her? Few, I fear, do so systematically ; else we should see fewer of these cases coming in later years to the out-patient room, groaning and panting, slung up with belts and trusses, the skin eczematous and ulcerated over the hernial protrusion, and wishing fervently that something had been done for them fifteen or twenty years before.

In all, their obesity is progressive and to be restrained must be dealt with *early*, yet this is quite the exception. Most are prolific, especially in the lower classes, yet how seldom is any attempt made to give them timely warning of the folly and danger of repeated pregnancy ! And when once a hernia has developed, how few are submitted to operation till the hour of grace has gone by ! When one day it has become the rule amongst us to regard excessive obesity as a disease, to study it in the same systematic manner as that in which anæmia, lymphadenoma, and myxœdema have been investigated, and to acknowledge to ourselves that it is a condition worthy of scientific study, and to wrest its treatment from the limbo of quackery and charlatanism in which it now wallows, then, and not till then, shall we be able to lay the foundation for the rational treatment of median hernia.

That the results of operations for median herniæ have not been all that could have been desired has been due, no doubt, at times to faulty technique; and this in its turn is certainly the result of the varying opinions as to which structure is of chief importance in the repair of the abdominal wall. The peritoneum, the aponeurosis, the musculature, each in its turn has been upheld, and still there is diversity of opinion.

The former is surely discredited as a structure of strength or reliability when we consider the readiness with which it will stretch, as seen in old hernial sacs, and its total inability to retain stitches in the face of the slightest tension. Its *rôle* is chiefly that of a lubricating membrane, and when efficiently closed it probably serves to prevent adhesion of the abdominal contents to the bare surface of the rectus muscle or its sheath. The fascial portion of the abdominal wall is, moreover, unless fully reinforced and backed by good muscular substance, quite unreliable as a bar to hernial protrusion. Like fibrous tissue in many other parts of the body, it will stretch when exposed to prolonged and undue strain, no matter how carefully it may be sutured. Muscular tissue, on the other hand, being a highly organised and elastic structure, is capable of powerfully resisting any attempt at protrusion, and provided its fibres are not separated up and attenuated, will not form any portion of a hernial sac; thus, even in the largest inguinal and umbilical herniæ, it is never seen in this position, being merely pushed to one side in the former or to either side in the latter. Even in cases of traumatic hernia of the abdomen (resulting from wounds, rupture of muscle-fibre, localised disease, etc.) it is not seen in the sac of the hernia; the stretched cicatrix fills the gap, and the muscle is forced to one side. This would seem to prove that it is upon the muscular portion of the abdominal wall that reliance must be especially placed in the operative treatment of median herniæ.

This being so, two courses are open to the surgeon; either he must take the case early, before wide separation of the recti muscles has occurred, or he must be prepared to make good the deficiency by the use of some material which will not stretch, in the later stages.

An unwise practice, born of the overcrowding of our hospitals and the not unnatural desire to place before our students an ever-fresh relay of clinical material, has been responsible for much of the recurrence of which we hear; this is the seriously curtailed period of convalescence in the recumbent position which is too often the rule in hospital. Wounds of the abdominal wall, no matter how perfect the apposition and rapid the union, are only completely healed throughout at the end of three weeks; at this date the union is composed of young fibro-plastic material which, if given time, will form tissue almost as good and as strong as the rest of the abdominal wall; but if, on the contrary, the patient be permitted to sit up or to propel himself about in an invalid chair, the union will inevitably stretch, and the foundation for recurrence, not for cure, is there and then laid. I have not the slightest doubt that such is the explanation of many of the failures which have done so much to bring the operative treatment of hernia into disrepute. It is better to have treated a few cases well than many imperfectly; and for the honour and credit of surgery longer convalescence and earlier operation, if fewer cases, should be aimed at.

Considerations prior to Operation.

Much, however, will depend on the manner in which the patient is prepared for operation, for there are few conditions for which so much may be done to help the surgeon in the weeks preceding the operation.

First, time permitting, the obesity should be dealt with systematically; and in the case of patients willing to undergo considerable dietetic privation and the discomfort of regular exercise the first and greatest difficulty will be overcome. The strictest dietary consistent with health and the utmost possible limitation of fluids, the performance and gradual increase of active exercise and the daily use of mild hydragogues in the poorer classes; and in the wealthier the practice of the Turkish bath (without, however, its attendant luxuries), and the excellent *régime* imposed at many of the continental watering-places, will work wonders in the hands of the firm practitioner. Secondly, an attempt should be made to reduce the size of the hernial mass during the last fortnight, and for this purpose recumbency is essential ; it may not be possible to reduce the whole of the mass, but since much of the bulk will be due to engorgement, reducible omentum, and at times flatulent bowel, much may be done by the use of the ice-bag, carminatives, enemata, and the rectal tube.

Thirdly, it is absolutely essential that a perfectly aseptic result should attend these operations ; for the readiness with which the abdominal fat breaks down and the loose areolar tissue becomes infiltrated by exudation renders this site of operation a particularly favourable nidus for bacterial growth, and one of all others where stitch abscesses are so frequently seen. The importance of asepsis here may be emphasised from another point of view. I have said that the perfection of the result depends especially upon the close apposition of the recti muscles ; the union of these must therefore involve the formation of the minimum amount of fibrous cicatrix. Now, if suppuration ensue, the very point of greatest importance is missed, and the wealth of fibro-plastic exudation forms a cicatrix which will stretch almost indefinitely.

Before determining upon any operation, the surgeon should endeavour to make out the actual amount of separation of the recti muscles which is present—a point not always easy, and at times very deceptive in fat subjects, what is taken to be the margin of the muscle frequently proving to be the thickened mass of omentum in an outlying sacculus, the true margin of muscle being considerably further out. In such cases, therefore, one should be prepared beforehand with any instrumental aid which may possibly help in bridging the gap, as such cannot be manufactured at a moment's notice.

Objections to existing Methods.

Operation viâ the sac of the hernia.—The practice, once common, now fortunately less so, of attempting to cure a median hernia by approaching it through an incision in the sac, is, to my mind, bad surgery, and for several reasons. It gives cramped access to the site of hernia and precludes the satisfactory exploration of the contents. The danger of puncturing the bowel which

may be adherent, or the greater probability of wounding the omental vessels, is always present in old-standing herniæ. The former presents a serious complication, while the latter, owing to the bleeding and consequent loss of time, and to the staining of the tissues, is inconvenient. The incision passes through skin which is less likely to be aseptic than that in the vicinity of the sac, as it is not possible to treat it with the same rigour in sterilisation. and it has possibly from time to time been ulcerated. It is much more difficult to expose the whole of the sacculi, if such are present, owing to the adhesions which the cicatrix has contracted with the subjacent tissues ; and when the operation is completed, either the skin-sutures must be placed through a redundant mass of devitalised material, or the cutaneous portion of the sac must be removed, thus involving a second and third skin incision to include the necessary ellipse, at best a clumsy method, and one involving loss of time.

The extensive nature of the operation necessary to afford a prospect of cure in these cases demands the freest exposure of the parts concerned, and this cannot possibly be done through the incision in question. It is true that no less an authority than the late Mr. Grieg Smith (1) advocated this incision, but that was ten years ago, and since then many of our methods have had to undergo revision. Ransohoff (2), on the other hand, advises free incision into the abdomen above the neck of the hernia, and with this advice I am in entire accord.

Simple approximation of the aponeuroses.—As usually performed, *i. e.* approximation from side to side, this method is only mentioned to be at once condemned. It is irrational to again entrust the guardianship of the site of hernia to a structure which has already proved itself untrustworthy. Such operations, when completed, amount to nothing less than a waste of time, a loss of opportunity, and the rendering more difficult of the operation which will assuredly become necessary within a very short period. An improvement is that of Warren(3), who in 1890 first practised the method of approximation from above and below. He points out that the great lateral strain is not here present, and that the hernial aperture lends itself especially to this method since it is wider laterally than in the vertical direction.

Overlapping of the aponeuroses—The method

just condemned is here elaborated, apparently with the idea that the incorporation of two thicknesses of bad tissue will produce one good one. Now, it is extremely difficult, especially in the presence of tension, to compel the complete adhesion, without the intervention of dead spaces, of the opposed surfaces of two wide strips of fascia : the exudation filling these spaces, as shown in the diagram (Fig. 1, x), serves to form fresh fibrous material, and as stretching will certainly take place where the

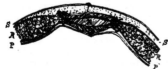

Fig. 1.—Showing "dead-space" x between over-lapped fasciæ of rectus muscle. Buried sutures have been used here. R. Rectus muscle. s. Skin. P Peritoneum. Transverse section.

repair is a purely fibrous one of new formation (Fig. 2), the result can be little better than in the method of simple approximation, the apparently better results reported by some surgeons being, I believe, simply due to the longer period required for the stretching of a thick mass of aponeuroses as opposed to a thin one. Again, the method of overlapping requires a very large number of buried sutures, and these in devitalised and avascular tissues are constantly sources of trouble ; and especially here, as they must be of stout material,

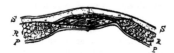

Fig. 2.—Showing commencement of stretching of fibro-plastic mass resulting from exudation in "dead-space," x. Transverse section.

with consequently large knots, and that in the presence of considerable tension. William Mayo (4) of Rochester, Minnesota, in 1901 advocated the application of a modification by him of Lucas Championniere's operation for the overlapping of the aponeuroses in inguinal hernia. This method, which he has adapted to the cure of median hernia, consists essentially in the opening of the abdomen transversely, removal of the sac and its omental contents in one piece, and the formation of an upper and lower flap from the fibrous aponeurosis,

the latter being drawn up by firm sutures beneath the former, and fixed between it and the peritoneum ; the free margin of the upper flap is then sutured down. It is reported to have given satisfaction ; but while confessing to an ignorance of its merits from practical experience, I cannot help thinking that there must exist a weak spot in the abdomen at each end of the overlapping portion, where a dimple must necessarily exist owing to the crossing of the flaps, and especially so in cases where the muscles cannot be approximated.

Methods involving Interference with the Recti Muscles.

By the term "interference" I mean the overlapping of the muscles, or the splitting of their fibres and eversion of their margins, in order to present a thicker mass of muscle in the median line. Both of these methods have been tried and advocated, but although in some cases they have undoubtedly resulted in success, I feel confident that such practices as routine methods are unsound. Recti muscles which can be made to overlap with the exercise of tension can obviously be made to meet with less or no tension ; and provided they are of good development, nothing further should be required to insure success; this method is that successfully followed by Gersuny (5).

Two grave objections to these methods present themselves. First, any interference with these important muscles is likely to convert their margins into fibrous cicatrix, the very last thing to be desired. For it is impossible to suppose that when the margins have been split, turned in and out, handled torn, and extensively sutured, their subsequent condition can be that of anything resembling healthy and elastic muscle. Secondly, the method of overlapping, while being, as I have said, unnecessary, tends to the formation of at least two serious "dead-spaces," as shown in the diagram (Fig. 3), and these must exist, one on either side.

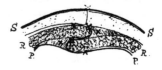

Fig. 3.—Showing "dead-spaces" xx produced by the overlapping of well-developed recti muscles. Transverse section.

throughout the whole length of the overlapped portion, one existing between the muscles of one side and the skin and the other between the muscle of the opposite side and the peritoneum. These operations, which involve great interference with the muscular tissue, give rise to considerable bleeding, and therefore the objection to these "dead-spaces" is a very real one. Meyer (6) and Blake (7), however, report good results, but the former draws attention to the difficulty of the operation.

Methods involving the Use of Mechanical Appliances.

These, some of which are among the most recent of surgical procedures for the cure of median herniæ, are the outcome of the gradual perfection of aseptic surgery, and for their success must depend upon the most rigid observance of its requirements. That it is almost impossible to close the great gaps which are left after the reduction of many median herniæ by means of even simple approximation aided by the exercise of great tension is an established fact ; and therefore, if a cure is to be effected in such cases, it must be done by replacing the separated muscles by some inelastic structure which shall remain as a permanent barrier to the extrusion of the abdominal contents. Such is to be found in plates of silver or other substance or in gridirons of silver wire.

The attention drawn by Crede to the powerfully antiseptic properties of silver has greatly aided the perfection of such methods as are now in use, and this metal is now the only one generally employed. It does not corrode, is extremely flexible, and does not easily break. It is, however, not often used in the form of plates, since such are less flexible than wire, and do not permit of complete incorporation with the tissues ; they are uncomfortable to the patient during the performance of abdominal movements, and frequently, acting as irritant foreign bodies, set up suppuration and have to be removed. In such an event the patient is no better, but rather worse.

These methods may be separated into two classes—viz. those in which a strong network of silver wire is woven into the gap during the performance of the operation, and those in which a gridiron or filigree of wire is manufactured previously and introduced ready made. Of the former method, perhaps Gersuny (5) and Schede (8) abroad and Barker in this country have been the chief advocates, and the excellence of the latter's results are well known. .Abroad, the second method has been chiefly pioneered by Witzel of Bonn(9), Göpel of Leipzig(10), Meyer of New York(11), and Willard Bartlett (12) of St. Louis. In this country the method has not yet received the support which is undoubtedly due to it, the first case so treated being the author's, which was shown to the Clinical

Society of London nearly two years ago (13), and which I may say is sound and well to-day.

Space will not permit me to enter into a discussion of the whole question of the use of silver wire in this connection, but references to much that has been written lately on the subject are given below : some conclusions, however, gathered from many sources may not be out of place. They are : (1) That herniæ previously deemed inoperable can now be dealt with by the use of silver wire, in the form of a carefully planned suture at the time of operation, or, what is infinitely preferable, of a ready-made filigree of the pattern devised by Bartlett. (2) Such herniæ are capable of really permanent cure, the reason for this being found in the complete incorporation of the wire in the tissues, and the impossibility of further stretching of the abdomen at the site of hernia. (3) The wire should be of very fine gauge, for, as pointed out by Bartlett, its flexibility must be perfect to insure comfort and to avoid causing irritation in the tissues. As gauges vary with different makers and in different countries, it will suffice to say that wire of the thickness of moderately stout sewing cotton will be found suitable. In those cases in which the wire has had to be removed, it has been due to one of two causes, viz. too stout wire, or filigree of too close mesh to permit of perfect flexibility. (4) The filigree should be at least half an inch larger than the muscular gap for which it is intended. (5) It should be placed *upon* the peritoneum and *beneath* the muscles : the omentum should be sutured into position where there is a deficiency of the former. (6) Except for the peritoneum, no buried sutures should be employed, removable deep sutures being substituted ; the method I have employed for some time and which I have elsewhere described (14) will, I believe, be found easily applied and as easily removed. (7) Where a "dead-space" is unavoidable, it should be carefully drained for twenty-four hours and then obliterated as much as possible by the careful application of padding. Perfect dryness of the wound is of the first importance. (8) Hardly any limit can be placed to the size of gap which may be closed if the foregoing points be borne in mind, and if sufficient peritoneum and sound skin are available.

With regard to the steps which should be followed in the performance of operations for the cure of median hernia, opinions, I know, differ greatly ; I would merely state therefore, with all due reserve, the method which I have found the simplest and most satisfactory in such cases as have come under my care. In the first place, my incision is made to commence in the median line above the neck of the hernia (the requisite amount of the skin of the sac being included in an ellipse), and to finish in the same line below it. Its extent is dependent on the size of the hernia and the stoutness of the patient, free exposure being, as I have pointed out, an essential of success. Through the upper portion of this wound the abdomen is opened, and, two fingers being introduced, the limits of the hernial aperture are explored. The whole of the external limits are next reached by dissecting back the skin and superficial fascia, and the neck of the sac is freely exposed. The abdomen is now opened below the neck, and, with two fingers to act as a director, an ellipse is cut out of the abdomen just wide enough to include the neck, and ending above and below at the upper and lower points of the skin incision, the sac and its contents being thus completely freed.

Where the aperture of the neck is so wide that this method would render the approximation of the peritoneum difficult, I modify it by removing the latter only over the limits of the aperture, and over the rest of the ellipse endeavour to save it by pealing it off from the superjacent structures; the omentum is then used to make up the deficiency. The contents of the sac are now turned out, any omentum present being removed, or if in good condition and required for the purpose, utilised as above. I next ascertain the inner limits of the margin of the recti muscles and open their sheaths along this margin throughout the whole length of the wound. It is now possible to see whether the muscles will come together (this will only be in the case of quite small herniæ) and if they are of good development. If so, and if no great tension is necessary to bring them together, I treat the case simply by very accurate closure of the abdomen in tiers, using numerous sutures of median catgut of undoubted sterility, and trust to the formation of a very close union of muscle to muscle, aided by sufficiently prolonged convalescence to secure the desired result.

But where tension would be required, or where no approximation is possible, I do not hesitate to use the filigree which has been mentioned. Placed for some time previously in ether, it is subjected to thorough boiling, and when required is taken straight from the steriliser, and, without being handled, is placed at once upon the peritoneum, which has been closed with a running suture of fine catgut; the muscles are then drawn together as much as possible over it by the removable suture already mentioned. The skin-incision is finally sutured, a fine gauze drain being left in the lower angle for twenty-four hours.

It will be seen that a certain amount of "dead-space" is unavoidable in this method of filigree implantation between the filigree and the superficial fascia; it is, however, but slight in stout patients, and can generally be overcome by judicious padding over the deficient area, and with absolute asepsis and temporary drainage is little likely to vitiate the result. Should slight suppuration, however, take place, it must not be supposed

that removal of the wire is essential; it will, as a rule, survive this *contretemps* with careful treatment, and it is as well such is the case, since one of the best recommendations of the efficiency of the filigree is that, once incorporated in the tissues of the abdominal wall, it is extremely difficult to remove.

A point of importance in securing a dry wound is the use of blunt round-bodied needles for the approximation of the muscles; anything of the nature of bayonet or Hagedorn's needles is to be avoided, since they cause free bleeding at times, which is difficult to arrest, and which may jeopardise all one's aseptic precautions. Again, in the closure of the abdomen without the use of filigree a "dead-space" may be formed which is frequently overlooked; for if the posterior sheath of the rectus is closed by the use of much greater tension than that which is required to close the peritoneum, the latter will sag as in the diagram (Fig. 4), and a

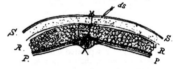

Fig. 4.—Showing "dead-space" x formed by sagging of loose peritoneum in presence of tighter posterior rectus sheath. Removable deep suture used here, *ds*. Transverse section.

three-cornered gutter will be formed which will contain quite a quantity of blood-serum. In conclusion, I would again urge, in the treatment of these herniæ, the more systematic attention to the reduction of obesity, the earlier performance of operation, the more extended use of the methods which have proved so successful abroad, and a considerable increase in the period of convalescence.

BIBLIOGRAPHY.

(1) Grieg Smith, 'Anns. of Surg.,' 1895.
(2) Ransohoff, 'Med. Record,' 1897.
(3) Warren, 'Boston Med. and Surg. Journ.,' 1903.
(4) Mayo, 'Journ. of Amer. Med. Assoc.,' 1903 ; cf. also Piccoli, 'Centralbl. für Chirurg.,' 1900 ; Sapiejko, 'Rev. de Chir.,' 1900 ; Blake, 'Med. Assoc. of New York,' 1901.
(5) Gersuny, 'Centralbl. für Chirurg.,' 1893.
(6) Meyer, 'Anns. of Surg.,' 1903.
(7) Blake, 'Anns. of Surg.,' 1904.
(8) Schede, 'Centralbl. für Chirurg.,' 1900.
(9) Witzel, 'Centralbl. für Chirurg.,' 1900.
(10) Göpel, 'Centralbl. für Chirurg.,' 1900.
(11) Meyer, 'Journ. Amer. Med. Assoc.,' 1902
(12) Bartlett, 'Anns. of Surg.,' 1903.
(13) McGavin, 'Clin. Soc. Trans.,' 1904.
(14) McGavin, the 'Lancet,' 1904.

December 18th, 1905.

THE CLINICAL JOURNAL,

CLINICAL RECORD, CLINICAL NEWS, CLINICAL GAZETTE, CLINICAL REPORTER, CLINICAL CHRONICLE AND CLINICAL REVIEW.

EDITED BY L. ELIOT CREASY.

No. 687.   WEDNESDAY, DECEMBER 27, 1905.   Vol. XXVII.   No. 11.

CONTENTS.

Specially reported for the Clinical Journal. Revised by the Author.

ALL RIGHTS RESERVED.

NOTICE.

Editorial correspondence, books for review, &c., should be addressed to the Editor, 51, New Cavendish Street, W., Telephone No. 904, Paddington ; but all business communications should be addressed to the Publishers, 22½, Bartholomew Close, London, E.C. Telephone 927, Holborn.

All inquiries respecting Advertisements should be sent to MESSRS. ADLARD & SON, Bartholomew Close, E.C. Telephone 927, Holborn.

Terms of Subscription, including postage, payable by cheque, postal or banker's order (in advance): for the United Kingdom, 15s. 6d. per annum ; Abroad, 17s. 6d.

Cheques, &c., should be made payable to THE PROPRIETORS OF THE CLINICAL JOURNAL, crossed " The London, City, and Midland Bank, Ltd., Newgate Street Branch, E.C. Account of the Medical Publishing Company, Limited."

Reading Cases to hold Twenty-six numbers of THE CLINICAL JOURNAL can be supplied at 2s. 3d. each, or will be forwarded post free on receipt of 2s. 6d.; and also Cases for binding Volumes at 1s. each, or post free on receipt of 1s. 3d., from the Publishers, 22½ Bartholomew Close, London, E.C.

MISTAKES.

A lecture delivered at the London Hospital.

By FRED. J. SMITH, M.D., F.R.C.P.,
Physician to the London Hospital.

GENTLEMEN,—These lectures are usually in the wards, but, unfortunately, in my beds at the present moment there are some cases which can be said to be of no particular clinical interest, and others of such interest that one cannot talk about them sufficiently in the ward. Therefore I had to look for some other subject. Dr. Andrews' article in the ' Gazette ' this month on "Common Gynæcological Mistakes" is a very excellent one, and I thought that, as mistakes are a very common incident in the life of most of us, I could not do better than talk to you about some of the commoner ones on the medical side.

As an introduction I will tell you the tale of almost the first professional fee I ever earned. A man came to me in great distress and asked me to see his wife. It was on a Saturday morning, and you will see presently that the date was important. He told me she had been confined on the previous Monday. On Tuesday she was in a considerable amount of pain ; on Wednesday she was in very great pain ; on Thursday a good deal worse ; and on Friday she said that if she did not have relief she would commit suicide. The man was in a great hurry, and, although it was not strictly in my line, I went. I asked the doctor what was the trouble. He said she had been confined on Monday, and had got acute inflammation of the womb. I did not know quite what that might mean, so I went in. As soon as I entered the room my nose was offended by a urinous odour. I turned down the bed-clothes and saw the abdomen enormously distended, with a huge tumour well above the umbilicus. This was the medical attendant's inflamed uterus. So I said to him, " Have you drawn off the water ? " He said :

"She is passing it freely." "Anyhow," I said, "that is a big bladder, and we will empty it before we go any further. Get a catheter." He brought a catheter, and I passed it and drew off an ordinary po quite full of urine. I do not know how much that would be, but I should think at least a couple of quarts. The natural result was that immediately all pain ceased, and the woman was perfectly well. What she had been suffering from was, obviously, retention of urine after confinement. She was a primipara. That tale—which, by the way, is perfectly true—is an illustration of mistakes. But you must not understand me to say that no man is ever to make a mistake. The man who says that he has never made a mistake in his life is certainly either a fool or a liar, and, very probably, a foolish liar or a lying fool. But, in any case, he is not a man to be trusted.

Well, there are various classes of mistakes. They may be of omission, or they may be of commission—that is to say, either negative or positive ; or, on the other hand, they may be what one may call simply neutral—you have not found what was the condition, but you did your best. And there are many matters upon which you may make mistakes—diagnosis, prognosis, treatment, and, in fact, any subject connected with medicine. In the next place, mistakes may be looked at from the point of view of the doctor or from the point of view of the patient. On the patient's side the mistakes may be of extremely serious consequences, even up to the loss of life, or they may be of no particular consequence. Again, mistakes may be serious from the doctor's point of view—that is to say, those involving loss of reputation. And let me tell you that reputations are far more easily lost than made, especially good ones. On the other hand, it may be that the mistake is not of very serious consequence except to the doctor's own self-esteem and to his conscience. He thinks, "Well, I made that blunder, it was a foolish thing to do, and I must try not to do it again." Of course the mistakes may be mere errors of judgment after taking every possible precaution to arrive at the facts. Between these extremes, of death to the patient and loss of reputation to the doctor, and mistakes which are of no importance whatever, there may be every possible grade.

For our present purposes I will divide them up into four or five classes, and we will go through those classes with illustrative examples and little bits of warning to you.

The first class is that of mistakes avoidable by knowledge, or, in other words, mistakes due to mere culpable ignorance. Let me give you a few illustrations. The illustrations which occur to one at the moment are those in which people, laymen particularly, rush into matters medical—*e. g.* spectacle-makers trying to correct sight. It is perfectly true that if—and that "if" has got to be spelt with a capital "I" and a very much bigger "F"—if there is nothing the matter but refraction errors I daresay the spectacle-maker will be as good as a doctor to the person applying. But you have to *know* that it is errors of refraction only that prevents the person from seeing properly. In the case of quacks of all sorts their mistakes, luckily for them, are buried in oblivion, because even in the case of death resulting the patient's friends do not like the ridicule which would be brought upon them by the knowledge that they preferred to go to a quack rather than to a regular medical practitioner. These quacks do make a tremendous number of mistakes from sheer ignorance. I may again mention that case which I gave you as a text, the instance of distended bladder following a confinement. The doctor said to me when we were going downstairs, "Is that common ?" I can only describe that honestly as culpable ignorance on his part not to know that retention of urine, especially in a primipara, after confinement is the commonest incident which you are warned about by everybody, it is the commonest thing to look out for, and it must be your first inquiry, "Did you pass your water this morning ?" Also, "Did you pass it voluntarily ?"— that is to say, was it merely an escape ? I said to him, "Just put your hand on the abdomen." If he had done that, he could not have made the mistake he did. It was culpable ignorance.

There is another frequent enough cause of mistake through sheer ignorance which a man has no business whatever to make, and that is in connection with the eye, in calling an iritis conjunctivitis. A practitioner looks at an eye with a very casual glance and without knowing anything whatever about the eye, says : "Yes, a little conjunctivitis ; put in a little of this lotion and you will be all right in a day or two." The results of such a mistake are most disastrous and may possibly lead to loss of sight. In more than half the cases of iritis which are mistaken for conjunctivitis the result is the loss of an eye, or, at any rate, some impairment of sight. Why do I say "culpable ignorance"? Because if you have a person with anything like severe inflammation of the eye your first duty is to see whether the iris reacts to light. I have not time to go into eye diseases, and I am not qualified to deal with them to any depth, but there is no doubt about that point. If the iris reacts to light, the probability is that the condition from which the patient is suffering is not iritis. If it does not react to light send the patient on at once to somebody who understands eye troubles ; do not tackle it yourself unless you know something about eye diseases and their treatment, or unless you are in the country and are obliged to do something for the patient. Do not let a person lose his eyesight through culpable ignorance on your part, through not knowing that the iris will not react to light when it is acutely inflamed.

One more example, because it has occurred to me in the last week. Those of you who are my clerks will remember that I was in the theatre on Monday to see a little boy operated upon. He had his leg amputated. One year ago he complained of pain in his left knee. His medical man saw it and called it rheumatism. I do not blame him for that, there is no particular mistake there. But your duty is, in such a case, to keep your eye upon the case ; for if a pain, as was the case here, remains for some months fixed to one knee, you may be quite certain it is not rheumatism, whatever else it may be. And do not be misled into the mistake of calling it rheumatism when you know, or ought to know, that it has remained fixed to one particular spot. The history makes it look worse still. After that doctor had treated him for several months and he got no better—he was not likely to—the parents were misguided enough to seek the advice of a homœopath. What you expect from homœopathy in the case of a knee-joint that has had pain in it for six months I do not know. However, the homœopath would not get anybody else's advice, the boy got very lame, and at length his mother brought him to me. I am not telling you because I think I can diagnose better than other physicians : I cannot. But one single glance at that knee was enough to convince me of what was wrong with him. There was the bottom end of the femur with a great bulge on it, and to

call that rheumatism, and to go on treating it with homœopathic remedies, was out of the question : in fact, I think one might say it was obviously wrong. Of course I told the child's mother the boy must either lose his life or his leg. He has lost his leg, and I hope he will not lose anything more. I admit that in this particular instance he might have had to lose his leg in any case, even if the condition had been properly diagnosed earlier ; still, it is quite out of the question to go on treating a pain localised for some months to one joint as rheumatism. Do not forget that.

The second group is those mistakes which are avoidable by the exercise of care—in other words, mistakes caused by carelessness, a very large class containing every grade of seriousness in the result. Let me give you one or two illustrations of this. First, as to diarrhœa and carcinoma of the rectum, or again, diarrhœa and typhoid fever. You may put it down as an aphorism that if a patient over forty-five years of age of either sex comes to you complaining of diarrhœa, you are distinctly negligent if you omit to pass your finger into the rectum. I will admit having made that mistake myself, and I was to blame. It was a serious mistake, made through hurry and carelessness. In other words, I did not pass my finger into the rectum. If I had done so I should have felt a distinct ring of carcinoma three inches in. But it taught me a lesson, and you should try to avoid neglecting that examination. I have mentioned diarrhœa and typhoid fever because you may, in your surgery, frequently enough get a patient coming to you and saying, "Doctor, I am very seedy ; I have had diarrhœa four or five days." Now, I consider it a very careless and negligent and bad mistake if you do not take that man's temperature. It is a very simple proceeding, and occupies about one and a half minutes. If his temperature is up I do not say the condition is necessarily typhoid—it is not the mistake of not diagnosing typhoid that I am speaking of, it is the mistake of not diagnosing "bed." That patient should be in bed who has diarrhœa and a temperature. That is where the negligence comes in, in not recognising that the first necessary step is to get him to bed.

Now let me tell you of another case which I saw some years ago now. A gentleman, æt. about 65 years, or at any rate who was getting on in years, was sent to me about July. The history he gave was that as long ago as the previous August—that is to say, for eleven months—he had been subject to periodic vomiting, and by that I mean he had not passed three consecutive days without vomiting. On many of those occasions he had vomited a large quantity. I stripped him, put him upon a hard couch, and laid my hand on his abdomen. I could feel nothing ; but before my hand had been there a few seconds I felt rising up underneath it a tumour, which in outline was like a Rugby football—that is to say, the man had a hugely dilated stomach. I do not quite know whether one ought to put that into the class of " carelessness," or whether one should not rather put it into the class of "ignorance," because that same tumour had been felt by his medical man for at least three months previously to my seeing him, and he had felt it frequently, and the patient had been told that he had got a big liver. There was this conjunction of things : periodical vomiting very nearly every day, or at any rate three days a week, and a big lump in the abdomen, which was not always there, but which one could feel rise up under one's hand, and he called it a big liver. I think such a case as that shows almost criminal ignorance. It is not as though it had been a small lump. In some abdominal cases, as I shall mention shortly, mistakes are unavoidable. So much for pyloric obstruction and distension of the stomach, and not atonic dilatation of it ; this man's stomach was still very strong, and was making frantic efforts to pass food through the obstructed pylorus, but it could not.

Another very common mistake I have put among the avoidable by care, or caused by carelessness, and that is, a patient comes to you in the surgery and complains of a cough, and you do not trouble to listen to his chest ; I mean just a brief examination, making him draw half a dozen breaths, and cough, and talk to you, not an elaborate routine one such as we conduct when we have an obscure case of disease of the lung. By neglecting that examination you may overlook early but easily diagnosable phthisis. That is a mistake which is rather serious, inasmuch as one has been forced to the belief—I have held it for a long time—that phthisis, in the early stages anyhow, is definitely curable, and especially with a certain amount of sanatorium treatment. By the way, I may say I believe that they make one great mistake in

sanatoria, and that is in spending their money in bricks and mortar when they ought to spend it in mere boards and a tin roof. Whenever a patient comes to your surgery with a cough and complains of the chest, do not merely prescribe a little physic without examination. I frankly admit that if you find it is phthisis you may equally well give him some squills and ipecacuanha, and things of that kind ; but you should know that he has phthisis, and then, having had time to read up phthisis, if you have forgotten it, or to take advice from somebody else on it, give him the best treatment for phthisis, and do not let him come back for another bottle of cough-stuff without giving him some appropriate advice about phthisis.

Another mistake, and not by any means an uncommon one, was really the object of one of the questions which we set in the last examination. A patient complains of sciatica. You will frequently, through carelessness, call it just simply sciatica. Let me tell you that there is one simple question which you should certainly put to such a patient, and if you do not put it it is a careless blunder : Is the pain confined to one leg, and is it worse at night ? If it is in both legs, or worse at night, do not forget to examine the abdomen and rectum and back for a growth. It is commonly enough called sciatica by the patient, but very few of those papers which I saw—certainly not half a dozen—gave one that straight tip about " sciatica." Of course, you may still be foiled, but those are niceties of diagnosis, and belong to the group of mistakes which are unavoidable. But frequently enough, through not putting these questions, you make a mistake which is distinctly avoidable with reasonable care.

One more of those instances of mistakes which are avoidable by a little care. It has reference to very much the same thing as rheumatism and sarcoma, which I spoke of just now as an instance of culpable and criminal negligence. It is epiphysitis and rheumatism. We had two of those cases of epiphysitis down in the operating theatre this week and neither of them was diagnosed straight off. That is no particularly serious mistake ; you cannot always diagnose them straight off. One was discovered, unfortunately, too late. But I do not know whether it is not always too late when you get a septic epiphysitis in a child ; I am afraid it is pretty nearly a fatal trouble, certainly it is fatal if the condition is not diagnosed quickly. There the mistake was made in the first instance by calling it rheumatism. And it is a very common mistake. But notice, you should clear that diagnosis in about three examinations anyhow. You will find that the pain is still in one spot, you will find it is the one joint only which is affected, and therefore, it is not rheumatism, whatever else it may be.

Now for the third group of mistakes, namely mistakes avoidable by delay, or, in other words, mistakes caused by impatience. These are chiefly mistakes in diagnosis in acute cases. Take, for instance, pneumonia and meningitis. On more than one occasion these have been confused. One instance is very fresh in my mind. I was sent for to see a boy of six or seven years of age, and I was informed that he was very acutely ill and likely to die of meningitis. Why? Because he had been vomiting very badly and had intense headache, and the doctor thought there was some retraction of the head. Now, such a case as that is good enough for wanting to have a second opinion, you would like somebody else to give you a hint in connection with it, or to look it up and see whether it is meningitis. Understand I am not blaming the doctor here, because it is a mistake which might be avoidable by delay, but sometimes the friends will not give you time but insist upon a diagnosis before it is reasonable. When I got there there was no brilliant merit to be attributed to me. His left lung was quite solid, and I therefore had no difficulty in saying, "It is a case of pneumonia and the probability is that the child will get well ; it is not meningitis." I am not talking about my superior cleverness : I am only talking about a doctor being compelled, or being very much pressed by the friends, to give a diagnosis before the facts warrant it. In other words, such a mistake is avoidable by delay. In a similar way almost any of the acute infectious fevers require time for diagnosis. A patient's temperature is 103° or 102°; what is the matter ? " Oh, I should think it is a bad cold, or measles ; " or " I do not think it is measles." That is because you rush in to make a diagnosis, possibly, as I say, because the friends insisted upon knowing at once what was the matter. More particularly is that true of typhoid as compared with acute tuberculosis ; for instance do not attempt to

be sure of typhoid before the seventh or eighth day, by which time you can reasonably expect some sort of rash. It is not always your fault, but it is a mistake which may cost you rather dearly, which may damage your reputation, if you say it is typhoid when it is not, or say it is not typhoid when it is. In neither case do you do your reputation or yourself any good. You should say " It is an acute fever of some sort, and you must give me a few days to tell you exactly what it may be." And if typhoid should cross your mind do not blurt it out ; wait for a day or two until you get more certain of it. Between typhoid and acute tuberculosis you may make blunders, and the mistake may remain till death. I advise you to read Fagge—I think the case is in all editions—under the heading of " Typhoid," and you will find there that sundry German professors examined a case for days very carefully, six or eight times, and each time they came they altered their opinion between tubercle and typhoid, and finally they guessed wrong.

There is just one other mistake avoidable by delay in that group, and that is poisoning by anything which is volatile. A very typical illustration of that happened the other day. I read the account, but I have forgotten what particular substance it was. It occurred at a fire, and there were some carboys burst, probably of nitric or hydrochloric or some other acid—it is really immaterial for my purpose—and four firemen were overcome with the fumes, and in consequence were taken into the hospital. In three or four hours they were very much better, and were allowed to go home. That is where the mistake comes in, letting them go home. Within the next twelve hours they were all brought back : two of them died and two of them managed to struggle through. These fumes had got into their lungs and caused acute bronchitis. I forget what the trouble was, but the fumes of the acid passed into the trachea and air-passages. The vapour of these volatile substances is dangerous and, therefore, any case of poisoning by these things should be most carefully watched for at least twenty-four hours. There is your mistake, in allowing them to go home because they do not seem to be very bad, and not particularly sick. Perhaps they will say in a few hours, "I am all right ; let me go home." I may mention another cause of poisoning, phosphorus, where you are likely to make a mistake by not delaying. In such a case keep the patient at least a week under observation and in bed, because of the possible secondary fatty degeneration which may come on in ten days or a week after the original symptoms have disappeared.

I made a mistake through impatience only this week in a nurse with rheumatism ; I mentioned it to you yesterday in the wards. It was a mistake in treatment. She was under salicylate and she got perfectly well as far as we could see. I had some suspicions of her heart, but as her temperature remained down for, I think, five days, I let her up. Next day she developed a temperature of 99°, and endocarditis, probably due to my letting her up too soon. At any rate, I must take the responsibility. Never let a patient in whom you have the slightest suspicion of endocarditis occurring on top of rheumatism get up for a fortnight after the temperature is normal. That is a mistake avoidable by delay. But it will not be your impatience only : it will also be the impatience of the patient. This nurse was very keen on getting on with her work, and I foolishly allowed her to get up. I could multiply such instances of mistakes through haste or impatience, but these will suffice to enable you to think of such for yourselves.

Now we come to a group of unavoidable mistakes. Remember I have divided mistakes into serious and non-serious, and although I call these unavoidable, they are still divisible into the serious and non-serious. And happy is the man who has taken every possible pains to avoid what was unavoidable and done his level best, so that let the result be ever so serious he has a clear conscience in the case. Now, in unavoidable mistakes you may put very many abdominal cases. They really are unavoidable. It is simply impossible with our present knowledge, and, I think, one may say with any knowledge, considering the variety of symptoms, to be certain, for instance, that a gastric or duodenal ulcer is present. Unfortunately, I have had experience of such mistakes after taking all the steps I could to ascertain the truth. One such I will mention to you. The wife of a medical man was sent to me from Southend. I had seen her about nine months previously, when she had symptoms of what I myself thought to be gastric ulcer. During the nine months' interval she had got rid entirely of all her symptoms, was able to eat anything, and

was perfectly happy. She was sent up to me to ask my opinion whether she might safely go with her husband on his holiday. I examined her as carefully as I could, inquired most strictly into the history of the nine months, and everything seemed to fit in very well. The pain had gradually disappeared, she had gradually been able to eat anything, and for three months had not had a symptom of any sort. I said I thought she would be safe in going for her holidays, as everything seemed satisfactory. But before she could start on her holiday she was dead with acute perforation of a gastric ulcer. Frankly I do not blame myself ; I think I had taken every possible step. But had her husband not been a medical man and known the difficulties of such cases, you can easily understand a thing of that sort would have been very awkward for me. To tell a patient she may be quite happy and go for her holiday without anxiety, and then for her to be dead before she could start, is not a pleasant thing to happen to anybody, and the husband is not likely to forget it.

Take perforation in typhoid fever. I have made several mistakes that way, simple mistakes in thinking perforation had taken place when it had not, and having the abdomen opened in accordance with my belief. In two of them I know there was no perforation found. The results were not particularly serious, because the typhoid itself was very bad, and the operation did not do any particular harm. But if a patient complains of an acute pain in the abdomen in typhoid it is extremely difficult to know whether perforation has taken place or not. I cannot enter into the diagnosis of that, but I can tell you the diagnosis is very difficult indeed. And yet, if perforation has taken place, the only hope for the patient lies in a surgical operation. If you let your patient die without that operation you will say, " What a pity ! " and if you open the abdomen and find no perforation you will say " What a pity ! " then also. All I can say is, it is unfortunate.

Let me mention phthisis and pneumonia. It is not a particularly infrequent history that a patient has pneumonia, the case seems fairly straightforward, and the patient gets a crisis, and then in a few days the temperature goes wandering about, and you think there is something else wrong, and ultimately it turns out to be a case of rapidly advancing phthisis. I think it is absolutely unavoidable omitting to detect the phthisis earlier. There are all the symptoms of pneumonia, all the physical signs of it, and the fact that the patient had had phthisis for some weeks, possibly even months, with no very obvious symptoms, could not be ascertained. You may have suspected it from the first, there is nothing more to be said about it.

Next, take stone in the kidney on the wrong side. Perhaps this is a surgical mistake, though such usually come first to a physician. There are too many cases on record for us not to recognise it as a mistake which is unavoidable. The patient complains of intense pain on the right side, passes blood and pus and all the rest of it. You say, "Yes, he has stone in the right kidney," and you have him operated upon. But you find his right kidney is healthy, and the trouble is all on the left side. The patient has always complained of pain on the wrong side, and that mistake is one which is quite unavoidable.

Abscess v. tumour in the brain is another unavoidable mistake, which I have made myself. I was asked to see a man, æt. about 45 years, who for the past ten or twelve years had had a constant discharge from his nose. In the previous few days he had developed cerebral symptoms rather acutely. The nasal discharge had ceased, and I made the mistake of assuming that he had cerebral abscess, and I therefore took him into the hospital with the view of having him operated upon. To show you that the mistake was probably unavoidable, I got Dr. Head to see him. He agreed with my opinion, but he said it was useless to operate, the abscess was too large. The patient died, and post mortem a small tumour was found in the left occipital region. The frontal lobe, which we thought was involved, contained no trace of anything wrong, there was no trace of abscess anywhere. I think that was an unavoidable mistake.

Then I want to say a word about pleuritic effusion and carcinoma of the lung. For your own satisfaction you may say this: fully 95 per cent. of primary growths or tumours of the pleura and lung will be called, and are, pleural effusions. The condition starts a pleural effusion. You put a needle in and draw off perhaps a couple or three pints of fluid, and it is only after you have done that that you are in a position to decide that the dulness and all the rest of the physical signs and symptoms, cough, and so on, were not due to pleural effusion,

but to invading malignant trouble. You will always call them pleural effusions until you have drawn off the fluid, and only when the chest does not clear up at all and the patient remains as pale as ever, and the temperature and other features such as local œdema develop, will you make a correct diagnosis. That is probably an unavoidable mistake.

Here is another unavoidable mistake. I was asked to see a little child with broncho-pneumonia. "How long has it been ill?" "It was taken suddenly ill the other day." I could not quite make the case out. I was told the child seemed to have been choked and I looked carefully at its larynx. To cut the matter short, it had broncho-pneumonia, came into hospital, and died. On post-mortem examination we found a piece of bone sticking in the trachea, below the vocal cords; this had caused suppurative inflammation, and so had set up an attack of septic broncho-pneumonia. How had he got this piece of bone into the throat? We inquired into it, and it appeared the child had been given some ox-tail soup and it had been noticed to choke, but nothing else had happened. He had only gone slightly blue, and that was probably due to coughing. I had looked at the throat and taken all the care I could, but could not discover the bone. I do not see how one could have avoided that mistake in diagnosis. That unavoidable group is a very large one; it embraces all the cavities of the body, as my five cases show.

I will now give you an illustration or two of classes of mistakes due rather to the nature of the case than to any attribute of the practitioner, mistakes which may belong to any of my groups.

Take, for instance, children in general, babies in particular, who are totally unable to speak. They will cry on account of pain, but you have to watch very closely, and trust to the mother's account, probably, for the localisation of the pain. A crying baby may not give you any clue and mistakes are sometimes unavoidable. You cannot find out why it is crying or where the pain is; but on other occasions a little abnormality, such as a swelling of a joint, or a swelling in the belly, or straining at stool, or passing a little blood per rectum, or a little swelling in the neck, or perhaps the child biting its thumb, suggesting pain in the gum through teething, will give you a clue upon which to work. But, as I have said, you may find absolutely nothing wrong, and even if the child loses its life you may find something post mortem which you could not possibly have discovered during life. Now, there is one special point to be observed about babies or children up to two or three years of age, and that is immobility of a limb—pseudo-paralysis. The healthy baby who is not crying, and not in pain, and not asleep, is scrambling about with both legs, and kicking somebody or something, and is using his arms on every possible occasion. But if you notice one arm or one leg is not being used, that is a thing which should put you at once on the track of two or three separate possibilities. And one of them is our old friend epiphysitis or osteomyelitis. Another is infantile paralysis. A third one might be an actual traumatic paralysis of the limb. Or it might be a congenital condition. You may have a hæmorrhage on the surface of the brain corresponding to the limb, a congenital paralysis or a birth palsy. Sometimes a little more observation and inquiry will enable you to see that that is the cause, or again, a little local examination may clear up your mistake. The same thing happens with tubercular disease in the joint. The child will hold such a joint still as far as he can because of the pain caused on moving it. And then there are startings at night. In the case of a child of six or seven he can tell you there is a pain in a knee, and as soon as he gets to sleep he will wake up with a jump, but in the case of a little child it is sometimes almost impossible to tell what is the matter with it. Again, fits in children, how easy it is to make a mistake there! I cannot enter here into the causes of fits, but one may mention some half-dozen common causes which have to be inquired into, and if you do not it is carelessness. But if you do you may get no satisfactory replies, and then it belongs to the class of unavoidable mistakes. For instance, there may be a genuine epileptic fit. There may be a fit due to teething, and the fact whether the child is or is not at the age for teething will give you an idea. Or the child may have a fit from the presence of worms. I think the most common cause of fits in children over a year old, or even under a year, is simple indigestion. A bad attack of indigestion in an adult, as some of you may have experienced in your own persons, will cause you considerable suffering, so that you can readily understand that

in the case of a little baby, with its very delicate nervous system, a fit could easily be started. The mistake may be made by impatience. The mother will want to know what is the meaning of this fit. Do not rush in at once and tell her it is so-and-so, but look around and say, " I cannot find any particular cause for it ; we must watch the child for a day or two." Perhaps you will at the same time give it a little santonin, or have its bowels washed out and tell the mother to look out for worms in its motions. You will also inquire about its food. You should do all that before you frighten the mother by saying it has had an epileptic fit or that it has serious trouble.

Then there is the "drunk or dying" group. Drunk or dying is the question which will perhaps more frequently occur than any other, and is more likely to get you into trouble if you make a mistake. And the mistake which you must avoid in that connection is not that of giving a wrong diagnosis, but in giving the wrong treatment—that is to say, sending the patient home and saying there is nothing the matter except that he is drunk. Act as though such cases were dying ; your mistake consists in not doing so. It is comparatively immaterial what is the matter with the man ; he is unconscious or semi-conscious, kicking up a row, and perhaps may be having fits; he may be paralysed anywhere ; it may be a case of diabetic coma ; it may be uræmia, or half a dozen serious conditions; it may be simply drunkenness. What does it matter about what is wrong if you take him in and care for him for twelve hours and have him watched ? Absolutely all you lose by it is a little trouble, and you probably will not sit up with him yourself—you will get a nurse—so it is not any real trouble to you. You cannot be blamed if you have taken the precaution of watching the case. You should say, "You tell me this man is only drunk, but I shall act as if he were dying, and treat him accordingly." It is probable that you may make a mistake about the diagnosis, but it is avoidable for you to treat a dying man as a drunkard, and put him into a cold police-cell.

Now, with regard to mistakes in prognosis. They belong very frequently to the unavoidable group, but they are a group in themselves that are just worth a few words in a clinical lecture, though, after all, I am afraid I shall have to tell you that your one way out of making mistakes in prognosis is to speak somewhat like a Delphic oracle of old did—saying if you are going to be successful you will, and if you are not going. to be you will not ; that is about what it comes to. A man will live if he does not die, and if he dies he will not live. But still, be very cautious, because a mistake in prognosis, although perhaps not serious for the patient, may be serious for your reputation. Take, for instance, heart-disease. I know no subject in medicine so difficult as the prognosis of heart-disease, absolutely none. There is no case of disease in which you will not make more glaring blunders than heart-disease ; do not commit yourself to a positive statement as to what is going to happen, but watch the case, and say : " It is going on very favourably, and I have every hope he may be restored, but I shall not tell you he will be." If you see him going downhill or remaining passive, and nothing seems to do him good, you can say : " I am not going to give up hope just yet. I feel extremely anxious ; he does not respond to remedies in the way I should like." Do not say : " I can promise you you will be all right in a week or two ; " never promise anything, especially about a heart case. It is much the same with a kidney case also, especially chronic kidney disease. Do not be too keen on prognosis. Again, with typhoid do not express a positive prognosis in that disease ever. I can tell you of a case which occurred to me in Gurney Ward some years ago. A young girl, æt. 26 years, had typhoid ; she was practically well, and I am not sure that she was not going out. The temperature had been down for some time, and one thought she would soon be out of hospital. But she only left it in her coffin. She suddenly got a perforation and died in less than twenty-four hours. There are always those possible chances in typhoid, and in giving a prognosis you will be sure to make a mistake if you speak too positively. There are very few diseases in which the prognosis is an absolute matter of certainty. I think one of the best conditions to be sure about would be myx-œdema, when treated by thyroid extract. I think you can speak more positively about the prognosis in that condition than in any other disease. Certainly in the case of disease of the lungs, where you may have phthisis at the bottom of it, the prognosis is a very serious matter to deal with, and I advise you not to be too rash about it.

We will finish with a few words about the commonest mistake, viz. that of drawing conclusions from imperfect premises, a mistake made by all who rush prematurely into print, partly intentionally, for mere advertisement purposes, and partly unintentionally, from enthusiasm. What I mean by that is this : You have a case of illness of any description, and give a certain drug, and the patient gets better. It is immediately said " Yes, he was cured by So-and-so by that drug." Of course it is very nice to feel it was the drug, and that it was you who gave it him, and that nobody else would have given it him. But if you make the mistake of drawing universal conclusions you will be led into serious errors of prognosis. You will get a case apparently exactly like the first one and you will say " Yes, I can cure him ; I cured Mr. So-and-so with this drug." You give it, but unfortunately the patient dies. Then your blunder is apparent and your reputation probably suffers material damage. Record the case by all means if you like—"I gave him iodide of potassium," for instance, "and he got well "—but do not be in a hurry to rush into print over it. I will give you an illustration. Quite recently I have had three cases of ulcerative colitis under my care, and they are all three still under care. In all of them I have had, or am having, mercury rubbed in very freely. They are all doing remarkably well. But I should be exceedingly foolish if I were to take a fourth case and say, " I will promise you I can cure you by rubbing in this mercury." It may be the case—I do not say it is, because there is no evidence of it—that my first two patients' conditions were due to syphilis, and therefore my unguentum hydrarg. did good because they were syphilitic cases. Or it may be that mercury has a specific effect upon the colon. I do not know ; I have not sufficient evidence on the subject to enable me to judge. I think it would be legitimate to point out the results I have obtained, and I intend to publish the cases and to state that I did have mercury rubbed in. But to immediately rush in and say that every case of colitis must have mercury rubbed in and they will all get well would be a very serious mistake, due to drawing rash conclusions from insufficient premises.

Gentlemen, I have concluded what I fear is a very imperfect sketch of mistakes, but my remarks may save some of you from a few unnecessary mistakes. I trust it may be so, and while remembering *Nemo mortalium omnibus horis sapit,* don't on that account be ignorant, careless, or impatient.

December 25th, 1905.

THE TREATMENT, ESPECIALLY POST-OPERATIVE, OF ACUTE ABDOMINAL CONDITIONS.

By J. H. BRYANT, M.D., F.R.C.P.,
Assistant Physician to Guy's Hospital.

GENTLEMEN,—I have chosen a very wide subject, and my remarks will necessarily be somewhat fragmentary. The acute abdominal conditions I propose to refer to are: appendicitis, general peritonitis from perforating gastric ulcer and appendicitis, and acute intestinal obstruction.

During the last few years a gradual change has taken place in the treatment of these diseases. I was brought up to the belief that opium in some form or other was the sheet-anchor, whatever that may mean, in cases of peritonitis, but I have long come to the conclusion that it is a snare and a delusion. A few years ago it was an almost unheard of event for a patient suffering from general suppurative peritonitis to recover, whether operated on in the early stages or not, whereas at the present time we are beginning to look upon it as quite an ordinary occurrence. One naturally reflects on the cause of such a change for the better. I admit great advances have been made in the surgical treatment of suppurative peritonitis, and it is now dealt with earlier and in a much bolder manner; but it is not enough to account altogether for such a marvellous improvement in prognosis, and I am convinced in my own mind that abstinence from the use of morphia before and after operation is one of the chief factors which has been instrumental in affecting this important change.

Morphia given in the early stages masks the symptoms, gives a false sense of security to both the doctor and the patient's friends, and misleads the surgeon; when administered at the time of the operation, or afterwards, it keeps up sickness, increases the tendency to paralysis of the gut, prevents the bowels being opened, and thus promotes septic absorption from the gut, a condition from which many of these patients die.

You may say it is imperative to give opium or morphia because the patient and those around him clamour for the relief of the pain which is frequently so intense and agonising in character, especially in the early stages. When satisfied the symptoms are due to general peritonitis it is best to combat the collapse with strychnine and to arrange for operative measures as soon as possible, and I would go still further and say that if in doubt it is far better to resort to surgery than to temporise with morphia. By hesitation and delay the golden opportunity is allowed to slip by and the life is lost.

I do not wish to give you the impression that I am so biassed against the use of morphia as to recommend that it should never be given. In some cases, especially in private practice, it is impossible to avoid it. Also, I do not wish to give you the idea that there is a very definite routine method of dealing with these cases. Each patient must be treated, not the disease. If possible, however, I am convinced it is best to avoid the administration of opium or morphia; but if it is absolutely necessary to deal with the pain and restlessness which may follow the operation, to substitute nepenthe (a derivative of opium which relieves pain and has no bad after-effects), in from 10 to 15 minim doses, administered *per rectum*.

The following case is an important justification for what I have just said:

At 1.30 a.m., on November 8th, I was summoned to Guy's Hospital to see a boy, æt. 14 years, who had just been admitted from Beckenham for pain in the abdomen. At 3 a.m. on November 7th he woke up with severe pain in his abdomen. His mother, thinking his trouble was due to wind, gave him a dose of castor oil, which he promptly returned. He remained in bed all day, and in the afternoon another purgative was administered, but as it did not act an enema of oil was given and his bowels were freely opened. As he still complained of pain, in the evening Dr. Butler was called in, who, finding his abdomen distended and tender all over, especially in the right iliac fossa, the temperature 101° and pulse 120, advised his immediate removal to Guy's Hospital for operation. No morphia was administered.

On admission the pulse was 130, temperature 101°. The abdomen was distended and tender, especially in the right iliac fossa, and the lower part did not move on respiration. The tongue was moist and clean. Nothing abnormal was found *per rectum*. The heart and lungs were normal. There was a leucocytosis of 30,000 to the cubic millimetre. On account of the severity of the onset, the rapid pulse, the leucocytosis, and the condition of the abdomen a diagnosis of gangrenous appendicitis and pelvic peritonitis was made. Mr. Steward was sent for and operated on him at 3.25 a.m. On opening the abdomen there were signs of acute peritonitis and practically the whole of the appendix was found to be in a condition of gangrene. It was removed and he was put back to bed. During the operation 4 minims of liquor strychninæ were injected. An hour after the operation his pulse rose to 140 and it was feeble, so 10 ounces of saline fluid were injected *per rectum*, but were not retained.

At 5.15 a.m. he became worse and the pulse was hardly perceptible at the wrist, so 3 pints of saline were injected into his right median basilic vein and 3 more minims of strychnine were injected hypo-dermically. At 6.30 a.m. he was much better, his pulse was 130, and he wanted to go to sleep. On the following day his abdomen was a good deal distended, and a *glycerine enema* was given, but with no result. On the 9th another oil and soap enema was given and his bowels were opened. He was given nothing by the mouth at first, but twelve hours after the anæsthetic he was put on small feeds of milk and barley-water and on the 9th on the ordinary milk diet of 5 oz. every two hours. On the 12th he was allowed other fluids and junket, and on the 13th farinaceous food. He is making a good recovery.

The promptitude of Dr. Butler in bringing this boy from Beckenham to the hospital in the middle of the night undoubtedly was the means of saving his life, for it was quite obvious from the appearance of the appendix that it would have very soon sloughed off and given rise to a most virulent general peritonitis. Morphia in such a case would have in all probability been the means of delaying the operation, and a delay would have lost the boy his life. This case also illustrates the important fact that there is frequently very little pain after abdominal section and that the routine after-treatment with morphia is quite unnecessary. The most important points in the after-treatment of this case were the injections of strychnine and the intravenous infusion of three pints of saline, but for which he would have died.

The importance also of making an early diagnosis in cases of perforating gastric ulcer cannot be under estimated, for there is no other but surgical treatment, and unless the patient is operated upon within the first twelve hours there

is very little hope of recovery. The two following cases illustrate, first, the satisfactory results which may be hoped for if the condition is dealt with promptly, and, second, the slight degree of general disturbance and collapse which resulted from the performance of the operation.

A strong, healthy-looking young stevedore, æt. 25 years, was admitted under my care on July 4th, 1903, for a severe attack of abdominal pain which had commenced suddenly at 9 a.m. that morning whilst he was at work in the docks. The pain was so intense, he felt so faint and looked so ill that his friends removed him at once to the hospital. For the last twelve months he had been troubled with attacks of vomiting, abdominal pain, and flatulence.

I saw him soon after admission. He was very pale and appeared to be suffering from acute pain in the abdomen, which was a little retracted, extremely hard and board-like, uniformly tender, and did not move on respiration. The pain was most marked in the epigastrium. Perforating gastric ulcer was diagnosed, and my surgical colleague, Mr. Dunn, operated on him at 2 p.m., five hours after the perforation had occurred.

A perforation was found of the anterior wall of the stomach close to the pylorus, and there was general peritonitis. The ulcer was closed by a purse-string suture, the peritoneal cavity was flushed out with a large quantity of sterilised water and a counter opening was made for the drainage of the pelvis in the median line between the pubes and the umbilicus.

He slept well after being put back to bed and had very little vomiting.

After-treatment.—Nothing was given by the mouth.

Large nutrient enemas (ʒviij) and salines 10 to 20 oz. were ordered every four hours alternately.

A mouth-wash containing glycerine and chinosol was ordered : ℞ glycerin ʒiij, sol. chinosol (1 in 1000) ʒxij.

July 5th.—At 4 a.m., as he was restless and in pain 15 minims of nepenthe were added to the saline enema. This relieved his pain and sent him to sleep. He was very comfortable all day. Sips of warm water were allowed him after 2 p.m.

On July 6th there was a natural action of the bowels.

On July 9th peptonised milk, ʒiij, alternating

with a similar quantity of equal parts of milk and barley-water, was allowed every three hours.

On July 11th the feeds were increased to ℨiv.

On July 12th a soap enema was administered with a good result.

On July 13th he was allowed custard and milk. The enemata were omitted.

From July 15th to 25th he was a little troubled with constipation, which was dealt with in the ordinary way.

On July 30th, twenty-six days after the operation, he was discharged and went to Swanley Convalescent Home.

His temperature was never above 100°, his pulse and respiration never above 84 and 24 respectively.

A warehouseman was admitted at 12 p.m., July 2nd, 1892, for acute abdominal pain and vomiting which had come on quite suddenly as he was seated in a train at Liverpool Street on his way to Yarmouth. He appeared to be so ill that his friends brought him to Guy's Hospital, when he was at once admitted. With the exception of constipation all his life and indigestion for the last four or five days he had enjoyed good health. I happened to be in the ward when he arrived. He was suffering from very severe pain in the abdomen, and his abdominal wall was contracted, rigid, and motionless. There was a good deal of tenderness, especially in the epigastrium. The pulse was 96 and of good volume. A diagnosis of perforating gastric ulcer was made, and I sent for my surgical colleague, Mr. Dunn, who agreed to operate at once. A small perforation was found in the anterior wall of the stomach near the pylorus, and was closed by means of a purse-string suture. The peritoneal cavity was flushed out with sterile water, and the edges of the wound were united with catgut sutures, a tube being left in the lower part as a drain.

He was got back to bed within three hours of the time of perforation. The pulse at the end of the operation was 104. As he was in a good deal of pain and there was no distension of the gut, a quarter of a grain of morphia was injected hypodermically at 3.30 a.m. Nutrient enemas, which were composed of starch solution ℨij, white of egg ℨj, bovril ℨij, peptonised milk ℨvj, were ordered every six hours. His mouth was frequently washed out with hot water.

July 6th.—The highest temperature was 101.°

Pulse 92. Respiration 32. He was feeling quite comfortable.

July 7th.—He was better, but felt a little sick. Highest temperature 101°. Pulse 92. Respiration 36.

July 8th.—Highest temperature 100·4°. Pulse 84, of good volume. His condition was excellent. He was ordered albumen water ℨj, water ℨss., to take every hour.

July 9th and 10th.—Temperature normal. Pulse 56. No abdominal pain, no distension. Albumen water ℨiij, water ℨij, every two hours. The enemas were omitted. He had been fed *per rectum* for three days.

July 11th.—Milk ℨiv, albumen water ℨij, every two hours. A soap enema was administered with a good result.

July 12th.—Milk, jelly, and custard ordered.

July 13th.—Drainage-tubes removed.

July 15th.—Bread and milk allowed.

July 16th.—Stitches removed.

July 19th.—Minced chicken and boiled fish allowed.

July 29th.—He got up after tea (twenty-four days after operation). The abdomen was tightly bandaged.

August 6th.—He was allowed to get up after dinner.

August 14th.—Discharged, thirty-nine days after the operation, feeling quite well.

On account of the short times which had elapsed between the times of perforation and the operation, three and five hours, there was neither collapse, nor loss of fluid, nor distension of the gut from paralysis to deal with, so that the after-treatment was comparatively simple.

In the first case pain and restlessness were relieved by 15 minims of nepenthe administered in a saline enema. I have found this preparation of opium very useful under similar conditions, and prefer its use to either opium or morphia, as there are practically no disturbing after-effects, such as headache, sickness, etc. In the other case one injection of morphia, gr. ¼, was all that was required.

With regard to the feeding, it is best to give the stomach a rest for as long as possible, and to rely on nutrient and saline enemata. Nutrient suppositories are useless. In my opinion it is best to give large nutrient enemata and saline enemata alternately every four hours. The rectum is much more tolerant if this method of alternating a simple saline enema with a nutrient enema is adopted, so that rectal feeding can be continued for a longer period, and thirst is allayed by the use of the saline enemata. For many years it has been customary at Guy's to limit the size of the nutrient enema to four ounces, but this idea has been revolutionised by Dr. Beddard, who in an article on rectal feeding in the 'Guy's Hospital Gazette,' October 12th, 1901, advocated the use of large enemata at longer intervals. To quote : "An adult will, as a rule, easily retain an enema of nine ounces if the following points are attended to—that the enema is at the temperature of the body, that it is run in slowly and continuously without squirting and without air, that it is spread over the largest possible surface of the large intestine, and that it is not allowed to trickle down in the rectum towards the internal sphincter, for the higher material is in the large intestine above the internal sphincter the less likely it is to set up a reflex act of defæcation."

The following are two examples of enemas recommended by Dr. Beddard : White of three eggs, salt gr. xl, peptonised milk, ad. ʒix, arrowroot ʒij, raw meat juice, ad. ʒix.

The amount of saline fluid (ʒj salt to a pint of water) should be 10 oz., or more if it can be retained and absorbed. If a difficulty is found in retaining these large enemata, it is better to give one every eight hours, and to supply fluid to the tissues by injecting saline fluid into the axillæ.

It is necessary to continue rectal feeding longest in cases of perforating gastric ulcer, but, as shown by the cases I have alluded to, it is soon possible to commence giving fluids by the mouth.

In the first case peptonised milk was given on the fifth day, and in the second case albumen water was given on the fourth day after the operation. If the peritonitis is the result of appendicitis, fluids may be given by the mouth as soon as vomiting ceases.

In order to give an idea of the manner in which desperately bad cases of general acute peritonitis are now dealt with I will read the following notes :

On November 2nd I saw, in consultation with Dr. Garbutt, a girl, æt. 18 years, who had been ill for a week and was suffering from vomiting and abdominal pain, distension, and tenderness. The temperature was 101° and the pulse 130. There was little difficulty in diagnosing general suppurative peritonitis, and the history of the illness pointed plainly in the direction of appendicitis as the cause. I advised her removal to the hospital with a view to immediate operation, and within two and a half hours she was operated upon by Mr. Lane.

General suppurative peritonitis was found, there being a large quantity of very foul-smelling pus in the pelvis. The appendix was gangrenous and had almost sloughed off close to the cæcum. It was removed, and the whole of the peritoneal cavity was flushed out with a large quantity of sterilised water. The flakes of lymph were peeled off the intestines, which were then returned to the peritoneal cavity. Gauze drains were placed in the pelvis and over the stump of the appendix. The wound was not sewn up, but pads of gauze were placed over the coils of intestine and the abdomen was then tightly bandaged with a sterilised towel. She was very collapsed before and after the operation.

Five minims of strychnine were injected during the operation and another 5 minims directly after it was over.

A coffee enema was administered at 4.30 p.m., but it was soon returned.

5.30 p.m.—A pint of saline fluid was injected into the axilla and another 5 minims of strychnine given and again repeated at 6.45 p.m., = 20 *minims in about two and a half hours*.

At 7 p.m. a turpentine enema was administered on Mr. Lane's suggestion, with a view to the relief of the abdominal distension. Four pints of saline fluid were infused through the median basilic vein.

At 9 p.m. four pints of saline fluid were infused into the left median basilic and another injection of strychnine was given.

Each time she improved after the injection of saline fluid and strychnine.

At 10 p.m. she was dressed, as the dressings had soaked through. An ounce of mag. sulph. was injected, in the form of a hot concentrated solution, into a coil of distended gut.

November 3rd, 12.30 a.m.—Five minims of strychnine were injected and two pints of saline were infused into the axilla at 1 a.m. The pulse remained feeble and rapid, and she suffered from severe vomiting.

At 1.30 a.m. another turpentine enema was

administered, and a good deal of flatus came away, affording considerable relief.

3 a.m.—The pulse was bad again, and four pints of saline were infused into the left median cephalic vein ; 5 minims of strychnine were also injected.

At 5 a.m. strychnine was again injected.

At 6 a.m. the pulse was still rapid, feeble, of poor volume, so a pint more of saline was infused into the right axilla. The wound was again dressed, and more concentrated solution of sulphate of magnesia was injected into the gut.

At 6.45 a.m. 5 minims of strychnine were injected.

At 8 a.m. she was fairly comfortable and the pulse was 116.

At 9 a.m. a glycerine enema was given, but with no result.

9.45 a.m.—Strychnine 5 minims.

At 10.30 a.m. I saw her and ordered calomel, gr. i, to be given every hour until the bowels should be opened. Small result at 3 p.m.—four doses taken.

At 2 p.m. Dr. Hale White saw patient and ordered a large enema consisting of 5 oz. each of olive oil and castor oil, which was given at 5 p.m. The bowels were well opened at 10 p.m.

At 4 p.m., as she was still vomiting, the stomach was washed out with hot water and a good deal of dark stale-smelling vomit was removed.

Thus nearly a drachm of Liq. strychninæ was injected in eighteen hours, and sixteen pints of saline in about fourteen hours were injected into the axillæ or veins.

At 2 p.m. a pint of saline fluid and 10 oz. enemas consisting of the white of three eggs, salt gr. xl, starch ℥ii, peptonised milk ℥viii were ordered alternately every four hours.

The bowels were opened in the morning. The wound was dressed in the afternoon under an anæsthetic, and the intestines were found to be much less distended. The intestines were then washed with saline solution and the wound was sewn up, except at the top and bottom, which were left open for the purpose of drainage. Five minims of strychnine were injected during the operation. In the evening she was fairly comfortable.

November 5th.—On the following day she was much more comfortable ; she was in very little pain and her bowels were opened twice.

November 6th.—The wound was dressed. A good deal of foul pus was evacuated.

November 7th.—Signs of bronchitis appeared.

November 8th.—She was not so well. The signs in the chest had increased, and she was evidently suffering from broncho-pneumonia, from which she succumbed on November 16th ; so that she lived for fourteen days after the operation for what appeared to be a hopeless condition.

The operation.—I have seen various operative measures adopted by different surgeons for dealing with general acute peritonitis, but am most impressed with the bold and effective methods of Mr. Lane. He makes a long median incision reaching almost from the tip of the ensiform cartilage to the pubes ; he then flushes out the peritoneal cavity with large quantities of water at a temperature of 110°, then wipes the peritoneal surface of the intestines from the duodenum downwards with sterilised pads of gauze, removing any lymph he comes across, wipes out the subphrenic spaces, and returns the coils of intestine to the peritoneal cavity. He makes no attempt to bring together the edges of the muscles, but covers the intestines with gauze which extends beneath the margins of the muscles that have separated to an extent proportionate to the intra-abdominal tension. To avoid any chance of the intestines protruding, the edges of the skin wound are brought together with horsehair except where a piece of the gauze is left for drainage. In this manner the distended intestines are quite relieved from the pressure, which if continued would of necessity cause death. In two or three days, when the distension of the intestines has subsided sufficiently, he brings the edges of the muscles together with sutures. I have seen excellent results follow this method of procedure, and my experience does not coincide with that of Mr. Barnard, who writes in the CLINICAL JOURNAL, September 30th, 1903: "I am strongly opposed to irrigating the general peritoneal cavity in these cases; for in the first place the toxin which was concentrated in the peritoneal cavity is well diluted and flushed into the general system."

It appears to me to be a good thing to wash away as much as possible of the results of the peritonitis and not to leave it behind in the peritoneal cavity, and I take it very little fluid would be absorbed during the process of irrigation through such a large incision. Mr. Barnard's method is to make a median incision above the pubes to reach the pelvic pouch and iliac fossæ, and one in each loin to reach the subphrenic spaces.

At the time of the operation should the pulse fail, still more liquor strychnine may be given, and I have sometimes had occasion to inject 10 to 15 and even 20 minims during this period. If the pulse does not react to the strychnine, it is advisable to infuse one, two, or three pints of saline solution into one of the veins of the arms.

In most cases of general acute peritonitis, whether due to appendicitis, perforating gastric ulcer, or other causes, and in cases of acute intestinal obstruction, whether peritonitis is present or not, the chief indications for treatment are to combat the—

(a) Cardiac failure and collapse,
(b) Loss of fluid from the tissues,
(c) Toxæmia,
(d) Tendency to paralysis of the gut,
(e) Pain,
(f) The condition of the mouth.

(a) Cardiac failure and collapse are best treated with strychnine. This drug should be pushed if necessary to its full extent, even up to the point at which twitching of the muscles commences. The dose of liquor strychnine is stated in Hale-White's 'Text-book of Materia Medica' to be from 1 to 4 minims if given hypodermically.

In cases similar to the one I have just described to you very large quantities of strychnine may and must be administered. The girl I allude to was given 55 minims in eighteen hours, i.e. half a grain of strychnine, which amount is stated to be the minimum fatal dose for an adult. A patient, æt. 22 years, who had been operated upon for appendicitis and pelvic peritonitis, and was put back to bed almost pulseless, was given 35 minims, spread over a period of less than twelve hours, but showed no signs of poisoning, and her tissues were so drained of fluid that during the same time she absorbed five pints of saline fluid from her rectum. A free supply of fluid to the dried up tissues is also an important aid to the stimulating effect of the strychnine.

(b) The loss of fluid.—In advanced cases of general peritonitis it is probable that for at least three or four days the patient has not retained any fluid which he has attempted to take by the mouth on account of the more or less constant vomiting

and in consequence it is obvious that there must be an enormous diminution in the amount of fluid in the tissues. The fluid so necessary for the life of the body and the needs of the circulation cannot, after an operation, be supplied by the mouth, nor in many cases can sufficient be absorbed by the rectum, so that it is necessary to resort to other means. In the case already alluded to nearly sixteen pints of saline were supplied by means of subcutaneous and intravenous injections.

Barnard in the same lecture which I have already alluded to strongly advocated the use of what he terms "massive saline subcutaneous transfusions," a method of treatment which was instituted by Kocher of Berne. Barnard uses the following apparatus. "About 4 feet of rubber tubing, weighted at the end, carries the saline from an ordinary ewer to a glass T tube, and this is connected by 2 further lengths of rubber tubing with 2 stout brandy-syringe needles which can be readily passed below the skin of the thighs." The strength of the saline solution in all the above methods should be 1 teaspoonful of salt to a pint of water. The water should be boiled and when used with Barnard's apparatus should be 115° F. when placed in the ewer, when used for intravenous injection the temperature should be 98°-100°. The ewer should be placed about a foot above the level of the thighs and it will then flow into the tissues at the rate of about 2 pints an hour. From 15 to 20 pints can, if necessary, be safely infused during the first 24 hours after an operation.

The chief effects of this free supply of fluid to the body are:

The sunken appearance of the eyes disappears and the face fills out.

The pulse is improved in volume and strength and becomes slower.

The secretion of salva is started again.

The tongue becomes larger and moister.

The discharge from the peritoneum is increased and the dressings become saturated.

The toxins are diluted and their elimination is promoted by the increased action of the skin and kidneys.

(c) Toxæmia.—I have already alluded to the effect of the large infusions of saline fluid on the toxæmia.

(d) The tendency to paralysis of the gut.—If the intestine becomes paralysed, the contents decom-

pose, tympanites follows from the resulting formation of gas, and the general toxæmia is increased.
It is therefore imperative to get the bowels to act
as soon as possible, and I know of no better
method than the hourly administration of one-
grain doses of calomel, assisted after a few hours by
soap, olive oil, castor oil, or glycerine enemata.
The addition of a drachm of boric acid to the
ordinary enema sometimes accelerates the action
of the bowels by stimulating the muscle of the
colon. Sulphate of magnesia given by the mouth
or injected into the gut at the time of the operation
is sometimes efficacious but cannot be relied upon
in all cases. It failed to act in the case I have
alluded to. Calomel also acts as an intestinal
antiseptic, and its action is important from this
point of view. Barnard states that in one case
72. grains were given. The following case of
intestinal obstruction is a good example of the
difficulty which is often experienced in securing
an action of the bowels.

A boy, æt. 9 years, was admitted under my care
on August 8th, 1903, for abdominal pain and distension. He became acutely ill on August 5th
with colic and sickness. He was frequently sick
the same evening, and the sickness continued, but
the vomit had not been fæcal. No food had been
taken and, in spite of various purgatives, the
bowels had not been opened for three days.

On admission the pulse was 120, respiration 22,
temperature 98·8°. The abdomen was tender,
rigid, and distended. Nothing abnormal could be
felt *per rectum* and there was no abdominal tumour.
Soap enemata were administered, but with no result.
Acute intestinal obstruction was diagnosed.

Sir Alfred Fripp was called in and performed
laparotomy, finding a peritoneal band stretching
between the great omentum and a caseous mesenteric gland which formed a loop, through which
the greater part of the small intestine had passed
and become twisted on its long axis. The gut
involved was deep purple in colour. The obstruction was relieved and the gut returned to the
peritoneal cavity. The patient was a good deal
collapsed after the operation.

Treatment.—Hypodermic injections of three
minims of Liq. strychninæ every two hours.

Saline and nutrient enemata alternately every
four hours.

August 9th.—11 a.m., calomel gr. ij. 12 a.m.,

calomel gr. ij. 3 p.m., mag. sulph. ʒij. 10.30
p.m., enema ; terebenth ʒj, acid. borici ʒj, enema
sap. ʒj. No result.

August 10th.—5 a.m., ol. ricini ʒj. 6 a.m.,
enema glycerin ; small result. 3 p.m. mag. sulph.
ʒj every hour ; no result. 10 p.m., acid. borici ʒj,
enema saponis ʒxvj ; a fair result.

August 11th.—Peptonised milk ʒij every two
hours. Injection of 3 minims of strychnine every
four hours instead of every two hours. Bowels
opened twice without medicine.

August 12th.—He was doing very well. Pulse 96.
Temperature 98·4°. Respiration 14. A copious
motion produced with another enema. Peptonised
milk and Benger's food now given. Injections of
strychnine every six hours.

August 13th.—The injections of strychnine were
omitted.

September 4th.—He was discharged, feeling
quite well—*i. e.* twenty-seven days after the operation.

(*e*) *Pain.*— In my experience pain is rarely
severe enough to call for the exhibition of morphia. I have myself found that it can be kept
under control by 10 or 15 minim doses of nepenthe,
given *per rectum*, as in one of the cases of perforating gastric ulcer. I have already given reasons
for abstaining from the use of morphia, but would
here reiterate its liability to increase the tendency
to paralysis of the gut.

(*f*) *The condition of the mouth.*—On account of
the dryness of the mouth and the increased liability
to bacterial infection, especially when the feeding
is entirely through the rectum, it is necessary to
allow the patient to swill out the mouth with hot
water, and for the nurse to frequently swab it out
with an antiseptic mouth-wash—*e. g.* glycerine and
chinosol, resorcin 10 grs. to the ounce, or formalin
(strength 1 minim to the ounce).

Finally, I would add, do not give up hope in a
case of general acute peritonitis ; on the other
hand, do not delay operation, and after operation
see that the patient does not want for saline fluid,
strychnine, and calomel, for if you tide him over
the first twenty-four hours there is a fair hope of a
favourable result.

December 25th, 1905.

THE CLINICAL JOURNAL,

CLINICAL RECORD, CLINICAL NEWS, CLINICAL GAZETTE, CLINICAL REPORTER, CLINICAL CHRONICLE AND CLINICAL REVIEW.

EDITED BY L. ELIOT CREASY.

No. 688.   **WEDNESDAY, JANUARY 3, 1906.**   Vol. XXVII. No. 12.

CONTENTS.

* *Specially reported for the Clinical Journal. Revised by the Author.*

ALL RIGHTS RESERVED.

NOTICE.

Editorial correspondence, books for review, &c., should be addressed to the Editor, 51, New Cavendish Street, W., Telephone No. 904, Paddington ; but all business communications should be addressed to the Publishers, 22½, Bartholomew Close, London, E.C. Telephone 927, Holborn.

All inquiries respecting Advertisements should be sent to MESSRS. ADLARD & SON, Bartholomew Close, E.C. Telephone 927, Holborn.

Terms of Subscription, including postage, payable by cheque, postal or banker's order (in advance) : for the United Kingdom, 15s. 6d. per annum : Abroad 17s. 6d.

Cheques, &c., should be made payable to THE PROPRIETORS OF THE CLINICAL JOURNAL, *crossed* "*The London, City, and Midland Bank, Ltd., Newgate Street Branch, E.C. Account of the Medical Publishing Company, Ltd.*"

Reading Cases to hold Twenty-six Numbers of THE CLINICAL JOURNAL *can be supplied at 2s. 3d. each, or will be forwarded post free on receipt of 2s. 6d. ; and also Cases for Binding Volumes at 1s. each, or post free on receipt of 1s. 3d., from the Publishers, 22½, Bartholomew Close, London, E.C.*

ACUTE INFECTIVE DIARRHŒA OF INFANTS.

By FREDERICK E. BATTEN, M.D.,

Physician to the Hospital for Sick Children, Great Ormond Street, W.

GENTLEMEN,—I feel that I owe you some apology for bringing before your notice to-day an affection which is essentially a disease of the summer months. My excuse must be that during the past three months, viz. July, August, and September, a ward in this hospital has been set apart especially for the nursing of infants suffering from diarrhœa, and I hope that the experience gained whilst in charge of the ward may be of interest and service to you.

In the first place, I would like to say a few words about the general management of such a ward ; for it is recognised that the congregating together of infants suffering from intestinal affections is by no means free from the risk of infection, not only to other children in the ward, but also to those in charge of such infants. During a previous summer, whilst in charge of a general children's ward, such an epidemic occurred and was primarily due to infection derived from nursing an unusually large number of such cases (seven) in the one ward without special precautions.

Nursing.—Without going into details, it may be said that the rules adopted were all directed to the one object, viz. the prevention of the conveyance of infection by the secretions or excretions of the children. All the cases were treated in the same way as a case of enteric fever so far as the nursing was concerned. In order to diminish, as far as possible, the risk of infection by means of the excreta two or more nurses, according to the number of infants, attended to the removal of the soiled diapers and did not feed the children.

How effectual these regulations were in the prevention of spread of the infection may be judged from the fact that no infant admitted for some other complaint was affected, and only one nurse suffered from a severe attack of diarrhœa and vomiting, which presumably was contracted in the performance of her duties, and three others from mild attacks which may, or may not, have been so contracted.

Classification.—One of the greatest difficulties in dealing with the question of diarrhœa in infants is to know how to classify these diseases, for at the present time it is impossible to form a classification on a bacteriological basis.

A classification based on the history of the case is obviously misleading, and one which sweeps all the diarrhœa into one class, under the term " summer diarrhœa," is of no value.

A classification based on the clinical features of the case together with the appearance of the stools is at the present time that by which we must be guided.

First.—What are the characteristic features of a case of acute infective diarrhœa ?

A disease, usually of sudden onset, attended by frequent vomiting ; frequent motions, of loose, watery consistency, which in the early stage contain neither mucus nor blood, are green in colour and not offensive ; producing a condition of collapse, so that the extremities are cold and cyanosed, the eyes sunken, the skin shrivelled, and the abdomen generally lax and retracted ; the pulse is feeble and small and the temperature is raised. The picture in the typical case is only too characteristic. This is the so-called " gastro-enteritis," the cholera infantum which is epidemic during the summer months.

Three other forms of diarrhœa and their characteristic features may here be mentioned :

The irritative diarrhœa, due to improper food or undigested food, and characterised by loose stools, bulky, green in colour, with the presence of white curds, often with a sour odour. This form is unattended by fever.

The catarrhal diarrhœa, due to prolonged indigestion, attended by the presence of mucus in the stools, which are brownish-green in colour and of foul odour. The temperature is rarely raised, and the children seldom so ill as in the former condition.

A third form, of which mention may be here made, is in my opinion much more rare, and there

has only been one undoubted instance of the disease in the ward during the present summer. This form is attended with considerable pain and with the passage of mucus and blood, and is due to ulceration of the large intestine and is described under the title of *ulcerative colitis*. It tends to run a prolonged course and is unattended by high fever.

I do not intend to-day to deal with the last three forms mentioned, but to limit my remarks to the first group.

During the past months some 120 infants suffering from diarrhœa have been admitted to the ward, and of these some thirty may be said to have presented the features of acute infective diarrhœa above described. I do not wish you to understand that in these cases all the features above described as characteristic of infective diarrhœa were necessarily present, but all presented the severe collapse associated with acute infective diarrhœa.

Now, of the thirty cases twelve recovered and eighteen died. With regard to those which recovered I shall have something to say later, but of the eighteen who died two groups stand out very sharply.

There are those which die in a few hours to a few days after admission to the ward, and those which recover from the acute attack and subsequently waste away in spite of all treatment and care ; and it is to this second group that I would particularly call your attention to-day, for it is a class of case which is but little understood. Of the eighteen infants who died, it may be said that no less than eight ran this prolonged course and died, without macroscopic evidence of organic disease ; most of these children lived four to five weeks after the acute attack, and one eight weeks. I will give you one or two examples of such a condition, taken from the cases which have occurred during the past summer.

(1) *Case illustrating the impaired digestive powers which follow an attack of acute infantile diarrhœa.*—The first case is that of a child, W. P—, æt. 6 months, who had been breast-fed for three months, and then fed by bottle with cow's milk and barley-water. He did not thrive very well on this, but when first seen in July was a healthy baby, with a sharp attack of diarrhœa, from which he quickly recovered and left the hospital in ten days' time. Some few days later the child was

brought to the hospital again and the mother stated that the diarrhœa and vomiting had returned, and it was obvious that the child was suffering from a very acute attack of infective diarrhœa. The motions were loose and green, not offensive in odour. The eyes were sunken, the temperature was raised, and the child had lost nearly a pound in weight in rather less than a week. The stomach and rectum were washed out and the child fed on albumen-water and brandy. The vomiting diminished and ceased altogether in four days' time and the diarrhœa became less. On the sixth day after admission white wine whey was given and by the tenth day the child was again taking milk diluted with barley-water. There was no vomiting, but the motions remained very unhealthy in appearance and contained curds and the child was losing weight. Raw meat juice was now tried, but the diarrhœa increased, and after four days it had to be discontinued. Various forms of feeding and modifications of milk were now tried. The child did not vomit, but the motions still remained loose and unhealthy, the child steadily losing weight. Signs pointing to some consolidation of the base of the left lung now developed, and it was considered probable that some tuberculous infection -of the lung was present. The emaciation steadily increased and the child died *eight weeks* after this acute attack. At the post mortem all the 'organs appeared healthy some collapse at the base of the left lung was present and accounted for the physical signs, but there was no evidence of tuberculous infection.

This case illustrates the fact that after a severe attack of infective diarrhœa the digestive powers may be so impaired that it is impossible to get the infant to assimilate its food, and the greatest care has to be taken with these infants in their return to a normal diet.

The following case illustrates termination with cerebral symptoms :

T. W—, æt. 7 months, was a breast-fed child. Three weeks before coming to the hospital the child had an acute attack of diarrhœa, from which he recovered. A second attack occurred in August, from which he again recovered after sixteen days, and was discharged well. Four days later another attack occurred, the temperature was 103° F. and the child was admitted extremely collapsed. From this he recovered, but the temperature again began to rise,

the child passing into a drowsy condition, with retraction of the head, and died ten days after the onset of this third attack. At the autopsy nothing was found to account for death.

The following case illustrates the occurrence of purpura :

T. H—, æt. 4 months, a bottle-fed baby, was quite well till July 23rd, when he had violent diarrhœa and vomiting. He was treated with barley and albumen-water, and under this treatment he improved, but on August 1st was not so well and was admitted to the ward. He was collapsed, with sunken eyes, passing green and watery motions. His temperature was 100°, on the following day it rose to 105°, and again on the next day to 106°. After this he began to improve, but on August 18th purpura appeared over the abdomen, disappearing again by August. 25th ; but the child never really improved, he gradually lost ground, and died on September 2nd, nearly six weeks after the acute onset.

At the post mortem nothing abnormal was found except superficial ulceration of Peyer's patches.

The purpura in these cases is a manifestation of the failure of nutrition and not of scurvy, for there was neither hæmorrhage from the gums nor beneath the periosteum.

Another case of this group exhibited albuminuria, and although it was in this case not the immediate cause of death, yet it was in all probability an important factor.

C. S—, æt. 3 months, was breast-fed for two months and then had Nestlé's milk. Diarrhœa and vomiting began fourteen days ago and on admission to the hospital the child was very bad, with loose green motions, without mucus, blood, or curd. After treatment the child improved, but six days later some œdema of the legs was present and on examination of the urine it was found to contain albumen and hyaline and granular casts. The child steadily lost ground, and died from a sudden paralytic distension of the intestine twenty-four days after the onset of the acute attack of diarrhœa.

At the autopsy there was very marked congestion of the small intestine for a distance of eight to ten inches and the kidney showed parenchymatous nephritis, both macroscopically and microscopically.

One more case which I believe is of considerable value as throwing light on the nature of these cases is the following :

R. C—, æt. 1 year and 11 months, suffered from an acute attack of diarrhœa and vomiting, which began three weeks before admission. Six days ago his face, feet, and hands began to swell, and the boy passed less urine. On admission to the hospital there was marked œdema of face, legs, and arms. The boy was not acutely ill, but passed a large green, offensive motion, with a quantity of mucus. There was flaccid paralysis of both legs, the weakness of the left being rather more marked than that of the right. There was wrist-drop on the left side. The knee-jerks were absent and stimulation of the feet would provoke but little movement of the legs.

The œdema gradually increased, the child became more feeble; the urine contained a trace of albumen, but this disappeared in a few days and remained normal. Œdema of the lungs supervened, and the child died.

At the autopsy there was some fluid in the left pleura and considerable consolidation of the left lung. There was considerable œdema of all the cellular tissues. All the organs appeared normal. The brain and spinal cord were removed, and except for œdema appeared normal.

On microscopic examination of the spinal cord, however, it was found that the walls of the vessels supplying the grey matter of the anterior horns showed very considerable fatty degeneration; this was most marked in the lumbar region, but was present also in the cervical region. There was an area of softening in the spinal cord of recent origin and another of longer standing, and it is therefore probable that the child had a previous attack of acute anterior poliomyelitis. On questioning the mother more carefully with regard to the past history of the child, she stated that when ten months old he had an attack of diarrhœa, from which after recovery weakness of the right leg was noticed, but up to the onset of the present attack the child had been able to get about with the aid of a chair.

The above cases illustrate some of the later effects of an attack of acute infective diarrhœa, the toxic effects of which may fall upon almost any system. It may affect the digestive, urinary, the nervous, or vaso-motor system. Why in different individuals it affects one system rather than another is most difficult to explain. In the last case it is possible to suggest that the nervous system had previously been attacked and its

powers of resistance had possibly been reduced. It is not difficult to speculate on the cause of these conditions, but my object in quoting these cases is that I wish to impress upon you that an attack of acute infective diarrhœa leaves behind it sequelæ of no less severity than those which we are accustomed to see after diphtheria, typhoid, or other specific fever.

Reverting now to the group of cases in which death took place in a few hours or days after the onset of symptoms. Out of the eighteen cases which died, five died within twelve hours of admission to the hospital. These children were moribund on admission and the infants failed to respond to any stimulation. The remaining five lived from four to ten days, and died from hyperpyrexia, convulsions, or cardiac failure.

I may say here that in none of these was any lesion found which would directly account for death.

Before passing to the final group, viz. those which recover, it may be well here to mention certain points in which these cases of acute infective diarrhœa differ from those of other observers, and more especially the American observers.

So far as my experience goes, it is rare for an infant with acute infective diarrhœa to pass blood in the motions; a streak may sometimes be found, but any quantity is of rare occurrence. In a paper on "The Etiology and Classification of the Summer Diarrhœa of Infants" by C. Dunn, he says that 42 per cent. of such cases pass blood. Now, among my present series of cases blood was only present in five, and in only two of these in any quantity. The following case is quoted in order to show that blood when present may be due to ulceration of the colon; this case was not regarded as a case of acute infective diarrhœa.

A child, æt. 10 months, who had been losing flesh for a month, had an acute attack of diarrhœa, with the passage of an offensive motion, mucus, and blood. The general condition of the child, together with the character of the motion, did not suggest to me the clinical features of an acute infective diarrhœa. Physical examination revealed no sign of disease. The temperature remained low, varying between 98 °and 100° F., but the motions continued to be undigested, contained mucus and blood, and were extremely offensive. During the five weeks the child was under treatment he steadily lost weight, though he rarely vomited his food.

At the autopsy an extensive ulceration of the whole of the large intestine was found which was not tuberculous in nature. This case belongs to the group colitis, and in all probability is closely related to infantile dysentery, to which the American cases would seem to stand in close relation.

Cases in which recovery took place.—In twelve cases out of the thirty cases recovery took place, and if we analyse the cases, it is at once apparent that recovery is due to the fact that they were cases of less severity and came under treatment early in the course of the disease. Though these two factors play a most important part in the number of cases which recover, yet the fact of recovery is certainly to be attributed to the treatment they received.

The following case illustrates well the effect of treatment on a child who was sent up to the ward as "moribund":

A. B—, æt. 3 months, had been fed on cow's milk and water. Seven days before admission to the hospital she was taken ill with diarrhœa and vomiting. On admission the child appeared to be dying, the eyes were open and sunken, the cornea was glazed, and the pulse extremely feeble, the temperature was 97° F. in the rectum. Hypodermic injections of strychnine were given, the stomach was washed out and a drachm of castor oil administered, and the child given albumen-water and brandy. The temperature rose in three hours to 104° F., but the pulse remained very feeble. A saline infusion of three and a half ounces was now given, and a definite improvement took place in the child's condition. The vomiting ceased, but the motions were very frequent, loose, and began to contain mucus. For four days the child took albumen-water and brandy only. On the fifth day one teaspoonful of citrated milk was added to the albumen-water; this was well taken and the child's condition steadily improved. The amount of citrated milk was now increased, and then gradually replaced by ordinary milk and barley-water. The child lost weight during the first week, but rapidly put on weight the second week, and left the hospital well on the eighteenth day after admission.

Such is the history and type of the successful cases.

I now propose to deal with the treatment of these cases; and though I could state the treatment which is required in a few words, yet I should leave you but little wiser and no more competent to deal with these cases unless I entered into some detail with regard to the methods employed. Shortly, may I say, treatment may be placed under the following heads, in their order of employment: (1) Hypodermic injections, (2) transfusion, (3) baths, (4) stomach wash-out, (5) rectal irrigation, (6) feeding, (7) stimulants, (8) drugs.

(1) With regard to hypodermic injections of strychnine, there is no doubt that this is one of the most valuable remedies which we possess in conditions of extreme collapse, and it is quickly and easily administered. If the child is bad, half a minim of the liq. strychninæ of the B. P. may be given and repeated in half an hour if necessary, and after that every four hours. I have myself on occasion seen strychnine-poisoning produced, but with the child under careful observation no harm will result from these doses. I would warn you against giving hypodermic injections of ether, because of the likelihood of such injections giving rise to an extensive sloughing of the skin. If the child recovers, one has this further complication added to those with which we have already to deal. Even subcutaneous injections of brandy are not desirable, though they are not so pernicious as injections of ether.

(2) *Transfusion.*—Two methods are possible, subcutaneous and intravenous, but I may say that only one is applicable; intravenous is difficult to perform and has no advantage over the easily performed subcutaneous injection. The apparatus needed is simple and consists of a rather long hypodermic needle, two feet of rubber tubing, and the cylinder of a glass syringe. A solution of salt (one drachm to a pint of water) at the temperature of 150° F in the body of the syringe is used.

The pressure under which the injection should be made is about 18 in., but in starting 24 in. may be required.

The injection is best made at the side of the thorax, the point of the needle being directed upwards to the axilla, and at least one and a half inches within the skin, otherwise the fluid tends to run out along the needle.

No benefit is derived from allowing more than about four ounces of the solution to run in, and this can safely be done with one puncture.

The length of time required varies greatly in different children ; in some cases the whole will run in in twenty minutes, in other cases it will take nearly an hour.

With regard to rapidity of absorption, again there is very great variation ; in some cases the fluid is absorbed almost as rapidly as it is injected, whilst in others it will take several hours before absorption is completed.

The proceeding is free from all danger, and the only complications which I have seen arise are subcutaneous hæmorrhage and suppuration, with the formation of an abscess ; and during the past summer, in which transfusion has been many times performed, no instance of either of these complications has occurred.

(3) *The hot bath.*—This is a most valuable remedy, and the only question is when it should be applied. If the child is not very bad, it may be given first of all ; but if the child is very bad, I would sooner transfuse the child than give it a hot bath. The temperature of the bath should start at 100° F. and should gradually be raised, and a child will stand a bath of 110° F. with benefit. Mustard should be added, as it stimulates the skin, dilates the vessels, and diminishes the peripheral resistance.

Are there any conditions under which it is inadvisable to give a hot bath ? From my experience I should say that if a child is very bad it is better not to give a hot bath, but to trust to transfusion and strychnine and local warmth, hot bottles, and warm-water cushions. I may say that I think pyrexia in itself is no contra-indication to a hot bath, and as an instance of this I may quote the following case :

A child, æt. 9 months, was admitted with an acute attack of diarrhœa. On the following day the temperature was 105° F., the eyes were sunken, the cornea hazy, and the child was extremely collapsed. A hot mustard bath was now given in which the temperature was gradually raised to 110° F. Immediately after the bath the child's temperature had fallen to 102° F. and she was less collapsed. Saline infusions were given and strychnine. The child took fluid readily, but vomited frequently. Improvement now took place, the child retaining first albumen-water and brandy, then peptonised milk, then citrated milk, then ordinary milk and barley-water, and she was discharged well eighteen days after admission.

(4) *Stomach wash-out.*—This should be done with a large size tube, No. 14, with a solid end, to which is attached twelve inches of india-rubber tubing. The tube should be passed through the mouth into the stomach. Some people endeavour to wash out the stomach by means of a nasal tube. Now, any nasal tube which will pass the nares of a child a few months old is so small that the curds and mucus soon block it. No harm ever results from the passage of the stomach-tube, even when the child is very bad, and the immediate effect is often strikingly good.

In one case only have I had any difficulty in passing the mouth tube in a baby, and in that child respiration stopped as soon as the tube was passed down. The tube was withdrawn and the child breathed naturally again. After an interval another attempt was made, with the same result, and on withdrawal the child breathed again. A nasal tube was now passed, and passed into the stomach and the stomach washed out. With this solitary exception I have never experienced any difficulty, and in this case no explanation of why the difficulty with respiration should arise was forthcoming. The stomach is washed out until the fluid which is used returns clear and moderately free from mucus. The fluid used has usually been a solution of sodium bicarbonate, two grains to the ounce.

(5) *The rectal irrigation* is performed in the usual manner with hot water, some six to eight ounces being allowed to flow in from a tube passed well into the rectum, about twelve inches being the pressure usually exerted. The irrigation is continued till the returning fluid is clear of mucus. In some cases the use of four ounces of $\frac{1}{2}$ per cent. solution of protargol after the wash-out be beneficial.

And now I come to the most important part of the treatment, viz. (6) the *feeding*, and I think that most observers are agreed that milk in any form should be entirely stopped. Numerous substitutes, such as barely-water, albumen-water, hot water, rice-water, may be used. During the past summer I have used albumen-water almost exclusively—the white of one egg with four ounces of water. The child, according to age, is given one to two ounces of that with ten to twenty minims of brandy every two hours. This diet should be continued for three days at least, and then into each two ounces of albumen-water one drachm of whey should be added ; this is gradually increased according to the general condition of the patient, until he is taking equal parts of whey and albumen-water. Usually at the end of the first week to this mixture one drachm of citrated milk, or of peptonised milk, may now be added. I have used citrated milk, for I find that in the majority of cases it is taken as well as peptonised milk and does not cause vomiting or curds in the motions, and I use the citrated milk of such a strength that there is one grain of sodium citrate to one ounce of milk. If the citrated milk does not agree or curds appear in the motions, peptonised milk may be substituted.

Having reached this stage, the further steps are simple ; the amount of citrated milk is increased and eventually is replaced by ordinary milk diluted to the capacity of the child.

Such may be said to be the lines on which these children should be treated, but in practice constant and often seemingly minute changes are called for.

With one set of preparations I have been most unsuccessful, and that is in the various forms of meat-juice. I have given raw meat juice, various proprietary preparations, and meat extracts, but almost all have been attended with failure, and in most the diarrhœa has been markedly increased. It must, however, be said that this form of feeding has been only tried in those cases which did not respond to the albumen-water treatment above described.

(7) *Stimulants.* — Ten to twenty minims of brandy, given every hour or two hours with the albumen-water, supplies all the stimulant which is necessary by the mouth.

Sherry in the white wine whey is also of use, but on the whole I prefer brandy to any other stimulant.

(8) With regard to *drugs*, during the acute stage castor oil and calomel are alone of much service. Objection has been raised to castor oil because it tends to make the infant vomit. My experience is altogether favourable with regard to castor oil. After the stomach has been washed out one to two drachms of castor oil are given and in only a few cases has it been vomited.

In the latter stages alkalies, acids, opium, bismuth, salicylates, creosote, cyllin, β-naphthol, all have their uses. Bromides are most useful in checking the restlessness of the child, and often seem to check the slighter form of vomiting.

In dealing with the after-effects of an attack of acute infective diarrhœa, each case needs individual treatment, according to the system most affected. In those cases in which the digestive functions have become impaired, the most careful regulation of diet is necessary, and this has to be continued for weeks ; even so improvemement is slow and relapses are frequent. One of the most fatal after-effects is the general œdema which occurs without obvious cardiac or renal lesions.

In conclusion, I trust I have made it clear that in dealing with acute infective diarrhœa one is not only dealing with an acute attack of diarrhœa and vomiting, but with a disease which leaves in its train well-marked sequelæ ; and it is the presence of these sequelæ which seems to me to furnish one of the strongest clinical facts for regarding this form of diarrhœa as a definite specific infection.

January 1st, 1906.

Laparotomy as Treatment of Puerperal Infection.

—Sourtille has treated four patients with severe diffuse puerperal peritonitis by mere laparotomy or posterior colpotomy, and succeeded in saving three of them. Removal of the uterus is a serious operation, and its record to date in puerperal infection is the reverse of encouraging The outcome proves it to be either a useless mutilation or else that the prognosis was inevitably bad. A mere laparotomy or colpotomy enables the exact condition of the parts to be ascertained and has direct healing value in itself. As it entails no shock, he urges that it should be done early in case of severe infection, without waiting for the woman to be touched by the wing of death, after failure of curetting or drainage of the uterus. Done systematically, in time it would enable the condition of the uterus and adnexa to be inspected, and if a threatening lesion were found, to have it removed while the patient's resisting powers were still able to cope with the major operation. He reports a number of cases in which laparotomy or colpotomy unmistakably saved the patients in diffuse puerperal peritonitis or post-abortion infection, and urges the general adoption of laparotomy with drainage as the routine procedure in threatening puerperal infection. Several surgeons have published reports of successful cases of this kind, but no one before, he remarks, has advocated this as the systematic technique for treating serious post-partum or post-abortion infection.—*Journ. A. M. A.*, vol. xlv, No. 24.

A CLINICAL LECTURE

ON

ACUTE INTUSSUSCEPTION.

Delivered at the London Hospital,

By JAMES SHERREN, F.R.C.S.,

Assistant Surgeon to the Hospital, Surgeon to the Poplar
Hospital for Accidents.

GENTLEMEN,—Of all the forms of intestinal obstruction, acute intussusception, if treated early, has the best prognosis. In children, in whom it occurs frequently in its most typical form, there should be no difficulty in its early diagnosis.

I have chosen this subject for my lecture to-day to draw your attention to the importance of early diagnosis and to acquaint you with suggested changes in its classification. The classification of this disease given in the surgical text-books consists of a list of what were considered to be the four varieties of intussusception, given in order of frequency—ileo-cæcal, enteric, colic, ileo-colic. It was pointed out, first, I believe, by Mr. Eve, that in many of the so called ileo-cæcal cases, the apex of the invagination was not the ileo-cæcal valve, but the caput of the cæcum. In a recent paper Corner has drawn attention to the frequency with which double intussusceptions occur; in his series of cases they were more frequently met with than single ones. By a double intussusception is meant invagination of an intussusception, the intussusceptum of the second invagination being the first intussusception. Of double intussus-ceptions the ileo-colic-colic—that is, invagination of a small ileo-colic intussusception into the colon —was considered by him to be the most common variety and to be the form most often met with of all varieties of intussusception; following this, the enteric-ileo-cæcal, meaning by this an enteric intussusception pushing the ileo-cæcal valve in front of it. It is evident, therefore, that under the heading "Ileo-cæcal" many varieties are in-cluded. Now that attention has been directed to the many forms of intussusception, a classification is needed that is more than a recital of varieties. Such a grouping is made by Sir Frederick Treves in the last edition of his book on Intestinal Obstruction. He divides the cases into three roups—

(1) Those that involve the ileo-cæcal segment of the gut.

(2) Enteric.

(3) Colic.

Group (1) will include all those cases starting in the caput of the cæcum, which in my series were the most common, the ileo-colic, ileo-cæcal, and the various double invaginations starting in this region. Another, and I think a better, name has been suggested for this group by Wallace. It is better, because there is no chance of confusion with the ileo-cæcal variety of intussusception, and because it is shorter; the name he has suggested is entero-colic, meaning thereby intussusceptions that involve both the large and the small intestine. I would suggest the following classification therefore.

(1) Entero-colic.

(2) Enteric.

(3) Colic. .

During the past two years I have operated on 22 cases of intussusception; of these 16 were males. This excess of the male sex over the female in acute intussusception in the young has been pointed out before, but no satisfactory explanation has been given.

Of these 22 cases, 16 were under the age of 1 year, the average age of these 16 being 6 months; 20 patients were under the age of 5, 1 was 9 years old, and 1, an exceptional case that I shall later relate in full, 49 years of age.

Over 75 per cent. (17) of these cases belonged to Group 1, the entero-colic, and of these, 7 were of the double variety. The most common form of intussusception met with, both in this group and in the total number of cases, was that starting in the caput of the cæcum; of the seven double cases the ileo-colic-colic was the most common variety, then the enteric-ileo-cæcal. Three cases belonged to Group 2, and two to the colic group.

Acute intussusception occurs most often in perfectly healthy breast-fed children. These chil-dren are usually the finest that are admitted to the surgical beds of the hospital, and it is rare to find any evidence or history of improper feeding.

It is evident from the nature of the disease that the condition is caused in some way by irregular peristalsis. Nothnagel from his experiments on animals suggested that a contracted portion of the intestine was "swallowed" by the segment below, and this is, at least, hinted at by conditions of the intestines found at abdominal operations for other affections.

In some rare cases intussusception has followed an abdominal injury or operation; the following is a good example of this.

A boy, æt. 9 years, was admitted to the Poplar Hospital on July 18th, 1904, having been crushed by a cart. I saw him two hours after the accident. His face and neck were blue with many ecchymoses, and he showed typically the condition known as traumatic asphyxia. He was very collapsed, his abdomen was rigid, and his pulse rapid and small. I opened the abdomen at once and found free blood in the peritoneal cavity due to a small rent in the spleen, which I sutured. His progress was uneventful till July 31st. On August 3rd I was sent for and told that he had developed signs of intestinal obstruction. He had been vomiting and his bowels had not been opened; no blood had been passed *per rectum*. I operated immediately and found an intussusception of the jejunum six inches long; this I reduced with difficulty. There were no adhesions present in the neighbourhood. The boy left hospital quite well four weeks later.

The following case in which intussusception followed injury to the intestine due to strangulation is most unusual. A few cases of intussusception following strangulated hernia are to be found scattered through surgical literature, but I have been unable to find the report of a case in which gangrene of gut was followed by intussusception and spontaneous cure.

A woman, æt. 49 years, was admitted to the London Hospital on March 3rd, 1903. She had had a small umbilical hernia for many years, but it had given her no trouble until the day before admission. That morning she was seized with violent abdominal pain and vomiting; the lump became larger and painful. A hernia was present in the umbilical region which was reduced on her admission to the ward. Immediately after its reduction she passed blood from the anus and became extremely collapsed; the vomiting persisted. Eight hours later I opened the abdomen; free odourless fluid was present in the peritoneal cavity and the great omentum presented, œdematous where it had been nipped in the hernial sac. The transverse colon was dilated and for about an inch, where it had been strangulated, was of a greyish-green colour

and had lost its resiliency; the remainder of the transverse colon from the splenic to the hepatic flexures was thin and congested, and showed a multitude of grey-green patches, varying in size from a pea to an almond. The blood supply of the colon was not interfered with. Her condition was so desperate that I closed the abdomen at once. In spite of saline infusion during the course of the operation, her state was so bad that I expected to hear that she had died on her way back to the ward. She, however, rallied, but was in a precarious condition for several days. The vomiting continued almost incessantly for seven days, but she was allowed to take as much fluid as she asked for. Diarrhœa set in on the third day and continued for three weeks. Nine days after operation she passed a cast of a portion of the large intestine measuring 18½ inches in length. Its inner surface was smooth and the outer rough and of a grey-green colour. Two days later she passed 3½ inches of large intestine with meso-colon attached; from the relation of its longitudinal bands, as well as from the presence of a mesentery, there is no doubt that it was transverse colon. She steadily improved from this time onwards and when she left hospital, on May 12th, seemed to be quite well, her bowels acting regularly. The operation wound healed by first intention.

She came again under my care in October, 1904, being sent to me by her medical man with a history of attacks of abdominal pain. She had never been quite free from pain since her discharge from hospital and had had several severe attacks, lasting two or three days, accompanied by vomiting. In the intervals her bowels were irregular, with occasional attacks of diarrhœa; there seemed to be no doubt that she was suffering from chronic intestinal obstruction.

I operated and found, just below the liver, an adherent mass consisting of intestine and omentum. The transverse colon stretched tightly across the abdomen; I traced it and the ascending colon into the adherent mass. It was obvious that the colon was obstructed at the site of the intussusception, probably as the result of these adhesions. I therefore performed ileo-colostomy and the patient left the hospital three weeks later with complete relief from all her symptoms.

I have related this case because it illustrates three points in connection with intussusception

(1) The onset of an intussusception after injury to the intestine.

(2) The method of spontaneous cure.

(3) The result of spontaneous cure in some cases.

Turning now to the symptoms of this disease, there are three which are of great importance in the diagnosis of the condition in children. They are, the sudden onset of screaming in a previously healthy infant, followed by vomiting and the passage of stools containing blood and often consisting of blood and mucus only, without any fæcal material, the symptoms occuring in this order. In a child they are pathognomonic.

The pain after its first onset is usually intermittent ; between the attacks the child may appear quite comfortable and give no sign of being dangerously ill. There may be nothing in the appearance or feel of the abdomen to make you suspect intestinal obstruction. A tumour is said to be present in about 50 per cent. of cases, but it is not a symptom to be relied upon ; as a positive symptom it is helpful, as a negative one it is of no importance.

Although the symptoms I have described are the usual ones in infants and sufficient for a diagnosis, yet in some children they may not be so definite, particularly when the intussusception belongs to the second or third group ; a good example of this is the boy whose history I related.

In adults acute invagination of the gut is so rare that it is impossible to lay down any rules with regard to diagnosis.

Most mistakes in diagnosis have been made, in the cases that have come under my observation, in respect to acute enteritis or colitis. Cases of intussusception have been sent to the Out-Patient Department or admitted on the Medical side of the hospital with this diagnosis. I need hardly point out the serious nature of this error, involving as it does delay in treatment. In acute intestinal inflammations the onset is never with the suddenness of invagination, diarrhœa is a marked feature, and if blood is present in the stools it is only small in amount and mixed with fæcal material ; after the disease has been present for some time the stools may consist of mucus and blood only. The opposite mistake, considering a case of colitis or enteritis to be intussusception, must be rare ; I have not seen or heard of it being made here.

In any case in which there is reasonable ground to suspect that an intussusception is present, exploration should be undertaken.

The treatment of intussusception admits of no discussion. Operation should be performed at once, the abdomen opened and the intussusception dealt with ; every hour lessens the chance of recovery. The incision is usually made through the right rectus muscle, as giving easier access to the region in which the condition is most likely to have originated. The invagination should be reduced by squeezing, as originally suggested by Mr. Jonathan Hutchinson, Senr., not by traction. The reduction of the terminal portion, especially in the ileo-colic-colic cases, may be difficult and it is justifiable in these cases to employ traction. If the invagination is irreducible or gangrenous, it should be left in infants ; I know of no recorded case where resection of gut, in this condition, has succeeded in a child under the age of one ; opening the gut above and establishing an artificial anus seems to be equally fatal. If the intussusception, therefore, is irreducible, the best treatment at present seems to be to leave the case to nature ; there is more hope of recovery taking place by spontaneous cure than after resection. Of course, in older children resection of gut has succeeded and should be employed.

The after-treatment is of great importance. Infants stand abstinence from food very badly and should be fed at once after the operation. The method in general use here is to start feeding with small quantities of a mixture of milk, water, and lime-water in equal parts ; this is given every 15 minutes until the child sleeps. The child is not then disturbed, but on awaking the amount and interval is gradually increased until the child is taking the usual quantity for its age. Restlessness may be combated with small doses of chloral.

The two principal factors in the prognosis are the condition of the intussusception, and its variety : of these the former is the more important. Of neither have we any means of gaining definite information before operation. But the first has a close relationship to the time since the onset. While no hard and fast line can be drawn as to the time at which intussusceptions become irreducible, I cannot go so far as some observers and say that there is no relation between the duration and irreducibility.

Of the 7 irreducible cases in my series all were over 30 hours' duration, 6 were over 48, 2 were of 50, and one each of 3, 4, 7, and 11 days' duration. All these cases died soon after operation. Of the cases reducible at operation one, a true ileo-cæcal invagination, was of 17 days', two enteric of 3 and 2½ days', and one caput cæci of 48 hours' duration. The remaining cases were operated upon within 26 hours of their onset. Of the 21 cases of intussusception treated by operation 10 died; of these 7 were irreducible. Of the three reducible cases which died, one had existed for four days, one for 48 hours, and one for only 18. In the first case the abdomen was markedly distended before operation; I always look upon this as of grave significance; few young children recover when the intestine is paralysed sufficiently to cause marked distension, drainage of the gut, the only admissible treatment in these cases, always proving fatal. In the second case, although the invagination was reducible, peritonitis had commenced and the gut was soft and ruptured during reduction. In the third case the temperature rose to 104° the morning following operation and the child died twelve hours later. At the post mortem nothing was found to account for death. From these figures I think we are able to say that cases operated upon within the first 48 hours stand a good chance of recovery, those operated on within the first 24, an excellent one. With regard to the variety of intussusception, those in which the intestine becomes nipped in the ileo-cæcal valve, the ileo-colic, and the ileo-colic-colic become irreducible early and the prognosis is less favourable than in the true ileo-cæcal, enteric, and colic, in which the strangulation may not be so severe. That this is the case is shown by the cases reducible at long intervals after onset, which I have just referred to.

I think sufficient has been said to indicate the necessity for early diagnosis followed by immediate operation if the results of treatment are to be improved. The fact that 7 out of the 21 cases were irreducible, and had existed for a considerable time before coming under observation at the hospital, points to a need of the wider appreciation of this contention.

January 1st, 1906.

REMARKS ON CONSERVATIVE GYNÆCOLOGY.

By CHARLES GREENE CUMSTON, M.D.,

Ex-Vice-President of the American Association of Obstetricians and Gynæcologists.

THE usefulness of the ovaries is no longer a matter of doubt, and they are certainly possessed of a regulating and dynamogenic function analogous to other glands of the body. I intend to discuss those lesions for which these glands have been removed, and endeavour to ascertain if a large number of females who have undergone irreparable mutilation might not have recovered and been mothers if other interferences or treatment had been carried out. In going over the literature from 1882 to 1892 it would lead one to suppose that there are few cases where temporisation and conservative treatment is justifiable. During this decade it is to be noted that operation was resorted to, not only in serious cases, but even for very trifling lesions. Not only were quantities of healthy ovaries removed, but mistakes in diagnosis led the most expert surgeons to remove healthy adnexa; and it is unfortunate, but yet true, that even at the present time ovariotomy and hysterectomy are still being done for simple metritis, catarrhal salpingitis, hydro- or hæmatosalpinx, bilateral or unilateral cystic transformation of the gland, ovarian neuralgia, so-called, generalised pains of nervous origin, hysteria, insanity, and even nymphomania and masturbation. Then, again, all types of prolapsus and displacements have been subjected to hysterectomy, which can hardly be called a rational procedure in these cases. In every other branch of surgery modern technique has resulted in conservatism, and it seems most curious that gynæcology alone is the exception to the rule, and that it has not followed this conservatism since the discovery of the antiseptic and aseptic technique. At the present time, instead of amputating, the surgeon endeavours to preserve the limb intact. Cavities are drained, abscesses and joints are curetted, and it is always the function and importance of the organ which guide the surgeon in his acts. To remove is not to save, and one should endeavour to obtain a satisfactory result by every possible means before undertaking an operation which, beside its inherent gravity, will place the woman in a condition of marked inferiority from a social point of view. Conservative surgery is, without any doubt, much more difficult and arduous and far less brilliant than the other, but it appears to me far more scientific and fruitful in its results. The future will, without doubt, show this, and so great an authority as Emmet hoped that future generations would not have to undergo castration, because he believed that surgeons would become better equipped for treating disease. It has been upheld that it is because the profession in general is not sufficiently well educated, skilful, or patient enough to treat their cases by simple means, and that they are in a hurry to have recourse to both violent and dangerous means.

On the other hand, although the operating surgeon has cause to complain of conservative treatment in many acute abdominal cases, and to reproach conservative operators for their lack of power in certain surgical conditions, it may be said in reply that this is still one more reason for endeavouring to improve a method which, in spite of its imperfection, or rather its non-perfection, has already given such splendid results, and which will enormously diminish the cases justifiable for ovariotomy or hysterectomy.

Although it has been held that many affections which are a despair to medicine are easily recovered from by surgical treatment, yet, in reply to this, it may be said that at the present time many diseases which were the triumph of surgery can be cured by medical treatment, and that not infrequently hot vaginal irrigations, revulsion, rest in bed, and simple means are quite sufficient for avoiding an operation which has been advised. For that matter, the greater number of surgeons who currently advise major interference are becoming more and more conservative, having experienced all the inconveniences and delusions, and they now only operate when absolutely necessary, in the first place endeavouring to treat the case by milder means. This tendency towards surgical conservatism is becoming more marked every day, and many prominent operators are endeavouring to preserve the physiological function of the ovaries.

The theory which gave rise to hysterectomy—that is to say, the formation of a large opening which would give issue to intra-abdominal collections of pus—is now giving way to curettement and drainage by incision through the posterior *cul de sac*. The pathogenesis of infection, being better known, has revealed the fact that the uterus is invariably the primary starting-point, and that inflammation of the ovaries, salpingitis, and generally speaking, all the various inflammations of the adnexa are merely the consequence of a metritis, or some uterine infection, which has developed from most varied causes. Whether the infection extends by way of the lymphatics, as is the present tendency to admit, and seems to be proved by the evolution of the process, or has followed the veins, as certain authorities still uphold, it has been demonstrated that if a curettement is done, and a careful antisepsis of the uterine cavity carried out, not only will the lesion of the uterus be cured, but the infectious phenomena by propagation are susceptible of subsiding little by little, and finally completely disappear. The salutary influence of a well-directed intra-uterine treatment—that is to say, conducted with every possible care and persistency from the very minute that the first sign of infection makes its appearance in the genital apparatus, cannot be too greatly insisted upon, and curettement, free dilatation, and drainage of the uterus represent a very effective treatment. It is not at all doubtful that when they are rightly handled the number of cases which have been considered as requiring the major interferences may be greatly reduced, and from our knowledge of the pathogenesis of lesions of the female genitals, it has been demonstrated that the therapeutics of affections of the adnexa are intimately united to pathologic processes in the uterus ; so that, under these circumstances, it is easy to understand how certain types of tubo-ovarian inflammatory processes, such as catarrhal salpingitis, purulent salpingitis at the beginning, and hydrosalpinx, may be greatly improved, or even completely cured, by simply treating the concomitant uterine lesions. It is only logical to maintain that in the treatment of periuterine inflammation serious interferences, such as laparotomy or hysterectomy, should always be reserved for those cases where it is manifestly impossible to resort to conservative surgery.

The uterus being the cause of infectious processes arising in the female pelvis, it was naturally logical to look in the first place for means of preventing this infection, or to control it if it had already developed, and all conservative operators have practically returned to the older procedures which had been abandoned. Hot vaginal irrigations, curettement, drainage, the various amputations of the cervix, and intra-uterine applications have been taken up, and haying applied some method to these various procedures, it was not long before all these conservative means were again adopted in current gynæcological practice. The best conservative treatment is that which does not allow the lesions to develop, and, consequently, the prophylaxis of the various forms of metritis will certainly diminish the number of cases requiring major interferences, but this teaching, although perfectly true in theory, is in my way of thinking very difficult to accomplish in practice. This may be accomplished in cases of metritis arising from post-puerperal infection, but those other cases which arise from causes of a more or less complex nature will always be met with. For example, the gonococcus shares largely in the pathogenesis of pelvic inflammation, and all the various microbic associations are quite capable at a given time of causing the various complications to make their appearance, which may be attributed to a kind of latent microbism, a sort of virtual affection waiting for some pathologic change to arise in order to develop. All reflex congestions produced by affections of the ovaries or tubes, excessive coitus, fatigue, and traumatism, are so many more causes quite impossible to prevent. As far as metritis is concerned, the results obtained by curettement are excellent, and it is well known that even when other infections do not exist it is nearly always a cause of sterility. The acid secretions given off by the inflamed uterus, the obliteration of its glands, the excessive proliferation of its epithelium, and by the mucous plugs obliterating the cervix, the organ becomes incapable of receiving the spermatozoid, and even if it should allow its entrance, it cannot preserve it alive in its cavity. And still more, when there is a metritis, it is almost always accompanied by a certain degree of salpingitis on account of the continuity and contiguity of the tissues. The question consequently comes up as to whether or not the lesion can be cured by the various means that I have mentioned, and if, for example, by destroying the uterine mucosa, the seat of the lesion, one might not permanently remove the power of gestation from the uterus. In reply to this, it may be said that besides the numerous instances of pregnancy arising after this treatment, and which have settled the question,

many authorities have experimented on animals and have found that the uterine mucosa is endowed with a surprising vitality, and that it is not long in becoming completely regenerated after having been removed by the curette. In dissecting metritis, which is a very rare lesion, where part of the muscular layer of the uterus is also eliminated with the mucosa, regeneration becomes an impossibility, but in all the other types of metritis, even when large strips of mucosa have been expelled, *restitutio ad integrum* occurs.

From the purely physiological and functional standpoint, the numerous writings of Schroeder, Martin, Durelius, Benicke, Henricius, and others, have demonstrated that after curettement conception can perfectly well take place, while gestation will undergo its regular evolution. Out of a total of fifty-six patients treated by curettement, Henricius found that sixteen became pregnant—in other words, 32 per cent. ; while de la Torre was able to obtain eleven pregnancies out of forty-eight interventions of this kind, which practically represents the same percentage. Among the patients treated by Henricius, pregnancy took place in two in five weeks and in one in eight weeks after currettement, which would seem to show that very little time is required for complete regeneration of the uterine mucosa. In thirteen cases of metritis complicated with catarrhal salpingitis, where the patients had been advised radical operation, I was able to obtain a cure by thorough curettement and antiseptic treatment, and three of these patients ultimately became pregnant and went to term. In several other cases of unilateral or bilateral purulent salpingitis, where I deemed removal of the tubes necessary, and where the operation was refused by the patients, I did a thorough dilatation and curettement and found that the tubes discharged by way of the uterus, and ultimately recovered perfect health, although I am unaware that any of these ever became pregnant.

The therapeutic results of curettement are too numerous and well known to require further discussion as to the value of this operation, but I would point out that when contrasting it with hysterectomy, it is far superior if the desired result is obtained by it, because it in no way disturbs the physiological functions of the organ and in certain cases even it appears to awaken them. Many cases of sterility might be quoted which have been overcome by this operation, and in my own notes I have two cases of women who had been married respectively three years and five years, who had remained sterile, and who conceived within four months after they were curetted. For example, in glandular cervical endometritis, which gives rise to hardly any painful phenomena, having no influence on the general health, and simply giving evidence of its presence by a slight discharge, or by a little mucous plug obstructing the cervix, finally leading to stenosis, pregnancy will frequently take place after curettement, dilatation, and removal of a portion of the cervical mucosa.

I believe that in cases which have reached the stage where they are giving rise to symptoms, there are several lesions in the genital apparatus and that the success obtained by operation depends entirely on the rational treatment of all the lesions met with. To this complex condition a complex treatment is required, and each element should be carefully treated, and if all the indications are not taken into consideration, an unsuccessful outcome will be the result. For example, the uterine mucosa and parenchyma must be attended to, the position of the uterus corrected if displacement exists, and intra-abdominal adhesions broken down if they are present. It was these very indications that caused Schroeder to invent his operation and Emmet to practise his well-known operation of trachelorrhaphy, for Bouilly to remove a portion of the cervical mucosa in order to open the deep-seated *culs de sac* and attend to the stenosis of the cervix or amputation of the cervix performed at different parts of the organ by all the well-known procedures. If, for example, we take a complete metritis, with laceration of the cervix and perineum, prolapsus of the vaginal walls, and backward displacement of the uterus, a cure can only be obtained by curettement, followed by Schroeder's operation, with a plastic operation on the vaginal walls, and some method of shortening the round ligaments. If one of these procedures is forgotten, the result will be that the patient will continue to suffer as she did before the operation, and I have come to the conclusion that a large number of cases considered as incurable, and where every conservative treatment had been tried without effect, have only been submitted to a major operation because the operator had omitted a certain point in the treatment which he considered perhaps as of too little consequence.

I have already pointed out that metritis exists rarely without some salpingitis ; and although the uterus is the starting-point of the infection, the process does not always remain localised to the mucosa of this organ, because it invades the tubes, and from the peri-uterine parenchyma it extends to the ovaries and peritoneum ; so that when this has taken place one will be dealing with a salpingitis, combined or not with inflammation of the ovaries and pelvic peritonitis, forming those cases presenting serious symptoms—in other words, a pelvic peritonitis. Now, it is just in these cases that I am of the opinion that a radical operation is far from being always indicated, and that more conservative measures may result in cures which can hardly be expected. I am firmly convinced that in the treatment of inflammation of the adnexa, whether this has or has not extended to the pelvic peritoneum, a certain proportion of patients may be cured by medical treatment, particularly so in the infection from the gonococcus, even when very severe peritoneal symptoms are present, which might lead the inexperienced surgeon to believe that the ultimate consequences would be serious. In point of fact, evidences of a former pelvic peritonitis will be met with in a very large proportion of autopsies, although the subjects have entirely recovered from the process which apparently has given rise to little disturbance during life. Experience demonstrates that a large percentage of patients presenting these conditions recover, and some even to such an extent that they not only have no discomforts from their affection, but they have even conceived at a later date and have been delivered at term. It would, however, be most illogical to suppose that each and every case will recover simply by *vis medicatrix naturæ* aided by conservative treatment.

Drainage in cases of metritis with inflammatory lesions of the adnexa has been a most effective treatment, and numerous recoveries without further operation have been recorded, and I have no doubt whatsoever that drainage of the uterine cavity with gauze may result in a cure of pyosalpinx in not a few cases, and that not infrequently the patients may ultimately conceive and go through a normal labour. Whatever material is used for drainage, be it silkworm gut, iodoform gauze, or rubber drains, it certainly favours the discharge of the muco-purulent secretions, and by acting favourably on the circulation of the uterus the muscular tonicity of the organ is awakened and the menstrual functions finally return and are carried on normally.

In a certain number of cases of encysted collections, surrounded by masses of dense false membrane, which might seem at first to require laparotomy or hysterectomy, they may in some few instances be recovered from by drainage of the uterus ; and on several occasions I obtained excellent results in cases of suppurating salpingitis by dilatation, curettement, and drainage of the uterus, the purulent collections in the tubes being emptied out through the uterine cavity, although this process has been denied by a number of eminent authorities. It was formerly thought that curettement should never be undertaken when lesions of the adnexa were present under the pretext that these lesions might be aggravated by the operation ; but on this point I cannot agree, as I have seen great improvement and even recovery follow this operative interference under these circumstances.

It may be questioned why one should be desirous of preserving the organs which, when patients are relieved of their pathologic process, will be of little or no use to the woman, because they are for ever afterwards incapable of accomplishing their functions. Now, it is quite certain that after a salpingitis the tubes do not always return to their normal state, and that by a fibrous or sclerous process their lumen becomes closed, so that a functional impotency results, producing sterility. Although this may be a general rule, I would point out that sterility does not appear to be an absolute consequence of salpingitis, and the tube may remain perfectly patent and never become obstructed. Even admitting that, following some suppurative process, the lumen of the tube becomes occluded, it may nevertheless be hoped that this mechanical or pathological obstruction may in time disappear as the lesion regresses. If the lesion is unilateral, as is often the case, it is evident that the healthy tube will continue its normal function, and no surgeon ever dreamed of removing both testicles when only one was the seat of an orchitis or an epididymitis under the pretext that the healthy organ would no longer be useful, and it is of every-day observation to find that after an inflammatory process the genital power has been preserved.

The pavilion of the tube may be compared to the epididymis, and in point of fact an analogy exists between tubo-ovaritis and epididymitis ;

and there is no doubt in my mind that certain lesions, such as catarrhal salpingitis, perisalpingitis, and perioophoritis, may be recovered from, the patient retaining her reproductive functions. I have notes of two cases, seen in consultation, of pregnancy following salpingitis where conservative treatment was used; so it seems possible that, under the influence of some conservative treatment, such, for example, as curettement and drainage, the uterine ostia of the tubes may become free of their obstruction, and by the action of the drainage the lesions regress sufficiently so that permeability of the lumen of the tube results. Assuredly, when in presence of serious suppurative processes in the uterus and adnexa, one should not be prevented from acting by a mere philosophical consideration; but such consideration, although no longer philosophical and in reality practical, is to be seriously considered when the suppurative process does not place the life of the patient in danger.

It is not my intention to consider all the various conservative treatments, because, given the great variety of pelvic suppurative processes, it at once becomes evident that one must make a choice of technique. I would, however, refer to posterior colpotomy in suppurative lesions, a subject to which I have given much thought, and with which I have had no little experience. The various changes this technique has undergone, and the brilliant results it has given at the hands of many operators, makes it at the present time a most valuable procedure. In the very acute cases, where it would be hazardous to open the abdomen with the purpose of performing any radical interference, drainage through the posterior *cul de sac* will relieve the patient of her septic symptoms and place her in a condition where later on she will be able to undergo a radical operation with all possible chance for a successful outcome.

Upon several occasions, where I have done an exploratory laparotomy, the result has been fortunate, and, although nothing radical could be attempted, abdominal incision followed by drainage has worked marvels. Many similar examples have been published by other operators, who, after having attempted removal of the diseased organ, were obliged to give up on account of the difficulties presented, and still, much to their surprise, within a short time the process disappeared, and the patients completely recovered. Whether or not the fact of opening the peritoneum has a revulsive effect on the lesions, producing a kind of irritation, greatly changing them, and even causing them to disappear, is an hypothesis which has been admitted, but not generally accepted.

As has been said, metritis is usually the direct cause of sterility, but it occasionally happens that this process gives rise to a retroversion of the uterus, and it is this displacement that is the hindrance to fecundation. Consequently, if the uterus is replaced surgically there may be some prospect of conception taking place.

January 1st, 1906.

THE FOOD FACTOR IN DISEASE. By FRANCIS HARE, M.D. In two volumes. (London : Longmans, Green & Co., 1905.)

The great question is, What are we to eat and drink ? There is nothing about which such a variety of opinions is expressed. Some say red meat, some say white ; some say vegetables only, some say mixed diet ; some say nuts, some say cheese ; some say take a moderate amount of alcohol, some say never touch the accursed thing ; some drink hot water, some drink cold ; some say never drink with your meals, some say never drink between. Indeed, it would be quite easy, in the course of half an hour to pick up such advice that if all of it were followed we should eat and drink nothing at all, and everybody is agreed this would be bad owing to the risk of starvation. This state of affairs is hardly creditable to the medical profession, and all arises from the evil habit of drawing conclusions from insufficient premises. Therefore we welcome Dr. Hare's book, comprised of two thick volumes, in which he attempts to show how far various diseases depend upon food. In the short space of this review we cannot discuss such a work in detail : we can only advise those interested in the question to read it, especially if they have recently read Professor Chittenden's work ; for while that attempts to show that we all take too much proteid, Dr. Hare believes that proteid is practically as essential in a hot climate and under sedentary conditions of life as in the opposite circumstances, but that under both external heat and diminished physical exercise the purely carbonaceous food-stuffs should be largely reduced.

DISEASES OF THE LIVER, GALL-BLADDER, AND BILE-DUCTS. By H. D. ROLLESTON, M.A., M.D. (Cantab.), F.R.C.P., Physician to St. George's Hospital, London. (Published by W. B. Saunders & Co.)

This is a text-book of the highest class, containing the ripe experience of many years of patient work at the subject, complete, well written, and well published. The whole work shows how laborious, patient, and conscientious its preparation has been. The literature is very full, and practically every view on the subject of hepatic and biliary disease has a patient hearing, but it is submitted to the searching criticism of one who has taken the trouble to investigate every question within the scope of his subject. The result has been a text-book which for many years to come will be the standard work upon this subject and which may be relied on to supply complete information on the rarest diseases of these organs and to elucidate the most perplexing cases. For instance, the writer was recently asked to explain the following case : A man with very obvious suppurative cholecystitis presented the signs of an acute nephritis, in addition his urine containing a considerable quantity of albumen and casts. The gall-bladder was drained and the nephritis immediately cleared up. The complication of suppurative cholecystitis by acute nephritis is fully treated of in this book. Dr. Rolleston is a skilled pathologist, and the figures which illustrate this book so fully are new drawings of his own specimens and microscopic sections. It is hard to find fault with such a book, and the only criticism we can make is that rarities are sometimes reiterated until they assume undue importance and get, as it were, out of focus. For instance, it must be extremely rare for a suppurating gall-bladder protruding from the end of a Riedel's lobe to simulate appendicitis. Yet this is again and again referred to under Diagnosis. A good many mistakes have escaped the proof-reader ; but this is almost inseparable from first editions, and such mistakes are usually obvious and seldom obscure the sense. This monograph can be strongly recommended as a complete and ultimate source of information on all medical and pathological aspects of liver and biliary diseases.

THE CLINICAL JOURNAL,

CLINICAL RECORD, CLINICAL NEWS, CLINICAL GAZETTE, CLINICAL REPORTER,
CLINICAL CHRONICLE AND CLINICAL REVIEW.

EDITED BY L. ELIOT CREASY.

| No. 689. | WEDNESDAY, JANUARY 10, 1906. | Vol. XXVII. No. 13.· |

CONTENTS.

* Specially reported for the Clinical Journal. Revised
by the Author.

NOTICE.

Editorial correspondence, books for review, &c.,
should be addressed to the Editor, 51, New Cavendish
Street, W., Telephone No. 904, Paddington ; but
all business communications should be addressed to
the Publishers, 22½, Bartholomew Close, London,
E.C. Telephone 927, Holborn.

All inquiries respecting Advertisements should be
sent to MESSRS. ADLARD & SON, Bartholomew
Close, E.C. Telephone 927, Holborn.

Terms of Subscription, including postage, payable
by cheque, postal or banker's order (in advance) : for
the United Kingdom, 15s. 6d. per annum ; Abroad,
17s. 6d.

Cheques, &c., should be made payable to THE
PROPRIETORS OF THE CLINICAL JOURNAL, crossed
" The London, City, and Midland Bank, Ltd., New-
gate Street Branch, E.C. Account of the Medical
Publishing Company, Limited."

Reading Cases to hold Twenty-six numbers of
THE CLINICAL JOURNAL can be supplied at 2s. 3d.
each, or will be forwarded post free on receipt of
2s. 6d. ; and also Cases for binding Volumes at 1s.
each, or post free on receipt of 1s. 3d., from the
Publishers, 22½ Bartholomew Close, London, E.C.

WITH DR. SAMUEL WEST IN THE WARDS OF ST. BARTHOLOMEW'S HOSPITAL.

NEW GROWTH IN THE UPPER PART OF THE RIGHT
LUNG.

THIS is an interesting man. He was sent in
having come under observation complaining of
weakness in his right arm and both legs. The
history is as follows : Thirteen weeks ago he had
diarrhœa for four days. During the last five weeks
he has been feeling weakness in his right arm and
both legs. The onset has been gradual, and he has
been steadily getting worse. That is all the history
when he came in.

If you will look at him you will see that he has a
puffy face. The case rather looked like one of
albuminuria. But he is not suffering from that ; he
has not any albumin. We proceeded to examine
him, and found that he had some œdema of
his right hand. There is no œdema of his legs,
nothing except weakness. So that we are on the
track of something interesting. It does not require
much observation to detect these little veins on the
chest, and there are some bigger veins also on the
abdomen. Then as to the blood-current, it is
running from above downwards. In the veins of
his neck there is a good deal of obstruction, and
they become more swollen when he coughs. All
these signs point to an obstruction high up—i. e.
to some interference with his vena cava. On percussing the chest we discovered that there was
great dulness from the upper part of the sternum
outwards over the whole upper part of the right
side. The heart is in its normal position. The
patient has not any temperature. Then, he has a
cough, and is hoarse ; but the larynx is normal, and
there is nothing wrong with the vocal cords. The
conclusion is that there is something on the right
side of his chest producing pressure upon the veins.

and preventing the blood coming back from the head, and neck, and right arm, which has caused the dilatation of the superficial veins. His pulse is weak. The air enters less freely on the right side than on the left, and there is one other thing to notice—viz. that there are enlarged glands in both axillæ. There is no reduction in his red-blood cells. The white cells show a slight increase, with a relative excess of polymorphonuclear, but there are no abnormal cells, and the hæmoglobin amounts to 70 per cent. He is not so anæmic as one would have expected in the circumstances. The cause of the weakness in the legs we leave for the present; it may be due to general causes, or be quite independent. The weakness in his right arm may be explained by the pressure on the vessels and possibly on the nerves too, though in the latter case there ought to have been pain.

This case presents several points of interest. It must be a mediastinal tumour, and yet it is not quite in the proper position for that, for it should be more in the middle line. Very often these mediastinal tumours run down the mediastinum and involve the parts over the heart. Or they extend down the posterior mediastinum and produce physical signs behind. In this case there are signs behind in the upper part of the back. The whole of the lung is more or less dull. I think there must be a tumour which apparently started near to the root of the right lung, and which has grown very considerably and come forward. If aneurysms develop in this place, they generally reach a large size, because there is practically nothing to interfere with them. But a new growth in that position is not very common. Why I had the blood examined was because I wondered whether there was any lymphadenomatous growth. The case is interesting because the condition of the chest was discovered solely by physical signs. The patient complained of nothing to draw attention to the chest, and was admitted simply for the weakness in the legs and right arm.

PERNICIOUS ANÆMIA.

This man came into the hospital for weakness and palpitation on exertion. In February last he had some attacks of giddiness and swelling of the feet. For nine months he had been unable to work, and had gradually been getting worse and losing weight. It is a case of profound anæmia;

that is the prominent symptom. He has not lost blood. There is no leucocytosis. So far as we can find out he has not any malignant disease. I do not think his condition has anything to do with his work. He has nothing to do with lead. The arteries are not thick, so that it is not granular kidney. Nor is it an aortic case. The patient's red cells are reduced to 1,600,000, the white cells number 6000. The hæmoglobin amounts to 45 per cent. That is rather excessive compared with the reduction of the red-blood cells. All this would fit in best with pernicious or grave anæmia. But we should be cautious in diagnosing anæmia because of the difficulty in excluding malignant disease. I have shown you two or three cases of that kind recently. In the present case we have not discovered any growth as yet, and his case looks like one of pernicious anæmia.

The treatment employed in such a case is rest, raw meat, and bone-marrow, with some arsenic. A case in the other ward is interesting because the patient took these things without any benefit, and she seemed to be getting worse. Her blood-tension was very low, so that we gave her 1½ drachms of adrenalin three times a day (1 in 1000 solution) and then she improved wonderfully. Her red-blood cells, which had been 900,000, went up to over 1,200,000. I suspended the remedy for a time and she went back. She is now taking it again and is improving; while taking it she at any rate feels much better. The woman was treated in the hospital for pernicious anæmia two years ago. She recovered and remained practically well for many months. Then the condition relapsed and she came back. Now she is getting better once more. It cannot be a question of new growth with her.

G. K—, æt. 50 years, came into the hospital yesterday with pain in the calves and back. He vomited and had a shivering fit. On admission his temperature was 103°; it went down to 101°. He was sweating profusely when he came in, and he is sweating profusely now.

As there were no physical signs yesterday, and the respirations were only 26, I thought that the case was probably one of influenza—a sudden attack, with fever, aching in the legs and back, and severe pains. But this morning he had developed signs of extensive pneumonia in his left lung. He is still going on sweating, and sweating is not a common phenomenon in pneumonia. Generally a case that sweats is a bad one. Judging by his pulse and respiration, you would not think that this man had pneumonia, but still the physical signs place the diagnosis beyond doubt.

He has another symptom which is useful for diagnosis when you cannot disturb the patient much for examination—I mean skodaic resonance. There is hyper-resonance on the left side, in the axilla, and in front, over the consolidation. Skodaic resonance is difficult to explain. If there were a large effusion there it might be said that the skodaic resonance was due to relaxed lung-tissue, just as the lung on the post-mortem table, relaxed and partially collapsed, gives a similar percussion note. But that cannot be so in this case. The only explanation I can suggest is that the altered note is due to loss of tone or tension, the result of impaired nutrition consequent on the inflammation. Sometimes a similar condition occurs on the opposite side as well. As long as it is unilateral it is not a serious sign, but where it is bilateral it is exceedingly grave.

The interest in this case is the sweating, and I presume we have a double infection, with the influenza bacillus and the pneumococcus. (Bacteriologically this was stated to be the case.)

ACUTE ASCITES IN CIRRHOSIS OF THE LIVER.

Here is a man who says he was well until fourteen days ago. Then his abdomen began to swell and he had pains in his shoulders. That is all the history at present. I think the case is one of cirrhosis.

I should like you to notice that the abdomen is very tight and round and not bulging at the flanks ; it is tense, resistant, hard. This shows that the ascites is of quite recent date. In ascites which has lasted for some time—weeks or months—the abdomen is flattened, bulging in the flanks, and not hard. That is to be explained by the condition of the abdominal muscles. In an acute case the nutrition of the abdominal muscles is not affected, and therefore when they get irritated by the distension they contract, whereas in a chronic case the muscles may be as thin as paper. If we measure the intra-abdominal tension in this case, which we will do when the patient is tapped, we shall find a considerable number of inches of water-pressure. (It proved to be 14 inches of water.) The high

pressure is causing considerable displacement of the diaphragm upwards and some dyspnœa. The patient is passing also a very small quantity of highly concentrated urine, which is loaded with lithates. The displacement of the organs, the dyspnœa, and the small amount of water passed are indications to tap as soon as possible, and this will be done as soon as we leave the ward.

MUCH CYANOSIS IN A CASE OF APPARENTLY SIMPLE MITRAL DISEASE.

This young woman is very dusky about the lips, cheeks, and ears. She has morbus cordis, with a loud double mitral murmur. There is also a little œdema of the feet and slight swelling of the abdomen, and the liver is enlarged. She has, then, all the signs of backward congestion, but there is much more cyanosis than the cardiac lesion will account for, and there is not enough bronchitis to explain it. The question is whether there may not be some congenital affection of the heart as well. Extreme cyanosis is only met with when the arterial and venous blood-streams are mixed.

There are two conditions under which extreme cyanosis is met with—emphysema and congenital heart affections. In congenital heart affections the blood-stream is mixed either through some malformation in the heart itself, such as a perforated septum, or through persistent fœtal vessels. In emphysema it is not so clear where the mixing takes place, but it is equally definite. The pulmonary arteries and the pulmonary veins and the bronchial arteries and bronchial veins all communicate and can be injected one from the other in a normal lung. These anastomoses are very minute under ordinary circumstances. But they provide a short cut when the circulation through the lung is greatly interfered with. The blood then takes that short cut ; it does not pass round through the lungs, but runs straight from the pulmonary artery to the pulmonary vein. The conditions, then, which determine cyanosis are exactly the same in emphysema and congenital morbus cordis.

Our next patient is this child, who was sent in on November 18th, with acute pneumonia accompanied with vomiting, restlessness, rapid breathing, and high temperature. In forty-eight hours after admission quite half the upper lobe on the left side was solid. The respirations were rapid (56) and the pulse was about 150. That respiration is not so very rapid for a child. There was another case in the other ward where the respirations ran up to 70 or 80. That case was one of pneumonia after whooping-cough.

The text-book accounts of broncho-pneumonia do not fit in with many of the cases which you meet with in your practice. It is not at all uncommon for babies suffering from pneumonia to get quite well quickly. Yet it is not at all common to get massive consolidation in children. There are many cases in which you get no massive consolidation. The description of broncho-pneumonia still found in many text-books applies to the cases which follow bronchitis. After bronchitis of some duration the temperature rises, inflammatory symptoms present themselves, and little patches of consolidation occur in different parts of the chest. The patient gets better, then has a relapse, gets better again, and has another relapse ; and so it goes on, it may be for weeks, though in the end the child gets well. In other cases there is exactly the same condition of things so far as the physical signs go, but the history is absolutely different. The little patches of pneumonia are as numerous and definite as in the other cases. The child is taken suddenly ill and has high fever. After a week's illness the temperature falls by crisis, and the child gets well just as quickly as if it had had typical pneumonia. What is to prevent you from saying that this latter class of cases is really a typical or pneumococcal pneumonia ?

Acute pneumonia, I hold, occurs in two forms— the lobar pneumonia, which is the massive form, and the lobular, which is the patchy, disseminated form, and this is very often multiple. The multiple or patchy form is common in children up to a certain age. The multiple, patchy form is rare in adults, but it does sometimes occur. The massive form is very common in adults and rare in children. But clinically both forms have practically the same clinical history and course, and we may conclude that they are both due to the same cause—viz. the pneumococcus. It is important to recognise the distinction in children, because in the one class of cases there is an illness which will relapse frequently and recovery be delayed, and in the other class an illness from which in the great majority of cases recovery is rapid. It may be a matter for discussion why pneumococcal pneumonia should take a different form in the adult from that which it takes in the child—why it should be liable to be disseminated and patchy in the child, and lead to massive consolidation in the adult, but the facts are indisputable.

January 8th, 1906.

THE
RÔLE OF THE HYPODERMIC SYRINGE IN THE TREATMENT OF SYPHILIS.

By CAMPBELL WILLIAMS, F.R.C.S.

THE comparatively modern practice of treating syphilis by instilling mercury into the tissues of the human body is, in its broad principle, far from being new. For chronological purposes its progress may be divided into three stages, namely the subcutaneous, the intra-muscular and the intra-venous methods. The idea of injecting mercury into the subcutaneous tissues was, if not actually conceived, at least advocated and practised, by Scarenzio, * of Milan, as long ago as 1864. He employed calomel suspended in glycerin or mucilage as his favourite therapeutic agent. In the same year Berkeley Hill † commenced to practise the "subcutaneous" method, using the bichloride of mercury in doses of gr. $\frac{1}{10}$ to gr. $\frac{1}{4}$ in 10 minims of distilled water. He also essayed the solution of mercuric cyanide, as well as the albuminised and peptonised solutions of Bamberger. These quickly gave place in his hands to Ragazzoni's formula of the red iodide of mercury in the presence of iodide of sodium. In later years he used the last named solution as an intra-muscular injection, but finally abandoned it in favour of the less pain-begetting sal alembroth. Lewin, ‡ of Berlin, was another of the earliest pioneers in this system of medication. He began in 1869 to treat all his cases with subcutaneous injections of a solution of perchloride of mercury, and stated that in over 3000 patients whom he personally injected there were only two cases complicated by abscess formation. Other names which are closely identified with the early advocacy and practice of instillation are those of Sigismund, Staub, Liégeois, Bamberger, Terillon, Ragazzoni, and Hürbringer. § The last named almost hit upon grey oil in that he injected metallic mercury subcutaneously. His results were not encouraging, and he abandoned the use of the preparation. In the early days of mercurial in-

---

* Scarenzio, ‘ Annali Universali di Medicina di Milano, 1864.

† Berkeley Hill, ‘ Lancet,’ May 5th, 1866.

‡ Lewin, ‘ Die Behandlung der Syphilis mit Subcutaner sublimat injection,’ 1869.

§ Hürbringer, ‘ Deutsch. Archiv. f. klin. Med.,’ 1879.

jections the subcutaneous tissues were always elected as the site for the infiltration of the drug. The *intentional* preference for the deeper or intra-muscular regions was not evolved until about twenty-one years ago. Its *raison de être* can be traced to an effort to lessen pain and also to minimise subcutaneous suppuration, which so frequently ensued at the site of the deposition. The intra-muscular method was brought pro-minently before the notice of the profession in England by Astley Bloxam,* who as far back as 1884 employed solutions of sal alembroth, in-stilling them deeply into the gluteal regions. Some of the first intra-muscular injections which I personally administered were given under his supervision at the Lock Hospital, Dean Street, in that year. Amongst those first in the field with the sozoiodol-mercury introduced by Schwimmer† in 1892 was Radcliffe-Crocker, who in the early nineties was using this salt upon his in-patients at University College Hospital. Originally he employed daily injections, the diurnal dose being about $\frac{1}{16}$ gr. In those days I was his assis-tant in the skin department and it was part of my duty to administer the injections in his absence, so I am able to testify as to the comparative free-dom from pain or other sequelæ which even the repeated "subcutaneous" injection of this salt caused. Small nodules did certainly supervene at the site of the punctures, but they caused no real discomfort and gradually became absorbed. After a short trial the subcutaneous plan gave place to the deeper and more satisfactory intra-muscular method, with larger doses, administered weekly. The modern school of "injectors" may be divided into advocates for the insoluble salts of mercury or into partisans of the intra-muscular and the intra-venous systems. The intravenous champions are necessarily, or rather should be, "solublists." Each faction can boast of certain advantageous points to favour their particular fancy. But there are likewise drawbacks which the "solublists" will urge against the insoluble preparations and *vice versâ*. Putting these differences aside, all injectors seem to be agreed upon certain conditions which they, not without reason or proof, claim for either the method as a whole or their individual preparations in par-ticular. These are :

* Bloxham, 'Med. Soc. Trans.,' 1888.
† Cotterell, 'Syphilis,' London, 1892.

(1) Accuracy and regulation of the dose of mercury administered.

(2) Rapidity of action.

(3) Certainty of absorption and consequently a fair chance of eradicating the disease.

(4) Non-impairment of the digestive functions.

(5) Comparative freedom from the grosser form of stomatitis.

(6) The mitigation, if not entire absence, of intestinal disturbance (?).

The solublists claim all the foregoing advantages, whilst the insolublists hold that the action of the drugs is so transient, and the mercury so quickly eliminated from the system, which is a debatable assertion, that it necessitates the giving of daily in-jections. They affirm that by giving an instillation of say either grey oil or calomel, that it remains longer *in situ* and is more slowly absorbed into the lympathic vessels as an albuminate of mercury, and that consequently it is only needful to give one injection each week or even every other week. But their opponents deny the necessity of more than semainal injections of certain of the soluble salts, and quote the undeniable fact that the usage of in-soluble mercurial preparations has in a few isolated instances been followed within a few moments of the operation by pulmonary infarction,* with all the distressing symptoms of embolism in the lungs. The most probable explanation for such a disaster is that the injections, although intended to be intra-muscular, were really intravenous, owing to the point of the needle having penetrated within the lumen of a vein. Such a contingency can always be guarded against by taking the simple precaution of either plunging the needle in separately or de-taching the syringe from it subsequently to penetra-tion and seeing whether any venous blood escapes from the aperture of the needle prior to injecting the insoluble salt. Professor Gottheil, of New York, has drawn attention to this necessary safeguard.

Lieut.-Col. Lambkin, R.A.M.C.,† has recently recorded his experience of 50,000 injections of metallic mercury suspended in the combined vehicles of lanolin and liquid paraffin. He states that he has never seen any untoward result follow the use of this preparation, which is really only a mitigated modification of the old injectio hydrar-

* Cooper, Sir Alfred, 'Syphilis,' 2nd edition, p. 453.
† Lambkin, 'Brit. Med. Journ.,' November 11th, 1905.

gyri hypodermica or grey oil,* and expresses the opinion that the reputed danger of pulmonary embolism, which is the bogey to the employment of the "insoluble emulsions," has not only been greatly exaggerated, but is, as far as his experience *proves*, non-existent. This view, if it be intended to include *all* the insoluble preparations of mercury other than his special grey oil product, does not exactly coincide with the observations of a large bulk of syphilographers as to the absolute absence of the lesser or greater evils which have been noted in connection with the administration of either the insoluble salts or even *basic* mercury itself. Moreover I fancy that the description of calomel in the article as a soluble salt † must be regarded as an oversight. The statistics of Alfred Fournier,‡ Professor of Venereal Diseases in the Paris Faculty of Medicine, certainly record a very different view as regards the intra-muscular injections of calomel. Although he speaks most highly of its rapid, nay, almost marvellous, action in clearing up various syphilitic phenomena, he nevertheless points out that the effects of the drug not only pass off quickly but that relapses are common. There are many drawbacks to its use, the chief of which are as follows: (1) Pain. This varies from little more than discomfort to bed-confining agony. It occurred to a greater or less degree in 50 per cent. of his cases; in fact, he remarks that scarcely a week passes without his having to discontinue its employment owing to the suffering it caused the patient. (2) Abscesses which occur in about 1 per cent. of injected cases, notwithstanding all "skilled" precautions. (3) Swelling and induration of the hip supervening in a day or two after the injection were present in a greater or lesser amount in 384 instances out of a total of 400 installations. (4) Nodes, varying in size from an olive to that of an orange, were not infrequent sequelæ. These usually disappeared in a few weeks, but some persisted for three, six, or even twelve months. (5) Pulmonary embolism has been noted by various observers. The attack comes on shortly after the injection, and lasts usually for three or four days. There is no accom-

panying rise of temperature. In one instance recorded the attack lasted for three weeks, with continuous bloody expectoration. In the case of grey oil, which is frequently exhibited in what is really a diluted liquid form of unguentum hydrargyri made with lanolin instead of lard, and to which is added a sufficiency of either a vegetable or mineral oil to give it the requisite fluidity, one is really effecting through the mechanical aid of a syringe that which a mercurial rubber essays to attain by manual labour. But herein lies the difference, that whereas one *actually* knows and can regulate the exact amount which *must* sooner or later be absorbed when it is injected, one must rely upon the energy of the operator together with the patient's dermal receptive power when absorption through the skin is invoked. Personally I hold inunction in the highest regard,* notwithstanding its dirtiness, erythema-exciting proclivities, and all its other drawbacks. For I have witnessed its great therapeutic value times upon times. But few cases can afford either the leisure and expense—the latter being greater than that of a course of injections—which a sojourn at a rubbing establishment entails—to say nothing of the publicity which so often ensues. Personal inunction is, in the majority of instances, unsatisfactory, and it is hardly fair to leaven the method as a whole by adding those failures which are really amateurish efforts.

No one who has had much experience of the instillation treatment, which is theoretically an ideal system, can deny that it holds forth a most reasonable expectation that a cure will be effected, provided that the injections be judiciously and regularly carried out over a sufficiently long period. We cannot, however, *guarantee* a cure with this or any other method. All we can say is, that people are undoubtedly cured of syphilis when treated with mercury. But it must not be assumed that either injections or inunction hold the record of such a much to be desired consummation. For countless numbers of syphilitic patients have been *really* cured by the antiquated oral method, which will continue to dispense health and freedom from all syphilitic sequelæ if the treatment be but adapted to the patient's individual needs. I am painfully well acquainted with many cases which have "gone

---

* Martindale's 'Extra Ph.,' p. 283, 11th edition.

† Lambkin, 'Brit. Med. Journ.,' November 11th, 1905, p. 1257, column 2, line 43.

‡ Fournier, 'International Clinics,' U.S.A., p. 105, vol. 14th series.

* Campbell Williams, "The Treatment of Tertiary Syphilis by Inunction," ' Lancet,' April 22nd, 1893.

to the wall" with the so-called parasyphilitic degenerations, or even tertiary mischief, who had been subjected to the oral *régime*. But on the other hand, I see patients from time to time who were primarily infected as long ago as twenty to twenty-five, or even thirty years, but who, notwithstanding that they only received the somewhat despised mouth treatment, are the fathers of healthy children and themselves free from any discoverable objective or subjective sign of syphilis. If they be not cured, they are at least content with that counterfeit which has brought them well through middle life and sees them, for aught they know to the contrary, in robust health. With injections, as with inunction, the element of finance will always prove an obstacle to many whom pain would not deter from invoking the needle's assistance. For a large majority of syphilitically injected people acquire the disease in those youthful days when spirits and erotic tendencies are in inverse ratio to the state of their exchequer. They could not afford, unless they received their weekly injections gratis, to embark upon a course of treatment which may have to be prolonged over the same number of months which is usually advocated for the personally controlled oral administration. The financial advantages certainly rest with the medical adviser when patients not only *desire* this line of treatment, but can likewise afford the weekly or fortnightly fee. It is superfluous for me to point out that there are other reasons, apart from a monetary consideration, which may deter a *private* patient from availing him or herself of mercurial injections. The fear of pain holds a chief place; many men who would without a second thought jump their horse over a five-barred gate, or in other ways unhesitatingly risk their lives, are abject cowards when it comes to a cold-blooded submission to even the most trivial physical suffering. I have met with patients who have courageously faced death from lead or steel, but nevertheless funked mercury and the needle's prick. The late Christopher Heath used to impress upon students the following motto : *Suaviter in modo, fortiter in re*, and I would add that one must always use worldly tact in dealing with one's patients—that is, if you do not want to lose them. If one makes the mercurial injection a *sine quâ non* in the treatment of *all* cases of syphilis, one will quickly find that a certain proportion of one's clients will find some

other surgeon who will treat them in the painless manner they desire, even though he might not think it the best method for them. Competition has many door-plates to your one, and it will equally militate against you should you fail to utilise mercurial injections as part of your armamentarium in treating syphilis. For them your methods may be styled as antiquated or inadequate, or it may be said that one's knowledge and practice has not advanced with the times. *Medio tutissimus ibis* ; therefore do not spurn any method. They all have good points. Occupation is another factor which operates against instillation. The nature of the patient's avocation may be such that the injection into the buttocks or elsewhere of any soluble or insoluble preparation of mercury might necessitate—through pain—its temporary discontinuation. A call to boot and saddle during the first two days following even a succinimide injection would hardly be hailed as tidings of comfort and joy by the gluteal regions of a cavalry officer. *Experto crede.* A patient's business, moreover, may make it imperative for him to be here to-day and there to-morrow, and consequently seldom in reach of his regular medical adviser and the remedial syringe. One can hardly expect the average syphilitic to travel about the country accompanied by all the paraphernalia necessary for an intra-muscular injection, nor that your patient will call upon various strange doctors armed with soft soap, spirit, syringe, solution, etc., for the purpose of getting them to carry out your treatment. There would be a decided element of risk in advising a layman, totally ignorant of anatomy, to administer the injections to himself in any of the various accessible sites. I think the reasons are too obvious to need discussion. I once had to cut down upon and remove a broken needle from Scarpa's triangle as the result of a self-administered injection, which was undertaken for the purpose of saving the injection fee.

Let us now assume that we have a patient who is either desirous or persuadable towards mercurial injections. One would first have to decide before urging their acceptance or employment that he or she really has syphilis. There must be no uncertainty as to the diagnosis. For if any element or query exists as to the nature of the primary lesion it should always receive the benefit of the doubt and all *constitutional* treatment be withheld until either the local sore declares its true nature through unmistakable induration, or by the evolution of glandular, dermal, or faucial corroboration. Many a patient has been *fully* treated for syphilis when he has never had it, owing to the wrongful diagnosis of inflammatory induration as a veritable specific hyperplasia. One cannot commence to treat syphilis too early. But of two evils, perchance the lesser is to err on the waiting side, until a roseolous rash, or some other indisputable sign, has placed all chance of error out of the question, rather than to unnecessarily drug a person for two years, or even longer, through a mistaken assumption. Before starting upon treatment, one should always find out if the patient is a "bleeder." For the hæmorrhagic diathesis is an absolute bar to mercurial injections, either owing to the formation of local hæmatoma or, as has actually happened, to its setting up hæmorrhage from the urinary tract from which the patient died.[*] The state of the kidneys must be examined, and should their power for elimination be found to be deficient, great care and watchfulness must be exercised in whatever way mercury is administered. More particularly is this statement applicable to the intra-muscular and intravenous methods since the renal apparatus is the principal channel by which mercury, thus employed, is carried off. In my opinion Bright's disease and kindred pathological changes in the kidneys are contra-indicative to mercurial injections. Again, diabetic subjects would not be suitable for this method. Tubercle complicating syphilis may also demand that we resort to less heroic measures. For, although mercury is a germicidal tonic and blood-maker when given in small doses, it has the reverse effect when the quantity exhibited exceeds the individual's needs or powers of elimination. The desideratum that should be sought after is to correct the toxic effect of the *Spirochæte pallida*,[†] which is the name of the latest suspected microbe of syphilis, and not to produce leucocytosis. The mouths of all patients should be put in order as soon as treatment is embarked upon, if such a course be possible, and all tartar removed. A small dose of mercury, no matter how administered, will cause inconvenience

[*] Fournier, Alfred, 'Internat. Clin.,' U.S.A., vol. iii, 14th series, p. 120.

[†] Schaudim and Hoffman, 'Arbeiten aus dem Kaiserlichen Gesundheitsamte,' 1905.

to the gums of dentally tartarous patients, which would not have the slightest effect upon the teeth or soft structures of those not subject to this complaint. Mercury often receives the full blame for conditions for which it is only partly responsible. I do not think that it originates Riggs' disease, although I fully admit that it acts deleteriously upon a pre-existing pyo-alveolaric state.

INTRA-MUSCULAR INJECTIONS.

The intra-muscular injection has entirely supplanted the more superficial or subcutaneous method. The usual and most convenient site for their administration is the gluteal region, the right and left buttocks being utilised alternately. The chosen spot for puncture should be above the level of the great trochanter, and at or about the junction of the *outer* and middle thirds of this area. In the erect position of the body the needle will either penetrate the upper fibres of the gluteus maximus or else engage the gluteus medius. The choice of this particular site has reference to the position of the great sciatic nerve, so that it may escape implication and the patient be saved from a traumatically acquired neuritis. On this ground I think a reference to the position of the nerve is pardonable. The great sciatic nerve leaves the pelvis through the great sacro-sciatic foramen in company with the pyriformis muscle and the gluteal sciatic and pudic vessels and nerves. Extending downwards from the lower border of the pyriformis muscle, it lies between the great trochanter and the ischial tuberosity, covered by the gluteus maximus. Superficially a spot corresponding to the junction of the *inner* and middle thirds of a line drawn from the posterior iliac spine to the great trochanter would mark the position of the gluteal artery, between which and the sciatic artery one finds the great sciatic nerve. An accidental instillation into the sheath of the great sciatic nerve may, apart from the intense agony it causes, give rise to transient paresis of the limb. It is therefore well to take all precautions to avoid it, both for your *own* and the patient's sake.

Having settled upon the site for the proposed injection, the next step is, not only to clean and sterilise one's own hands, but also to pay similar attention to the patient's buttock. It should first be thoroughly cleansed by scrubbing it with soft soap. It is next washed in either ether or alcohol.* The ordinary commercial methylated spirits of wine does admirably. It is pure spirit and the wood oil which it contains, to meet the requirements of the Excise, is in itself, through being one of the turpentine series, no disadvantage in that it possesses both cleansing and mild antiseptic properties. Personally, I never irritate the skin more than necessary and regard the extra application of lotions, such as a solution of $\frac{1}{100}$ hyd. perchlor., as superfluous when the part has already received a thorough spirit-washing. The patient is now ready for the injections. The syringe, having been filled with the prescribed solution or emulsion, is attached to its needle. The latter should be sterilised immediately prior to usage by being held for a few seconds in the flame of a spirit lamp. Having allowed the needle to cool, it is plunged into the tissues, at a right angle to the same, until it is judged that the requisite depth has been reached. This necessarily varies with the amount of subcutaneous fat present. The desired spot is usually from three quarters to one inch below the surface of the skin. If emulsions of the insoluble salts or the metallic base are to be instilled, one should take the precaution to see that the point of the needle is not engaged within the lumen of a vein by detaching the syringe and ascertaining whether any blood escapes through the needle's channel. This manœuvre is unnecessary with the soluble solutions, since they can be injected intravenously without the danger of causing pulmonary infarction. All being well, the piston rod is *slowly* pressed down and the injection infiltrated into the intra-muscular tissues. The needle is now withdrawn and gentle finger massage is employed to disperse the fluid. The puncture wound is finally sealed by means of a fragment of antiseptic wool saturated in collodion. Should any blood ooze from the skin prick, it may be arrested by applying gentle pressure for a few moments. One little device which I employ prior to plunging in the needle is to draw up the skin slightly, so that the dermal and deeper puncture tracts do not coincide. There is thus no direct continuity between the air, the surface of the skin, and the intra-muscular region. It is simply the

old tenotomy dodge of making the skin act as a valve.

THE CHOICE OF A SYRINGE AND NEEDLE.

A syringe which will admit of thorough sterilisation, by means of boiling, without marked deterioration, is the best. One that will allow of this procedure has a barrel • piston rod, and washer entirely of glass, whilst in others the washer is made of indiarubber. Such can easily be taken to pieces for cleansing processes, and a faulty or worn-out indiarubber washer can be replaced by a fresh one in a few moments. Needles constructed of platino-iridium are to be recommended in that they do not rust or corrode nor do they quickly become blunted by repeated boilings as steel ones will do. Some people prefer a syringe which has a glass barrel with vulcanite mountings. But frequent boiling is apt to loosen the nozzle mount should it be retained in position by shellac, and thus cause the instrument to become leaky and inefficient. One of the foregoing styles of syringe is absolutely necessary when the greasy emulsions are being used, because, owing to oil's tenacity, it is impossible to rapidly wash out either the needle or the syringe with water or even saponifying soda-water. Consequently there would be sufficiently long contact of the retained mercury with the metal mountings of an ordinary syringe or steel needle for the formation of an amalgam or to effect corrosion. In the case of soluble solutions one can practically circumvent this action by not filling the syringe until the instant one is going to use it, and by carefully washing it and the needle out with warm water the very moment after it has been withdrawn from the tissues. All that is required to prevent a steel needle from rusting or eroding is to plunge it into pure spirit and then hold it for a few seconds in the flame of a spirit lamp. This device both dries and sterilises it effectually. In the case of a steel needle one should carefully examine it each time before usage to see it is not eroded lest it chance to break when plunged into the flesh.

MERCURIAL INJECTIONS.

Practically all the salts of mercury, soluble and insoluble, together with the metallic base itself,

* The *ether soap* of the ' Extra Pharmacopœia ' (p. 470) or the same preparation with mercuric iodide combine the soap, ether, and the alcohol in a handy solution ready for use.

• Syringes of this nature can be obtained from Martindale, 10, New Cavendish Street, London, W.

have been impressed into the service of the hypo-dermic syringe in the search after a preparation which shall be more than transitorily efficacious and at the same time comparatively painless and not prone to be followed by local or visceral complications.

The following catalogue has been compiled more for descriptive purposes than practical utility. Many of the preparations have signally failed to sub-stantiate those advantageous claims which their respective advocates have put forward upon their behalf. The schedule is divided into salts soluble in water, which include certain salts which though not naturally soluble can be rendered such by the presence or addition of various substances, and insoluble preparations that require an oleaginous medium for their suspension. Benzoate of mercury, owing to its practical insolubility in water, has been included in the latter group.

Soluble, or else convertible into a soluble prepara-tion, administered in water :

(1) Sal alembroth : Ammonio-mercuric chloride.

(2) Hydrargyri cyanidum.

(3) Hydrargyri oxycyanidum.

(4) Hydrargyri iodidum rubrum c̄ sodii iodido (Ragazzoni's solution), mercuric iodide with sodium iodide.

(5) Hydrargyri lactas.

(6) Hydrargyri oxidum c̄ asparagin (mercuric oxide with althein).

(7) Hydrargyri oxidum c̄ formamido (mercuric oxide ,with the amide of formic acid).

(8) Hydrargyri perchloridum (mercuric chloride or corrosive sublimate).

(9) Hydrargyrum sozoiodol (mercury combined with di-iodo-para-phenol-sulphonic acid).

(10) Hydrargyri succinimidum (imido-succinate of mercury).

(11) Hydrargyri et sodii disulphocarbolas (her-mophenyl).

Insoluble preparations, administered in liq. paraffin, vegetable oil, or lanolin and oil :

(1) Hydrargyrum (metallic mercury : injectio hydrargyri hypodermica : grey oil).

(2) Hydrargyri oxidum flavum (yellow mercuric oxide).

(3) Hydrargyri salicylas (neutral salt).

(4) Hydrargyri tannas.

(5) Hydrargyri thymolacetas (mercury thymol ˙etate).

(6) Hydriodol. (cypridol : mercuric iodide oil).

(7) Hydrargyri benzoas (mercuric benzoate).

(8) Hydrargyri subchloridum (calomel).

Let us now review the above formidable list and briefly append to each preparation its drawbacks and advantages, if any should exist. Allow me to say once and for all that every intra-muscular in-jection is more or less painful. The pain is only a matter of degree, which varies with different preparations and the individuality of the subject operated upon.

The soluble or quasi-soluble preparations :

(1) *Sal alembroth.*—This is a reliable prepara-tion. It consists of two molecules of ammonium chloride to one of mercuric chloride. One grain of sal alembroth would therefore contain two thirds of a grain of corrosive sublimate. The usual dose of the standard solution is 10 m̃. This should convey half a grain of the ammonio-mercuric chloride to the tissues. As the preparation does not seem to be eliminated from the body with marked rapidity, it will usually suffice if an injection be given once every fifth or seventh day. The salt is fairly rapid in action, but is rather of the pain-producing order. Abscess formation *may* follow its induction, notwithstanding all precau-tions.

(2) *Hydrargyri cyanidum.*—This salt has been used intravenously as well as intra-muscularly It is, excepting possibly mercuric ethylene-diamine sulphate—otherwise sublamine—one of the *most poisonous* of all the mercurial salts. It is apt to give rise to severe diarrhœic symptoms, whilst albuminuria has frequently been noted to have ensued after its administration. Moreover, it is rapidly excreted from the system, necessitating injection either daily or every other day. The sole point in its favour, when used intra-muscularly, is that it is one of the less pain-begetting preparations.

(3) *Hydrargyri oxycyanidum* is the outcome of an effort to produce a salt resembling the cyanide, but which, whilst being richer in mercury, should possess less toxic properties. It mimics the cyanide product, when used intravenously, in being an intestino-renal irritant. It has, therefore, fallen into disuse in the hands of its original advocates.*

(4) *Ragazzoni's solution* of mercuric iodide, or

* Barthelemy and Levy Bing, ' La Syphilis,' February, 1905.

the modifications thereof, are again coming into favour on the Continent. Intravenous injections of the biniodide of mercury are recommended by Barthelemy and Levy Bing.[*] They have instilled it into the veins in doses of 1, 2, and 3 cgm. per c.c. They state that it has never given rise in their hands to any toxic symptoms. When used intra-muscularly it is decidedly painful, but the advantage is that a weekly injection of 10 ℳ of the solution, conveying about ¼ gr. of the salt, is sufficient. Mercuric iodide alone is almost insoluble in water, but freely so in solutions of other iodides.

(5) *Hydrargyri lactas.*—The lactate of mercury, which is soluble about 1 in 7 of water, is one of the least irritating of all the mercurial salts. It may be instilled as an intra-muscular injection in doses of ¼, ½, or even ¾ gr. One of the drawbacks urged against its use is the rapidity with which it is eliminated from the body. This necessitates closely repeated injections. The salt, which is rich in mercury, containing over fifty per cent. of the base, does not seem to exert such a powerful controlling action over symptoms as certain other preparations will do. But it is to be strongly recommended on account of its safety and comparatively painless after-effects.

(6) *Hydrargyri oxidum c̄ asparagin.*—This preparation is the yellow oxide of mercury in the presence of asparagin, which is also known as althein.[†] An aqueous solution of althein will dissolve the mercuric oxide, which is otherwise insoluble in water. I know of no special advantages which can be claimed for this preparation. Althein in itself is a diuretic.

(7) *Hydrargyri oxidum c̄ formamido* is a similar essay to transform yellow mercuric oxide into a soluble preparation by combining the salt with formamide—the amide of formic acid. I place it in the same category as the preceding product.

(8) *Hydrargyri perchloridum.*—This is the salt originally employed by Lewin, of Berlin, as a subcutaneous injection. Solutions of corrosive sublimate have been used both intravenously and intra-muscularly. When instilled into the latter region it is excessively painful, possibly

owing to its power of coagulating blood-serum, apart from its inherent irritative property. Nodes frequently follow at the site of injection, or there may be diffuse brawny induration of the buttock. It has been injected in a strength of $\frac{1}{31}$ gr. to 10 ℳ of water, but it is too painful a process for the majority of patients, and cannot, therefore, be advised. Von Zeissl,[*] of Vienna, used to inject ½ gr. at a sitting!

(9) *Hydrargyrum sozoiodol* is a combination of mercury with di-iodo-para-phenol sulphonic acid. It is one of the more favourite salts, owing to its safety, efficaciousness, and the comparative absence of local pain following its injection. Personally I instil as much as ½ to ¾ gr. at a sitting—or rather standing—and find that this amount suffices for five to seven days. The standard solution of the sozoiodol of mercury contains twice the weight of iodide of sodium as of the mercuric constituent. The addition of the soda salt is for the purpose of creating and maintaining solubility. The solution is at its best when freshly prepared, and, accordingly, it is advisable to order only small quantities at a time from one's chemist.

(10) *Hydrargyri succinimidum.*—The imido succinate of mercury is very freely soluble in water, and possesses the great advantage of being one of the least irritating or pain-begetting salts of mercury. Its power for coagulating albumen when exposed to it in a *test-tube* is feeble. But it does not necessarily follow that a correspondingly imperfect transformation into an albuminate of mercury will ensue when it is subjected to the reaction of Nature's laboratory. It is rapidly absorbed and eliminated from the system, since its presence can be detected in the urine shortly after it has been injected into the muscles. This is assumed to be a disadvantage, as theoretically it entails the administration of daily intra-muscular injections. My own experience is that an injection every fifth or sixth day of ½ gr. of the succinimide in 15 ℳ of water suffices to remove symptoms and to keep them in check. I can strongly recommend the salt as a safe and comparatively non-irritating agent.

(11) *Hermophenyl*, or hydrarg. et sodii disulphocarbolas, has been injected hypodermically, intra-muscularly, and intravenously in doses of ¼ to

---

[*] Barthelemy and Levy Bing, 'La Syphilis,' February, 1905.

[†] To make the solution the yellow oxide must be *freshly* precipitated

[*] Von Zeissl, 'Pathology and Treatment of Syphilis,' p. 372.

½ gr. A brief trial of the preparation convinced me that its therapeutic value was less than that of several other preparations.

The insoluble and quasi-insoluble preparations :

(1) *Hydrargyrum.*—Metallic mercury is administered in the form of grey oil. The original formula for oleum cinereum, which is also known as injectio hydrargyri hypodermica, is as follows : Mercury 39, mercurial ointment 2, vaseline oil 59. The foregoing preparation has not met with continued favour owing to its irritant properties. These may in part be due to the fact of the prepared suet or lard having undergone butyric acid changes. The many drawbacks which attended its use led to the appearance of various modifications which are intended to admit of the *base* being conveyed to the tissues under more propitious "probabilities." To this end vegetable and mineral oils, sterilised or even carbolised, have been advocated as the medium for suspension. A mercuric cream—10 per cent. of mercury—has been largely used in Vienna. Another formula for grey oil is that contained in Squire's 'Pocket Companion.'* The ingredients are—mercury 39, mercury ointment 2, white vaseline 19, liquid vaseline 40, all by weight. It contains 40 per cent. of metallic mercury and is administered in a dosage of 1 to 2 ℳ. Colonel Lambkin† gives his preference to the following preparation : Mercury 1, anhydrous lanolin 4, petroleum oil (carbolised 2 per cent.) to 10. It will be seen by comparing this product with the two previous grey oils that the amount of metallic mercury which it contains is 10 per cent. as against the other preparations' 40 per cent. The dose of the lanolised grey oil is 10 ℳ, conveying 1 gr., given weekly. Most of the modern variations of oleum cinereum combine 10 per cent. of the metal with either albolene, olive or almond oils. They all require violent trituration before usage so as to re-suspend the mercury—precipitated by its own weight—otherwise an under- or a poisonous over-dose may be injected. The advantage claimed for these preparations is that metallic mercury is slowly absorbed from the tissues, and that the therapeutic effect of an individual injection is therefore protracted. This is to my mind a tacit acknowledgment that a complete transformation of the base into a negotiable albuminate is a most laborious effort on the part of Nature. The therapeutic value should, therefore, be of an equally remedial order. I do not think sufficient stress has been attached to the presumption that mercury and its salts become changed into albuminate of mercury when introduced within the living body. The logical deduction from the foregoing assumption is that the therapeutic activity of a mercurial preparation is, in direct ratio to its proclivity and celerity for combining with albumen.

(2) *Hydrargyri oxidum flavum.*—The yellow oxide of mercury has been given as an insoluble (*vide* Hydrargyri oxidum flavum c̄ asparagin vel formamide) preparation suspended in oil. It is painful and can claim no special advantage.

(3) *Hydrargyri salicylas* (neutral salt). This preparation, which must not be confounded with the basic salicylate of mercury,* has been most favourably commented upon by Dr. Gottheil,† of New York. He states that personally he has never seen embolism follow its employment, although he acknowledged that "one or two cases have been recorded in which death is supposed to have happened in consequence of the treatment." The formula which he advocates is—Neutral mercury salicylate 1, liquid albolene to 10. The dose given varies according to the necessities of the case. Thus from three to ten drops may be injected, making the amount of the salt $\frac{3}{10}$ to gr. 1, either weekly or fortnightly as may be required. Dr. Gottheil recommends it upon the following grounds : "It is non-irritant, only slight stiffness being noted on the day following the injection, and it is as effective as any of the insoluble salts." My own personal acquaintance with the drug empowers me to endorse his statements.

(4) *Hydrargyri tannas.*—Tannate of mercury has been used, but it does not seem to possess any claim for distinction.

(5) *Hydrargyri thymolacetas.*‡—The thymol acetate of mercury has been employed as an intramuscular injection—1 of the salt being suspended in 10 of liquid paraffin. I am not personally acquainted with the preparation.

---

* Squire's ' Pocket Companion to the B.P.,' 1904.

† Lambkin, ' Brit. Med. Journ.,' November 11th, 1905, p. 1256.

* Martindale's ' Extra Ph.,' p. 293, 11th edition.

† Gottheil, " Hypodermatic Treatment of Syphilis," ' Internat. Clinics,' U.S.A., vol. iii.

‡ ' Pharmaceutical Journal,' 1888, p. 427 ; 1889, 341, 607.

(6) *Hydriodol.*—This is better known under its commercial name of "cypridol." It contains 1 per cent. of mercuric iodide in sterilised oil. I do not use it.

(7) *Hydrargyri benzoas.* — The benzoate of mercury is practically insoluble in cold water and for all intents and purposes may be reckoned as an insoluble salt. It has been used as an injection, both intravenously and intra-muscularly, but I have no experience of its value.

(8) *Hydrargyri subchloridum.*—More local after-pain follows the intra-muscular injection of calomel than with any other mercurial preparation. On the other hand, its remedial effects are more rapid and temporarily complete. Pain is the bar to its continuous acceptance. As an heroic measure, which is how I regard it, I know of no mercurial preparation which exerts such a marvellously rapid action upon syphilitic symptoms. It is, in my opinion, the remedy *par excellence* for endarteritis and its sequelæ. But it, like every other drug at our command, is not infallible. Moreover it has not sustained its reputation as a panacea for all syphilitic troubles, which its more enthusiastic advocates originally claimed for it. Relapses are common even in cases where it has been employed with every early indication of success. Perhaps the best vehicle for its suspension is sterilised olive oil, as follows : Calomel 5 gr., sterilised olive oil 100 ℳ. Dose, 10 to 15 or even 20 ℳ, according to the needs of the case. This would mean a respective dosage of $\frac{1}{2}$, $\frac{3}{4}$, or 1 grain. With calomel, as with all other mercurial products, one has to *know* and *consider* the renal state of the patient, and also "the personal unit of idiosyncrasy as to mercurial toleration." What would *poison* one person would not affect another deleteriously. Injections are given every seven, ten, or fourteen days, according to requirements. The preparation must be thoroughly stirred and shaken before being sucked up into the syringe.

A perusal of the foregoing list should show that the spirit of research has not been lacking amongst syphilographers. Many of the salts scarcely survived a brief trial by their respective champions and have been relegated to obscurity. In the following schedule will be found those preparations which have a favourable reputation either amongst solublists or insolublists. Personally, my leaning is towards the soluble preparations, when I con-

sider an injection *régime* necessary, in that they are devoid of that *infinitesimal* risk inseparable from the use of either the metal itself or its insoluble compounds. One has to remember in private practice that *one* fatality following the injection of an insoluble mercurial preparation might possibly ruin the well-meaning but unfortunate operator, whilst the occurrence of a gluteal abscess is not calculated to enhance a patient's confidence in his medical attendant. As one is able to gain ameliorative or curative results with safety by restricting one's choice to the less pain-begetting soluble preparations, I see no overwhelming advantage or necessity for habitually employing the insoluble products, even when it is deemed impossible to cure an *ordinary* case of syphilis by orally administered drugs—a view in which I do not concur. In my opinion intra-muscular injections are not so immeasurably superior to a scientifically conceived and enforced oral *régime.* Personally I reserve the use of *calomel* as an injection for those urgent or desperate cases where one knows that the patient's powers of absorption from the alimentary tract or the skin are not to be trusted, and one is, so to speak, fighting against time, and needs to deal a sharp and decisive blow. Let me once more repeat the warning, if one be using either the base or its insoluble salts, that you should be sure that you are not injecting them into the venous system instead of into the intended intra-muscular regions. If one will but take this simple precaution, then their use becomes comparatively safe for the patient and, in private practice, decidedly remunerative for the surgeon.

INTRAVENOUS INJECTIONS OF MERCURY.

The intentional injection of mercury directly into the veins was first advocated by Barcelli in 1893. The method soon gained a number of adherents amongst the more adventurous of Italian surgeons, but it remained to Mr. Ernest Lane to bring the practice before the notice of the profession in England. In 1896 Mr. Lane read a paper upon the subject at the third International Congress of Dermatology,[*] giving the results of his primary experience and practice. Apparently the system has not appealed to the profession at large, if one is able to judge from the absence or paucity of

---

[*] Lane, ' Brit. Med. Journ.,' 1896.

records bearing upon the method which have been published since then. Latterly, however, it has had a more extended trial upon the Continent. But the evidence of various experimenters as to its assumed superiority over the simpler and less fear-begetting intra-muscular plan is far from convincing. The system is not one that is ever likely to find general favour or acceptance, either with surgeons or patients, nor could its habitual adoption be advised. The advantages which have been claimed for the procedure are :

(1) Absolute painlessness, when an intravenous and not perivenous injection is effected.

(2) Smallness of the dose which it is necessary to administer, and the ease in regulating the same.

(5) Violent dysentero-diarrhœic symptoms or polyuria and even albuminuria.

(6) The possible occurrence of pyæmic infarction.

(7) The necessity of a daily injection.

(8) Uncertainty as to whether the method guarantees a greater chance of cure or freedom from relapse than the intra-muscular system or even the oral mode.

Let us now review those points *seriatim*. No pain beyond that due to the primary prick of the needle is noted when a successful administration has been effected. But it sometimes happens, notwithstanding all skilled precautions, that the fluid is ejected into the perivenous tissues. This occurrence may be sequent upon failure to enter

FAVOURITE PREPARATIONS.

Soluble Salts—Aqueous Medium.	Insoluble Salts—Oleaginous Medium.
℞ Hydrarg. sozoiodol . . . grs. 2½ Sod. iodidi. . . . . grs. 5 Aq. dest. . . . . . ℳ100 Dose 10 to 15ℳ, containing ⅓ to ½ gr. of the salt.	℞ Hydrarg. salicylatis neut. . . . grs. 10 Paraffin liq. . . . . . ℳ100 Dose 3 to 10ℳ, containing respectively ⅒ to 1 gr. of the salt.
℞ Hydrarg. succinimid. . . . grs. 2½ Aq. dest. . . . . ℳ100 Dose 10 to 15ℳ, containing ⅓ to ½ gr. of the salt.	℞ Hydrarg. . . . . . grs. 10 Adipis lanæ anhyd. . . . . grs. 30 Paraffin liq. (carbolised 2 per cent.) . ℳ100 Dose 10ℳ, containing 1 gr. of the *base*.
℞ Hydrarg. lactatis . . . . grs. 2½ Aq. dest. . . . . . ℳ100 Dose 10 to 15ℳ, containing ⅓ to ⅔ gr. of the salt.	℞ Hydrarg. subchlor. (calomel) . . grs. 5 Ol. olivæ (sterilised) . . . ℳ100 Dose 10 to 15 or even 20ℳ, containing respectively ½, ¾, or 1 gr. of the salt.
℞ Sal alembroth . . . . grs. 5 Aq. dest. . . . . . ℳ100 Dose 10ℳ, containing ½ gr. of the salt.	NOTE.—The larger quantities must be given most cautiously. The intense pain following its injection may necessitate a local hypodermic of ¼ gr. morphia.

Any of the above can be obtained in sterile bottles from Martindale, 10, New Cavendish Street, London.

(3) Certainty of absorption and rapidity of action, together with the absence of dyspeptic symptoms.

(4) Freedom from salivation, or at most slight gingivitis.

The drawbacks which have been noted in connection with its use are :

(1) Difficulty in getting a patient to allow of its employment.

(2) Possible failure in making the vein stand out with requisite prominence.

(3) Perivenal instillation, followed by great pain and possibly abscess or dermal ulceration.

(4) Thrombosis at the site of puncture, particularly when injections are used *cold*.

the lumen of the vessel or to the fact of the point of the needle having transfixed the vein. When such a *contretemps* ensues the operation is transformed into a *subcutaneous* injection and is immediately followed by considerable suffering. To this swelling, cellulitis, abscess, or even sloughing of the superjacent skin, may possibly be added later on. It must be obvious that a considerable amount of manual dexterity is needed for the successful performance of this little operation, and that any movement on the part of the patient at the critical moment of puncture is liable to upset the best of anatomical intentions. The smallness of an effective dose, together with its almost mathematical regulation, has been urged as a point in favour of this method. But a similar advantage has been claimed for the less terrifying intra-muscular mode, which can also boast equally of the certainty of absorption, rapidity of action, and the absence of dyspeptic sequelæ. Freedom from salivation or gingival symptoms is to my mind dependent upon the dose of mercury employed rather than upon the method invoked. Having considered the presumed advantages, let us next review the drawbacks. First and foremost amongst these is the fear with which the preliminary application of the ligature inspires the patient. Moreover the very idea of sticking a needle into a vein is apt to upset the average layman's nerves. They do not like the thought, and will in many cases refuse to submit to the procedure. I do not blame them. But assuming that one has persuaded a client to be rubbed, scrubbed, sterilised, and ligatured, it may turn out that these necessary preliminaries are all in vain, since we cannot make the selected or any other vein stand out with that prominence requisite for an intravenous injection. Should, however, this contingency be absent and all goes well, one still has to face the possibility of venous thrombosis ensuing. This is a complication which not even the precaution of warming the solutions will always prevent. One must also remember that antiseptics are not infallible in anybody's hands, and, like the proverb of the pitcher and the well, the possibility of mishap must always attach itself to an intravenous injection, and that your most carefully planned or rigidly conducted precautions for asepsis may fail, and pyæmia ensue therefrom. There is no absolute safety in statistics or numbers, and the fact that you have given a great many injections without a fatal result in nowise guarantees that the very next one which you administer may not have a lethal termination. With every man's system there is an average, and it is only a matter of time before one discovers what that average is. Another great disadvantage of the method is the fact, which is admitted even by its champions, that injections are requisite either daily or every other day. Apart from financial considerations, few people would have sufficient courage, or shall I say temerity, to subject their venous system to this oft-repeated ordeal, more particularly so when one cannot conscientiously guarantee them any greater therapeutic benefit therefrom than can be obtained by other means. I do not favour the procedure, and unhesitatingly advise the general practitioner to shun it. He should remember that England is not the Continent, and that there are such public proceedings as coroner's inquests and also High Courts of Justice in this country. The following is the technique which has been advised for intravenous injection. The preferential site for an instillation is the flexor region of the elbow-joint, the vein which is usually selected being the median basilic. But any superficial one will do, provided that it can be made prominent by means of pressure applied above, and that it be not varicose. Injection into varicose veins is almost certain to be followed by trouble, which is usually attributable to the impaired nutrition of the overlying skin. Having carefully sterilised one's own hands and instruments, the patient's skin is subjected to most thorough antiseptic precautions. It should first be scrubbed with soft soap and subsequently with ether or spirits of wine. It is next swabbed over with some disinfectant lotion. The ligature, which is either an ordinary or an elastic bandage, is now applied about the upper level of the humeral condyles, the force exerted being sufficient to allow of arterial flow whilst insuring hindrance to the return of blood from the veins, and thus rendering them prominent. As soon as the previously disinfected tourniquet is operative, the needle is introduced obliquely through the skin into the prescribed vein. The next step is to release the venous compression and thus re-establish the vascular current. When this has been effected the piston-rod of the charged syringe is pressed upon and the mercurial solution expressed directly into the blood-stream by which it is immediately carried away. The needle having been withdrawn, the superficial puncture wound is sealed up by means of a fragment of antiseptic wool steeped in collodion. As before remarked, the little operation should, apart from the skin-prick, be painless when it is successfully performed. It is important to remember that all solutions should be *warmed* to a temperature of 100° F. *prior to being injected.* This precaution minimises the chance of thrombosis following venous puncture, but it does not invariably prevent its occurrence. Only the aqueous preparations of the mercurial salts should be used intravenously. The introduction of the *insoluble* ones, or the *base*, would probably be followed by disastrous results. I am of the opinion that when pulmonary trouble follows the administration of either metallic mercury or its insoluble compounds it is not due to fat embolism, but to a molecular transference of the base or salt to the lungs, where the chemical irritant sets up a similar inflammatory action as is met with, say, at the gluteal site of primary deposition. If these cases of embolism were of the fat order, one should meet with them when the soluble preparations are employed as intra-muscular injections. The answer is that one does not. Consequently one would deduce that it is the drug and not an adipose globule which is at the bottom of the mischief. Solutions of the following salts have been tried, namely mercuric cyanide, oxycyanide, biniodide, succinimide, and perchloride. Barthelemy and Levy Bing[*] are of opinion that "a radical cure cannot be effected by intravenous injections," whilst Gravagna has abandoned the practice owing to the severe enteric

---

[*] Barthelemy and Levy Bing, ' La Syphilis,' 1905.

disturbance which it sets up. This quasi-dysenteric condition would seem to supervene, more or less, with all the preparations that have been tried. It has been a marked feature in many cases where either the cyanide or oxycyanide has been injected. Lane's experiments were made with a 1 per cent. solution of mercuric cyanide. He injected 20 ꟽ or ¼ gr. of the salt either daily or else every other day.

SEROTHERAPY IN SYPHILIS.

The injection of animal serum into the human body has been tried as a remedy for syphilis. Up to the present time all the recorded efforts have proved futile. My old friend the late Edward Cotterell made a series of experiments with dog's serum, but with negative results. The idea which dominated this line of treatment was that as certain animals seemed to be immune to syphilitic inoculation their blood necessarily contained some product or antitoxin which was inimical to the development of the syphilitic poison. It remains to be seen whether the discovery of *Spirochæte pallida*, the organism which Schaudinn and Hoffmann suspect to be the microbe of syphilis, will lead to the production of a remedial antitoxin serum.

I will now bring this somewhat lengthy article to a conclusion with what may be termed a " confession of faith." I do not believe in the practice of intravenous injections, nor am I of the opinion that they are therapeutically superior to either the intra-muscular or even the discarded subcutaneous system. I likewise believe that it is necessary and advantageous to resort to the use of intra-muscular instillations in certain cases, such as syphilo-dyspeptic glossitis, intestinal intolerance of orally administered drugs, cerebral endarteritis, and cases which do not react to remedies taken by the mouth or skin. But I consider that an ordinary straight-forward case of syphilis can be treated perfectly as well by a thoughtful and appropriate oral *régime* as by any other method. But when one relies upon mouth medicines to effect a cure it is necessary to remember that the human stomach is a highly selective and fastidious organism, which ofttimes needs a deal of humouring. One should not treat it either as a crucible or as a penny-in-the-slot machine into which one needs but to drop any kind of pill to cause the figure to work. The chief causes of failure in mouth-treated cases are the prescribing of preparations unsuitable to the individual's internal economy, together with the patient's personal disregard of instructions. Conversely the secret of success lies in the individual's power for absorbing some form of mercury in such dosage that it not only clears up symptoms, but also through regular continuation holds all further developments of the disease in check until such time that one may, from experience, reasonably assume that he or she is cured. My unshaken belief in the "obtainable" efficacy of the oral *régime* is not due to inexperience of other methods, for I have employed them all, time after time, during twenty-one years of close acquaintance and practice in the treatment of syphilis. Finally, I know of no drug or method which will cure syphilis in a patient who persists in remaining a chronic alcoholic.

January 8th, 1906.

PARALYSIS AND OTHER DISEASES OF THE NERVOUS SYSTEM IN CHILDHOOD AND EARLY LIFE. By JAMES TAYLOR, M.A., M.D., F.R.C.P. London : J. & A. Churchill.

AN understanding of the functions of the nervous system of children is of such importance that a book of this kind cannot fail to be useful. Dr. Taylor's long connection with a hospital for children has afforded him ample opportunities for observation in this direction ; and although there is, doubtless, a good deal in the diseases of childhood which is common with those of adults, there is also much that is different to be considered, and Dr. Taylor successfully points out the peculiarities which have to be borne in mind. While the degenerations special to childhood are interesting from a diagnostic point of view, it is, perhaps, to the functional diseases of childhood that many will turn, since so much of their future depends upon their recognition and adequate treatment at an early stage, and an interesting account of these will be found.

In the treatment of chorea Dr. Taylor considers that hygiene and diet are among the most important weapons at our disposal for combating the disease, and while fully acknowledging the benefits obtained from arsenic in many cases, he does not consider that large doses of the drug should be given.

The book is well illustrated, and will be found most useful and interesting.

PSYCHOLOGICAL MEDICINE : A MANUAL ON MENTAL DISEASES FOR PRACTITIONERS AND STUDENTS. By MAURICE CRAIG, M.A., M.D. Cantab., M.R.C.P.Lond. London : J. & A. Churchill.

THIS is a very suitable book for practitioners and advanced students. The symptoms and medico-legal aspects of the insane are clearly laid down, and a chapter on normal psychology forms an interesting introduction, while at the end the directions for case taking and treatment are equally useful. Throughout the student is strongly advised to approach the study of mental disease in the same attitude of mind as he would engage upon the study of medicine and surgery, and so learn to recognise and treat the earliest manifestations of disorder, when they are most likely to be curable. There are numerous excellent illustrations of pathological conditions, especially in connection with general paralysis of the insane.

THE CLINICAL JOURNAL,

CLINICAL RECORD, CLINICAL NEWS, CLINICAL GAZETTE, CLINICAL REPORTER,
CLINICAL CHRONICLE AND CLINICAL REVIEW.

EDITED BY L. ELIOT CREASY.

No. 690.　　　　　WEDNESDAY, JANUARY 17, 1906.　　　Vol. XXVII. No. 14.

CONTENTS.

*Specially reported for the Clinical Journal. Revised
by the Author.
ALL RIGHTS RESERVED.

NOTICE.

*Editorial correspondence, books for review, &c.,
should be addressed to the Editor, 51, New
Cavendish Street, W., Telephone No. 904, Paddington; but all business communications should
be addressed to the Publishers, 22½, Bartholomew
Close, London, E.C. Telephone 927, Holborn.*

*All inquiries respecting Advertisements should be
sent to MESSRS. ADLARD & SON, Bartholomew
Close, E.C. Telephone 927, Holborn.*

*Terms of Subscription, including postage, payable
by cheque, postal or banker's order (in advance): for
the United Kingdom, 15s. 6d. per annum: Abroad
17s. 6d.*

Cheques, &c., should be made payable to THE
CLINICAL JOURNAL, *crossed
"The London, City, and Midland Bank, Ltd.,
Newgate Street Branch, E.C. Account of the
Medical Publishing Company, Ltd."*

Reading Cases to hold Twenty-six Numbers of
THE CLINICAL JOURNAL *can be supplied at 2s. 3d.
each, or will be forwarded post free on receipt of
2s. 6d.; and also Cases for Binding Volumes at 1s.
each, or post free on receipt of 1s. 3d., from the
Publishers, 22½, Bartholomew Close, London, E.C.*

A LECTURE

ON

THE EARLY DIAGNOSIS
OF PULMONARY TUBERCULOSIS.

Delivered at the Hospital for Consumption and
Diseases of the Chest, Brompton.

By F. J. WETHERED, M.D., F.R.C.P.,
Physician to the Hospital; Assistant Physician to the
Middlesex Hospital.

GENTLEMEN,—The importance of an early diagnosis in pulmonary tuberculosis can scarcely be
overrated. It is an accepted fact that the prospect of cure in this disease varies in proportion to
the stage at which the malady is recognised. It
behoves us, therefore, as medical practitioners to
use every method in our power in order to detect
the disease in its earliest stages. I propose this
afternoon to give a brief résumé of the various
methods which may be adopted to achieve this
result. I can only deal with the most common form
of pulmonary tuberculosis—namely that known
as the fibro-caseous type. The method which we
follow is to study the history of the disease, to
examine the symptoms and physical signs exhibited by the patient, and also in some cases to
make use of certain auxiliary means which have
more recently been introduced.

A study of the history of the patient is synonymous with ascertaining his predisposition to the
disease. This predisposition may be hereditary or
acquired. The significance of a family history of
pulmonary tuberculosis, perhaps, has lost some of
its importance since the discovery of the tubercle
bacillus. Nevertheless in any particular patient
in whom the signs of the disease are doubtful, the
fact that he comes of a tuberculous stock must
always be taken into consideration. The nature of
this hereditary process is uncertain. The actual
disease is certainly not transmitted from the parent
to the child, but the second etiological factor of

tubercle—namely a diminished resistance, a suitable pabulum, or whatever you may like to call it—may certainly be the result of heredity. Some observers would have us believe that heredity consists in the transmission from the parent to the child of specific toxines, reaching the fœtus.

Next, as to an acquired predisposition. Certain infectious diseases seem to diminish the natural resistance against tubercle. If it were not for this natural resistance the human race would long ago have become extinct. These diseases are, more particularly, pleurisy, pneumonia, typhoid fever, and influenza. In children also measles is frequently a starting-point of pulmonary tubercle. It is remarkable how many cases suffering from pulmonary tubercle give a history of pleurisy in previous years. In a large number of instances the pleurisy has been accompanied by effusion. This fact is now generally recognised by insurance companies, so that when a person presents himself for life insurance giving a history of pleurisy with effusion in past years, an addition will most probably be made to his life.

Other circumstances also tend to produce an acquired predisposition. Amongst the most important of these are alcoholism, and certain occupations, notably those which produce a considerable amount of irritating dust. In addition to the above are certain conditions other than infectious fevers which are also of value when examining doubtful cases. Amongst these I may mention enlarged glands in the neck or scars of the same. Some observers believe that adenoids predispose to tubercle. Professor Dieulafoy maintains that adenoids form the first stage of a cervical glandular tuberculosis capable of invading the lungs. The prolonged existence of anæmia also, according to some authorities, diminishes the resistance to attacks of the tubercle bacillus. Dr. Turban of Davos maintains that the enlargement of the thyroid gland is frequently noted in those individuals which may be considered predisposed to tubercle. Another significant feature is a persistent frequent pulse without any organic lesion to account for it.

To pass on to the history of the illness. As we know, the onset is very insidious, and it is often difficult to ascertain exactly how long certain symptoms have existed. Cough is usually the first thing that is noticed by the patient, but different classes of patients give their history with varying exactitude. Patients of the well-to-do class are usually more accurate than those of the working class, and more reliance can be placed on their assertions. A working man, owing to his circumstances, dates his illness, not from the time of the commencement of symptoms, but from the time when he has had to give up work ; consequently on cross-examination we find that the length of time in which his symptoms have lasted is usually much longer than his first statement would lead us to believe.

I would here give the caution that in cases of acute diseases, more particularly in those involving the lung, tuberculosis must never be forgotten. For instance, in children general tuberculosis may resemble typhoid fever or broncho-pneumonia. Further, in adults, the onset of malignant disease may resemble tubercle, but the course of the former is usually more rapid, and when there is a neoplasm of the lungs dyspnœa may be out of proportion to the physical signs. This latter fact is an important one.

The onset of pulmonary tubercle may be obscured by following on acute diseases, especially those I have mentioned above, namely pleurisy, pneumonia, or influenza. Pulmonary tubercle is also difficult to recognise when it becomes engrafted on emphysema. At one time emphysematous patients were considered to be very free from an attack of tuberculosis. More recent investigations have shown, however, that such is by no means the case, and we now recognise a distinct type of tuberculosis, namely the emphysematous, and in such cases the prognosis is usually favourable.

I now come to consider the symptoms and physical signs of pulmonary tuberculosis, and as a preliminary I would urge you to remember the phrase introduced by the late Sir Andrew Clarke, that in order to detect pulmonary tuberculosis we must have an assemblage of signs and progression of symptoms. Numerous errors are made by diagnosing the disease on one symptom or one sign ; and as a matter of fact my experience has shown me that errors in diagnosis are more common in commission than omission—that is to say, that the disease is not so often missed as diagnosed when it is not there.

Cough, as I have already said, as a rule first gives rise to suspicion. It is only of value when taken in conjunction with the other symptoms, for cough is common in many circumstances. Some patients complain that they have had cough all their lives ; these seldom yield corroborative signs of pulmonary tubercle. In children the presence of adenoids frequently gives rise to persistent cough, which may be very troublesome at night. Pharyngitis, especially in smokers, also gives rise to an intractable cough. Bronchitis too yields the same symptoms and patients suffering from chronic catarrh of the stomach frequently complain of a troublesome cough, probably due to accompanying pharyngitis. The characteristic cough in early pulmonary tubercle is dry, with difficult expectoration, often occurring in paroxysms, and may disturb the patient at night. Frequently, however, it is scarcely noticed by the patient and its existence is only acknowledged after close questioning.

Expectoration is often absent in the early stages of the disease, a fact to be regretted since its examination frequently gives valuable diagnostic aid. In advanced cases the sputum is more characteristic, but then other signs of the disease are obvious. There is a peculiar sweet odour of the phlegm and sometimes of the breath which, if recognised, tells its own tale. The microscopic examination of the sputum for elastic tissue may yield valuable help.

Hæmoptysis is a symptom seized upon by the laity and quite rightly so. The more one sees of pulmonary tubercle the more does one become convinced that in cases of true hæmoptysis—that is to say, when the amount of blood exceeds one drachm—if cardiac disease and liver disease can be excluded, in the huge proportion of cases the case will prove to be one of pulmonary tubercle. If a rise of temperature accompanies the blood-spitting, then the probability of tubercle is even more certain. In some cases, however, there may be no physical signs for some time. To give an illustrative case, a gentleman was sent to me some years back with a history of having for a period of nearly two years had several attacks of slight hæmoptysis. His temperature had never been raised and between the attacks there was absolutely no cough. There had been no loss of weight and no corroborative sign of pulmonary tubercle. He had seen several other physicians, all of whom considered that pulmonary tubercle was not present. Some time afterwards I was called into the country to see him and learned that he had had another slight attack

of hæmoptysis, and there were then crepitations to be heard over the upper part of the right lung and tubercle bacilli were found in the sputum, thus rendering the diagnosis undoubted. He went to a sanatorium and made a good progress, with eventual arrest of the disease. A person naturally becomes alarmed when he or she has an attack of blood-spitting. The majority of these cases, provided the disease is not far advanced, generally do well—so much so, that in " hæmorrhagic cases " a favourable prognosis may generally be given. Indeed, the hæmoptysis may be considered a blessing in disguise, as it draws attention to the disease in an early stage, whereas if the hæmorrhage had not occurred the malady might have advanced to a further stage before the disease was recognised, when the chances of cure might not have been so favourable. Slight hæmoptysis may occur under other conditions. Anæmic girls often find that in the morning the pillow may be stained with blood, and on first waking a little blood-stained fluid may be ejected. On closer examination this is simply found to be saliva tinged with blood, the source of the bleeding being the gums. The amount of blood is so slight that during the day it is not noticed, but it collects in the mouth during the night and becomes mixed with the saliva and so gives rise to the symptoms I have mentioned. As in anæmia there may be slight cough, such occurrences naturally give rise to considerable alarm on the part of the patient and her friends, and great care is required in the investigation of such cases Occasionally varicose veins are observed in the throat and may give rise to minute hæmorrhages. I have myself seen a small quantity of blood actually exuding from such a vein. Malignant disease of the lung may give rise to hæmoptysis which is very dark in colour, looking something like prune-juice. The hæmoptysis due to cardiac disease, especially mitral stenosis, or hepatic disorders, may be recognised by the physical signs proper to those affections.

Loss of flesh is, of course, also of importance, but only when taken in conjunction with other signs and symptoms. Many conditions give rise to emaciation, more or less marked, and in some no definite diagnosis can be made. But there are two conditions which we must particularly be on the look-out for, namely malignant disease and neurasthenia. In some instances of the latter malady I have seen most profound wasting rapidly developing.

The investigation of the patient's temperature in cases of suspected tubercle is of the utmost importance. It is not sufficient to take it at 8 o'clock in the morning and 8 in the evening. It should be taken every four hours and also at about 2 p.m. and 5 p.m., rise of temperature in tuberculous subjects being often noted at those hours. More modern investigations have shown that there is considerable variation of temperature even in healthy individuals. But in tuberculous subjects there is one peculiarity of temperature which is, perhaps, not sufficiently appreciated—namely that it is extremely unstable. It is very easily affected by exercise. The patient then should be allowed to take a certain amount of exercise and his temperature should be taken immediately afterwards and again about an hour afterwards. In healthy people the temperature is raised sometimes as high as 103° after active exercise but falls very rapidly, so that in about half an hour or even less the normal is again reached. When tuberculosis is present, however, a rise of temperature takes place, but does not subside for an hour or more. In doubtful cases, especially in winter-time, the rectal temperature gives more reliable information than the mouth temperature.

Pain in the chest.—This may be present or absent and is not a symptom upon which any reliance can be placed. It is more common in advanced disease than in the earlier stages. Occasionally over the affected area there may be hyperæsthesia, but personally I do not place much reliance on this symptom, pain being so common in many varying conditions.

The occurrence of night-sweats is of some significance, but profuse perspirations frequently occur under other conditions—as, for instance, they accompany a failing heart; so that the value of this symptom is only of any account when considered with the occurrence of other symptoms.

I now pass to a consideration of the physical signs which occur in pulmonary tuberculosis.

Inspection.—In the early stages this is not so important as in the more advanced cases, for when there is only slight infiltration no falling in of the chest is apparent. The shape of the chest may be suggestive. Pulmonary tubercle is especially liable to be found when the chest is long, narrow, with a small costal angle and broad spaces between the ribs. The scapulæ too are frequently prominent. On the other hand, tuberculosis is also seen in perfectly developed chests and, as already mentioned, in emphysematous chests.

Palpation.—This sometimes enables one to distinguish the differences of expansion between the two sides which is not apparent to the eye. Also information may sometimes be obtained by standing behind the patient and placing the fingers over the shoulders so that the tips are in the supraclavicular fossæ; one apex of the lung may sometimes be felt to rise higher than the other. The observation of the vocal fremitus must also be tried, the normal differences being duly recollected. If the fremitus is more easily felt on the right than the left side, no definite deduction can be made, but if the fremitus is more marked on the left than the right side, then suspicion of disease in the left lung is thereby arrived at.

Percussion.—Here again the normal differences in various parts of the chest must be remembered and allowed for. In itself I do not consider this method of physical examination to be of value to the same extent as are the other methods. There is much of the personal equation in it that somewhat detracts from its value. In order to secure the best results the pleximeter finger must be laid perfectly flat on the chest and percussion made very lightly. Slight differences are the more easily appreciated in this manner than when heavy percussion is employed. The phenomenon known as myoidema is by some considered to be of value. It is brought out by sharp percussion over the muscles of the chest and the production of a small swelling about the size of a split-pea, which rapidly subsides. After trying this test in a very large number of patients I have come to the conclusion that it is more frequently found in tuberculous subjects than in others, although it may occasionally be elicited in any wasting disease. On the other hand, I have frequently failed to elicit it in advanced cases of pulmonary tubercle.

Auscultation.—Again, we must be careful to remember the normal differences that exist in various regions of the chest. I have frequently known students to diagnose a cavity at the right apex and when asked their reason for doing so state that they heard bronchial breathing above and below the clavicle. Their observation was right, but the deduction wrong. In many cases typical bronchial breathing is heard in that region in perfectly healthy people, and therefore without corroborative signs the diagnosis of excavation must not be made simply because bronchial breathing is heard in that region. Bronchial breathing is also heard in the healthy chest opposite the spines of the scapulæ, and again the same precautions hold good. A diagnosis cannot be made from one sign, but only from an assemblage of signs. Weak breath sounds at one apex is a suspicious phenomenon. It may, however, be caused by a quiescent lesion and not by a recent one. Wavy breath sounds are only of significance when confined to one portion of the lung. If heard over both lungs, they are probably due to nervous influences. Prolonged expiration over a limited area is also to be taken notice of, but if general, as in emphysema, the same importance cannot be ascribed to it.

Adventitious sounds.—The occurrence of crepitant râles over one apex, especially if elicited or increased by cough, is one of the most important signs in the diagnosis of pulmonary tubercle. It may, however, be simulated by what is known as the emphysematous crackle, by pleural creaks, or by fascial creaking. The influence of cough on these phenomena may distinguish them from the râles. I will again impress upon you the importance of always remembering the significance of "assemblage of signs," but the existence of crepitation apart from the other signs always raises a suspicion of serious pulmonary trouble.

I now come to consider certain auxiliary tests which may be of the greatest assistance at a diagnosis. The most important of these is the examination of the sputum for the tubercle bacilli. I do not propose to describe the process which is adopted, but will merely say that the sputum ejected in the early morning before any food has been taken is the most satisfactory to use for purposes of examination. A positive result is, of course, of the utmost significance, indicating the existence of tubercle somewhere in the respiratory tract. A negative result cannot be taken as indicating that tubercle is not present, and in suspicious cases at least three examinations should be made. Even then if all these should prove negative pulmonary tubercle cannot be excluded. To illustrate this I would say in one case I examined the sputum nineteen times with a negative result. On

the twentieth tubercle bacilli were found. On the twenty-first a negative result again was experienced. The case proved fatal and post mortem showed miliary tubercles of the lungs.

The use of tuberculin has been recommended by some as a diagnostic test. Koch's original tuberculin is generally employed. In making the test it must first be ascertained that the patient's temperature is normal. He should therefore be kept in bed for forty-eight hours, the temperature being taken every four hours. If the temperature during that time proves to be normal and the patient be not very weak, one milligramme of tuberculin may be injected. If there be a rise of temperature of one degree or over within the following twenty-four hours, the reaction is positive. But if there be only a rise of half a degree the same dose should be repeated after an interval of two days, when a more marked reaction may take place. If there should be no rise of temperature after the first or only a slight rise after the second injection, two milligrammes should then be injected. If a doubtful reaction occurs, the dose should be repeated after a short interval. If still no definite reaction takes place, five milligrammes should be injected. If after that doubt should remain, ten milligrammes may be injected twice. In the case of a child or of a weakly subject the initial dose should not be greater than half a milligramme. Any marked rise of temperature is accompanied by some constitutional disturbance, shown by a feeling of malaise and pain in the back and limbs. Although the value of a positive reaction from a diagnostic point of view is very great the test is not infallible, as exceptional reactions occur in non-tuberculous patients. When the test is thoroughly made and no reaction occurs, it is extremely improbable that the case is one of tubercle.

The Roentgen rays have in recent years been used to attempt to assist diagnosis in early cases. The general impression, however, seems to be that it is only in exceptional cases that tubercle can be diagnosed by the rays when no physical signs exist. They do, however, show the extent of the disease, and may be of value in the emphysematous type, when the physical signs of local disease are masked by those of the surrounding emphysema. The rays may also indicate the existence of an old lesion in one apex and thus corroborate doubtful infiltration in other parts of the lung. Sometimes, too, the diaphragm working better on one side than on the other suggests the existence of tubercle in the latter.

Quite recently examination of the respiratory exchange has been suggested as an aid to diagnosis. It has been stated by some observers that the respiratory exchange is higher in tuberculous subjects and in those predisposed to tubercle than it is in healthy subjects. The reports of various observers, however, differ so greatly that at present I do not think any reliance can be placed on this.

The interest attached to the early diagnosis of pulmonary tuberculosis has naturally given rise to numerous attempts to add to or improve our methods. The majority of these auxiliary means, however, are too delicate or too elaborate to be of general acceptance. In the vast majority of instances therefore the old measures to which I have referred must remain. But certain of the newer procedures may, as I have explained, be of value in special cases.

January 15th, 1906.

GASTROSTOMY.

By WILLIAM SHEEN, M.S.Lond., F.R.C.S.,
Surgeon Cardiff Infirmary, Consulting Surgeon
Seamen's Hospital, Cardiff.

GASTROSTOMY when done for cancer of the gullet, as in the case that I am about to relate to you, is a palliative operation ; the real disease remains untouched and is bound to be fatal in the near future. We can do good by removing a source of irritation of the growth and by providing an avenue for nourishment. Apart from the immediate dangers of the operation, we can do harm by leaving a leaking opening out of which the irritating acid gastric juice flows, reddening and excoriating the skin, producing intolerable itching, rendering life a misery and death a happy release. *Nil nocere* is the first motto of the surgeon ; it behoves us, therefore, in these cases to make the opening valvular, so that fluid cannot flow out. Numerous methods have been devised by surgeons to achieve this object.

Following the early methods of simple opening, often in two stages, which always resulted in leak-

ing, came the vertical splitting of the rectus devised by Howse. Later a cone of stomach wall was drawn upwards under the skin and its apex fixed and opened in a separate incision—the method of Frank. Finally the stomach wall itself was folded round a tube to form an oblique opening—the method of Witzel. These methods have been variously combined and modified, so that the names of numerous surgeons are associated with the operation. In the method that I am about to describe all the three above indicated were employed, so that the operation is called the Hacker-Frank-Witzel operation.

FIG. 1.

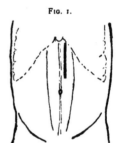

FIG. 2.

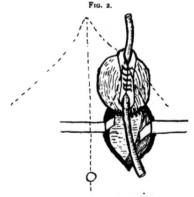

In performing it I followed the description in Kocher's 'Operative Surgery' and I have attempted to illustrate it by a few rough diagrams, some of which are modified from Kocher's book.

E. E—, æt. 60 years, a ship's carpenter, was admitted to the Seamen's Hospital, Cardiff, on August 28th, 1905, and was seen by me at the request of Dr. Dewar, the resident Medical Officer, a few days later. The man had the ordinary symptoms of œsophageal obstruction; he was thin, coughing, and spitting out all his saliva;

FIG. 3. '

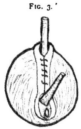

all bougies were arrested fifteen inches from the lips; only small amounts of fluid could be swallowed, with a great deal of hawking and coughing;

FIG. 4.

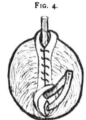

pain was complained of over the trachea in the lower part of the neck. The condition did not improve and the man lost weight, so on September

FIG. 5.

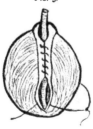

28th I performed gastrostomy, Dr. Cyril Lewis giving the anæsthetic and Dr. Dewar assisting. A vertical skin incision was made to the left of the middle line and when the rectus sheath was opened

the muscle was displaced outwards; this is Hacker's method and is preferable to splitting the muscle which cuts off the internal fibres from their nerve supply, so that they atrophy. The posterior part of the rectus sheath and peritoneum were then incised, the stomach found, drawn out of the wound, and

FIG. 6.

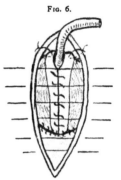

a cone of it near the cardiac end fixed at its base by a purse-string suture to peritoneum and fascia of abdominal wall. A rubber tube was then laid vertically along the stomach wall, which was stitched over the tube, the serous coat and some

FIG. 7.

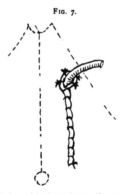

muscle being picked up, for a distance of rather more than half an inch. Immediately below this tunnel a puncture was made through all the coats of the stomach and the lower end of the rubber tube passed through it, the part of tube then left exposed was buried by a further folding over of the superficial parts of the stomach wall. Finally the outer stomach opening was fixed in the uppermost part of the wound and skin and superficial structures stitched over the projecting portion of stomach, this last procedure representing Frank's part of the operation, (see diagrams). The tube was fixed by means of a stitch and the wound sealed with gauze and collodion.

The man bore the operation well, the wound healed by primary union, and the valvular action of the fistula was perfect, so that three weeks after the operation all dressings were left off. Improvement subsequently was rapid, he became much stronger, gained weight, learnt to feed himself through the fistula, and went home to Cardiganshire on November 29th. Previous to leaving the hospital he was able to swallow his saliva again and could take a little fluid by mouth, although his main nourishment was through the fistula. The valvular action remained perfect. There was a slight tendency to contraction, for which he wore a solid bit of rubber tubing. I commend this method of gastrostomy. It produces a short upwardly directed subcutaneous oesophagus which opens into the stomach, as Witzel says, "in the same manner that the ureter opens into the bladder."

January 15th, 1906.

The Relation between Anthracosis and Pulmonary Tuberculosis.—Jonathan M. Wainwright and Harry J. Nichols, in considering this subject, refer to the most frequently mentioned theory that has been advanced to explain the observation that anthracotic lungs are less susceptible to tuberculosis than the normal organs, namely that it is due to the germicidal action of the coal-dust. The writers have found from various tests, however, that coal-dust has no germicidal action whatever. The writers think that the coal-dust in the lungs does exert a true protective influence against the tubercle bacilli, and that it is due to the stimulating effect of the coal-dust on connective-tissue growth. This growth is the way in which Nature overcomes the tubercle bacilli. It is well known that coal-dust causes stimulation of connective-tissue growth. The writers have performed some interesting experiments on guineapigs in relation to the effect of anthracosis on tuberculosis, and as far as they have gone the experiments have been affirmative.—*Medical Record,* vol. lxviii, No. 26.

A LECTURE
ON
SOME PHYSICAL ASPECTS OF CARDIAC FAILURE.

Delivered at the North-East London Post-Graduate College.

By DAVID FORSYTH, M.D., M.R.C.P.,
Assistant Physician to the Evelina Hospital for Children and to the Tottenham Hospital.

LADIES AND GENTLEMEN, -- The treatment of heart disease is a subject so large, and extends its boundaries over a field so wide, that it would be unprofitable to discuss in a single lecture more than one or two of its aspects. I shall therefore restrict my remarks to a feature of the disease which is to my mind of great importance, but which lacks emphasis in the text-books. I want you to consider with me some of the purely physical as distinct from the physiological principles of the circulation, and to inquire in what way they may be unbalanced or even suppressed by disease. The information we collect in this survey will enable us to formulate principles to guide us in treatment.

A healthy heart can cope easily and well with the ever-changing conditions of circulation, but once disease lays hold of it embarrassments spring up on every side. At first the ventricles strive to sweep away besetting obstacles by calling on their reserve fund, the power of compensation, and for a time are successful. But capital is not inexhaustible, and the heart's credit grown low and its difficulties multiplied, there comes a day when the harassing demands of the circulation can be met only by painful effort. One by one the functions of the heart fall into disorder, and the disastrous sequence of symptoms comprised under the term "cardiac failure" run riot through the body.

To a heart thus stumbling under the increased strain of disease we can, fortunately, give valuable assistance to rid it of its impediments and to reinstate it in its former position, and our efforts must be marshalled along certain main lines. Our first endeavour will be to curtail the duties of the heart by lightening the work of circulation. Next, the beneficial result that will follow such release must be amplified by the use of appropriate drugs that will encourage and stimulate the heart to renewed activity. Lastly, by recognising the additional strain imposed by a too generous diet, we shall be led to adopt such depletive measures as will relieve the arterial tension without unduly weakening our patient.

No treatment can be regarded as efficient that is not planned on this triple foundation. It must, however, be realised that the three factors are not of equal value. The two former that I have mentioned could be used successfully, unaided by the third, and the cases are not rare which improve when no drugs are given; but without rest you can effect but little. Rest stands foremost in our treatment, and it alone will accomplish more than both the others. Although I do not intend this afternoon to discuss the administration of cardiac tonics, nor the relief to the heart of depleting the system, yet you must bear in mind both these lines of treatment, in addition to the one on which I shall chiefly dwell. Remember that in the treatment of heart disease the three cardinal virtues are rest, drugs, and depletion, and the greatest of these is rest intelligently applied. It is not enough to send your patient to bed and to think you have given the heart all the repose it can obtain. You have not. Though this measure affords relief, its benefits are limited. Without doubt there will be a marked decrease of œdema, but other and distressing symptoms—sleeplessness, vomiting—may persist unmitigated. You will have to find additional means of lightening the heart's work, for, after all, to relieve œdema is not even half the battle, and your patient would probably rather keep his swollen legs and have a good night's rest than be neat-ankled and count the chimes till dawn. It is only by close attention to the little signs and signals hung out by the heart in distress that you will discover how further to succour it. For these appeals are commonly made in divers remote parts of the body—a few râles at the lung-bases, a headache, veins over-full—which have to suffer for the heart's incompetence to cope with the physical exigencies of the circulation. We shall do well, therefore, to study the conditions of the healthy circulation to learn how their abeyance will be revealed. By the title of my lecture, I am restricted to the failing heart, the heart that is staggering beneath its over-heavy burden, worn out by ever-increasing difficulties, or stunned, almost at

a blow, by acute disease. We are not concerned to-day with the heart that, after suffering temporary slings and arrows, recovers in the end and goes happily ever after. Our text includes only those more serious afflictions which, if not necessarily, are at any rate commonly mortal. Yet inevitable though the termination of such cases may appear, it is not for us, as doctors, to stand by to let events hurry to their close. However gloomy the prognosis, we have the satisfaction of knowing that by the exercise of skill there can be added a few to the number of the remaining days, and still more certainly is it the privilege of our art to rob those days of much of their pain and suffering.

Regarded at its simplest, the mechanism of the normal circulation consists of a force-pump, the heart, propelling liquid through a system of closed tubes. This primitive conception is, however, rendered much more complex by the occurrence of other factors influencing the blood-flow. For example, the tubes are not of uniform calibre. The more remote from the heart, the smaller do the vessels become, but at the same time the greater is their united cross-sectional area, and just as a river flows sluggishly where its banks have receded to widen its channel, so the velocity of blood-flow in the little vessels is considerably less than in the main arterial trunks. In the minutest vascular tubes the velocity has been estimated to be only one two-hundredth of that in the aorta, and it is obvious that much of the propulsive force of the heart will be lost in this meshwork of countless capillaries, leaving very little power to impel the blood on still further along the veins back to the auricles. Normally the ventricular systole is sufficient to complete this circuit unaided, but even in health the great work this would entail on the heart is lessened by the action of another force which is of such prime importance that I shall venture to remind you of its action. I refer to the movements of respiration, which, by the alterations they produce in the physical conditions of the thorax, play an essential part in the normal circulation.

The two pleural cavities, being air-tight, possess an internal pressure quite independent of the atmosphere without. Each contains one lung, and provided neither air nor liquid be admitted, the existence of a vacuum—abhorred by Nature—can be avoided only by the lung bulging out until viscer and parietal pleuræ are everywhere in contact. But the lung hides in its tissue a quantity of elastic fibre which, like all elastic material, resists stretching, and this opposition expresses itself as a pull of the visceral pleura away from the parietal. In other words, there will be a negative pressure in the pleural sac, and the more distended the lung the greater will be this pressure, because the more vigorous becomes the elastic pull. We find accordingly that while the pressure at the end of expiration is about — 2 mm. of Hg., — 30 mm. is the figure reached after a moderate inspiratory effort.

An every-day example of the very real force exercised by this pressure is afforded by the misshapen outline of a rickety child's chest, whose soft and flexible ribs, unable to withstand the inward pull of the pleural sacs, bend in to produce a characteristic deformity.

Now see what effect this negative thoracic pressure will exercise on the circulation. You have a closed thoracic chamber at a pressure below zero; you have the blood in the veins and capillaries at a positive pressure. You know it to be an axiom of hydrodynamics that fluid will always flow from a level of higher to one of lower pressure, and the blood, obedient to the law, must therefore run from periphery to thorax. The chest will act in such a way as to suck back the blood from abdomen and extremities to the right auricle. The accelerated motion thus imparted to the blood trickling through the capillaries is of very great assistance indeed to the heart in helping it maintain a brisk circulation.

Within the thorax, exposed to its pressure, lie the great arteries and veins, the auricles and ventricles. The musculature of the last and the strong coats of the aorta and pulmonary arteries are firm enough to stand against this pressure, but the thin walls of auricles and veins alike are too feeble to resist, and they must become dilated, sucked open, whenever the negative pressure is at all great. On the other hand, if at any time the thoracic pressure should become positive—the change occurs in coughing or on making a forcible expiration with the glottis closed—the tenuous coats of the veins will be compressed and the flow within them impeded, if not altogether dammed back. This is a not infrequent occurrence pathologically, and leads, as we shall find, to the very serious embarrassment of the heart.

We see, then, that the circulation depends largely on the efficient action of two forces. Behind is a force-pump, the heart, impelling the blood onward, and a suction-pump, the respiratory movements, in front, aspirating the blood to the right auricle. If either of these be impaired, extra work will be thrown on its fellow, with consequent confusion to the circulation.

The practical application of this conception of the circulation I hope to explain in a moment, but before going further I want you to give thought to another physical factor—a very potent one too— which, Janus-like, faces both ways in its action, either aiding or impeding the heart. This attribute is the property of the power of gravity. Leonard Hill, who has done more than any other to unravel the influences of this force, says that gravity must be regarded as a cardinal factor in circulatory problems, and his pronouncement is particularly true when the problem has to be solved in erect-going man, in whom power must be provided not only to drive the blood through the resisting arterioles and capillaries, but to raise it to considerable heights against the action of gravity. For example, the left ventricle has to expend in its systolic effort enough energy both to propel the blood through the capillaries of the brain and to sustain the column of fluid extending from the root of the aorta up to the skull. Similarly in the case of the legs, blood must be pumped up from the feet to the auricle, a height perhaps of four or five feet, and all this entails a very considerable amount of work. It is true that gravity will aid the return of blood from the head and facilitate its distribution to the lower limbs, but this slight assistance is no compensation for the additional obstacle it sets in the way we have just discussed. Indeed, were it not for the support the column of fluid derives from the surrounding vessel wall, the blood would gravitate to the dependent parts of the body, there to stagnate. Illustrations of the truth of this will occur to you all. The particular vein in the body whose thin wall, unsupported by fascia or by muscle, has to bear the longest column of blood, the internal saphenous vein, is of all the most prone to yield beneath the pressure, and the area it drains or fails to drain grows œdematous, congested, ulcerated. In the case of the splanchnic vessels the support of their walls is dependent on the efficiency of the vasomotor mechanism; and, since the abdominal veins are capacious enough when distended to hold all the blood of the body, we reach this important conclusion, that one of the great natural opponents to the impeding action of gravity is the integrity of the vasomotor control to the splanchnic area. When this influence is interfered with the result must necessarily be serious, and even if the loss of control be only momentary the effect is marked. Those of you who have been confined to bed for a few days together will recall the sudden giddiness that clouded your senses when first you put foot to ground. During the days you lay horizontal the effect of gravity on your circulation was at a minimum, but at the moment you stood erect a sudden pressure was thrown on your splanchnic vessels, and they, taken unawares, distended to accommodate more blood than was proper—result, too little blood to the brain, cerebral anæmia, giddiness.

It is unnecessary for me to emphasize the great help a horizontal position confers on the heart in overcoming the effect of gravity, for it is obvious that, *ceteris paribus*, the circulation will be carried on at a minimum expenditure of labour when the trunk and limbs lie in the same horizontal plane. Further, that by elevating any part of the body above the heart-level the difficulty of supplying blood to it will be increased but the return flow expedited.

We are now in possession of the most important facts bearing on our subject. Let me recapitulate briefly before applying them to treatment.

We have seen how the circulation is maintained, partly by the pumping action of the heart, partly by the suction of the respiratory pump, as it is called. We have seen how this suction is strongest on deep inspiration, when the diameters of the thorax are greatest; that it is less when the chest falls in on expiration; that it is abolished when the thoracic pressure becomes positive, as in coughing. We have recognised that in gravity the heart has to contend with an impeder, an obstructionist, but that by intelligent dealing this force can be won over as an ally. Lastly, we have realised that without proper vaso-motor control efficient circulation is impossible, and the results the most widely felt depend on the condition of the splanchnic vessels.

What, now, are the circulatory diseases which we can hope to relieve by applying these principles? How are we to recognise when a failing heart is embarrassed by a disturbance or opposition of these principles? And what measures are we to adopt to liberate the heart from its impediments, and to lessen the work thrown upon it?

In answering these questions it would be best to divide our cases of failing heart into two main groups. Firstly, there will be those in which the failure is acute, appearing in the course of, at most, a few days; and secondly, those in which the failure has been slow-growing but progressive, usually the result of chronic endocarditis. Under the first heading we must include such conditions as acute pericardial effusion, syncope, asphyxia, cardiac failure under anæsthetics, etc.

Within the limited time at my disposal I shall not be able to give an account of all these conditions, since their physical features vary so widely and include factors other than the two I have described. The treatment of acute pericardial effusion and of syncope, however, depends on the points we have just discussed, and it is to these conditions that I shall draw your attention.

I am unable, of course, to bring an example before you in person, but I have here an abstract from the report of a case of acute pericardial effusion which will serve to illustrate my remarks.

A schoolboy, æt. 12 years, was admitted into hospital on November 12th for difficulty in breathing. From his history we learnt that two years before his tonsils had been removed for recurrent sore throat, and that since about that time he had suffered from vague joint-pains. That is to say, he was rheumatic. He was under-sized and anæmic-looking, and had palpable glands in his axillæ as well as along both sterno-mastoids.

When I first saw him there were pains in the knees, a cough, and sore throat. The cardiac impulse lay in the sixth left space, as far out as the nipple-line, though the beat was visible for two inches around. The cardiac dulness covered an area bounded by the third rib, the right edge of the sternum, and a line just external to the nipple; at the apex was a systolic bruit traceable into the axilla, and a mid-diastolic which sometimes appeared presystolic. The second pulmonary sound was accentuated. As far as the lungs were concerned there was little amiss, except for a few rhonchi on the left side.

For a week the patient showed no change, but on November 19th his cough became worse and he expectorated much thin sputum coloured brightly with blood. The note over the right apex in front became impaired and many moist râles developed. From this date until the end—six days later—he went rapidly downhill. The right lung became full of râles and rhonchi, and the left was but little better. The noise thus produced, together with the cough, now incessant, masked the valve-sounds, but it was clear the condition of the heart was growing worse, as the cardiac dulness began to still further encroach on the surrounding lung resonance, and the pulse grew so fast and feeble as scarcely to be counted. On one occasion ,it was noted as 132. The respirations increased to nearly 60, and associated with the cough were further hæmoptysis and attacks of cyanosis. At times it was now possible to distinguish a pericardial rub over the right ventricle. Twice on the 23rd the patient suddenly collapsed ; the pulse could not be felt, the lividity was profound and the dyspnœa urgent. He survived, however, for another twenty-four hours, and then, after a period of gasping for breath, died. For the last few days he found relief from being propped up by pillows.

Post mortem, the pericardium was distended with six ounces of serous fluid. The heart, which was dilated, showed old endocardial changes (the mitral valve contracted and its chordæ thickened) together with small, recent vegetations. The right lung felt solid, but this was due, not to any pneumonic change, but to an intense œdema ; its appearance was that of a backward-pressure lung. The left lung showed the same changes but to a less degree.

Examined in the light of our discussion, this case is most instructive. There can be no doubt that the pericardial effusion was the cause of death, and its fatal effect was due to a mechanical interference with the circulation. Six ounces of fluid were rapidly poured out around the heart. The strong fibrous coat of the pericardium was too rigid to relax for its accommodation, and a sac large enough to contain only the heart was now occupied by heart and effusion. The result was a positive pressure in the pericardium, leading to compression of the thin-walled venæ cavæ and obstructed return of blood to the auricles. The pulmonary veins shared the fate of their neighbours, and their blood was stemmed back until the lung capillaries

grew over-swollen. This led to œdema of the lungs and a copious exudation into their alveoli of serum and even blood, the irritation of which stirred up violent attacks of coughing. The coughing raised the intra-thoracic pressure still higher, and the diastolic filling of the heart became a matter of difficulty. This again aggravated the lung condition, and so the vicious circle went round—heart, lung, lung, heart—with the pericardial effusion for its centre. Doubtless the ventricles put forth all their energies to accomplish the impossible, but enfeebled as they were by old disease the pace told, and at times they almost ceased to beat and not a flicker could be felt at the radial artery. Finally and with increasing frequency the blood in the veins was unable to make its way back to the heart—its channels were blocked—and surrendering its oxygen to the tissues, showed livid through the skin.

This case possesses no feature that is rare ; it is an ordinary example of what you all are meeting with from time to time, and its treatment must therefore be of interest.

Pericarditis is almost invariably associated with greater or less inflammatory change in the myocardium, which must interfere with the force of the heart-beat, and this you will try to antagonise by employing cardiac stimulants. But with that your interference should merely begin, not end. The whole energy of treatment must not be bent only to whip and spur the heart, the symptoms being interpreted as evidence of the failure of the ventricles to carry on their duties. Thought must be given to the more powerful assistance that it is possible to offer. Drugs often fail notably to improve the heart's action in cases of pericarditis. Medicinal treatment may be admirable enough if regarded as accessory to other measures, but alone how can it relieve the *fons et origo mali* ? We have to remember that large pericardial effusions kill by the pressure they exert on neighbouring parts, and no treatment that ignores this fact is sound. There are two clear indications to bear in mind, the one to relieve the ventricles of as much work as possible, that they may economise what energy is still theirs, the other to minimise the pressure effects of the effusion ; and we must keep this twofold purpose clearly before us, since it will not always follow that a means of relief to the one is a source of help to the other.

The patient will, of course, be kept confined to bed, and that will do much to realise the first indication. It is best, at any rate at first, to keep him lying absolutely flat unless the attitude distresses, but I shall say something further on this point in a few minutes. He must be allowed to make no unnecessary muscular effort. To insure this may need constant watching, for it is often a matter for comment how much less ill a patient with early pericarditis will feel than the seriousness of his affection would suggest. I know an instance where a man, a doctor too, overtaken by what later proved to be pericarditis, attempted to shake off his malaise by setting out on a walking tour, and though he was frequently attacked by faintness, it was a matter of a week or more before he finally gave in. The food, which must be liquid or semi-liquid, should be offered from a feeding-cup with spout, so that there shall be no occasion for the patient to raise his head. From the first every care must be taken to prevent straining when the bowels are opened. Any difficulty in this direction will be doubly injurious. Not only will the greater muscular effort required throw a severe and sudden tension on the heart, but the straining will perforce require a deep inspiration followed by a strong muscular movement of expiration with the glottis closed. The negative thoracic pressure will disappear, to be supplanted by a marked positive pressure of perhaps 60 mm. of Hg. or more, and the venous blood will be held back at the very gates of the thorax and the circulation incommoded. This disturbed pressure is of even more moment than the muscular effort, and if constipation be allowed to occur, constitutes a very real danger, not only in the condition we are considering but in other diseases as well. Many a man, for example, has been struck down by apoplexy from this very cause—straining at stool—whose degenerated cerebral arteries were too weak to withstand the sudden pressure thrown back on them from the veins through the capillaries. Never neglect, then, to inquire not only if the bowels have acted but also the degree of effort entailed. The best purgatives to use are naturally those which lead to a watery evacuation. From half to one drachm of the compound jalap powder overnight answers well, and may be followed if required by a saline draught the next morning.

Our second indication is to relieve the pressure effects of the effusion. In the early stages, when the quantity of fluid is still only slight, the pressure symptoms will not disclose themselves; but later, as the fluid accumulates and the pericardium grows distended, the signs will develop, their gravity depending on the quantity and rapidity of formation of the fluid effused. The cardiac dulness spreads, often rapidly, the pulse grows quick and feeble and the patient begins to show he is suffering from the addition made to the contents of his thorax. The earliest changes are often to be found in the lungs. Numerous râles and rhonchi express their œdematous condition—the result, not so much of right-sided failure as of compression of the pulmonary veins — and the alveolar exudation is expelled by a frequent cough. Further characteristic signs may now be heard in the left lung behind. The patient lying supine has the whole weight of his pericardial contents pressing back on that lung, which becomes compressed, and over an area around the angle of the scapula signs of consolidation develop. Thus new respiratory difficulties are produced which may be further aggravated if, as sometimes happens, a pleural effusion follows the pericardial. Finally, as the effusion grows in volume, the pericardial sac comes to occupy so considerable a share of the thorax that the negative pressure tends to disappear, and with it the suction action of the chest. When this condition is present in the left half of the thorax it is often revealed, especially in children, by a distinct protrusion of the intercostal spaces or a general bulging of that side of the chest. The left bronchus or the bifurcation of the trachea may be pressed on, and even the free-way down the œsophagus interfered with. The great veins are well nigh occluded, the circulations both greater and less, blocked, and the superficial veins stand out distended, while the lips grow livid and the legs œdematous. A veritable air-hunger seizes the patient, whose alæ nasi, with all the other accessory muscles of respiration, join in futile attempts to respire. The heart, unable to stem such odds and poorly supplied with but indifferent blood, comes gradually to a standstill.

This, then, is the train of pressure symptoms which we must expect and which we must attempt to evade. We will suppose that the heart has been relieved of as much work as possible along the lines I have sketched and has been encouraged with such stimulants as are advisable. What steps must be taken to release these pressure symptoms? Serious as the condition of such a patient now is, we can without doubt do great service. Our efforts must be directed towards three ends. We must so dispose the patient that the oppressive weight of the heavy pericardium bears on no vital structure; we must encourage the efforts of respiration so to assist the circulation; we must finally, as a last resource, relieve by paracentesis the thorax of what is practically a large tumour.

Early in the course of the disease you kept the patient on his back, but now the time for this posture to be of good has passed, and he will probably show signs of distress unless he be moved. Roll him, therefore, slowly to his left side and there support him by pillows. The weight of the pericardium will be taken by the bony thoracic wall, and the whole of the right lung and the greater portion of the left will be released from pressure. This position often brings quite a considerable amount of ease, the dyspnœa is relieved and the feebleness of the pulse improved. After a while, as the effusion is added to, these symptoms may recur, and then you will obtain fresh benefit by rolling the patient still further over, so that the pericardium comes to rest upon a more anterior part of the ribs and freer play is given to the lungs. Take care, however, that there is no impediment to abdominal respiration. Much depends on the efficient movement of the diaphragm. You will sometimes be gratified to discover that after the patient has been moved as far over as possible, the signs at the angle of the scapula will disappear. This alone will show the good that the altered position may bring.

It is not, however, all cases that will derive benefit from the lateral position. Many suffer from such marked orthopnœa that they must be allowed to sit up in bed. This change will, of course, add somewhat to the work of the heart since the effect of gravity becomes more prominent, but other factors more than counterbalance the objection. The pericardium will now press directly downwards on the diaphragm, depressing its left cupola, so that the capacity of the chest will be increased at the expense of that of the abdomen. The thoracic pressure will therefore tend to fall and the abdominal to rise, both factors helping on the circulation. Some of the text-books are rather prone to dwell on the serious results that may follow if you sit your patient up. One of them tells us that it is "highly dangerous to place the patient in the sitting or erect posture; such disturbance may even prove immediately fatal." Well, I should be inclined to agree with that only with reservation. If you are going suddenly to change your patient's posture from the supine to the sitting, I can quite understand the necessity of the warning. But no one who understood anything of the physics of the circulation would dream of such abrupt action. He would take care that every alteration of position was carried out with cautious slowness. The complete turning of a patient to his side must be a gradual process, and no patient should be suddenly sat erect, but as his dyspnœa increases so pillow after pillow should be placed behind his back.

Our second object was to encourage the movements of respiration. As a rule it is not the ribs that are impeded but rather the diaphragm. Any abdominal distension will raise the height of the muscle and hinder its descent in inspiration. This defect will be obviated in part by the special attention to the bowels which I have already mentioned, but in addition the nature of the diet must receive consideration. This is particularly necessary because your patient will be restricted to a milk diet, and the lumpy curd produced by the gastric juice is often difficult of digestion and apt to provoke abdominal distension. In such cases the feeds should be diminished in size but increased in number and the ordinary diluents of milk should be tried—barley-water, lime-water, rice-water. Another method of overcoming the difficulty is to produce a very fine curd in the milk before it is taken. To do this, heat the milk with a little of the juice of a lemon, when the caseinogen will be precipitated by the acid. Strain off this curd from the whey and forcibly squeeze it through the meshes of a muslin bag. On adding this to the whey you will have all the constituents of milk, but the caseinogen will be as a flocculent cloud easy to digest.

Finally we have to discuss the advisability of removing the pericardial effusion. Once the action of this fluid is realised no two opinions can be held on the question of paracentesis. When an effusion has become large, perhaps is still increasing, and its obstructive effects have become marked, removal of the effusion is the only method that can possibly give relief. It is a thousand pities that the truth of this is not more widely appreciated. Yet that it is not acted on is obvious, for how often do you hear of a pericardium being tapped? And when the operation is performed, has it not usually been deferred until the patient was almost *in extremis*—past help of any kind? Too often this delay has made success impossible, and the operation suffers disrepute. This is unfortunate, for were the paracentesis to be undertaken earlier, when the odds against were not so heavy, more satisfactory results would be obtained. Just as a pleural effusion is removed as soon as it embarrasses the breathing, so paracentesis pericardii should be performed early, if there are signs that the circulation is becoming obstructed. If that grave stage is reached, every hour's delay lessens the chances of recovery. Once you have made the diagnosis of pericardial effusion you must be ready at any moment to aspirate the fluid. I would give these as indications for the operation : (1) spreading cardiac dulness, (2) progressive enfeeblement of the pulse, (3) increasing dyspnœa, especially of the air-hunger variety, (4) distended veins, (5) cyanosis. I would not advise you to wait for the appearance of all these signs before deciding on tapping, otherwise you may be too late. The first three indications alone justify the use of an exploring needle, and as they are commonly the earliest in appearing, to accept and act on their evidence will improve the prospects of success.

Of course, if you believe the effusion to be purulent—often a diagnosis of great difficulty— you must wait not an hour before having the pus liberated and free drainage provided.

Where should the pericardium be opened? There are two sites for the operation. The needle may be passed through the fifth left intercostal space, either close to the sternal edge or an inch and a half removed, at both of which positions the internal mammary artery will be avoided. The objections to this route are that there is very considerable danger of your trocar wounding the heart itself, and that the opening does not give access to the back of the sac where the fluid chiefly is, nor does it reach its most dependent part—both obstacles to a complete removal of the fluid. The alternative route is through the left costo-xyphoid angle. If your needle be inserted in that angle, near

but not too close to the junction of the seventh costal cartilage with the sternum, and be passed upwards, backwards, and slightly inwards behind the sternum, it will enter the pericardium at its lowest part after travelling from two to two and a half inches. Personally I believe this method the better of the two for both serous and purulent effusions. In the latter especially, prolonged drainage has to be provided for, and this is much more likely to be efficient with an opening from below than when a rib has been resected and the drainage-tube passes to the region of the sac in front of the ventricles.

It is, of course, all important to regulate the speed with which you draw off the fluid. Sudden relief of the intra-pericardial pressure will so profoundly alter the conditions of the circulation that this danger must be guarded against by only slowly liberating the fluid. The fact that the effusion may be under pressure and will spurt from the cannula makes caution all the more necessary. The immediate effect of the operation is often wonderful. Within a few seconds the bulging veins of face and neck become smoothed out, the horrid livid tint yields to a less unnatural pallor, and soon the veil of half-consciousness, the muttering delirium that obscured the patient's mind, lifts to give him back his intelligence.

In addition to pericarditis as a cause of cardiac failure I mentioned certain other conditions, but as I explained, in some of them the physical causes of the failure are so different from those of failure from pericardial effusion that in the few minutes left to me I should be unable to discuss them adequately. For the present at any rate, I must defer their consideration, and rest content with saying a few words about syncope, the treatment of which depends largely on the principles we have already formulated.

In syncope the heart is suddenly dealt a paralysing blow by some inhibitory impulse and ceases its beat without warning. In the majority of cases of course, this fatal accident befalls only the diseased heart—its muscle-fibres impeded by excessive fat, its aortic orifice regurgitant or its nervous mechanism deranged by toxins—for a healthy organ has its rhythm so deeply ingrained that it needs some very serious cause to abolish it. But instances of a healthy heart ending by syncope are not rare. Occasionally a patient with pleural effusion dies from sudden cardiac failure—probably from altered conditions of pressure in the thorax or dislocation of the heart—but in others absolutely nothing pathological is found. One such case was brought to my notice only recently. Three little girls returning from Sunday school were alarmed to find themselves followed by a ruffianly-looking man. Reaching the outskirts of the town, they came to a cross-roads. Their shortest way lay along a lonely lane, but, timorous, they stood a moment to debate their route. Before they had reached a decision the fellow had overtaken them, and guessing the cause of their hesitation, gruffly ordered one of them to follow the lonely road. Without a word the terrified child fell dead. Post mortem every viscus was healthy; death must have occurred from inhibition of the heart by fright.

Death by syncope of an apparently healthy person is so awful that we should make every effort to restore the victim before it is too late, and it is in just such instances as the one I have quoted that success may be looked for, provided remedial measures can be applied without delay. Remember that for a heart to have ceased its beat does not necessarily imply that it is incapable of resuming its pulsation. A heart as highly organised as a mammal's can be excised some time after death, and, suitably stimulated, induced to begin once again its rhythmic action, and probably all of you have seen at least one instance of a human heart that had failed, gradually recover under appropriate treatment. What, then, is the best stimulus to apply? The best stimulus—it goes without saying— is the natural stimulus, the stimulus which normally provokes the systole of the ventricles. Normally, the chief factor that starts each ventricular systole is the tension of blood within the ventricular cavity; that is to say, once the chamber is full of blood, its walls become stretched open and its muscle-fibres respond by sudden contraction. We must seek a means whereby we may help on this intra-ventricular tension. Fortunately we have a means not difficult to employ and always ready to hand wherever we may be. By means of artificial respiration we can help to fill the heart with blood, and so provide it with the stimulus it wants. Each inspiratory movement will suck blood to the chest and so to the lungs; each expiratory movement will press blood out from the lungs to the left auricle and so to the ventricle.

Although, like other methods of treatment, artificial respiration in cases of cardiac failure will not always be successful, still it is the rational course to adopt, and, with massage of the heart, the only rational course. The movements should be persevered with even if no immediate result is obtained. More than once a man apparently dead, whose heart had been stopped by contact with strong electrical discharge, has recovered only after many hours of such treatment.

In conclusion, ladies and gentlemen, if I have impressed nothing else upon you in this lecture, remember, at any rate, how powerful an auxiliary the respiration is to the circulation. Remember when next you come to treat a failing heart the existence of a respiratory suction-pump as well as of a cardiac force-pump, and let your efforts be directed to improving and expediting the action of the former, in addition to stimulating and restoring the latter. Those of you who are interested in tracing the effects of physical forces on the course of disease will find it not unprofitable to apply our principal theme of this afternoon—the respiratory movements—to diseases other than circulatory, for there are not a few conditions which either modify or are modified by these forces.

January 15th, 1906.

THE treatment of backache in women is complex and often unsatisfactory. Toxic and lumbar backaches are treated with laxatives, diuretics, and colon irrigation. To the congestive type are administered ergot, digitalis, strychnine, and bromides. The anæmic are given iron and tonics. Temporary relief is afforded by the use of local counter irritation. For neurasthenics the rest cure is advised. Surgical measures have for their object the sewing up of lacerations, the correcting of malpositions, and the removal of diseased organs and tumours. Krusen emphasizes the value of the drinking of large quantities of water in these cases. Frequently a rheumatic diathesis is associated with pelvic disease. Pains may be due to the lithæmic diathesis, and a certain proportion of backache is due to traumatism. The fact that women are habitually constipated and that they drink small quantities of water are two factors to be borne in mind in treatment. Hydrotherapy plays an important part in the relief of symptoms.—*Journ. A. M. A.*, vol. xlv, No. 26.

THE CLINICAL JOURNAL,

CLINICAL RECORD, CLINICAL NEWS, CLINICAL GAZETTE, CLINICAL REPORTER,
CLINICAL CHRONICLE AND CLINICAL REVIEW.

EDITED BY L. ELIOT CREASY.

| No. 691. | WEDNESDAY, JANUARY 24, 1906. | Vol. XXVII. No. 15. |

CONTENTS.

* *Specially reported for the Clinical Journal. Revised by the Author.*
ALL RIGHTS RESERVED.

NOTICE.

Editorial correspondence, books for review, &c., should be addressed to the Editor, 51, New Cavendish Street, W., Telephone No. 904, Paddington; but all business communications should be addressed to the Publishers, 22½, Bartholomew Close, London, E.C. Telephone 927, Holborn.

All inquiries respecting Advertisements should be sent to MESSRS. ADLARD & SON, Bartholomew Close, E.C. Telephone 927, Holborn.

Terms of Subscription, including postage, payable by cheque, postal or banker's order (in advance): for the United Kingdom, 15s. 6d. per annum; Abroad, 17s. 6d.

Cheques, &c., should be made payable to THE PROPRIETORS OF THE CLINICAL JOURNAL, *crossed* "*The London, City, and Midland Bank, Ltd., Newgate Street Branch, E.C. Account of the Medical Publishing Company, Limited.*"

Reading Cases to hold Twenty-six numbers of THE CLINICAL JOURNAL *can be supplied at 2s. 3d. each, or will be forwarded post free on receipt of 2s. 6d.; and also Cases for binding Volumes at 1s. each, or post free on receipt of 1s. 3d., from the Publishers, 22½ Bartholomew Close, London, E.C.*

CLINICAL REASONING.

A Lecture delivered at St. Bartholomew's Hospital.

By C. B. LOCKWOOD, F.R.C.S.,
Surgeon to the Hospital.

GENTLEMEN,—I do not know whether you can remember that in December of 1903 I began my course of clinical lectures with an introductory one which dealt with clinical methods. Clinical methods are only the methods of obtaining something which the mind has got to use. It is of no use having clinical methods unless you have got a mind which can turn their products over, can extract their essence, and convert that essence into a quintessence which ought to be your diagnosis. The methods which I advised you to use were, first of all, methods which applied to the observer, to the person who is trying to make the diagnosis. First you must use your eyes. I think most people would manage with their eyes if they never used anything else; if the other sense organs were abolished the eyes would usually suffice. The hands I advised you to use with great care, and your tongue with still greater care. Please do not believe or assume that I do not think the tongue can be used with effect—I mean in diagnosis. The tongue will extract very important information from educated people who have some intention of speaking the truth. Now, with regard to the patient, I advised you to cultivate the habit of looking at the whole patient. We have had some instructive instances of the importance of looking at the whole patient. I am quite sure that the child who is in Coburn Ward, and which some of you may have seen, owed its life to the fact that the person who saw it was in the habit of looking at the whole patient, and was in the habit of drawing rapid conclusions from what he saw. In that ward, in a cot, was a wretched child which looked as if it had an enormous head, the reason being, of cause, that its body was small, being wasted by illness. In the next place, it was exceedingly anæmic ; it had no colour in its face at all. The poor little creature was so anæmic, and its muscles so flaccid, that it sat in its cot in a sort of hump and supported itself wearily with its arms. The muscles of the neck are strong muscles, and they ought to support the head of the person erect and keep it straight upon its shoulders, but in this child the muscles were so exhausted that its head hung down upon its chest. I inquired whose patient it was and I was informed that it was mine. I asked what was the matter with it, and I was informed that it had cellulitis of the scalp. I remarked, "There is no such disease as cellulitis." The disease in this child's case was ascertained by the pathological laboratory, and the report came that the child had streptococci, and some form of staphylococcus in its scalp, probably in its hair-follicles, and above all things, they informed me that it had diphtheria bacilli in its scalp. As soon as that was ascertained the child was put upon anti-diphtheritic serum, and began to mend, and after- great dangers in consequence of paralysis—it had paralysis of the various muscles supplied by cranial nerves, paralysis of the bladder, and so forth-—it began to mend, and ulimately got well. I am sure it would have died if the person who saw it had not been keenly alive to the importance of looking at the whole patient, and drawing proper conclusions from the appearance of the whole patient. You will remember the next rule. After looking at the whole patient you are advised to examine both sides of the human body. I had a most striking instance of the troubles which may accrue from that rule being neglected. I was asked to see a friend of mine—I will not specify further, because it does not reflect credit upon those who saw him. He was said to have great trouble inside his chest, which had resulted in the formation of matter, and that the matter was pointing behind the angle of the right scapula. One naturally asked to be shown the abscess which was pointing near the angle of the right scapula. After examining the abscess I said, "I cannot open this abscess, because the abscess happens to be the rhomboideus major." This statement of course excited some amount of interest and he said, "Why do you say that ?" He put his left arm into a similar position, and the left rhomboideus major assumed a similar position to what was thought to be an abscess on the right. Obviously the muscle had been mistaken for an abscess ; perhaps the man was supporting himself in bed with his right arm. Now came the question, What were we to do? I want you to observe now the methods of clinical reasoning. I may be quite wrong in regard to my methods of clinical reasoning ; but as I advise you to doubt everything and to grow up rational human beings, I assume as a matter of ordinary fact that you will doubt my clinical methods and my methods of clinical reasoning. Should any gentleman doubt my methods and see serious cause to consider that they are wrong, I myself should feel to him under an eternal debt of gratitude if he came to tell me that they were wrong. I should merely ask him to do one thing further and state his reasons for thinking that I was wrong. Now, these were the steps in reasoning. First of all, it was quite clear that the disease was of an inflammatory nature. This may seem to you a very elementary proposition. But it is a very important point if you are sure of it. I could adduce cases which had been assumed to be of inflammatory nature, but turned out to be malignant. I can bring plenty of examples of things which were supposed to be malignant and have turned out to be inflammatory. So if you are certain of that particular fact, which is one you will often have to decide, you will have proceeded a long step of your way towards a correct diagnosis. Next, the temperature chart demonstrated a continuously high temperature. Next, the pulse record was continuously high ; it was usually 108 or 110. Further, assuming that this disease was inflammatory, it was inside the chest, it was not outside. I had been called up to open an inflammatory disease outside his chest, so it was of not inconsiderable importance to get it inside. The next step was to tell whether the inflammatory affection inside the chest was solid or whether it was fluid. If it was fluid and composed of pus, one must have pursued the ordinary surgical methods and let it out. If it was solid, one would wait a little while and see what happened to it. Pus is more likely to increase than it is to depart, but a solid inflammatory swelling of the pleura or lung will as often as not take its departure. The voice sounds could be heard, and it was clear that the sound was proceeding through something which was solid. A slight fall in the temperature and in the pulse rate told that this solid inflammatory trouble inside the chest was beginning to get better. There was a small but continuous drop in the temperature and in the pulse rate, and over and over again the preliminary to recovery in an inflammatory affection is a slight drop, either in the pulse rate, or in the temperature. I think the pulse rate usually falls before the temperature. When the temperature has been high—102° or 103°, a small drop in the pulse rate, say from 96 to 90, has told me, and in future I hope it will tell you, that the patient as a matter of fact is getting better rather than that he is either at a standstill or getting worse.

I remember another case illustrating the importance of seeing everything, and being quite sure of what you see, and I relate it to you because I think I may assume that of the gentlemen in this theatre many are not going to be occupied either in amputating at the hip-joint or in opening the abdomen several times a day, or, in fact, in doing that very rare kind of surgery which is called "major." I think you will be occupied in other pursuits. I remember a friend of mine coming to me in a state of great distress to say that he had attended a patient in her confinement, and that at the end of five or six days she had a very high temperature and very rapid pulse, and he feared she had got what I think he called puerperal fever, which is, of course, another word for sepsis. Now, this was not exactly a surgical case, but to help my friend I went to see this patient. I saw a woman with a temperature of 103°, and whose pulse was high, but when one examined her abdomen and pelvis one found nothing to account for her high pulse and temperature. I was told as part of her clinical history that she had been vomiting, or I think the expression used by the person in attendance was that she had been " bringing something up." Curiously enough, difficulties were placed in the way of my seeing what was brought up. But I insisted on seeing what the people said had been brought up by this patient, and after some trouble I obtained a pot in which was obviously pneumonic sputum. On further examination dulness was found at the back of the right lung. From this one was able to say that the young woman had got pneumonia of one lung, and it was not apparently getting worse, and that therefore it was almost certain to end in recovery. You cannot tell what weight of anxiety and care that lifted from the mind of my friend, because he was engaged in practice, and had other midwifery cases to

attend, and as an honourable man he could not attend other midwifery cases if he had already under his care a patient suffering from puerperal sepsis.

As regards the importance of the next step in examination of the patient, the examination of the whole of the diseased structure, we have at the present moment in Lucas Ward a patient who is a very good illustration of the importance of examining the whole diseased structure. She has in both her posterior triangles of the neck a quantity of enlarged lymphatic glands. These lymphatic glands were diagnosed as being lymphadenomatous, whatever that may be. The enlarged glands in the posterior triangle of the neck having been seen, the examiner was not led to proceed further and say, " I have examined and found enlarged glands in the posterior triangle of the neck, and I will proceed to examine the lymphatic glands in all parts of the body." In this particular instance the lymphatic glands were enlarged in the arm-pits and groins, and further, she has enlargement of the lymphatic tissues in the other parts of the body, namely of the lymphatic tissue in the spleen. It is thought by some that if you name a disease everything is clear. To me it is not so at all. To me lymphadenoma is a phrase. We removed one of the glands from the posterior triangle, and we were disputing as to its nature, as to whether it was lymphosarcoma, or whether it was lymphadenoma. In lymphadenoma I would go so far as to accept this as a true statement, that the large endothelial plates can be seen in the enlarged lymphatic glands. I do not know what they mean, and I do not know what the disease is or how it arises, neither do I know what the end is; but I know that the patients not infrequently die of it. The only thing which would shake Dr. Andrewes was my statement that she had considerable enlargement of her spleen. If she had lymphosarcoma that growth, he thought, would not occur in the spleen, but more likely in the lungs, or possibly in the liver.

Now, I will endeavour to go a step further with our processes of reasoning. And obviously when a person looks at a patient, if it is a tumour or a surgical disease there is something to be seen, and there is something to infer from what is seen. If you go into Kenton Ward, there is an excellent case for you to practise your powers of seeing and also your powers of inference. You may possibly come to a correct conclusion about the nature òf the case. The man in Kenton Ward has a large tumour occupying the left parotid region and the upper part of the posterior triangle of the neck upon the same side. Between the parotid tumour and the tumour in the neck there is a rather deep groove. Naturally you would say this about the case, that the patient has a tumour of the parotid gland and that the swelling beneath the groove in the posterior triangle of the neck is a group of enlarged glands related to the growth in the parotid gland. That would be the natural thing to say. I think I should also say that, if I had not a little knowledge which one derives from experience, and which could not very well have been known by the members of my class ; and it is that a parotid tumour has a curious habit of descending into the neck. I have seen a tumour almost in the anterior triangle of the neck, and low down on the sterno-mastoid, and which was a parotid tumour which had descended down the anterior border of the sterno-mastoid and lodged where it was seen in the upper part of the triangle of the neck. With that knowledge I was a little reluctant to assume that the tumour in the triangle of the neck was in the lymphatic glands. I rather inferred it was a portion of the tumour which had grown down ; that is what it was because there was complete continuity between the tumour in the parotid region itself and the tumour in the upper part of the neck. There are many other points about that case which you should pay attention to. In looking at the whole of it it is very important that you should reason anatomically ; the important points would be overlooked if you did not. For instance, in that parotid region, besides the blood-vessels which pass through the parotid gland there is a very important nerve—the nerve of expression, the facial nerve. Many members of my class did not observe that the man had facial paralysis. If one of the class had proceeded to operate upon that patient and had removed the tumour, and had not observed the left facial paralysis, or the patient's friends had noticed it after his operation, what would the position have been ? They would have said, "In removing this tumour you have done it badly, because you have divided the facial nerve." As a matter of fact it had been destroyed before during an attempt which had been made to remove the

growth. There is another important matter in connection with that man. The tumour of the parotid gland may pass along the prolongations of the parotid gland, especially the portion which inhabits the parotid fossa. He could not open his mouth very well, so perhaps the tumour had passed into the glenoid lobe of the parotid gland. Also the tumour was exceedingly fixed below, as if it was anchored by some prolongation. But if this growth was malignant it might have penetrated in various directions and gone through the jaw or into the pterygoid fossa, or through the temporal bone into the middle ear and so forth. So we ascertained the hearing. If any person were to undertake to remove the tumour and afterwards the patient found that he was deaf, he might reasonably say the operator had injured his ear. The patient happened to be deaf on the side where he had a tumour, and not on the other side. Perhaps the operator who had already made an attempt to remove the tumour may have injured his hearing. A man in a humble position in life would not be very particular about that, perhaps, but more educated people would consider it a serious ground for offence, and I think perfectly rightly too. In drawing inferences from what you see and from what you know the patient has got, you must be exceedingly cautious. I am always making mistakes in the matter of inferences. I do not think people make so many mistakes in their observations. Their eyes are educated to see, but the human mind is almost an absurdity ; it is always jumping to wrong conclusions, it is always telling you untruths. The mind is an exceedingly idle possession ; it hates thinking carefully and taking trouble. Whatever the ego is, it has to kick the human mind along to make it take enough trouble and prevent it from deceiving the ego. The other day I was asked to see a lady who was supposed to have had an abscess in her left kidney. The reason for thinking she had an abscess in that kidney was this, that she had got a great deal of matter in her urine. In addition to that I was told, as a positive fact, that the left kidney had been enlarged and tender. I was called in to see the lady with the view to the removal of her left kidney, which was the kidney which was supposed to have in it an abscess, and which was thought to be a useless organ, and, moreover, a source of danger to the patient. I had to ask myself, "What do my senses tell me about this patient?" The only thing which I knew for a fact was that I had seen a quantity of pus, say 10 per cent., in her urine. Next, I think that that pus must have come from her kidney or her ureter, for a very simple reason. If the pus is from the bladder it is usually mixed with mucus—in other words, it is muco-pus. The pus which comes from the ureter behind the kidney, or from the kidney itself, is not mixed with mucus, and looks, when it is in the urine, almost like a granular precipitate. I had a further report concerning this, namely that the pus was associated with the presence of the colon bacillus, which is very common, and further that the histological appearances indicated that there were some renal cells in it. I had been told all that, and I think it was probably true. I thought that that pus must have come from the left kidney, relying upon the evidence. But in reasoning about the patient it became clear that we had very little to go upon—merely the presence of pus in the urine and the assumption that it came from the left kidney; so before I proceeded to perform nephrectomy, which is a serious operation, I should require further evidence, and for that purpose it would be necessary to examine the patient under an anæsthetic to see what both kidneys were doing. The patient was given a dose of methylene blue. I confess I am not very learned in regard to methylene blue, but I believe that if you take methylene blue the kidney epithelium itself selects it from your blood and passes it out into the urine. Obviously, if on one side or the other of the body you have not kidney substance which is working, that side will not pick methylene blue out of the urine. The first thing which happened under an anæsthetic in this case was that the endoscope showed that the mouth of the left ureter—that is to say, the one we are speaking about—was red. You may look upon the mouth of the ureter as a sort of optic disc of the kidney—that is to say, that the ureter bears the same relation to the kidney as the optic disc does to the brain. You are aware that when it is some question of disease of the brain—I am putting it into very popular language—you may see the end of the brain in the eye, for the end of the optic nerve is, developmentally, a prolongation of the brain. If that looks red and inflamed, it is a fair

inference that the brain is red and inflamed also. If it is swollen and full of venous blood, you may assume that the brain also is full of venous blood. The mouth of the ureter is very much in the same relation to the kidney, therefore, as the optic nerve is to the brain. With the endoscope we could see the urine descending the ureter in question. So you would have said "There is enough evidence to go upon." You have got the history of a swollen and tender left kidney, you yourself have seen the pus which comes from the swollen and tender left kidney, and you have seen the red end of the ureter of the left kidney, the right not being red or inflamed. If you think about it as a matter of reasoning, you will see that that is not quite enough. You are engaged now upon a difficult quest in reasoning. That is not definite, clear evidence. There is a fallacy—you have never seen the pus coming from that left kidney. We proceeded further, and put the separator into the bladder. In a few minutes this is what happened : from the right side of the bladder the urine came out full of pus and deeply stained with methylene blue. From the left side of the bladder a little perfectly clear, watery fluid came out slowly, drop by drop. It was obvious that what had happened to the patient was that she had had a violent attack of septic inflammation of her left kidney, that when I saw her that septic inflammation had ceased and had left a damaged left kidney, so that it could not excrete methylene blue and urea, and that the pus which was seen in the urine was not coming from the left kidney at all, but was coming from the right. Needless to say, no nephrectomy was done, her left kidney is still there, and I believe the right kidney is improving under ordinary measures, such as washing out with diluents and by using urotropin, and, best of all, going to live by the seaside. I have described that case rather quickly and hastily, but you will observe it affords a great deal of food for reflection.

I now propose to tell you of another case which, in my opinion, is a very good instance of correct clinical reasoning. I wonder if the gentlemen here, if I give them the facts, can reason correctly from them. About February or March last year I saw a stout lady who had had repeated attacks of appendicitis. I need not go into the clinical symptoms of the repeated attacks of that disease, but I think that, from a clinical point of view, there could be no doubt as regards the nature of her illness. The attacks had been typical. By that I mean she had the general symptoms of temperature and pulse. Her temperature had been up to 102°; her pulse had not been really known, but she had had a rigor, which always means some serious form of septic absorption. You may always look upon a rigor as a danger-signal. In addition, she had had very violent vomiting during the attack, and also she had fainted from the pain which occurred during the attack. Although she was improving when I saw her a year after the commencement of the disease, she had not got well, so I concurred in the opinion that the appendix should be removed. I removed the appendix, which was very long, very inflamed, and very adherent. After she had recovered from the operation I saw her in the month of June, which was the fourth month after her appendix was removed, and she was then of opinion, and I think everybody was, that she had made a perfect recovery, and she was very much better than she had been for a long time. So, clearly, we were upon the right tack. I heard nothing of her until January of this year, when I was asked to go and see her. I was told that in the month of December she had been seized with pain in the region of her liver. In addition to that she had had shiverings, and, beyond that, her pulse had been rapid, so that it was when I saw her, I believe, 120 or 130. In addition, her temperature had ranged continuously high, and it was almost 103°. She was exceedingly ill, and quite evidently was going to die unless something occurred. I proceeded to reason in the following way. First of all I said, "The patient's present illness, whatever it is, is obviously caused by serious septic absorption. If you doubt that fact, look at her pulse-rate and her temperature. But I think I ought to have a little more information, which can be easily obtained; I should like to know what her blood count is." Afterwards I was told that her leucocytosis amounted to at least 20,000, and I think a little more. So we were getting clear evidence of a serious septic absorption. The next step in the reasoning was this, Where has the sepsis been absorbed from? You could get one step further in ascertaining this because she was exceedingly tender over the region of her liver. So I went a step further with my reasoning, and I said that the sepsis was in some way associated with the liver. Next, as the tender-

ness was so much greater at the situation of the gall-bladder, the septic absorption was probably taking place from empyema of the gall-bladder. Dr. Hooper May, a man of great experience and acumen, agreed with that, and said that he had observed very much more tenderness in the region of the gall-bladder. Do you observe that I have not told you I felt it? I am very chary about feeling gall-bladders—indeed, about feeling anything. So there the case stood. Would you now proceed to the rational treatment? which is to give an anæsthetic and remove the sepsis from the gall-bladder. I was reluctant to do that, because of something which was brought to my notice, namely that near the angle of the tenth rib, on the right side, there was a very tender and rather hard swelling. How shall you reason from those facts—I think they are facts—profound sepsis related to the liver, most probably related to the gall-bladder, and then a lump upon the angle of the tenth rib, which was tender and inflamed? Some might have assumed that the patient was septic, and had a septic periostitis in connection with the tenth rib. However, I said this about the patient:—Observe that we are now coming to another branch of surgery altogether; and I wish to draw your attention to this other branch, and that is surgical strategy; it is an exceedingly difficult branch, which you have to learn and apply. In this instance I said, "We can explore the lump upon the angle of the tenth rib, and if that lump proves to be a mere septic periostitis, it is reasonable to go on and see what has taken place in the gall-bladder. But if that lump on the tenth rib proves to be of a different kind, we shall still know what we ought and what we ought not to do." An anæsthetic was given and I made a cut down on the rib. It was quite dramatic. First of all, the lump to the naked eye was obviously inflamed. When touched it fluctuated, and on being opened a fluid like pus came out. By means of the finger bare bone was felt, but it was red. A piece of the wall of that apparent abscess was given to Mr. Shaw, and in three minutes I saw the most perfect specimen of columnar-celled carcinoma I ever saw in my life. How did she become infected with carcinoma? I say infected because I cannot help feeling that it was so. I have been looking with extreme care and interest at the vermiform appendix to see if I could discover anything which might be a source of infection. In the first place, we may say she had no tumour there; but a cancerous infection need not necessarily imply a tumour which is obvious to the unaided senses. We know that a little while ago a patient had a tumour removed from her breast of such a size that it might have been covered by a threepenny-piece, but the tumour in her axilla was a huge mass. I have seen patients with minute ulcers on the tongue but masses of cancerous glands underneath the jaw. There were curious things in this appendix. Of course, when I speak of cancer I am talking about an unknown disease. Nothing is known about the origin of cancer, and it will not be known until people recognise that fact. The appendix was distended with material which may be mucus or it may be colloid material. It had no tubular glands. Next, the epithelial lining of the lumen was proliferating, and it had become converted into mucous or colloid material. At the gap in the appendix through which the little arteries and nerves pass into the meso-appendix you can see this material passing through the gaps into the muscular wall, through the submucous coat, and filling up the spaces in the meso-appendix. I cannot see any epithelium in the fluid or in any of the stuff in the meso-appendix. If you saw epithelium there it would be evidence in favour of cancer, but altogether to my mind it is a curious state of things and suspicious. Of course, if a post mortem. had been made you might have found a carcinoma in some part of the intestine or in some part of the alimentary tract.

I would now draw your attention to the great danger we are always in of drawing wrong inferences. You may have seen a patient yesterday in the theatre; if not, go to Lucas Ward and you will see an old lady, æt. 73 years, who yesterday had laparotomy performed. She was seen by Dr. Champneys, and she had in her pelvis a tumour which felt elastic and hard. The sense of touch was very fallacious. Dr. Champneys declined to express a clear opinion as to its nature, but he was of opinion that it was so likely to be malignant that it would not be advisable to operate upon an old woman of seventy-three. I saw this patient myself, and by the vagina I felt the uterus fixed; I could not move it, which was, of course, a suspicious fact. I felt behind the uterus and found there was a very hard, rather elastic swelling, which I could not move. Of course it is likely you may not be able to remove a tumour if you cannot move it on examination. *Per rectum* I could feel it hard and fast, in my opinion, and I

think I was right, to the left wall of the pelvis, another suspicious circumstance. A malignant tumour growing from the ovary was infiltrating the broad ligament and had begun to infiltrate the pelvis. However, the inferences which you would draw from things which you merely feel are so apt to be fallacious and incorrect that it is desirable they should be confirmed by the sense of sight, and I proceeded to look and see whether my inferences about the fixity of this tumour were correct or not. Yesterday the abdomen was opened and a tumour with thick walls was found filling up the pelvis. The tumour was of a curious black colour, and inflamed throughout the whole of its extent. It was stuck to the back of the uterus, to the left broad ligament, to the left side of the pelvis, and also to the intestines which overlay it. These adhesions were easily undone, and I ended by withdrawing from the pelvis a small ovarian tumour with thick walls and full of ancient blood-clot, due to the fact that it had had a hæmorrhage in it in consequence of its pedicle having been twisted. When a vascular pedicle gets twisted, at the beginning the thin-walled veins are blocked, so that the blood cannot return, while the thick-walled arteries keep open, so that there is a discharge of blood into the capillaries, and, as in this case, into the interior of the cyst. I have said before that if the human blood becomes extravasated into any part of the body it begins by clotting and causing its surroundings to inflame. That was the case here. It was an apoplectic ovarian cyst, very easily removed, and I could not doubt, or at all events I feel confident, that the patient will make a good recovery. My confidence happens to be based upon reasoning, because the old lady had a very good nervous system, an excellent heart, excellent lungs, excellent kidneys, and so forth. I saw the contents of her abdomen and they looked exceedingly good. The thing which was bad about her was this apoplectic ovarian cyst which has been removed, so I think it is only reasonable to say she will get better.*

Next week I shall go on to talk of the same subject, and it is a subject which may be of great trouble to you in practice. Please do not think I can make it clear to you, but I will try to make you think about it. The subject is the course of abdominal inflammation. Because it will happen to you all. "We know this patient has got an inflamed appendix. I wish I knew what was going to happen. Is the case going to get better, or is it going to get worse, or has it reached a point at which I ought to intervene?" These cases are very difficult to solve. Next time we meet I will try to tell you the kind of reasons which compel me to operate upon these cases of intra-abdominal inflammation.

January 22nd, 1906.

---

* She made a rapid convalescence.

CONGENITAL MALFORMATIONS
OF THE HEART.

A Clinical Lecture delivered at the Brompton Hospital for
Consumption and Diseases of the Chest.

By W CECIL BOSANQUET, M.A., M.D.Oxon.,
F.R.C.P.Lond.,

Assistant Physician to the Hospital and to Charing
Cross Hospital.

GENTLEMEN,—Congenital malformations of the heart are due to arrest or perversion of the normal process of development ; and in order that we may understand the nature of the different lesions it is necessary to have a rough idea of the changes which take place in this process. The earliest process by which the organ is divided into right and left halves, for which purpose it is necessary that a partition should be formed down the middle of both cavities. This is not done by a single process, but separate partitions or septa develop in the auricle, in the ventricle, and in the conus arteriosus respectively (Fig. 4). The auricular septum starts first, tending to produce a condition similar to that existing in the frog, in which there are two auricles and one ventricle. Almost immediately afterwards a similar septum begins to form in the ventricle, starting from the apex and growing towards the auricle, whereas the auricular septum starts from the upper margin (supposing for the sake of clearness that the heart lies as in the diagram, with the ventricle pointing downwards) and grows to meet

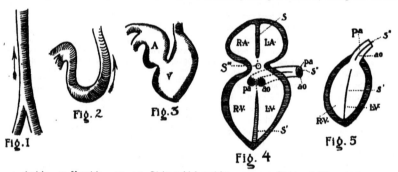

A. Auricle.   v. Ventricle.   R.A., L.A. Right and left auricles.   R.V., L.V. Right and left ventricles.
P.A. Pulmonary artery.   AO. Aorta.   s, s', s'', s'''. Septa between auricles, ventricles, arterial
trunks, and auriculo-ventricular orifice respectively.   (The figures are diagrammatic.)

stage of all in the development of the heart is seen in the formation of two vascular tubes representing the two primitive aortæ. These fuse together, giving rise to a single vessel, having afferent channels or veins entering it from behind and efferent trunks or arteries leaving it in front (Fig. 1). This tube next becomes bent upon itself, so that the afferent and efferent vessels approximate to one another (Fig. 2). Coincidently the tube becomes widened at two points into two separate chambers, representing the future auricles and ventricles respectively (Fig. 3), having a narrow channel of communication between them. The heart now corresponds roughly with the heart of a fish, possessing one auricle and one ventricle, with a single aorta leaving it. Now begins the the ventricular partition. At the same time a septum develops in the efferent vessel, also starting distally and growing to meet the others (Fig. 5). The point at which the various septa meet and fuse corresponds with the upper margin of the interventricular septum, and is necessarily the seat of a somewhat complicated process. Here in normal hearts the septum is thin and membranous and is often spoken of as " the undefended spot."

Now, we have to bear in mind that in fœtal life the right side of the heart receives the stream from the placenta which exercises the function of purifying the blood. The circulation could not be kept going if there was a complete division between the right and left sides of the heart ; some arrangement has therefore to be made for a temporary channel of communication. For this purpose there de-velops in the interauricular septum an opening known as the foramen ovale ; this is a secondary for-mation, arising as a number of small perforations in the septum, which afterwards coalesce into one orifice. Provision has to be made for the subse-quent closure of this opening, after birth, and for this purpose a flap or valve grows out over it in the left auricle, permitting the blood to pass freely from the right to the left side, but not in the re-verse direction. When, however, the pressure in the left auricle becomes equal to that in the right, as occurs in post-natal life, this valve closes and the opening is gradually obliterated.

The various septa are formed by the outgrowth of processes of the endocardium, and the valves of the heart are formed in the same way.

During fœtal life the course of the blood is as follows : The umbilical veins bring blood from the placenta, and this stream divides into two chan-nels, one of which passes through the liver and by the hepatic veins to the inferior vena cava ; the other constituting the ductus venosus, and joining the vena cava directly. The blood from the vena cava is directed from the right into the left auricle by the Eustachian valve, and from the left auricle passes to the left ventricle and thence is distri-buted to all parts of the fœtus. The venous blood is returned partly by the inferior cava, mixing with the placental blood ; partly by the superior cava, this portion passing from the right auricle to the right ventricle and thence to the lungs. As, however, the lungs are rudimentary and functionless, the greater part of the blood passing through the pulmonary artery joins the aortic stream by means of the ductus arteriosus.

After this preliminary sketch of the development of the heart and of its functions in fœtal life, it will not be difficult to understand the various malfor-mations and defects which may be produced by arrest or disturbance of this process. We are not now concerned with defects of the pericardium or of the chest-wall, which may alter the general relations of the heart. Since, however, the heart is originally a mesially situated organ, there seems no particular reason why it should so regularly occupy a position on the left side of the body. As a matter of fact we do occasionally come across cases in which it is placed on the right-hand side, this condition being generally accompanied by

similar displacement of the other viscera, so that the liver is on the left, the spleen on the right, and so on. In other instances the displacement of the heart is less considerable, so that it merely lies in the middle line instead of on the left side.

Arrest of development at a comparatively early stage may leave the heart with only one auricle and one ventricle, as in fish, while at a rather later period of fœtal life it may be left with two auricles and ventricle, as in the frog. In the heart, as in other organs, the animal to some extent " climbs up its own genealogical tree," passing through the different stages of development through which its ancestors passed in bygone ages. The existence of such defects as those just mentioned constitutes practically a reversion to an ancestral type in respect to one particular organ.

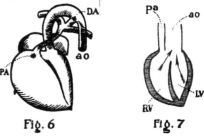

Fig. 6   Fig. 7

Stenosis of pulmonary artery. Small pulmonary artery and large aorta. AO. Aorta. PA. Pulmonary artery. DA. Ductus arteriosus.

The high degrees of malformation just mentioned are not compatible with any extended post-natal life, and are, therefore, of little clinical interest. The more important conditions embrace defects in the septa, in the great vascular trunks, and in the valves. One of the commonest varieties con-sists in a *narrowing of the pulmonary artery* (Fig. 6) either at its orifice alone or throughout its course. The former condition may arise from intra-uterine disease affecting the valves and orifice during their growth, the latter from displacement of the septum which divides the aorta from the pulmonary artery. If this septum develops rather to one side of the original vascular trunk, then one of the great arteries will be narrow and the other unduly large. It is more often the pulmonary artery which is small and the aorta large, but the reverse condition may occur. A defect of this nature is almost necessarily accompanied by other abnormalities, in order that the circulation may be maintained. If the stenosis of the pulmonary artery is slight, it may constitute the only defect, but usually there is along with it either a *communication between the two ventricles* permitting of free passage of blood between them, so that the aorta is supplied by both ventricles (Fig 7) ; or there is a *patent foramen ovale,* allowing communication between the two auricles ; or there is a *patent ductus arteriosus* .by which the blood reaches the right and left pulmonary arteries, and so the lungs, by passing from the aorta to the bifurcation of the pulmonary trunk. Often two or more of these conditions are combined in a single case. Each of the last-mentioned defects may exist alone, constituting special forms of congenital malformation.

Other forms of malformation which may be found are transposition of the aorta and pulmonary artery, the former arising from the right ventricle and the latter from the left, and defects in the valves, especially those in the pulmonary or aortic ostia, two or four being found instead of three, or the cusps being adherent one to another. A form of tricuspid stenosis met with along with mitral stenosis in a certain number of cases seems also to be due to congenital defect.

Malformations such as have just been mentioned necessarily result in alterations in the shape of the heart and in the size and relations of the four cavities. Thus, in cases of stenosis of the pulmonary artery of comparatively slight degree, so that no other gross defect exists simultaneously, the right ventricle is hypertrophied and dilated as a result of the effort needed to force the blood through the narrow orifice, the dilatation met with being probably due to failure in this effort. On the other hand, when the aorta subtends both ventricles, a free communication existing between them, one of the ventricles may atrophy, the other doing all the work. It is apparently more often the left ventricle which wastes and loses its function, the right becoming correspondingly hypertrophied. In the common form of defect, in which there is some narrowing of the pulmonary artery with communication between the ventricles or the auricles, the right side of the heart is usually enlarged.

We have not time this afternoon to consider the anomalies which may be met with in the arrangement of the great vessels, but one of these may be alluded to as being closely connected with cardiac malformations, namely stenosis or obliteration of the aorta occurring at the site of junction of the ductus arteriosus. This condition is rare ; it is accompanied by great dilatation of the anastomosing arterial trunks, so that enlarged, tortuous, pulsating vessels are visible on the front of the chest and elsewhere, conveying blood from the first part of the aorta to the lower extremities and the rest of the body. Patency of the ductus arteriosus is another vascular defect which must be considered along with cardiac malformation.

CAUSATION.

Two great causes have been assigned for the production of cardiac malformations, namely germinal defect and intra-uterine infective disease. There is no reason to doubt that the toxins of rheumatism may affect the heart of the fœtus along with or even apart from that of the mother, and in a certain number of cases evidence pointing to such infectious endocarditis during intra-uterine life has been brought forward. Opinion, however, at the present day is tending to regard this mode of production of congenital defects as comparatively rare. The greater number of such defects are now assigned to developmental peculiarities such as result in malformations of other parts of the body. In favour of this view is to be set the not infrequent coincidence of other malformations along with those of the heart. Thus, for example, two cases are reported by Krausse, in one of which along with pulmonary stenosis and patent foramen ovale there were found a trilobate condition of the left lung and absence of the spleen ; while in the second case, in which there was a single auricle and single ventricle, with aorta and pulmonary artery combined into one trunk, while the long axis of the heart lay from left to right, the spleen was absent and the kidney was of horse-shoe shape. The occurrence of numerous cases of congenital heart-lesions in members of the same family is also evidence of this mode of origin. Thus De la Camp records six cases of patent ductus arteriosus in one family, and other writers recount observations of similar import. Congenital cardiac malformations are thus to be placed in the same category as hare-lip, cleft palate, imperforate anus, and persistent Meckel's diverticulum. Of course the existence of these developmental errors itself needs explanation, and this is not easy to give. Probably any cause which lowers the vitality of the parents predisposes to such errors, such as alcoholism or advanced age at the time of procreation ; but there is some evidence to show that syphilis is a specially important factor. Thus De la Camp records the case of two sisters who suffered from congenital lesions of the heart, and whose parents were both evidently syphilitic ; and the same view is enforced by Cautley.

CLINICAL PHENOMENA.

The most striking feature of congenital disease of the heart—the cyanosis or blueness of the face and extremities which gained for the affection its old name of "morbus cæruleus"—is too well known to need any detailed account here. The cause of the phenomenon is, however, as yet unexplained. The view that it is due to admixture of arterial with venous blood, owing to communication between the two sides of the heart, is not tenable, since the cyanosis is not invariably present along with such communication, while it may be well marked in other congenital lesions. That it is connected with insufficient aeration of the blood is probable, and such a condition may well be present in all such cases, since the heart must be working at some disadvantage ; but the cyanosis occurs apart from evident signs of failure of the heart. The intensity of the blue colour is probably connected with another peculiarity of the blood in these patients, namely its concentration or richness in corpuscles and consequently in hæmoglobin. If a concentrated blood is venous owing to its containing excess of CO_2, the colour will naturally be darker than that of a normal specimen. The cause of the concentration is, however, unknown. Gibson has attributed it to diminished wear and tear of corpuscles, but there is little or no evidence in favour of this suggestion. Others have suggested that the excess of corpuscles is a compensatory phenomenon, an attempt to make up by numbers of oxygen-carriers for the deficiency of oxygen resulting from defective pulmonary circulation.

The clubbing of the fingers in these patients is perhaps due to slowness of circulation in the extremities ; but a very similar condition is met with, not only in cases of chronic pulmonary disease, such as bronchiectasis, empyema, and tuberculosis, in which circulatory disturbance might be supposed to occur, but also in some cases of hepatic and other abdominal disease in which this factor is apparently absent. Hence it has been suggested that some toxæmia is at work, possibly derived from intestinal absorption. This, it may be remarked, is now becoming a fashionable explanation for many conditions of which the pathology is obscure.

Along with these signs, cyanosis and clubbing, there is generally present a murmur in the cardiac area. The time and character of this sound will vary somewhat with the particular lesion present, but a systolic murmur audible practically all over the chest is perhaps the most frequent phenomenon. Diastolic and presystolic murmurs also occur. In some cases, however, no murmur is audible, and the absence of one must not be allowed to negative a diagnosis of congenital cardiac disease.

Patients suffer chiefly from dyspnœa on exertion, the most characteristic sign of cardiac trouble of all kinds. They also feel the cold severely, owing to bad circulation, and they readily "catch cold" and are very liable to pulmonary tuberculosis. In a certain number of instances no symptoms of disease arise in the first few years of life, but later the characteristic phenomena become apparent. Graham records a case in which an infant was apparently quite well for the first six months of life : afterwards it developed cyanosis and dyspnœa (lesion similar to that in Fig. 7). It is not uncommon to detect a cardiac murmur pointing to this malady accidentally in examining a baby for some other trouble.

DIAGNOSIS.

As regards diagnosis two questions arise. In the first place we have to decide whether a patient is suffering from congenital malformation of the heart, and in the second what is the nature of the lesion. Cases which present the typical clinical features of the disease, viz. cyanosis, clubbing of the fingers, and a cardiac murmur, offer no difficulty with respect to the former problem. In other cases, however, these signs may be absent, or at least may not occur in combination, and yet we may be led to make a diagnosis of congenital defect. A cardiac murmur alone occurring in a small baby within the first two years of life is very suggestive of such a lesion, since there has not been much opportunity for it to acquire the ordinary form of cardiac disease. If along with the murmur there is a thrill or signs of enlargement of the heart, the diagnosis is almost certain. Apart from these latter phenomena it is not easy to be sure of the condition present, for functional hæmic murmurs are not unknown in infancy. Indeed, I believe that they are much commoner than a perusal of most textbooks of medicine would indicate ; certainly, well-marked murmurs may be present in an infant at one time and have entirely disappeared a month or so afterwards. It is not impossible, however, that slight congenital malformations may occasionally exist at birth and may afterwards disappear by a natural process of obliteration.

We have to remember that defects may be present and give rise to no signs at all. Sometimes, as previously noted, symptoms may arise later on in life, the condition being latent for some months or perhaps even years (Morse). In other cases, again, congenital cyanosis may be present without any definite signs of cardiac disturbance ; a provisional diagnosis of congenital heart-disease may be made in many of such instances.

In after-life, apart from the characteristic cyanosis and clubbing, a diagnosis of malformation may be made occasionally in the presence of cardiac conditions which do not conform to the well-known clinical types characteristic of acquired disease. Thus, a loud, harsh, basal, systolic murmur, most clearly audible in the pulmonary area and conducted to some extent all over the chest, may be quoted as an example of such a condition, especially if it is accompanied by a thrill and if anæmia and aneuryism can be excluded : enlargement of the right ventricle would be a confirmatory phenomenon.

Diagnosis of the actual deformity present is often impossible and always, perhaps, open to some doubt. Certain signs have, however, been associated with particular lesions. Thus a basal systolic murmur, audible most intensely on the left of the sternum and accompanied by a thrill, as well as by cyanosis and clubbing of the fingers, is suggestive of pulmonary stenosis. A systolic murmur, generally without these last-mentioned signs, may be due to a patent foramen ovale or ductus arteriosus ; but in case of the latter lesion the murmur is often prolonged into the diastolic period of the heart's action and may begin after the systolic sound, so that it may constitute practically a

diastolic murmur, while the bruit due to an open foramen ovale may apparently be presystolic rather than systolic in time. Such at least may be gathered from a case reported by Mendez, in which along with occlusion of the tricuspid orifice there was patency of the foramen ovale and a communication between the ventricles at the undefended spot. Systolic and presystolic murmurs were present, and in view of the ordinarily accepted explanation of the murmur of mitral stenosis as due to auricular action, the presystolic bruit in this case must be assigned to the passage of blood from one auricle to the other during auricular systole. In stenosis of the pulmonary artery the pulmonary second sound is usually weak. Exaggeration of this sound is generally attributed to patency of the ductus arteriosus, increased pressure being produced in the pulmonary circuit by this communication with the aorta. Burke, however, denies this inference, and believes that the sign is more likely to be due to patency of the foramen ovale. Stenosis of the aortic orifice is signalised by the well-known signs—a systolic murmur at the base, most audible to the right of the sternum, along with hypertrophy of the left ventricle, 'and tricuspid insufficiency by a systolic murmur best audible at the lower end of the sternum, cyanosis and pulsation of the jugular veins and sometimes of the liver.

PROGNOSIS.

The outlook in cases of congenital cardiac defects is always unfavourable, since few patients in whom the condition can be recognised reach middle life. The graver forms of defect generally lead to death within the first few months of extra-uterine life, but the case reported by Mendez, and referred to above, lived twenty-five years, with total occlusion of the tricuspid valve and patent foramen ovale and undefended spot. If the patient survive the first few years of life, two great dangers are to be feared. On the one hand, there is reason to believe that hearts which are the subjects of congenital defects are more liable to be attacked by endocarditis should rheumatism occur, and such supervening lesion will probably lead rapidly to a fatal issue. On the other hand, these patients, especially those who suffer from pulmonary stenosis, are very liable to tuberculosis of the lungs which runs a rapid course.

TREATMENT.

It is generally said that congenital defects of the heart are beyond the reach of treatment; and as far as the actual deformity goes this is true enough. But patients who suffer from these conditions are in urgent need of constant medical supervison. The most important service which can be rendered to them is in the direction of prophylaxis—in warding off the risk of intercurrent rheumatic attacks and of tuberculosis. For both reasons careful attention to clothing is requisite and thoughtful guidance as to selection of a place of abode. Damp, low-lying spots and all clay soils must be rigorously avoided. Life in the open air in a sunny locality is to be aimed at. Wintering abroad is often advisable, if the sufferer can afford it, high altitudes being avoided as a rule. Heart-failure, should it occur, must be treated, on the usual lines, with digitalis and stimulants, along with rest in bed and careful feeding and nursing.

REFERENCES.

BOURKE, 'Buffalo Med. Journ.,' August, 1902.

CAUTLEY, 'Edinb. Med. Journ.,' 1902, p. 250.

DE LA CAMP, 'Berlin klin. Woch.,' January 19th, 1903.

GRAHAM, 'Arch. of Pediat.,' March, 1902.

KRAUSSE, 'Jahrb. f. Kinderheilk.,' 1905, Bd. lxii, Hft. 1.

MENDEZ, 'Abstr. in Zentralbl. f. innere Med.,' 1905, p. 19.

ROBINSON, 'Bull. of the Ayer Clin. Lab.,' 1905, No. 2.

MORSE, 'Arch. of Pediat.,' October, 1901.

January 22nd, 1906.

WE have received a copy of Wellcome's 'Photographic Exposure Record and Diary, 1906.' The 1906 edition, whilst retaining all the important features which have contributed to the success of previous issues, has been brought right up to date. The exhaustive revision to which the whole book has been subjected is of special importance in the speed table. This comprises a list of English, Continental, and American plates and films, giving the latest speeds to be used with Wellcome's Exposure Calculator. The monthly light tables, as in the 1905 issue, face the mechanical calculator affixed to the inside of the back cover.

THE VASO-MOTOR FACTOR IN THE PAIN OF MIGRAINE.

By FRANCIS HARE, M.D.,

Late Consulting Physician to the Brisbane General Hospital; Visiting Physician at the Diamantina Hospital for Chronic Diseases, Brisbane; Inspector-General of Hospitals for Queensland.

IN an article entitled "The Food Factor in Migraine," published in the CLINICAL JOURNAL, October 11th, 1905, I briefly reviewed the evidence which can be brought to support the view that (1) migraine in some cases depends upon "hyperpyræmia"—that is, an accumulation in the blood of unoxidised or imperfectly oxidised carbonaceous material which is beyond the capacity of the physiological "decarbonising" processes; and that (2) the recurrent paroxysms may be regarded as pathological functions—as ultra-physiological or pathological reinforcements of inadequate physiological function—adapted to disperse hyperpyræmia, the humoral condition on which they depend. In the present article I propose to discuss the mechanism of the well-known pain of migraine.

The view that migraine is of humoral origin and depends on a gradual accumulation in the blood, leads naturally to the view that the pain depends proximately on a variation of vaso-motor action. Such a view has been widely entertained. Du Bois Reymond, noting chiefly the constricted condition of the temporal in his own case, was led to conclude that the pain depended on the vaso-constriction which he ascribed to a "tetanus of the sympathetic."[*] Möllendorff, noting chiefly the dilated condition of certain cranial arteries, was led to conclude that the pain depended on the vaso-dilation which he ascribed to a paralysis of the sympathetic.[†] The seeming incompatibility of these divergent observations and views led to the suggestion, widely accepted in Germany, that there are in reality two distinct types of migraine, the one characterised by vaso-constriction, the other by vaso-dilation. But I shall argue that any such fundamental division is unjustifiable and has originated from an insufficiently comprehensive

---

[*] 'Megrim and Sick-Headache,' Ed. Liveing, 1873, pp. 295, 296.

[†] *Ibid.*, p. 307.

view of the vaso-motor phenomena of migraine. I shall attempt to show that the special variation of vaso-motor action responsible for the pain of migraine is by no means limited to the cranial area, that both vaso-constriction and vaso-dilation occur in all cases, that these contrary variations are correlative, that their united action results in an intense vascular distension of some cranial area, and that this vascular distension is the proximate cause of the pain.

VASO-CONSTRICTION.

During a paroxysm of any severity there is palpably a widespread vaso-constriction of the cutaneous area, most marked in the extremities. This is shown by the intense chilliness of the surface (Anstie),[*] by the icy coldness of the hands and feet (Möllendorff).[†] In several of my cases shivering amounted to distinct rigor. The radial artery is small and wiry (Anstie), and William Russell has demonstrated hypertonus of this artery in more than one case of headache.[‡] But other arteries are often affected. In Du Bois Reymond's case the superficial temporal artery of the painful side was always constricted, and Lauder Brunton has frequently seen the anterior temporal reduced to the size of a piano wire.

Some of the premonitory symptoms of migraine are explicable by vaso constriction. Sometimes there is early polyuria, and this could be explained by a generalised vaso-constriction in which the renal arteries did not share.[§] Various paræsthesiæ could be explained by vaso-constriction localised in the cerebral centres or at the periphery. Yawning is a common premonitory symptom ; and yawning has been noted by Hughlings Jackson to depend on cerebral vaso-constriction.[‖] Cerebral vaso-constriction and consequent anæmia would explain the drowsiness which in some persons invariably precedes a migraine paroxysm.

[VASO-DILATION.

The vaso-dilation of migraine was pointed out by Möllendorff. Not infrequently it is conspi-

cuously visible. Wilks says that while the radial is small, the carotid on one side is larger, and with its branches throbs inordinately.[*] Möllendorff saw the background of the eye on the affected side bright scarlet red, the optic papilla red and œdematous, the arteria and vena centralis retinæ enlarged.[†] I have myself frequently seen the various branches of the temporal markedly dilated on the painful side during a migraine attack.

THE MUTUAL RELATIONS BETWEEN VASO-CONSTRICTION AND VASO-DILATION.

The interrelationship between the vaso-constriction and the vaso-dilation of migraine can readily be understood if we view the vasomotor and vascular systems as a whole. To do so, however, it is essential that we be permitted to extend certain fundamental physiological principles into the domain of pathology,

It is admitted by all that during life the general or aortic blood-pressure tends to be maintained at an approximately uniform mean height. But it is known that countless and ceaseless variations of calibre are occurring in all parts of the vascular system. It follows that "every variation in one part is compensated by a simultaneous and contrary variation in another part" (Leonard Hill).[‡] This common knowledge may be applied to the vascular conditions in migraine. There is, as pointed out, a more or less generalised area of vaso-constriction and a more or less localised area of vaso-dilation, and these two contrary variations for the most part arise and subside simultaneously. Consequently we may regard them as correlative or mutually compensatory, the vaso-constriction tending to prevent a fall of general or aortic blood-pressure from following the vaso-dilation, the vaso-dilation tending to prevent a rise of general or aortic blood-pressure from following the vaso-constriction. Thus there tends to be maintained uniformity of general or aortic blood-pressure. But such general uniformity is manifestly attained at the expense of uniformity of localised blood-pressure. For it is certain that the local blood-pressure peripheral to the vaso-constriction is reduced, and

---

* 'Neuralgia and its Counterfeits,' 1871, p. 29.

† 'Megrim and Sick-Headache,' Lieving, 1873, p. 311.

‡ 'Lancet,' June 1st, 1901, p. 1522.

§ 'The Food Factor in Disease,' Francis Hare, 1905, vol. ii, p. 182, et seq.

‖ 'Lancet,' January 21st, 1905, p. 174.

* 'Lectures on Diseases of the Nervous System,' 1878, p. 427.

† 'Megrim and Sick-Headache,' 1873, p. 310.

‡ 'Text-Book of Physiology,' E. A. Schäfer, vol. ii, pp. 81, 82

that the local blood-pressure peripheral to the vaso-dilation is increased. In less technical terms the blood is in great part shut off from wide superficial areas and turned on with concentrated force and in greater quantity to some part of the cranial area. Thus is produced a vascular distension or determination of arterial blood in the latter. And this vascular distension *depends upon the generalised vaso-constriction not less than upon the localised vaso-dilation.* This point, which seems to me incontrovertible, has not, so far as I know, been brought out by any of those who adhere to vaso-motor theories of migraine. Nevertheless, it is of primary importance. For unless it is fully realised, it is impossible to understand the *rationale* of most of the various means of relief from the pain of migraine or the results which sometimes follow the paroxysm.

CLINICAL EVIDENCE IN SUPPORT OF THE PREFERRED THEORY.

On the view propounded above, the pain of migraine depends simply on vascular distension of the painful area. In this vascular distension there are plainly four essential factors : (1) a localised vaso-dilation ; (2) a generalised vaso-constriction ; (3) the work done by the cardiac systole ; and (4) the amount of blood in circulation. It follows that anything which increases any or all of these factors will tend to increase the pain, and that anything which diminishes any or all of these factors will tend to diminish the pain. These deductions will. be found adequate to explain the action of most, if not all, of those agencies which have been found by observation and experiment to be effective in exacerbating or relieving the pain of migraine.

Conditions affecting the localised vaso-dilation.— In some cases, presumably those in which the dilated area is situated in the scalp or pericranium, hot applications locally serve to increase the pain, doubtless by increasing the vaso-dilation. On the other hand, the vaso-dilation, and hence the vascular distension and pain, may be controlled by the application of cold lotions or the ice cap. Authorities in support of these statements are hardly required.

Conditions affecting the generalised vaso-constriction.—Exposure of the general surface of the body to cold, air or water, has often precipitated a migraine paroxysm ; it never fails to increase the pain of existing attacks. This is well known to all sufferers. On the other hand, exposure to heat of the general surface of the body, or of any part *other than the dilated area,* is an efficient means of relief. Toasting the feet at the fire (M. Piorry),[*] immersion of the feet and legs in hot water (Graves),[†] sitting over the fire (Haig), [‡] are all followed by relief, but I have found that a full-length hot bath is a more effectual measure.

All these act by reducing the generalised vaso-constriction. But to such means we may well add measures which reduce the localised vaso-dilation. A general hot bath, air, vapour, or water, combined with cold to the head in the form of cold douche or ice-cap, is the most efficient of all thermal measures ; it rarely fails in my experience to give complete though temporary relief from the pain of migraine.

The generalised vaso-constriction may be relieved by drugs also. Amyl nitrite was found by Lauder Brunton in some cases to relieve the pain, and nitro-glycerine is praised by Gowers as one of the most beneficial drugs in migraine.

Conditions affecting the work done by the heart.— Anything which increases the force of the heart-beat is liable to increase the pain ; hence ammonia usually, and alcohol sometimes, is immediately aggravative, but alcohol may relieve the pain. This is probably to be explained by the fact that alcohol, which in the first place stimulates the heart, acts also as a general vaso-dilator. On the other hand, anything which reduces the force of the heart-beat relieves the pain. Nausea and vomiting are commonly associated with reduced systolic force, and in many ' patients the onset of these digestive symptoms is the signal for the abatement of the paroxysm. In one of my patients marked faintness often terminated the pain. The rapid relief which follows antipyrin is probably to be explained by reduced systolic action.

Conditions affecting the amount of blood in circulation.—It is not, of course, possible to estimate the influence of an increase in the amount of blood in circulation upon the pain of migraine. But the influence of a decrease thereof is readily demonstrated. In certain cases—some of those in which

[*] ' Megrim and Sick-Headache,' Liveing, 1873, p. 470.
[†] ' Clinical Med.,' New Syd. Soc., vol. ii, p. 350.
[‡] ' Uric Acid in Disease.'

the vascular distension trenches upon the nasal mucosa—the migraine paroxysm is complicated by epistaxis. In these the result in all cases is the rapid alleviation—usually the termination—of the pain. The same result follows hæmorrhage from any other part, as in venesection (Graves),[*] hæmorrhage from piles,[†] etc.

Digital compression of arteries.—But the vascular distension of migraine may be reduced more effectually by shutting off the supply of blood to the distended area through digital compression of the supplying trunk artery. And it has been shown by Parry [‡] in the first instance, and later by Möllendorff,[§] that pressure on the common carotid of the affected side disperses the pain in practically all cases. These observers also showed that immediately the pressure was relaxed the pain returned and after a few pulsations resumed its former severity. My own observations on the effects of compressing arteries during the migraine paroxysm have been recorded in 'The Food Factor in Disease.' [||]

* 'Clin. Med.,' New Syd. Soc., vol. ii, p. 357.
† 'The Food Factor in Disease,' Francis Hare, vol. ii., pp. 88, 89.
‡ 'Megrim and Sick-Headache,' Liveing, 1873, p. 297.
§ *Ibid.*, p. 309, *et seq.*
|| "(a) In unilateral migraine pressure on the common carotid of the corresponding side invariably at once and completely removes the pain. (b) In bilateral migraine pressure on either common carotid removes the pain on the corresponding side and increases the pain on the opposite side; by alternately compressing the right and left common carotid the pain may be rendered hemicranial on the left and right sides alternately. I have not tried the effect of compressing both common carotids simultaneously. (c) In a case of bilateral occipital migraine immediate relief was afforded by compressing both occipital arteries, and the pain was rendered unilateral by compressing one occipital. (d) In a case of intense pan-cranial migraine complete cessation of all pain followed simultaneous compression of both temporals and both occipitals; the pain was rendered unilateral by simultaneous pressure on the temporal and occipital of one side, or by pressure on one common carotid; it became limited to the posterior portion of the cranium by pressure on both temporals and to the anterior portion of the cranium by pressure on both occipitals; finally, pressure on any one of the named arteries relieved the pain in the area of distribution of that artery. (e) In a case of severe frontal bilateral migraine the patient discovered for herself that pressure on both angular arteries (which were throbbing violently) gave very great, though not complete, relief; she would sit for hours compressing the root of the nose between her finger and

Results of vascular distension.—Most of the so-called complications and sequelæ of migraine may readily be explained by vascular distension in various localities. In many cases there is intense soreness and tenderness of the scalp, a symptom which may persist for several days, and be so severe as to preclude combing the hair. There has been observed œdema and even ecchymoses *at the seat of the most intense pain* (Gowers). The conjunctivæ are sometimes ecchymosed (Labarraque). Tissot noticed extravasation of blood, rendering the skin of the forehead, eyelids, and even cheeks black and blue (Liveing). Epistaxis has been already referred to. Fatal apoplexy has occurred during a headache indistinguishable from migraine (Hilton Fagge). The ocular tension may be increased during a " bilious headache " (Lauder Brunton), and acute double glaucoma has occurred during an attack of migraine, which affection had been previously recurrent.[*]

Finally, there seems no room for doubt that the long recurrent distension of any special artery during migraine paroxysms may conduce ultimately to distinct arterio-sclerosis of the vessel. Gowers noted this condition in the right temporal artery of a woman æt. 50 liable to right-sided migraine from youth,[†] Thoma noted it in the left temporal in a case of severe left-sided supra-orbital neuralgia, [‡] and I have myself seen two similar cases.

January 22nd, 1906.

thumb; and she had thought of devising a special padded clip for this purpose. (f) In many cases general compression of the painful area of the scalp gave much relief; this has been noted by many writers; cases so relieved are doubtless pericranial." ('The Food Factor in Disease,' vol. i, p. 283, Longmans, 1905.)
* 'Brit. Med. Journ.,' " Epitome," March 24th, 1900.
† 'Dis. Nerv. Syst.,' 1893, vol. ii, p. 848.
‡ Allbutt's ' System of Medicine,' vol. vi, p. 617.

Spirochetes in Syphilis.—Hoffmann's experience now includes three hundred cases of syphilis in which the *Spirochæta pallida* was found. Its discovery in fresh, dubious lesions was always followed by the development of the lesions into the unmistakable syphilitic type. He has never found it in non-syphilitic affections, and doubts the accuracy of the technique in the few instances in which others claim to have found it in non-syphilitic lesions.—*Journ. A. M. A.*, vol. xlv, No. 27.

THE CLINICAL JOURNAL,

CLINICAL RECORD, CLINICAL NEWS, CLINICAL GAZETTE, CLINICAL REPORTER,
CLINICAL CHRONICLE AND CLINICAL REVIEW.

EDITED BY L. ELIOT CREASY.

No. 692.   WEDNESDAY, JANUARY 31, 1906.   Vol. XXVII. No. 16.

CONTENTS.

* Specially reported for the Clinical Journal. Revised by the Author.

NOTICE.

Editorial correspondence, books for review, &c., should be addressed to the Editor, 51, New Cavendish Street, W., Telephone No. 904, Paddington; but all business communications should be addressed to the Publishers, 22½, Bartholomew Close, London, E.C. Telephone 927, Holborn.

All inquiries respecting Advertisements should be sent to MESSRS. ADLARD & SON, Bartholomew Close, E.C. Telephone 927, Holborn.

Terms of Subscription, including postage, payable by cheque, postal or banker's order (in advance) : for the United Kingdom, 15s. 6d. per annum : Abroad 17s. 6d.

Cheques, &c., should be made payable to THE PROPRIETORS OF THE CLINICAL JOURNAL, crossed "The London, City, and Midland Bank, Ltd., Newgate Street Branch, E.C. Account of the Medical Publishing Company, Ltd."

Reading Cases to hold Twenty-six Numbers of THE CLINICAL JOURNAL can be supplied at 2s. 3d. each, or will be forwarded post free on receipt of 2s. 6d. ; and also Cases for Binding Volumes at 1s. each, or post free on receipt of 1s. 3d., from the Publishers, 22½, Bartholomew Close, London, E.C.

THE COURSE OF INTRA-ABDOMINAL INFLAMMATION.

A Clinical Lecture delivered at St. Bartholomew's Hospital.

By C. B. LOCKWOOD, F.R.C.S.,
Surgeon to the Hospital.

GENTLEMEN, — Last week I endeavoured to show you that the diagnosis of a clinical case included various steps. First, there is the process of making clear observations with your own senses, above all with your eyes, and to some extent with your hands. Next, that from those observations inferences were to be drawn. And then, when you had collected all the inferences that could be drawn from the case you ought to reason from those inferences, and that the ultimate end of the reasoning brought about the diagnosis. To perform all these mental acts correctly requires, of course, a long period of training. You get this training by seizing every opportunity of using your eyes and other senses, and the correct methods of inference you can acquire by watching the process as performed by others and continually correcting your own mistakes. Of course the process of drawing a general conclusion from your inferences necessitates considerable mental aptitude, and you will only acquire that by long and continuous reflection.

To-day I propose to endeavour to draw your attention to a very important matter, and that is the course of intra-abdominal inflammation. Observe, I have purposely taken a general subject. It does not want much effort of the human mind to deal with a few trifling particulars, but it is a great effort of the human mind to be more general, and I am myself quite aware of my own deficiencies. But, remember, it is a process which you ought to expect from all who pretend to teach you—that is to say, to teach you to think. I tell you why I have chosen the course of intra-abdominal suppuration for my subject. It is that the course of intra-abdominal suppuration, in the vast majority of cases, can be quite correctly surmised. But if you are incorrect in your surmise as to the course which intra-abdominal inflammation is to pursue, there will be some dreadful disaster to the patient who has committed himself or herself or itself into your care, and in addition there will be some dreadful disaster to your own reputation and to your own fortunes. I cannot help often recalling seeing a youth of about twenty years of age who had had intra-abdominal inflammation for at least ten days. Incidentally I had heard that it was proceeding to a safe issue. But I was asked, one morning early, to see this youth and found him with his hands and feet cold, and a cold sweat on the surface of his body. His pulse could hardly be counted—I should think it was 150 per minute—his abdomen was rigid, and he was obviously dying. I do not know that he knew he was dying, because those who have the abdomen full of septic material are fortunately in a state of intoxication, so that their eyes are bright, their minds are alert, and often they are happy, and will laugh and talk, and they will have no conception that they are about to die. I cannot help feeling that this condition of septic intoxication is one which often leads to mistakes, as I shall tell you directly. Why had this youth got into his parlous condition? It is true he was known to have intra-abdominal suppuration, it is true it was supposed to be running a safe course, but I do not think that the exact site or situation had been correctly diagnosed, and those who were watching him were not aware of a collection of pus in the pelvis which could be felt *per rectum*, and that its course almost inevitably was to increase and at last burst and infect the general peritoneal cavity, and in all human probability to kill the patient. Another distressing case I recall was that of a young woman who had not long been married. She was seized with a pain in the lower part of the abdomen. There were speculations as to the cause of this pain, but a very shrewd man who saw her said he thought she was beginning to have an acute attack of appendicitis. For some reason, she was placed in other hands, and was watched from day to day. She had a continual high temperature, a continuously rapid pulse, and there was considerable tenderness in the lower part of the

abdomen. At length the day came when the collection of pus at the brim of the pelvis burst and infected the rest of the peritoneal cavity and slew the patient. When I went into the room to see her, her hair was quite glossy and like the hair of a healthy person, her eyes were bright, she smiled when one entered the room, her mind was quite alert, and at any light remark she laughed. Apparently she had not the slightest conception that she was dying or going to die. I think many of those who were looking on did not know that. But one glance at her abdomen, distended, tender, rigid, especially if one had one's finger on the pulse for a moment (for the pulse could barely be counted) and her cold hands and feet at once told the observer that the end of that unhappy person was approaching. I am sure that those poor wretches ought not to have died in that way. I am not sure that they ought not to have died, but they ought to have died after a better attempt had been made to save their lives. I can recall some splendid successes of people who must have been saved from death by the methods which were adopted for evacuating the pus and other septic material which was present. Dr. Bridges, an old house-surgeon of mine, rang me up one night at a quarter to seven, and said he had that moment seen a child whom he believed to have an exceedingly acute attack of appendicitis, and further, that he thought it was the kind of case that I would operate upon if I saw it. I requested him to get an anæsthetist and nurses, and have a room prepared, and that I would arrive by a quarter to nine. At the appointed time I entered the house and saw the child, and before 9. 30 p.m. we had extracted from its abdomen a gangrenous appendix, and given exit to a quantity of exceedingly septic matter. The night before that child went to bed perfectly well. At five o'clock in the morning it was awakened by a pain in the abdomen. At breakfast time—that is to say, about eight o'clock—the mother gave the child a dose of calomel—a piece of domestic medicine. It got worse during the course of the day, and Dr. Bridges saw it at a quarter to seven, and I saw the patient at a quarter to nine. The child was lying in bed, and I believe it was reading a book. It did not look very ill, but had acute tenderness over the lower part of the abdomen, and its pulse was 120 per minute. Also I was struck by the appearance of the child.

You cannot always define—from want of education in my case—the signs which convey impressions to the mind. But the child was very pale, it had a curious livid appearance, and I remember my remark to my friend Ernest Bridges, namely, " I am absolutely certain that that child has got something horrible proceeding in its inside, and I shall not be happy until I have seen what that is." I looked, and found a gangrenous appendix. The next day the child was better, and the day after that we told the friends we thought it was on the point of convalescing, and that they might now cease to be anxious about it. It was a rapid course of events altogether. Abdominal inflammation is over and over again overlooked because a rectal examination is omitted. I remember a child whom I saw in the country who had been seen by a friend of mine in London. The latter had considered that the child was merely suffering from colic, or some ailment of that kind. The child was allowed to go into the country, where the pain returned. But at that period the child had become worse, with a heightened temperature and pulse. It was a deceptive case, and the reason was that its inflammation was proceeding in the pelvis and Douglas's pouch. Now, had a rectal examination been made on that child when it complained of so-called stomach-ache, it would have been ascertained that it had extreme tenderness in Douglas's pouch, and that there would have been a hard, tender swelling there. And the person who performed that examination would have been certain in his own mind that that child had something very serious proceeding in its pelvis. As a matter of fact that child had a perforated appendix removed from its pelvis. It also had an abscess in its pelvis, and it ultimately got an exceedingly acute form of sepsis, and died in a few hours. It had got some form of septicæmia. The history of this case seems clear. The child had an appendix hanging into its pelvis and containing a concretion. The concretion grew and was accompanied by chronic ulcerative appendicitis. This had gone on to perforation or gangrene and a pelvic abscess. The next stage was removal of the appendix and general sepsis. To my mind that is a perfectly clear sequence of events. I was struck with the next thing that happened in that family. A cousin was at school, and looked very ill and pale. He was doing the ordinary work at a public school, but continually complained of pain in his abdomen. That pain might very well have put anybody off the scent. In the first stage of bad abdominal pain I should think it a safe rule to say it is always felt in the middle of the abdomen, hence the silly expression "the dry belly-ache." But if the pain in the middle of the abdomen is accompanied by vomiting, especially vomiting of bile, then it may be called a " bilious attack." This boy had not, when I saw him, a pain in the centre of the abdomen, but one which was entirely on the left side, underneath the ribs. His mother suspected—I do not know why—he might be like the cousin who died of sepsis due to pelvic abscess. How would you proceed with a patient of this description ? I have got, now, a routine method of treating these doubtful abdominal cases, and I consider every person with pain in the abdomen doubtful until I know what is causing the pain. This boy was treated in the ordinary manner, the routine way. First of all he was put into bed. I shall mention some very elementary and rudimentary facts to you which do not occur to those who are immersed only in hospital work. So much of the work is done for you in hospital by sisters and nurses, and you come across so many interesting and good cases, that you are little aware of the kind of case which you may have to deal with later on in your careers. I am going to tell you of an absolutely typical case. Why is the boy put to bed? For a great variety of reasons. The general and local symptoms of inflammation in that boy's case were absent. I only knew that he had pain underneath the left costal margin and some tenderness there. He had no rigid or tender spot in his abdomen, and I think most people who had examined that boy's abdomen with an unprejudiced mind would have said there was nothing the matter with it. First of all he was put quietly into his bed, so that it would be possible to get the correct reading of his pulse and temperature. You can never read a person's pulse right if he is walking about or going up and down stairs. The correct pulse-reading, in my idea, in a case of this sort, is taken when the patient is asleep in bed and by an intelligent nurse. A visit by the doctor will send up an ordinary person's pulse ten per minute. So it is obviously important that these patients should be kept quiet when the readings are taken. You will never get a proper reading by the thermometer unless the patient is quiet. If the person gets up and walks along the corridor, sits in a draughty water-closet, and then walks back to bed, you cannot get the proper reading. It is clear that such a patient should use the bed-pan when the bowels act, which entails a skilful nurse. You may be tempted to say that these are trivialities, but they constitute correct medical practice. For several days the boy's pulse and temperature were normal, and then suddenly the pulse gave a jump, and simultaneously the temperature went up. Being in bed and properly nursed gave us another opportunity of investigating this boy; we knew what went into him, and we saw what came out. There came out a quantity of mucus streaked with blood. Therefore it was clear that he had something odd going on in his colon. He had colitis, whatever else he had. We watched him for nearly three weeks. A friend of mine (Dr. John Harold) looked after him, and one day he said, "Come and see that boy." I went up to see him. And they said, "You have a pain, have you not?" "Yes." "Where is it?" "It is here, on the right side." Altogether he had been going on in this way with these "bilious attacks" for six years; his abdomen was opened, and an inflamed appendix was extracted from behind his colon. That ulcerated and septic appendix was full of fæcal concretions. I guess that boy had had an escape. But why did he get that dreadfully dangerous appendix removed? Simply because he was put on what I strongly recommend for these patients with doubtful conditions, a period of probation.

I have referred to some of the signs of intra-abdominal inflammation. If any gentleman in this theatre, after what I have said, is deluded by that pain in the middle of the abdomen, he is past forgiveness. The ordinary place for abdominal pain to begin is in the centre of the abdomen. If it is appendicitis, the patient will place it after a while in the right iliac fossa. If the patient has inflamed Fallopian tubes, or an inflamed uterus, or an inflamed ovarian cyst in the pelvis, then, after a while, the patient will place it low down in the abdomen. If it is a septic gall-bladder, the patient will probably place the pain under the right costal arch. Or if it is a septic kidney, with an inflammation of that organ, the pain will be placed after a while in the flank. And in almost all the

instances I have given you there is a period in the disease when the patient refers his pain to the centre of the abdomen. There is an obvious reason for that, which is founded upon a correct appreciation of the anatomy of the solar plexus, a portion of the anatomy of the human body which is singularly neglected, and which will repay any gentleman to work for his thesis. The locality of the pain may continue doubtful although you have tried it many times. I recall the case of a lady whom I saw yesterday, who was supposed to have had a septic gall-bladder and gall-stones, and which was afterwards found to be true. She was asked where the pain was, and she put her hand anywhere down the right side of the abdomen. But if I had been asked where she put it most, I should say at the region of the appendix. Occasionally, if she was pressed, she put the pain more towards the right flank. After thinking a great deal about the pain of that patient, I should have said she put her pain anywhere down the right side of the abdomen, travelling down the course of the ureter, for all I know. There were peculiar circumstances. She had never had an attack of jaundice, she had passed a renal calculus, a uric acid calculus. There was good evidence of that. Whether she had ever had appendicitis I could not tell. As regards her tenderness, it was very difficult to make out where her tenderness was. It might have been in the gall-bladder, over the kidney, or over the appendix, or down the course of the right ureter. I will tell you why I think her tenderness was so difficult to elicit. You will notice I am drawing a distinction between tenderness, or pain on pressure, and the pain which the patient says she feels. I think one of the reasons why the tenderness was so very difficult to locate was that she was exceedingly stout; probably the fat on her abdominal wall was nearly two inches thick. There is not one here who will not be deceived by a fat person. He will be deceived in this way, that he may think the person has fluid in the abdomen, or abscess when she has not; in addition, he will think such a patient has not got pain and tenderness when she has. The human mind cannot help being sceptical about the existence of pain if it is not accompanied with a corresponding degree of tenderness. I remember being called to an hotel not very far from here, and this was the reason of my being called. They said there was a man in the hotel who had had a very bad attack of abdominal pain and diarrhœa, but that he had recovered and they did not think that it indicated anything serious, but as his friends were far away it was desirable that somebody should share the responsibility of a decision. We found there a very stout person, sitting upon the edge of the bed. He did not look very ill. He had had his breakfast, he had walked across the room, had stood up at the looking-glass and shaved himself, and had just returned to the edge of the bed when I saw him. When he laid down it was difficult to tell whether the rotundity of his abdomen was due to distension, or whether it was due to a huge layer of fat which enveloped it. He said his pain was better. That is a very common story and it is sure to deceive. No particular amount of tenderness could be elicited in the front of the abdomen. But he had a pulse of 130, and since the diarrhœa he had passed nothing from the bowels, neither fæces nor flatus. He was a dying man. The person who does not pass flatus from his intestines is, unless something happens, going to die. What did it all mean? That case was cleared up at once. First of all the pulse being at 130 per minute excited intense suspicion. The finger passed into the rectum could feel peritoneum, with nothing intervening between the peritoneum and the finger except the rectal wall. When the peritoneum was touched it nearly made the man leap out of bed. There is no more tender structure in the human body than the inflamed parietal peritoneum. Perhaps the exposed pulp of a tooth is about as painful, but the peritoneum when inflamed is certainly the most exquisitely tender structure which the body contains. His abdomen was opened and it was found to be full of pus and contained a gangrenous appendix. He died, not many hours after the operation, from septic intoxication. I remember another circumstance in connection with that case. After the operation, at night, his relatives appeared on the scene, and I said: "I am going to take you to see your relative. He has had his operation performed, his abdomen has been cleared of the septic material, but he is going to die. Do not be deceived; he may laugh and talk to you with a good voice and be cheerful, but he will suddenly collapse and die. I regret to have to tell you this." I knew this because he had a pulse which was continuously ascending after the operation. If it had fallen one might have felt

hope, but it ascended to 140, and it was certain that his heart would not long endure that strain, and it was equally certain that his cheerful demeanour was due to septic intoxication. I could quote other cases in which the situation of the pain had been ambiguous. But remember that you must be very careful not to assume that tenderness is absent, for the presence of fat will obscure it, and it may only be elicited by rectal examination.

Now I shall tell you of something else which will hide the local tenderness and which will make it most difficult for you to say whether the patient has got an actually inflamed organ situated in some particular part of the abdomen. Not very long ago I was asked to see a patient who had been exceedingly ill for several days. It was obvious that she was suffering from some form of septic absorption, because she had a continuously high pulse and temperature. No doubt if we had had the Pathological Department present they would have found she had a continuously high leucocytosis. Her abdomen was distended uniformly; her bowels had passed nothing for at least thirty-six hours, no flatus nor fæces. The front of the abdomen was comparatively free from pain and tenderness. It could be moved and pushed and indented; but she had intense tenderness in Douglas's pouch. Directly the finger was passed into the rectum it became obvious that we were dealing with an intensely inflamed pelvic peritoneum. There were two reasons why her abdomen was not painful in front, and this is a point which may deceive you very much. First of all her abdomen was fat, though not inordinately so. Next it was distended with wind. Now, if the inflamed structure, let it be kidney, appendix, or pelvic abscess, or inflamed ovarian cyst, or inflamed uterine fibroid, or any inflamed structure in the abdomen, be hidden by distended intestines, how can anyone elicit tenderness? Why, it is like feeling through a thick air-pad! How, then, shall you elicit tenderness in a structure which is at the back of the abdomen, behind a layer of fat and a cushion of air? The diagnosis in that case was an acutely inflamed and septic organ, either tube or appendix, situated near the right brim of the pelvis, and a septic and perforated appendix was removed, after which she got well. It is sometimes most difficult to decide when to operate upon such cases, but in this the decision was arrived at upon simple and obvious signs. Almost always in such cases it is possible to fix upon what I shall call a determinant symptom. The determinant symptom of this case was that the patient had not passed any flatus for thirty-six hours, and could not be made to do so with enemas; she had inflammatory intestinal obstruction, and though she was not vomiting it was highly probable that the obstruction would continue, and if it did continue she would die. How shall you tell whether obstruction is complete or not? It is very simple to find that out. An irritating enema was given—in fact, I think two of them were given—but there was no passage of anything, not even flatus. So, as these enemata were carefully given, it was quite clear that her obstruction was complete. From the abdomen was removed a quantity of pus, and a gangrenous and perforated appendix, which lay far back at the pelvic brim. It was never felt *per rectum*, though the inflamed pelvic peritoneum about it was felt. Sometimes the vomiting may be a determinant feature. For instance, there are degrees of vomiting. I take vomiting in its anatomical order. If a person merely vomits the contents of the stomach, it is clear that the vomiting is not of a very severe character. If he vomits up the contents of the duodenum—that is to say, if the vomited matter contains bile—it is more severe. If it begins to get down to that black material which inhabits the jejunum, it is a decidedly serious form of vomiting, and is of great import. I suppose some people will proceed to allow vomiting to go on to such a degree that at last it gets to the contents of the ileum, in which case it is called fæcal. I do not think to-day such a thing would occur, but I have known practitioners who have said, " I did not think it necessary to send for you before because the vomiting had not become fæcal." I will not refer to the next alteration of function, namely distension, but you know the function of the intestines, besides dealing with the contents, is to propel them. Inflamed structures do not perform their functions properly, and if the intestines do not propel their contents there will be distension, and intestinal obstruction, which are inevitable. I wonder if any gentleman can tell me where the intestinal gases come from. Obviously they are manufactured by the intestinal bacteria. If you grow the colon bacillus in gelatin, you will find over each

colony a little balloon of gas, and if you can carry your mind to countless millions of colonies growing in the intestines, and feeding upon the intestinal contents, such as pieces of vegetable which the patient has been allowed to eat before the illness or during it, you can imagine what a quantity of gas they will produce. But I have often doubted whether that was the whole truth, because I have seen a patient one hour comfortable, and without any trace of intestinal obstruction, and an hour afterwards with the abdomen tightly distended. Where did all that gas come from in such a short time? There must be other factors besides bacteria in producing flatulent distension, but I think you may safely say that that is the most important as far as you are concerned. And you guard against this danger in the preliminary treatment of all abdominal operations by clearing the intestines of the food which the patient has taken, and not allowing him to have any other food placed in his alimentary canal shortly before the operation, and in addition by taking care after the operation to see that an accumulation of intestinal gas does not take place.

Now I shall refer to another symptom of intra-abdominal inflammation which is a source of fallacy to you. It is the muscular rigidity which accompanies any inflammation of the peritoneum, whether visceral or parietal. That muscular rigidity, doubtless, is a protective rigidity. Everyone here has seen, during an inflammation of the hip or knee or any other joint, how firmly the joint becomes fixed. The muscles become rigid and taut and tend to prevent the inflamed structures of the joint being moved or stretched. Exactly the same thing occurs in the abdomen. The muscles of the abdominal wall become rigid to protect the inflamed tissue underneath. In consequence of that muscular rigidity curious mistakes may occur. I have often seen the protective rigidity which takes place at the upper end of the rectus mistaken for the gall-bladder and for tumours of the pylorus. When this muscular rigidity occurs on the right side of the abdomen it is not unusual for it to be mistaken for appendicular abscess. I think most of these mistakes can easily be avoided, first of all by remembering how fallacious these signs may be, and secondly, by an examination under anæsthesia. Also, if there were a gall-bladder there you might possibly find dulness, but carcinoma is also a dull thing ; appendicular abscess is as a rule, but it may not be.   I think if you exercise a little caution you will not be deluded by that.   But when you encounter this abdominal rigidity, which indicates so clearly that there is something inflamed underneath, do not be too sure of the nature of the structure which is underneath. I have seen some very curious mistakes made. On Friday there was a patient whom we knew had a septic kidney.   We knew that because there was pus in his urine ; we could see the pus emerging from the left ureter.   We saw the retraction of the left ureter, which is also an indication.   And then when the patient was placed upon his back and his abdomen was felt, we at once came upon a huge hard mass, which I think I am correct in saying none of us had felt before.   So the rigidity had protected the inflamed septic kidney from pressure. And the rigidity in this case was very great because the peritoneum over the kidney was inflamed too. I know that because I have seen it.   Curious instances of mistakes due to this form of protective rigidity occur.   I saw a very stout woman in the country, who had been seen by a friend of mine, and he concluded that as she was rigid in the abdominal wall on the right side and it was very tender, she must have acute appendicitis.   It was a fair assumption to make as the pain was in the right side.   It was clear she had intra-abdominal inflammation, and the pain and tenderness and rigidity were all in the right place for that condition.   I was a little more cautious, because I had not seen that inflamed appendix. All I said was that she had some inflamed structure on the right brim of the pelvis, and that as her temperature was continuously high, and her pulse had become increasingly rapid and she had rigors, it was clear that unless she had something done she would probably die.   The moment she was placed under an anæsthetic a tumour was felt with a line of resonance between it and the right crural arch. Also we could feel the rounded margin of the tumour.   My next question to the medical man was, " Has she any uterine fibroids ? "   I thought she might have some uterine fibroids which had become septic.   He said, " No, I am sure she has not." I said, " Then she must have a twisted or suppurating ovarian cyst." Her abdomen was opened, and it was found that she had a suppurating ovarian cyst, which was

bulging the right broad ligament. It was very fixed and exceedingly difficult to remove.   Clearly in that case the cautious inference was the right one. When you encounter muscular rigidity remember it sometimes protects malignant growths.   What is the common course of malignant growth in the alimentary tract? First ulceration of the malignant growth, then sepsis from the intestinal contents, and then extension of septic inflammation to the visceral and parietal peritoneum, and to the abdominal wall, with the formation of abscess.   The abdominal abscess may be opened by a thoughtless person, who may be surprised to find a fæcal leak which will never heal.   Therefore, when a person has a rigid area do not merely say it is due to septic inflammation pure and simple, such as from an appendix or from some other organ.   You ought to weigh all the possibilities very carefully, and you may ultimately conclude that it is perfectly true you have to do with septic inflammation of the peritoneum, but behind that septic inflammation you may find carcinoma of the colon, such as we saw the other day in the operating theatre, or of the pylorus, or of some part of the alimentary tract.

My time has come to an end.   This is a very great topic.   Supposing you are brought into contact with a very chronic and mild case of intra-abdominal inflammation, I think the issue is easy. You put the case to bed and give it a period of probation.   But the more fulminating cases are more difficult to manage.   You will have to decide quickly whether the inflammation is increasing or diminishing.   If it is diminishing, the pulse and temperature and leucocytosis will fall and the local symptoms also will diminish.   I so often observe that gentlemen do not know how to tell whether the local area of rigidity and tenderness is diminishing or not.   If there is any question about it, place the tip of your finger on the abdominal wall where the local tenderness is and give a sharp prod with the tip of your finger at one place.   The patient will perhaps say that does not hurt him.   Move it about an inch away and do the same, and he will perhaps say it does hurt.   Then draw your line round the area of tenderness as ascertained in that way.   Next day you will be able to judge accurately whether the tenderness is an inch or two less, or whether it has spread beyond the line.   There you have a determinant symptom.   Simultaneously the pulse rate and the temperature will rise.   Supposing the patient vomits extensively, you have a determinant symptom. Or if no passage of wind has taken place, you have a determinant symptom; and I think, instead of taking days as your period of probation in order to ascertain the progress or otherwise of the case, you should take a few hours only. If the patient is getting worse, you will have some determinant symptom to tell you so, and that will be your guide as to whether there should be operation or not.

You may have observed in the two lectures I have given you that I have not mentioned any details of operative surgery. My reasons for this omission are simple. To order an operation in the case of grave abdominal disease is very much the same as ordering a dose of medicine, and upon my word it often requires just as much general knowledge and as much trained judgment to order a dose of calomel for a person with serious abdominal disease as it does to order an exploratory incision. As regards you gentlemen, you will see plenty of operations performed, and my advice to you is to give the greatest possible care and attention to that which goes before the operation and to that which comes after it—that is to say, the preliminary diagnosis and the subsequent treatment.

January 29th, 1906.

Fever during Menstruation as Early Sign of Tuberculosis.

—Franck announced four years ago that a rise in temperature preceding or during menstruation is a strong presumptive sign of a morbid process somewhere in the body. It points especially to tuberculosis, and if the woman is anæmic and thin, with a tendency to sweat and to catch cold readily, the physician will do well to inaugurate antituberculosis treatment or to recommend a sanatorium, superfeeding or a course of cinnamic acid or iron and arsenic. He is convinced that the normal limit of the temperature is $37 \cdot 5°$ C. ($99 \cdot 5°$ F.), measured in the rectum, and that even a fraction of a degree above this is fever. Sabourin and Kraus have also recently pointed out the importance of fever during menstruation as an early sign of tuberculosis. Measured in the rectum, a fraction of a degree above normal may be due to the hyperæmia of some inflammatory affection in the adnexa, but, if such can be excluded, then the assumption is in favour of tuberculosis.—*Journ. A. M. A.*, vol. xlvi, No. 1.

THREE LECTURES

ON THE

SYMPTOMS AND TREATMENT OF GOUTINESS.*

By LEONARD WILLIAMS, M.D., M.R.C.P.,
Physician to the French Hospital ; Assistant Physician to the Metropolitan Hospital.

LECTURE I.

GOUTINESS is a sufficiently common and sufficiently well understood term, but, inasmuch as it is also a very elastic one, I must begin by explaining the limitations which in these lectures I intend to apply to it. In dealing with common ailments, I have endeavoured, as far as possible, to avoid treating of subjects which are adequately noticed in the text-books, and to this rule I intend to adhere in dealing with goutiness. First of all, then, we must exclude acute articular gout and those forms of subacute gout, such as tophaceous, as are usually described, for I have nothing to say on these subjects which has not already been well said. Neither need we employ our time in considering such conditions as renal and hepatic calculus. These are, in many cases at any rate, truly gouty in origin, but then they are also in the nature of classical complaints whose symptoms, diagnosis, and treatment are fully set forth in the text-books. With these exceptions, the whole field of troubles caused by the gouty diathesis is open to us, but I may as well say at once that I do not propose to try and exhaust it. I shall, however, endeavour to include the most important points, and shall seek to lay stress upon those which seem to me to require emphasizing.

In considering any question connected with gout, one is immediately brought face to face with the numerous and very divergent theories which have been expressed by very competent observers on the subject of its causation, and one finds oneself forced to confess that very little is really known concerning it. Fortunately, however, that does not prevent us from obtaining a very fair working estimate of it from a clinical standpoint, nor from being able to treat it with a measure of success. Gout, it is generally agreed, is due to

* Delivered at the Medical Graduates' College and Polyclinic.

insufficient or perverted metabolism, leading either to the formation of material which is foreign to the healthy economy or to the inadequate discharge of normal excreta. Whichever of these views is correct matters nothing for our purpose; what we have to realise is that there is a something circulating in the blood which, in its endeavours to escape, may project itself, so to speak, upon any organ or tissue, and that the form which the gouty manifestation will assume will depend upon the organ or tissue selected. What determines that selection in any particular case it is quite impossible to say. Thus, the "something" may project itself into the neighbourhood of joints, causing a chronic gouty arthritis; it may project itself into the sheaths of nerves causing a gouty neuritis; it may project itself on to the integument to cause a gouty eczema, a gouty psoriasis, and, what is contrary to general belief, a furunculosis. It may attack the air-passages to cause pharyngitis, laryngitis, bronchitis, or asthma; it may find its way to the stomach and cause dyspepsia; it may select the brain and give rise to irritability, somnolence, and disinclination for work; it may provoke a cystitis and, according to some, even a urethritis. There is, in fact, no part of the body which can be said to be free from the liability to invasion by the gouty poison,* and fortunate indeed is he who, being obliged to suffer manifestations of the diathesis in any situation, suffers them in some painful and easily recognisable shape rather than in the painless, insidious, but far more inexorable, forms of arteriosclerosis and kidney-disease.

The main thing, then, to remember about gout is not to forget it. In the presence of a disturbance of any sort in any part of the body it is wise to ask ourselves the question, "Is this due to gout?" Many of us who do not forget the question are, perhaps, too liable on insufficient grounds to answer it in the affirmative, but such an attitude is less liable to lead to disaster than omission to remember it. The points upon which a correct answer to such a question depends are too numerous to enter into here. They involve such matters as heredity, habits, aspect, slight manifestations in other organs, and the like, which can in reality be acquired only by clinical observation and experience. There are, nevertheless, some points in connection with the condition of which the most experienced may profitably remind himself, some of which we will now briefly consider.

Gouty symptoms are rare before middle life, and when that period is reached they are commoner in those whose youth has been athletic. Our national pride in outdoor sports might well be tempered by the consideration that the habit of body which these sports engender is very apt to lead to gout in those who, having once indulged in them, are ultimately condemned to a sedentary existence. The boy is father of the man, and the man is apt to suffer if he is unable to continue the catabolic activity to which the boy has accustomed the organism. It is said that women do not suffer from gout. This is true only in so far as acute "big-toe" gout is concerned; for women certainly suffer very frequently from irregular gout, especially in the form of headache, neuralgia, and bronchitis, and, after the menopause, they exhibit a very decided tendency to conform to the types, such as chronic arthritis, skin affections, and dyspeptic troubles, which are so common in men.

The chief cause of gout, in whatever form it may appear, is want of balance between intake and output. Either the intake is too great or the output is too small. Not infrequently both factors are in operation. So far as the intake is concerned the excess is not necessarily one of quantity. Meat foods and alcohol, even when taken in what is usually considered moderation, by a predisposed person leading an inactive life, are very powerful producers of gout; and in the same way a man who takes a great deal of exercise may be very gouty if he indulges too freely in the pleasures of the table. The discovery of a gouty manifestation, then, immediately provides two cardinal indications: the one is to check the source of the poison, the other is to aid and hasten its elimination. The first of these is met by prescribing and insisting upon a suitable dietary, the second, by increasing metabolism, and invoking the active aid of all the emunctories.

In the matter of diet the most important point is the reduction of the alcoholic drinks. Beers and wines in contra-distinction to spirits are often spoken of as peculiarly productive of gout. It is, no doubt, true that the beer-drinker is more liable to gross and obvious forms of the malady than the spirit-drinker, but to argue from this that spirits are harmless to a goutily-disposed person is to play

---

* *Totum corpus est podagra.*—SYDENHAM.

the part of the ostrich. Spirit-drinking, though it may not provoke arthritis or eczema, is in the highest degree calculated to cause arterial degeneration and granular kidneys, and these, though less strikingly, are no less truly gouty in origin than the others. That spirits, not being productive of gout, are therefore harmless and even "wholesome" to gouty people is a heresy which would be ridiculous were it not so pernicious, and no words of condemnation are too strong for him who aids in its dissemination. Alcoholic drinks of all sorts are in the highest degree harmful to the goutily-inclined, and the larger the percentage of the contained alcohol, the greater is the harmfulness of the beverage. The first thing to do, then, with a gouty person is to make him, if you can, into a teetotaler. Impress upon him the "ostrich" view of the question, and bring home to him that it is practically impossible to check the manufacture of an article except by stopping the supply of the raw material. It is said that some light wines have very little influence in provoking or maintaining the gouty state. This may be so, though I do not believe that it is. I have had opportunities from time to time of sampling some of them, and each recalled more forcibly than the last a story which used to be told about a distinguished statesman who was much afflicted with gout. To him a firm of wine-growers sent a parcel with a letter assuring him that the accompanying wine would "cure" his gout The parcel, from one bottle of which a small quantity had been taken, was shortly returned, with the following note : "Lord D— presents his compliments to Messrs. C— and begs to return the parcel of wine the consumption of which was to have cured his gout. Lord D— prefers the gout."

If we have, happily, succeeded in making the gouty patient into a teetotaler, our next endeavour should be to convert him into something approaching a vegetarian ; for, after alcoholic drinks, the ingestion of meat foods takes the highest place in the production of the malady. In the times of our forefathers there was a saying that the gouty patient should have three meals a day, "one of fish, one of flesh, and one of neither." This may be a useful formula for a recalcitrant patient whom we are trying to persuade into the paths of physiological righteousness ; but it is far, indeed, from being a counsel of perfection. The three meals of a person with definite manifestations of goutiness

in any form (I am not now referring to such as are merely goutily disposed) should consist of one of fish or flesh and two of neither. Even the one of fish or flesh represents, in my judgment, a concession which we are frequently obliged to make to the weaker brethren, for the less nitrogenous food of animal origin which a patient can be induced to take, the more rapidly and the more completely will he get rid of his troubles. There are, of course, nitrogenous foods *and* nitrogenous foods, and there seems no doubt whatever that those which, roughly speaking, are obtained without the sacrifice of life are less deleterious to gouty people than those which entail such sacrifice. For instance, milk, cheese, eggs, and the pulses (peas, beans, and lentils), though rich in nitrogen, are, compared to flesh—poultry, fish, and game—very poor in the constituents which help in the elaboration of the gouty poison. It is from the former, then, that the gouty patient should be encouraged to draw his nitrogenous supplies, and it should be made clear to him that in the presence of a manifestation, however slight, the latter will prolong the attack and militate against the action of remedial measures.

It used formerly to be believed that sugar was productive of gout. Although this is now very generally recognised as fallacious, there seems to be some measure of truth in it, inasmuch as sweets are very liable to upset the stomachs of gouty people. This they do more especially when introduced into that organ without having been thoroughly insalivated. Gouty people who are afflicted with a "sweet tooth," as the saying is, should therefore be warned against indulging it unduly ; and it should be explained to them how they may indulge it with the best prospect of doing so with impunity—namely by efficient mastication.

Another question, closely connected with diet, which has been engaging a considerable degree of attention during the last few years, is the part played by common salt in what we may call the indirect causation of many morbid conditions which are associated with faulty metabolism and insufficient excretion. It has been recognised since 1850 that the chlorides are retained in the body during acute illnesses, to be discharged *en masse* as soon as convalescence sets in. It has also been known for a long time that œdematous fluid contains a very large percentage of common salt, which is excreted by the kidneys as soon as the œdema disappears. Another fact which has been recognised for some time is that the amount of NaCl contained in the blood itself is always the same under all normal circumstances quite irrespectively of the amount ingested—that is to say that if more is ingested the surplus is immediately excreted. Now, Widal [*] has shown that in many conditions which are associated with renal inadequacy, of which goutiness may be taken as a type, that inadequacy first shows itself by an undue retention of chlorides. The common salt passes out of the blood-vessels into the tissues. Here it attracts to itself fluids, and œdema is the result. This œdema is at first visceral and deep-seated, so that clinically it is not easy to detect except by careful comparison of the patient's weights. And, as one would suppose, among the first of the viscera to be attacked are the kidneys. They become œdematous and, consequently, to their inadequacy in the matter of chlorides there is superadded a general inadequacy. Thus it is that chlorides, though not poisonous in themselves, very easily lead to the retention of other matters, and of these other matters many are highly toxic. Widal has, in fact, shown that in kidney affections uræmic symptoms may be provoked or suppressed at will by largely increasing or greatly diminishing the amount of common salt ingested. Now, in view of these facts it is obvious that chloride of sodium constitutes a very grave potential danger to the goutily disposed, and we should be particularly careful to warn them against the habit of adding large quantities of salt to their food. For the same reason highly salted foods such as bacon and sea fish are better avoided, and those natural mineral waters which contain large quantities of NaCl (and a great many of them do) should not be recommended as habitual laxatives. Widal's work teaches us a further lesson of importance, namely that the amount of chlorides in the urine offers a very fair gauge of the functional renal capacity of the patient, thus helping us to a very early diagnosis of renal inadequacy.

Having by these dietetic regulations so arranged matters that the supply of the poison shall as far as possible be checked, our next care is to aid in

* 'La Presse Médicale,' June 29th, 1903, and 'Compt. Rend. Soc. Biolog.,' 1904; see also 'Treatment,' August, 1903, and an article in 'Practitioner,' August, 1905, by J. H. Bryant.

the disposal of that which has been already formed. To this end a vigorous appeal must be made to all the excretory organs to aid in ejecting the invader. Now, it is to be remembered that no appeal to the excretory organs is ever successful which is not accompanied by a liberal supply of fluid. An abundance of water is necessary to the action of each and all of them, and to ask them to excrete poisons without fluid is to ask them to make bricks without straw. It is said by those who wish to belittle the spa treatment of gouty conditions that this treatment is successful only because of the large quantities of fluid which the patients are made to consume. It is not necessary to give adherence to this suggestion in order to learn a lesson from it. If the ingestion of large quantities of water, as water, is beneficial at health resorts, it should be equally beneficial at home ; and certain it is that if a gouty patient can be induced to take, say, from two and a half to three pints of H_2O in the twenty-four hours, he is materially aiding his recovery in a most essential particular.

So much being established, let us see when and how the water is to be taken. First and foremost it should be taken before meals, and not with, or after meals. Half a pint may be taken half an hour before breakfast, about half a pint at 11 a.m., the same quantity half an hour before luncheon and again at 4 30 p.m., before dinner another similar amount, and before bedtime a full pint. This is a large quantity, but if all the excretory organs are to be kept working vigorously, it is not too much. The question of how the water is to be taken, whether hot or cold, whether plain or with additions, must be left to individual tastes and peculiarities to decide. Some people will take water hot when they will not take it cold ; some will take water in which tea has been infused or to which some fresh lemon-juice has been added when they will not take it plain ; others, again, will attach virtues to a water poured from a bottle which they will deny to that which is drawn from a tap. These are largely matters of fancy on the part of the patient and of diplomacy on the part of the doctor ; the only suggestions on the subject which I have to make are that still waters are preferable to sparkling waters, and that lightly mineralised waters are preferable to those which are strongly charged. Inasmuch as fresh lemon-juice is believed by some observers whose opinion is entitled to respect to have a beneficial influence upon some, at any rate, of the gouty manifestations, it is well to encourage its use, for even if it has no other merit—and, as will appear presently, I am one of those who believe that it has—it can certainly claim to render the dose more palatable.

Of drugs which possess a general influence in aiding the elimination of the gouty poison, iodide of potassium stands pre-eminent. There is no gouty manifestation which does not yield in a large measure to its intelligent employment. And by intelligent employment I mean its association with other drugs or measures specially directed against the particular manifestation present. The mistake which is usually made in connection with it is fear of large doses. The B. P. initial dose of two grains is much too small. If the drug is given at all, it should be given in doses which commence at ten grains; and, curious though it may seem, the larger quantity is infinitely less liable to produce coryza and the other symptoms of iodism than the smaller. If there is any suggestion of a rash appearing in consequence of its administration, a few drops of Fowler's solution added to the mixture readily prevents further trouble.

Another drug which is very valuable in counteracting the gouty poison, and one which resembles iodide of potassium in the fact that the exact nature of its working is still hidden from us, is guaiacum. The two may very suitably be given together in cachet form:

R. Pulv. guaiaci ⎫
　　Potass. iodide āā grs. x. ⎰ M. ft. cachet.

　　Sig.: One, three times daily.

If the guaiacum causes purging, the dose must be reduced, or five or ten grains of creta præp. added to each cachet. In any case, the cachet should be followed by a draught of water. It is not desirable to give guaiacum in a mixture. Patients readily rebel against it on account of its unpleasant taste and objectionable consistence.

The salicylates, while regarded by some writers as excellent remedies in gouty conditions, are loudly condemned by others, notably in France. The objections urged against the salicylates, especially that of soda, are that they are depressing, and that they have an irritating effect upon the kidneys. There may be some truth in this, but my personal experience with aspirin (grs. x to xx) has so far been quite favourable. It is, however, well

to remember the renal charge which is, on the Continent, very actively brought against it. Many people complain that the salicylates are inert. When this is true, it will usually be found that they have been combined with alkalies, and I find, in point of fact, that the combination of salicylate of soda and bicarbonate of soda is a very favourite one. When salicylates are given they should be prescribed either alone or in conjunction with such a drug as nux vomica, which does not influence their chemical medium, for in the body they play the part of acids, and it is in virtue of this part that they do good.

Another acid whose virtues in the gouty state have recently been attracting considerable attention on the Continent is phosphoric acid. According to the experiments of Joulie,* it would seem that gouty manifestations are due to the retention in the blood of matters whose escape is favoured, not by alkalies, but by acids, and the acid which he has fixed upon as most potent in this connection is phosphoric acid. I believe there is a large measure of truth in his contentions; at any rate, I have been successful in giving relief with dilute phosphoric acid where iodide of potassium and guaiacum had failed me.

Citric acid, in the form of lemon-juice, has often been lauded in the management of the gouty diathesis. This drug, when taken in large doses, say half an ounce in the course of the day, undoubtedly renders the blood more fluid by dissolving out the calcium salts. What it does with these salts is a matter which I understand still awaits investigation; at any rate, they disappear from the blood, thus rendering the fluid more mobile and better fitted for its purpose of bathing and flushing the various tissues, and so promoting efficient excretion. I believe citric acid to be a most useful general corrective to the gouty tendency.

January 29th, 1906.

* "L'Acidité Urinaire," par M. H. Joulie, 'Revue Générale de Chimie,' Paris, 1901; see also " La Médication Phosphorique," Dr. Jean Nicolaidi, Paris, Octave Doin, 1904.

MAYER reiterates that sixteen years of experience with Pirogoff's method of treating erysipelas have confirmed him more in his high opinion of it. He gives, every hour or second hour, '15 gm. triturated camphor, with hot drinks to promote sweating, and the usual external measures.—*Journ. A. M. A.,* vol. xlvi, No. 1.

CHRONIC DYSPEPSIA IN OLDER CHILDREN.

A Lecture delivered at the Hospital for Sick Children, Great Ormond Street, London.

By HUGH THURSFIELD, M.A., M.D.,

Assistant Physician to the Hospital, and to the Metropolitan Hospital.

GENTLEMEN, — Of the whole number of out-patients at this hospital above the age of two years I believe at least half are brought owing to a failure in the digestion of food and a consequent diminution in general health. A chronic indigestion is not in these children of the same serious importance as in the younger infants, for it does not lead to the atrophy of the mucous membrane of the digestive tract, which is the cause of the fatality in infants ; but, on the other hand, it stunts their growth, renders them liable to a number of diseases which a more healthy child would escape, and causes an amount of suffering which it is hard to estimate.

The causes of the condition are varied. That which is most obvious, and most easily remedied, is a carious condition of the teeth. The teeth of the children of large towns in this country are deplorably bad, and habitual neglect of them adds in many cases to the original evil. The causes of the inherent deficiency in the teeth I will leave to the dental surgeons to explain, merely mentioning here that rickets and malnutrition in infancy have much to do with the future condition of the teeth in childhood. But it would matter comparatively little if the teeth were merely decayed ; when they are neglected in addition there is an accumulation of foul and putrid material in the mouth, which has a most harmful effect upon the tissues and functions of the digestive tract.

In the next place associated with the chronic indigestion is a chronic hypertrophy and catarrh of the lymphatic tissues of the fauces and pharynx. Sometimes one is tempted to believe that this condition is brought about chiefly by the neglect of the teeth and gums, and the consequent slow poisoning of the lymphatic tissues, but in other cases it appears that these tissues are themselves deficient in powers of resistance, and that the hypertrophy of the tonsils and follicles arises from causes with which we are not as yet familiar. I need only remind you in this connection of those cases of sudden death in well-fed and well-developed infants, in whom is found at the post-mortem examination hypertrophy of the lymphatic structures throughout the body. Whatever the immediate cause of the hypertrophy, it is certain that it is found in association with chronic indigestion in a large number of cases, and that attention to the improvement of the condition is a chief factor in successful treatment. But the main cause of indigestion in these children is certainly unsuitable feeding. Among the children of the well-to-do the food is often too rich, and too little care is exercised both as to the quantity and the regularity of the meals. In out-patients at the hospital there is more usually a deficient quality of food, and an excess of carbohydrates, while at the same time tea and sugar form an additional portion of the diet, taken in the intervals of the more regular meals.

However, when we have reviewed the possible causes of indigestion we are forced to recognise that there are a considerable number of children whose digestions are not normal—who cannot, that is, assimilate thoroughly the ordinary materials of a healthy child's diet—and it is in these cases that the greatest difficulty is found in treatment. It is no longer the custom to talk of hereditary diathesis ; but in these children there are obscure metabolic processes which are not obviously related to the physical conditions or to the nature of the food, and though we do not now speak of the gouty or scrofulous diathesis, it is necessary to recognise that there are conditions, both hereditary and acquired, as, for instance, following diphtheria or typhoid fever, of which we cannot even guess the causes.

Leaving these speculations, we must study the clinical symptoms of children who are the subjects of indigestion, and here we are confronted by manifestations of the most varied character. One symptom alone is constant, and that is the failure to grow, or, in the usual words of the mother, the failure of the child to "get on." The children are always thin and wasted, their muscular development poor, their skins dry and harsh, and usually show a considerable degree of anæmia. They are often round-shouldered, with flattened chest and protuberant abdomens ; they are easily fatigued, both physically and mentally ; they are drowsy by day and restless and sleepless by night ; their appetite is capricious, at times ravenous, at others there is absolute anorexia. Their bowels are sometimes perfectly regular and normal, more often irregular, with alternate diarrhœa and constipation. In some cases there is a large quantity of mucus passed in the stools, a point to which I shall recur. So much for a general picture of the disease : some particular symptoms must be described in greater detail.

In the first place one is often told by the mothers that the children have "fits" of pallor, or "fainting fits" as they are sometimes called. The child does not lose consciousness, but quite suddenly turns white and is collapsed for some seconds and then slowly regains his natural colour. What these attacks are it is impossible to say, but it has been suggested that they are closely related to epilepsy, and are the result of a general vaso-motor disturbance originating in the cerebral centres. Apart from their general significance they are not of great consequence, but it is important to realise that they do not imply any lesion of the heart, although in some cases the heart rhythm is found to be irregular and the cardiac area of dulness slightly increased. The mention of epilepsy brings to mind the fact that sufferers of *petit mal* are not infrequently the subjects of indigestion, the chief symptom in their case being a sudden attack of abdominal pain, occasionally accompanied by vomiting, but more often not. In cases, therefore, where attacks of abdominal pain occur at frequent intervals, still more when they occur in groups, it is well to remember that they may be merely manifestations of *petit mal*. Abdominal pain sometimes accompanies the "fits" of pallor, and sometimes occurs quite independently of any other symptom. Occasionally, no doubt, it is due to a spasm of the intestinal muscle, but more often it is probably of the nature of a chronic uneasiness, due to a distension of the intestinal tract, rather than to any acute spasm. On the whole pain is comparatively a rare symptom in these children. So also is vomiting. In the infant any gastro-intestinal disorder is apt to be accompanied by vomiting, but in the children of four to ten years whom I am considering one finds a very considerable degree of intestinal complaint without vomiting. If it does occur at all it is at long intervals. There is, however, a type of case, which was described some years ago by Dr. Gee, in which attacks of vomiting,

apart from all other symptoms of indigestion, recur at intervals ; the attacks are so severe as to endanger the life of the patient. To this disease the name "cyclic" vomiting has been assigned, and it is certainly a neurosis, not a gastric disorder.

Constipation is more frequent than diarrhœa ; the stools are large and offensive, and consist of scybalous masses, often with portions of undigested food. Attacks of diarrhœa occur at intervals, and both in the case of diarrhœa and constipation it is not infrequent to find a large quantity of mucus, which is described by the parents as "jelly" or "slime." Dr. Eustace Smith has made a special category of these cases, to which he has given the name "the mucous disease." His theory is that in certain conditions the intestines and the mucous membranes generally are stimulated to an overproduction of mucus ; that this prevents digestion of food, promotes constipation, and provides a convenient breeding-place for the worms which are so often present in these patients. This theory serves to explain the appearance of some of the symptoms, but in many cases of chronic indigestion there is no evidence of the presence of an excess of mucus.

When there is diarrhœa it often occurs in a peculiar fashion. One will be told that the child can never eat any food without at once having a loose motion. The nervous and muscular mechanism of the intestines is in so irritable a condition that the presence of food in the stomach at once sets up peristalsis in the intestine, with the result that the food is hurried through in an undigested state, and no doubt tends to increase the irritability of the mucous membrane. This form of diarrhœa, which is not uncommon in children of from four to ten years, is called "lienteric diarrhœa." It is fortunately, as a rule, amenable to treatment, a small dose, 1 to 2 minims, of Fowler's solution, given three times a day, usually correcting the tendency at once. If Fowler's solution fails to produce the desired effect, recourse can be had to opium, bismuth, and an extremely restricted diet for fortyeight hours, in order to give as much rest as possible to the intestine.

In many of the cases of chronic indigestion there is at frequent intervals slight fever. Usually the temperature does not rise above 100°, but it is sufficient to render the child miserable and fretful and the parents anxious. More rarely the temperature may rise somewhat higher, and, together with the dry, furred tongue and the presence of some distension of the abdomen, give rise to a suspicion of an attack of typhoid fever. In such cases a calomel purge is often sufficient to dispel the suspicion, and it is a remedy which is perfectly safe in the first week of the febrile attack. But the more usual course of the fever is that it recurs at intervals, the child being noticeably more ill at these periods than in the intervening times.

Among the most marked symptoms of this complaint is the occurrence of an irritating cough, which is, one is often told, worst in the morning, but is always present. It is, of course, not directly due to the condition of the patient's digestion, being caused solely by the condition of congestion and hypertrophy of the lymphatic tissue of the pharynx, and it is hardly worthy of much notice, except that it often leads to errors in diagnosis, and is regarded by many parents as an index of the ability of the doctor; if it improves under treatment, the doctor will be given the opportunity of proceeding with the cure of the indigestion ; if it persists, the child will be hurried off elsewhere.

But I have probably indicated sufficiently the chief symptoms of the complaint, and I must say a few words about diagnosis. The most frequent mistake, both among doctors and parents, is to regard the children who are merely suffering from chronic indigestion as victims of tuberculosis of the lungs. It is easy to see how the mistake arises ; the wasting, the cough, the ease with which the child sweats, the lassitude, and the general restlessness and irritability are all symptoms which are met with in "consumption"; and there is often sufficient catarrh in the respiratory passages to mislead the doctor who is not on his guard. The slight attacks of fever are also a further support to the suspicion. In the majority of cases a careful examination of the lungs will reassure the doctor, and he will be able to remove the parents' doubts. A sign which is of the greatest importance in the early diagnosis of pulmonary tuberculosis is the limitation of movement of the sub-clavicular region on one side, or its lagging behind the opposite side. This is best appreciated when one stands behind the child and watches the breathing with the forefingers of the two hands placed upon the clavicles. If the lagging is detected, a more minute comparison of the two

sides by means of percussion and auscultation will often reveal confirmatory signs, such as slight impairment of the percussion note, or crepitant râles after a cough or deep breath. But even where one finds reason to suspect the existence of a lesion at one apex, it is wise to suspend sentence until you have had a second opportunity of examining the patient after he has been under treatment for indigestion for a fortnight. The second examination should be made, if possible, unbiassed by the first, and if the former results are confirmed the suspicion of tuberculosis becomes almost a certainty. I may say here, in parenthesis, that personally I have been able to obtain no help from the use of X rays in these cases. If one takes these precautions, one finds that the number of cases which are said to be tuberculous is enormous, but that those in which that diagnosis is ultimately made are very few. With the exception of pulmonary tuberculosis, there is no other disease which is closely simulated by chronic indigestion. Occasionally a doubt arises as to whether there may not be a tuberculous peritonitis, but abdominal examination, as a rule, quickly settles the point.

Prognosis is as a rule good ; it is usually possible to correct the varied mistakes which have been made, and in a comparatively short time to re-establish the health of the patient. In a few instances treatment must be continued over many months ; but the only thing which will cause any real anxiety will be the intercurrence of some infective disorder, which, acting on a constitution weakened by the prolonged malnutrition, may run a more dangerous course than it otherwise would tend to do.

The general principles of treatment are quite clear : the first indication is the removal of possible causes of the complaint—e. g. carious teeth or chronically inflamed tonsils ; next, attention to clothing, ventilation, regularity of habits, and sufficiency of sleep and exercise ; and, thirdly, the careful regulation of the diet and of the functions of the bowel. With regard to the first two points I have nothing especial to say, except that the physician must never forget that fresh air and exercise are of even greater importance to the growing child than to the adult. With regard to diet it will suffice to lay down a few general principles, and to elaborate these for each individual patient. It is probable that a considerable number of the cases of chronic indigestion are due to the irregular and injudicious meals allowed by the parents, and to the habit, almost universal at the present day, of sweet-eating. Among the poorer classes in London the extent to which sweets and sugary confections have displaced the more ordinary foods is remarkable. A child who is unable to consume any breakfast is given a halfpenny by its mother and buys sweets, with the aid of which it proceeds to destroy any appetite it would have acquired for its dinner. A prolonged indulgence in this habit leads to chronic indigestion in a severe form. With the children of the better class sweet biscuits, rich pastry, jams, and chocolates often form too large a portion of the diet. The first requisite, therefore, in treatment is to forbid absolutely sweets, rich cakes, sweet biscuits, chocolates, and similar dainties, not only between the meals, but even at the meals. Such articles must be reserved for rare occasions. Secondly, nothing must be taken between meals, unless it be a cup of milk. Thirdly, new bread, potatoes, pickles, fried fish, and the coarser kinds of vegetable must be forbidden, and lastly, all meals must be taken at stated and regular intervals. There is often some difficulty experienced in suggesting a diet and a number of meals appropriate to a child of a given age, but it may be broadly laid down that after two years of age the number of meals should not exceed four in the day, and that the material should consist largely of milk and milk-products, such as rice-pudding, etc., with the addition of other articles according to the age of the child. Except for special reasons meat should not be given more than once in the day. Thus, for a child of about six years of age the meals should be at 8 a.m., at 12 noon, at 4 p.m., and at 7 p.m., and of these the only large meal should be that at mid-day, while the last meal should be nothing more than milk or bread-and-milk. Now, in severe cases of chronic indigestion it may be necessary to modify this diet in both directions, to give the meals more frequently, of course in smaller quantities, and to remove practically all farinaceous food from the diet for a time, using milk, eggs, cooked fruit, and meat and fish, with a very little toast or stale bread. But in the majority of instances abandonment of the richer and more complex articles of food is sufficient in itself.

Having thus regulated the diet, and taken the first step towards restoring the injured organs to their natural functions by giving them only the simplest work to do, one can proceed to attempt to give assistance by the use of drugs. And in chronic indigestion drugs are of the greatest possible value. Whether Dr. Eustace Smith's theory of the mucous origin of the symptoms be true or not, it is quite certain that the treatment founded on the theory is of great service. An alkali, with a few minims of tincture of nux vomica, given before meals, will serve to stimulate gastric digestion, and to give an appetite. Or, if it be preferred, a similar remedy can be given in the form of a powder, consisting of sodium bicarbonate and bismuth. Whether there is constipation or not, it is further advisable, at any rate in the initial stages of the treatment, to give aperient medicine, either in the form of rhubarb, or senna, or one of the aperient salts. In many cases instead of the alkali an acid mixture with a little arsenic or tinct. ferri perchloridi will be found to be as efficacious as the alkali, though the administration of iron should always be deferred until the bowels have been well opened and the tongue is clean. Another drug that is of well-proved value is mercury, used either in the form of grey powder or as calomel, and, personally, I believe that it is best to give the mercury in small repeated doses, and add to its effect by the use of salts. In those cases where the stools are large, whitish in colour, and offensive, calomel, given three times a day, with a morning dose of magnesium and sodium sulphates, usually quickly restores the intestine to its normal functions.

When the child's bowels are acting naturally and its tongue is clean, when the restlessness and irritability are lessening and its appetite returning, iron and cod-liver oil, or one of its substitutes, should be employed. Alcohol is an unnecessary drug in these disorders. I have only indicated here the broad outlines of treatment, but, in the majority of cases, nothing further will be required. Special symptoms, such as repeated vomiting or marked pain after meals, during the progress of digestion must be met by special measures adapted to the circumstances, but, fortunately, children's recuperative power is so great that these complications are rare. The text-books on children's diseases recount much that is of interest regarding the rarer disorders of gastric and intestinal digestion, but these also may be passed over at present. Lastly, it will be found that if in a particular case progress appears slow or unsatisfactory a visit to the country or to the seaside will often make an enormous difference to the child's general condition, a difference which is usually permanent

January 29th, 1906.

THE CLINICAL JOURNAL,

CLINICAL RECORD, CLINICAL NEWS, CLINICAL GAZETTE, CLINICAL REPORTER, CLINICAL CHRONICLE AND CLINICAL REVIEW.

EDITED BY L. ELIOT CREASY.

| No. 693. | WEDNESDAY, FEBRUARY 7, 1906. | Vol. XXVII. No. 17. |

CONTENTS.

NOTICE.

Editorial correspondence, books for review, &c., should be addressed to the Editor, 51, *New Cavendish Street, W., Telephone No.* 904, *Paddington ; but all business communications should be addressed to the Publishers,* 22½, *Bartholomew Close, London, E.C. Telephone* 927, *Holborn.*

All inquiries respecting Advertisements should be sent to MESSRS. ADLARD & SON, *Bartholomew Close, E.C. Telephone* 927, *Holborn.*

Terms of Subscription, including postage, payable by cheque, postal or banker's order (in advance) : for the United Kingdom, 15s. 6d. *per annum ; Abroad,* 17s. 6d.

Cheques, &c., should be made payable to THE PROPRIETORS OF THE CLINICAL JOURNAL, *crossed "The London, City, and Midland Bank, Ltd., Newgate Street Branch, E.C. Account of the Medical Publishing Company, Limited."*

Reading Cases to hold Twenty-six numbers of THE CLINICAL JOURNAL *can be supplied at* 2s. 3d. *each, or will be forwarded post free on receipt of* 2s. 6d. ; *and also Cases for binding Volumes at* 1s. *each, or post free on receipt of* 1s. 3d., *from the Publishers,* 22½ *Bartholomew Close, London, E.C.*

ON SOME COMMON SYMPTOMS OF DISEASE IN CHILDREN.

A Lecture delivered at the Hospital for Sick Children, Great Ormond Street, W.C.

By ROBERT HUTCHISON, M.D., F.R.C.P.,

Assistant Physician to the London Hospital.

LADIES AND GENTLEMEN,—On one or two previous occasions, when it has been my turn to lecture here, I have taken up some aspects of disease in children from what one may describe as the symptomatic standpoint ; that is to say, I have selected certain common symptoms, and then tried to make out what their diagnostic significance was. I believe that to be an exceedingly important way of treating a subject. It is essential for you to have your medical knowledge "indexed both ways " ; in other words, you should be able at examinations, given a certain disease, to tell what are its symptoms, and you should also be able at the bedside, given certain symptoms, to say what is the disease. The training which fits you to reply to the one set of questions does not always enable you to reply to the other. I make no apology, therefore, for taking up some more symptoms in the same manner and trying to arrive at an idea of their diagnostic value, and shall deal to-day with some symptoms relating to the alimentary system.

ABDOMINAL PAIN.

Abdominal pain is a very common symptom in children, and its cause is often difficult to determine, because if there be, as there often are, no objective signs of disease, you have very little to go upon in forming your diagnosis. A child is unable to tell you exactly where the pain is, when it comes on, what is its character, and so forth ; and hence you find lacking in children those guides to diagnosis which are often present in the case of abdominal pain in grown-up persons. There is all the more reason, therefore, why you should study carefully what the possible causes of abdominal pain are, so that you may proceed to your diagnosis by the method of exclusion.

The first thing I would remark about abdominal pain in childhood is that it may be due to causes which are outside the abdomen altogether. I would therefore group the first set of causes as *extra-abdominal*—that is to say, cases in which pain is referred to the abdomen, although its site of production does not really lie in the abdominal cavity at all. One fairly common example of such an extra-abdominal cause of pain is *spinal caries*. The pain of spinal caries, travelling along the intercostal nerves, is very often referred by the child to the epigastrium, and the first piece of advice I would give you is, that when pain is complained of in the epigastrium, you should never omit carefully to examine the vertebral column for signs of disease. Another extra-abdominal cause of pain is *pleurisy*. Dry pleurisy is not common in children, but when it does occur the child often refers the pain to the pit of the stomach. It may therefore be necessary, in order to exclude this cause, to examine the bases of the lungs carefully for friction sounds, because it is only when the pleurisy is of the dry variety that sufficient pain is produced to give rise to symptoms. Another possible cause of pain referred to the abdomen, but really due to causes outside it, is *hip disease*. In a few cases the pain of hip disease is referred by the child to the iliac fossa, and you are apt to be misled, and to think you are dealing with appendix mischief or something of that sort, when all the time the seat of the trouble is in the hip. All these causes you may have to satisfy yourself as to the absence of, before you conclude that the pain is truly intra-abdominal in character. Before leaving this part of the subject I should mention that abdominal pain seems sometimes to be of *rheumatic* origin, although it is uncertain whether its seat in such a case be really intra-abdominal or merely in the abdominal wall. The pain comes on paroxysmally, starting usually below the costal margin on either side and lasting for a few minutes. There may be several such attacks in the course of the day, and after lasting for a few days they may culminate in acute rheumatism.

Passing now to the causes of abdominal pain which are due to disease inside the abdominal cavity, I would point out that pain of intestinal origin is certainly commoner in children than pain of gastric origin. In other words, any pain in the abdomen is more likely in a child to be due to something wrong with the intestine than to some disorder of the stomach. The reason is that children do not often suffer much from organic disease of the stomach. Functional dyspepsia, I need hardly say, they do suffer from to a great extent; but such organic diseases as ulcer or carcinoma of the stomach children do not exhibit, except in rare cases. Now, you know that functional dyspepsia does not give rise to severe pain; it causes discomfort, distension, sensations of sinking, and so on, but not real pain. With regard to intestinal pain, I should say that the most common cause of it is colic, in one or other form. Such intestinal pain is often very deceptive, for the reason that it may come on immediately after the taking of food. You will constantly see children—they are usually about five to ten years of age—who are brought with the complaint that there is pain in the abdomen which comes on immediately after eating and you will naturally think that the pain must be due to some condition in the stomach itself. But you must not allow yourselves to be deceived in that way, because it would seem that the entrance of food into the stomach often excites peristaltic contractions in the intestine, particularly perhaps in the colon, which contractions give rise in certain patients to a pain which is colicky in character. The most conspicuous example of such excitation of peristalsis in the large bowel is found in the case of lienteric diarrhœa. In that condition, as soon as the child takes food there is an immediate tendency for an action of the bowels to occur. The food has excited a peristaltic contraction in the colon, and that leads to defæcation. Similarly, in certain cases, the entrance of food into the stomach gives rise to contractions in the bowel, such as produce colicky pain. Sometimes a very small amount of food will cause it. I have even known cases in which the taking of a little milk gave rise to severe distress. The pain may be so severe, for instance, that the child has to rise from the table and lean against some hard object, such as the back of a chair, in order to get relief. Further, you will find that in many cases the kind of food that the child eats does influence the pain, that it is worse after eating hard and comparatively indigestible foods. I suppose that is because such bodies stimulate the interior of the stomach more powerfully than the blander forms of nourishment do and so give rise to more powerful reflex impulses. At any rate, all these things taken together—the fact that the pain comes on immediately after eating, and that it is influenced by the nature of the food—are apt to lead you into error, and make you think it cannot be pain of intestinal origin, but that it must be due to some disorder of the stomach. But I advise you not to be so deceived, and to remember the possibility that you are dealing with a purely intestinal pain. Another point about these intestinal colicky pains in children is that they frequently come on when the child walks quickly. Perhaps the commonest circumstance in which they come on is on hurrying off to school after breakfast; such a pain is usually referred to the right iliac fossa and may be so severe as to necessitate sitting down. I do not pretend to be able to explain why it is that exertion brings on pain of that sort, but I think most people suffer occasionally in that way, and must have experienced the fact that violent exertion, or even hurrying after a meal is apt to produce what is popularly called "a stitch in the side," usually on the right side, in the region of the cæcum.

Slight *chronic appendicitis* may be a cause of abdominal pain. The position of the pain will draw your attention to its possible cause. Appendicitis in childhood is by no means a common event. It does occur undoubtedly, but it is relatively not so common as it is in later periods of life, and the younger the child is the less likely is it that you are dealing with any form of appendicitis, and the more likely is it to be colic. In trying to confirm or exclude this cause you will have to palpate the appendix region with special care, and note whether there is a point of special tenderness between the umbilicus and the anterior superior spine on the right side—that is to say, over the site of the appendix. If you find there is a tender spot there, and particularly if the child has recurrent febrile attacks, your suspicion that it is appendicitis will have been confirmed.

Another cause of occasional pain in the intestines undoubtedly is the presence of *worms*, particularly, I think, of round worms. Now it would be a mistake to suppose that to be a common cause; still, one does every now and then meet with cases in which a child has suffered from intestinal pain,

often referred to the region of the umbilicus, in which relief has only been experienced after the passage of a round worm, either by the bowel or by vomiting. And I think one is bound to conclude that such a cause may account for the pain, and that the worms have sometimes acted in the way in which a lump of indigestible food would act.

Passing from these intestinal causes, one has to mention another possible source of abdominal pain which you are apt to overlook, namely pain which is produced in the *urinary tract*. By that I mean the pain which arises on the passage of uric acid or small stones down the ureters. The pain due to this cause may closely simulate intestinal colic. It comes on irregularly; it is referred usually, if the child be able to refer it to any spot, to the lateral region of the abdomen, and it often passes down into the groin. But in some cases all these aids may be absent, and it will be necessary for you to make a careful examination of the urine for the presence of uric or oxalic acid crystals, before you can exclude this cause of obstinate abdominal pain.

There remains, lastly, for consideration the pain that is of *gastric origin*. I will put a query against that on the board, because I am not certain whether pain of gastric origin occurs at all in childhood. Still, one does meet with cases where the results of treatment seem to show that the pain has been of this nature, cases in which the child has complained of pain, as a grown-up person does, a short time after food, perhaps one to two hours afterwards, and where the pain has been relieved by giving drugs which are directed to exert either a soothing effect upon the stomach or to neutralise hyperacidity. I had such a case not long ago in the person of a little girl who complained of pain in the stomach shortly after meals. Examination revealed nothing definite, but I treated her with carbonate of magnesia, and the pain at once disappeared. I think there is reason to suppose that such pain is due to the over-production of acid, just as may happen in an adult. But I believe such cases are uncommon in children, and in the majority of cases you will be wise to suspect that pain arising soon after meals is not of gastric but of intestinal origin, and inasmuch as colicky pains are more common, it is of their treatment that I wish more particularly to speak to-day.

The first thing to be done in dealing with intestinal colic is to see that the diet is adjusted in such a way as not to produce much fermentation in the intestine, and you should therefore see that the food does not contain those ingredients which tend to produce large quantities of gas—I mean such articles of food as are rich in cellulose, which is the source of marsh gas in the intestine.   You will therefore eliminate green vegetables, restrict or abolish the consumption of fruits, and limit all the starchy things in general, whilst you may have to increase the amount of animal food in the diet so as to compensate for the restrictions in other directions, and insure that the child is sufficiently nourished.   So much for the dietetic treatment.

Now, there is no doubt that some of those cases are aggravated, if not actually caused, by chilling of the abdomen.   It is always wise, therefore, to order that the child should wear a warm flannel abdominal binder.   Lastly, you will have to consider the question of drugs.   Many—perhaps, indeed, the majority—of these patients suffer from constipation.   Even when there is no apparent constipation it is advisable to begin the treatment by administering laxatives, and it is well to combine with these such drugs as belladonna or hyoscyamus which have the power of diminishing intestinal spasm.   I have found a combination of cascara and belladonna in the following form very useful : · fluid extract of cascara 5 to 10ɱ (the dose being graduated according to the condition of the bowel), tincture of belladonna 5ɱ, aromatic spirits of ammonia 15ɱ, syrup of ginger half a drachm, and peppermint-water to a couple of drachms. The child takes this dose three or four times a day, after meals.   You will find that the effect of a medicine of that sort is to cause a gentle laxative action, and in addition belladonna tends to prevent any griping, and with some such treatment as that you will, in the majority of your cases, meet with success.   Sometimes, however, you will find that the pains persist in spite of all you can do, and if you are face to face with a case of that sort you may be compelled to fall back upon opium.   Two grains of Dover's powder night and morning, or two grains three times a day if necessary, will be found sufficient in most cases to allay the pain. The disadvantage of opium is its constipating tendency, and the fact that it has often a depressing effect upon the digestion.   But it is curious that where opium is needed, and where it is doing good,

the constipating tendency is often in abeyance. The opium seems to act in such cases simply by relieving the irregular peristalsis and spasm of the bowel, and not by causing a cessation of the peristalsis altogether.

DYSPHAGIA.

I want now to pass on to speak briefly of another symptom, one which is far less common, though of considerable interest, and which will sometimes puzzle you and occasion you a good deal of trouble in practice ; that is, dysphagia in children.   Difficulty in swallowing is a subject which you do not read much about in books which deal with diseases of children, but you will find that it is not a very uncommon occurrence in little babies and in children up to, though not often beyond, the age of three. By dysphagia I mean a difficulty in carrying out the act of swallowing.   The mother will tell you that the child takes a mouthful of milk, and when it gets to the back of the throat it seems to lodge there, the child makes an abortive attempt at deglutition, but the milk comes back again out of the mouth, very little going down the throat. Your advice is sought as to the cause of this, and how it is to be put right.   The first thing to do in a case of this sort is to make sure that there is no mechanical obstruction in the throat.   The most common mechanical obstacles are *congenital adenoids*—which I have repeatedly known to cause difficulty in swallowing—and *cleft palate.* I saw, not long ago, a baby in whom this symptom was very well marked.   For a time it puzzled me.   I examined the throat by rather an indifferent light and I thought I saw nothing wrong, and I could not understand what the difficulty in swallowing was due to.   But next time the child was brought to me I had a better light and I saw that there was a bifid uvula.   I have no doubt that was a sufficient cause for the difficulty in swallowing in this case.   You will frequently find difficulty in swallowing in children who suffer from *mental deficiency.* The act of swallowing, like most other co-ordinated muscular acts, is acquired with difficulty by these children, and if you can see no local cause for the dysphagia you should bear in mind the possibility that you are dealing with a child who is mentally defective.   In older children you may find difficulty in swallowing result from *paralysis of the palate,* which may be one of the sequelæ of diphtheria.   It may also be seen in children in whom the throat is very irritable and congested, and where there is some enlargement of the tonsils. You may find in such a case that as soon as a crumb or anything solid gets into the child's throat it excites hawking and retching movements and the child cannot swallow it. Some of these cases are exceedingly troublesome, and I remember one in which the use of purely liquid food had to be persisted in so long that the child became rickety. In some cases difficulty in swallowing is due, I believe, to what one must describe as *perverseness* on the part of the child, or pure "cussedness." Many children who are accustomed to the bottle, especially if they have been allowed to have it too long, very much resent the transition to solid food, and they show their resentment by hawking and coughing, and spitting out any solid food which is given to them. I had a case in private the other day where the mother was very alarmed at this difficulty. The only plan in such circumstances is firmness, to insist again and again, no matter how often the food is rejected, on the child taking it. Sometimes you can overcome the difficulty by gradually increasing the consistence of the food ; you can begin by thickening milk with farinaceous material and get it gradually thicker, until it is practically solid. At any rate, I am sure that perseverance in such cases can always overcome the trouble.

VOMITING.

It will be convenient to consider this symptom (1) as it occurs in young babies, and (2) in older children. The commonest cause of vomiting in young babies is some error in feeding, a maladjustment of the food to the digestive power, the giving of too strong a milk mixture being the commonest. On the other hand, the mixture may be right in its proportions, but the vomiting is due to its fermenting in the stomach and producing acidity. The commonest cause of this is the use of a tube bottle. It is always well to bear in mind, however, that vomiting may be the sign of more serious disease, and one thing which you have to exclude early if you can is *congenital stenosis of the pylorus.* Congenital stenosis of the pylorus is a rare condition, but still it is probably commoner than is generally believed. It is doubtless often overlooked. It consists, as you know, of an overgrowth of the muscular and fibrous structure of the pylorus, leading to difficulty in passing on the stomach contents. Whether this malformation be the result of prolonged spasm is not known, but in a typical case the usual history is that there was little or no vomiting until the child was two weeks old, when vomiting began and has persisted ever since. You will find that all sorts of foods have been tried, that each food suited for a day or so, and that then the vomiting began afresh. You will find, further, that the vomiting is usually associated with constipation, and that, of course, there has been progressive loss of weight. When you examine the child there is usually no sign of organic disease other than distension of the abdomen, but if you are lucky you will be able to see what is the diagnostic sign, namely a wave of stomach peri-

stalsis, which begins below the left costal margin, and travels towards the umbilicus. The peristaltic wave often occurs in two portions separated by a sulcus, so that the stomach stands out like an hourglass. Sometimes, too, you can feel the thickened pylorus by pinching up the abdominal contents a little above and to the right of the umbilicus.

Intussusception is another possible cause of vomiting in infants and should always be thought of when the vomiting has come on suddenly.

Lastly, vomiting in young babies may be *symptomatic.* Some cases of meningitis, for instance, begin with vomiting, and so may the acute specific fevers.

(2) Passing now to the question of vomiting as it occurs in older children, here again the symptomatic causes are not to be lost sight of. The older the child the more likely is vomiting to be of symptomatic causation. ᐧ It occurs especially in febrile disorders, such as pneumonia and scarlet fever ; or it may occur at the onset of tuberculous meningitis or in cases of cerebral tumour or uræmia, and it may be necessary to look for the other signs of those conditions. Vomiting in older children may also be the result of *acute gastritis,* the so-called accidental dyspepsia. If the vomiting be periodic, you have to think of the possibility of *migraine,* which is not uncommon in children. A child will be brought to you who has "bilious attacks, " as the mother says, and you will often find that such a child is really the subject of migraine. Sometimes you have to deal, not with the typical form of the disease, but with "masked migraine," in which headache is not a prominent symptom, but where the chief symptom is vomiting. These cases are to be dealt with by removing all possible causes of cerebral strain, particularly correcting errors of refraction in the eyes, and by the habitual administration of aperients. Recurring gastritis may simulate migraine. In children who suffer from slight chronic gastritis one finds that every now and then, after a little chill or indiscretion of diet, the condition flares up into an acute or subacute attack. You will recognise such cases by the fact that they are nearly always febrile, the child has fever and a furred tongue, and these are generally absent in true migraine.

Lastly, there is the recurring periodic form of vomiting in nervous children which is termed *cyclical vomiting,* which can be recognised by its periodicity. It occurs at very regular intervals, is very little influenced by the kind of food the child takes, and will often go on even when the stomach is empty. Cases of this sort are not very common, but one meets with them every now and then, and they have to be treated by attention to the nervous system, the continued administration of bromides and aperients being perhaps the best method of dealing with them.

February 5th, 1906.

SURGICAL NEURASTHENIA,

WITH SPECIAL REFERENCE TO POST-OPERATIVE CASES.

A Lecture delivered at St. Thomas's Hospital.

By EDRED M. CORNER, M.A., B.C.Cantab.,
B.Sc., F.R.C.S.,

Surgeon to Out-patients, St. Thomas's Hospital; Assistant
Surgeon, Hospital for Sick Children, Great Ormond
Street; Consulting Surgeon, Wood Green
Hospital.

GENTLEMEN,—The object of this lecture is 'to bring more prominently into notice the subject of post-operative neurasthenia. The occurrence of neurasthenia as the result of disease or accident is now well known. But hitherto little or nothing has been said of its relation to operations. Considering the increasing amount of operative surgery done in modern times, the subject must and will become of greater importance in the future than it is at present. It is a curious fact that some of the most general and common results of injury and disease should have received so little attention. I propose to draw attention to one, the best name for which is "surgical neurasthenia."

Neurasthenia is a condition of exhaustion of the nervous system, which renders it susceptible to stimuli, both from within and without, to which it would not react if in a normal state. The way in which this exhaustion is produced may be briefly sketched. Every movement of the body is accompanied by some expenditure of nervous energy, the amount of energy expended varying with the character of the movements. For instance they may be passive, active, or resistance movements.* The more slowly they are performed the less the effect produced on the nervous system. Thus when employing physical exercises to improve the health, slow movements are always used at first. Quick movements cause a far greater loss of energy. Hence it may be laid down as an axiom that slow movements affect the muscles and quick ones affect the nervous system. The nervous expenditure in slow-moving animals is far less than in quick ones. Again, quick and slow actions of the mind influence the nervous system in a way similar to that in which the muscles do. Slow, stolid thinkers expend far less nervous energy than their more nimble-witted "nervous" brethren; so long as it is the healthy exercise of function no harm is likely to result. It is the unhealthy or improper exercise of function, such as the ecstatic and artistic emotions, which do the harm. It is not healthy thinking but unhealthy worry which brings about nervous break-down. Thus, this catastrophe is seen more frequently in the upper and educated classes than amongst the lower and less educated masses. The prolonged stress of worry, whether in the shape of disease or accident, on account of the vast output of nervous energy which it causes, is liable to produce the condition of neurasthenia.

To return to the surgical aspect of our subject, it is necessary to distinguish between the mental shock immediately consequent on an operation or accident and the more prolonged mental symptoms of neurasthenia. We know that every bodily action is accompanied by some nervous expenditure, just in the same way that every injury inflicted on living tissues, unless it kills them, excites within them the process of repair. The mental shock which follows immediately on an operation or accident may be justly compared to the healing of the wound. If the union takes place by first intention, the mental condition will pass away. On the other hand, should the mental repair not take place at once, or be deficient for the needs, then the symptoms will persist. Thus, the neurasthenia of surgical cases may be looked upon as examples of delayed psychical healing.

As instances of this condition I shall cite certain typical cases. For this purpose it is necessary to employ some classification. I shall divide the causes of "surgical neurasthenia" into three classes—those consequent upon injury, operation and disease.

The first class, in which the nervous condition is consequent upon injury, is the one which is best known, and I shall give three illustrations of it. The first illustrates a condition which used to be called "railway spine," or "spinal concussion." The absurdity of the first name has become apparent now that we find the same malady following mishaps other than those which occur on a railway. Further, I shall endeavour to show that disease and operations may produce similar mental effects.

* See article "Physical Exercises," Clifford Allbutt's 'System of Medicine' (Macmillan), new edition, 1905, pp. 382–421.

Case of traumatic neurasthenia.—An Austrian citizen, æt. about 52 years, in June, 1903, was seated in a car on a Canadian railway when the train in which he was ran into another coming in the opposite direction—a kind of accident called a head-to-head collision in railway parlance. The cars were going at about twenty to twenty-five miles an hour, causing the trains to telescope for four feet. The man was seated at the back of his car, so receiving no direct shock from the accident. He was thrown on to the back of the seat in front, which he says was splintered. He did not lose consciousness, and crawled out of the *débris* without assistance. He was lame on account of a bruise on his left leg. In spite of this and other injuries he helped the other sufferers and, an hour later, walked home, a distance of about a quarter of a mile. That night he had company in his house, and stayed up later than usual. Next day he resumed his business, merely feeling that he had sustained "a bad jar." Some time later, as he found that he did not throw off these feelings, he consulted a doctor, who unfortunately told him that he had injured his spine, his left shoulder and tibia, his stomach, and his bowels. This verdict threw away the little healthy nervous capital he had left, and he quickly developed "diarrhœa-like pains in his stomach without passing stools." He improved under a course of gastro-intestinal antiseptics. When I saw him he complained that his left side was defective, he suffered from flatulence and eructations, unaccompanied by dyspepsia or sickness. His weight had fallen from 192 to 175 lb., he felt a stupor over him, felt shaky and tremulous, could not concentrate his mind nor finish a book which he was writing, he left the last half of his words unwritten, he slept badly, etc.

His speech was slow and stumbling, he wandered in his sense and lost his words. His gait was tottering, his handwriting bad. His back and spine, plus his left tibia, were tender, but not so when his attention was not directed to the examining hand. His abdomen was distended by gas. His tongue was furred and tremulous. His reflexes were exaggerated. There were no signs of any injuries to the bones. Under treatment, he slowly improved, and set about an action for obtaining damages from the railway company. A few months later he had improved in every way, finished his book, etc., but was still nervous, tremulous, and uncertain.

This case is typical of the so-called railway spine and of what was previously termed "spinal concussion." The man was not hurt badly at the time of the accident; his illness and troubles came on afterwards, and were perfectly genuine. His doctor's very depressing statement completely upset him and started the train of gastro-intestinal symptoms which formed so prominent a trouble later.

There are two further points about this type of case. First, the claimant for damages always makes a number of wild and foolish allegations. He does so because he estimates the importance of all events and sensations from the low level of a neurasthenic. Thus his conclusions show a complete want of mental perspective, and much of the matter given in his "pleadings" is nonsense. But this very nonsense may be a symptom of his mental state. Secondly, at the beginning his mind is worried about his injuries and his slow recovery from the accident. Next, he worries about his claim for damages, which retards his recovery greatly, so much só that, as medical men, we must often advise the companies to settle the claim at once. The patient's mind is relieved, and allows him to recover. Sometimes he recovers with such rapidity that, unless he was known beforehand, he must appear to be a malingerer. In the very case I have related to you the company refused the man's claim; and in consequence, although he had improved in all respects, fifteen months after the accident he was not well. Moreover, he won't be well until the claim is settled; the longer the delay, the more the company will have to pay.

My second example is an instance of a similar condition, the result of an accident, which did not take place on a railway.

A married woman, æt. between 30 and 40 years, about a year before she was seen, was thrown out of a dog-cart, hurting her back against the wheel. The injury was in the lumbar region, situated over the lower vertebral spines. At first there was paralysis of all four limbs, then she walked a few steps, after which she remained more or less paralysed for eight weeks. She was seen about a year after the accident, her attention having been re-directed to her back by a strain whilst lifting a box. She complained of pain in her back whilst walking, but chiefly that her left leg "wouldn't work properly." She was a highly nervous subject, showing great cutaneous tenderness. The lower part of the lumbar spine, the sacrum, and coccyx were tender. A most excellent skiagraph was taken, which showed a normal lumbar spine. With rest, massage, and exercises under medical superintendence, she improved enormously.

Considering that the injury was over the lower part of the cauda equina, whilst the paralysis was four-limbed, and that there was a brief interval of power in the course of the paralysis which was immediately followed by its resumption, there can be no doubt of the neurasthenic origin and nature of the symptoms.

This case, like the first, teaches the lesson how unwise it is of the medical man to give the laity diagnoses which cannot be proved. In the first case it was "injury to the spine, left shoulder, tibia, stomach, and intestines"; and in the second "injury to the spine, muscles, and nerves, with fracture of a vertebra." Such diagnoses do an infinity of harm when there is any chance of a neurasthenic condition being present.

There is one more case in connection with this which I must mention, as it illustrates how the sufferer, an old soldier, with an excellent record and character, in his neurasthenia, made obviously foolish claims against a company which had treated him well.

It was the case of a man who had served with great distinction in the Austrian army, and was working in a large factory, where he bore an excellent reputation. In his employment he met with an indubitably severe accident, which was due to his own misfortune rather than to any fault of his employers. During his illness the latter treated him very well, when a third party incited the neurasthenic to try to obtain damages. In his claim he referred to many injuries which he was stated to suffer from—for example, loss of sight, particularly in the left eye. Examination showed "old age" changes in both eyes, which must have been proceeding for the last few years. As is well known, these changes do not proceed equally in the two eyes. In his case they predominated in the left. He stated that he had left-sided facial paralysis. There was no trace of this. In fact, all of the *objective* complaints had little or no foundation. Unfortunately, we could only with difficulty and uncertainty test his *subjective* ills. Apparently these rested upon as little

foundation as the others. Here was a man of good character making foolish and obviously untrue statements about himself, partly on account of the depressed condition of his nervous system and partly with a view to damages. Practically the only true ill which could be found in his case was traumatic neurasthenia, of which his foundationless complaints were themselves symptoms.

The important question to be considered is the amount of roguery. If the neurasthenia predominates, it is better to advise that the claim be settled; for then the neurasthenic often recovers with surprising rapidity. On the other hand, if roguery plays the more important part, it becomes a question for the lawyers to decide whether it is worth while to go to the court or not.

It is sometimes a very difficult decision to have to make, and every medical man will be called upon to do so. More than this, in doing so he may do great harm to his own reputation, and, whichever view he takes, will make enemies of the one side or the other. Yet, curiously enough, the subject is one to which little or no attention is directed.

It comes as rather a surprise to find that disease, operation, and emotion may produce a condition similar to that caused by a railway or other accident, and to which the names of "railway spine" and "spinal concussion" have been given. Yet it is a fact that an operation or any other shock can bring it about. It sounds particularly silly that a patient who has appendicitis also has "railway spine" when he may not have taken a journey for years! It becomes a matter of the greatest importance that this should be considered before recommending an operation, for one would scarcely recommend a railway accident. When an operation has been performed it may be necessary to treat the neurasthenia and prolong the convalescence. This subject cannot escape the attention of medical men. How often do they find that, although the immediate aim of the operation is attained, yet there are complaints, and the patient recovers but slowly if at all.

It is not an easy question to decide how the nature of the operation affects the occurrence of surgical neurasthenia. The severer operations have the longer convalescence and after-treatment.

This is important, because we know that those, whose injuries received in a railway accident necessitate their remaining in bed for some time, escape the so-called railway spine. On the other hand, we know that those who are not laid up by the accident, and who go about their business, later begin to fail. Hence, it is quite comprehensible that those who have had severe operations escape on account of their long convalescence, whilst those who have slighter operations are apt to become neurasthenic. Thus it is not the big abdominal operation which causes most trouble. If one was to select any class of procedures which would seem most prone to be followed by neurasthenia, one would suggest operations on the genito-urinary organs of both sexes, and particularly small operations.

Secondly, the question of the employment of anæsthesia must be considered. It is not that chloroform, ether, or any other agent disposes of or protects from, neurasthenia, but whether the anæsthetic should be employed at all. Most people are more frightened by the anæsthetic than by the operation ; yet they would be most frightened at the prospect of an operation without an anæsthetic. These remarks apply to general and not to local anæsthesia. Local anæsthesia is a great advantage in suitable cases, but its limitations are so many that its use is very restricted. The prolonged mental anxiety and strain which are present during the whole operation when local anæsthesia is employed prevent its use in many subjects. General anæsthesia serves to reduce the shock.

The personality of the patient is the most important factor. Post-operative neurasthenia is far more frequently seen amongst the educated upper classes than amongst those who attend hospitals. On a rough estimate it would seem to be more frequent among the males of the upper classes and the females of the lower. The mental character of the patient is by far the most important factor in this connection. For instance, as surgeons we know that some people have poor tissues, which offer little or no chance of a cure resulting from an operation, say for hernia. To very few is it given to have a body like Hackenschmidt's, and to still fewer to have a mind like that of Huxley. As with the body so with the mind, and it must never be forgotten that severe neurasthenic results may be inflicted on the mind by a small operation. In the

hospital little is seen of this, as patients are not followed much afterwards, but in private practice it will soon be found that the condition is forced upon your notice. For these cases are often the very people who stick closely to you, their hearts full of gratitude, unconsciously and perchance heaping coals of fire on your head.

The neurasthenic effects of an operation may be subdivided into immediate and remote. With the former this lecture has no concern. But I would like particularly to mention vomiting. The symptom is usually attributed to the anæsthetic, unless peritonitis or the like is present. The early vomiting after an operation probably is due to the anæsthetic, but often the persistence or recurrence of it is due to a nervous condition. Instances of remote neurasthenia following operation are most various and varied—so much so that it will be best to cite to you in brief form a number of cases.

A man, æt. 21 years, was operated on in August, 1903, for a right inguinal hernia. It was a peculiar case, and presented certain features which rendered it advisable that he should be careful for some time afterwards.[*] By these means it was hoped that his " radical cure " might be a good one. The wound healed *per primam*, and he left the home happy. Three months later he was very depressed and his father came secretly to say that his son was very unhappy. He complained of pain and weakness over the scar, which was perfectly firm and sound. He had given up all outdoor amusements, ate and slept badly. Under advice this condition improved, and ten months after the operation he was happier and only felt pain in the region occasionally. Twenty-two months afterwards he wrote to say that he had no trouble from the site of the operation, which appeared to be a radical cure. Then he continued : " I fear that you may think I am somewhat neurotic, but may I take this opportunity of saying that for some time past I have had a number of spots on my back and face, which I suppose is due to an irregular circulation of the blood, which might be indirectly connected with the operation." So the condition still persists in a very mild form.

A young man, æt. 21 years, was operated on in 1903, for a left varicocèle and a right reducible inguinal hernia. Both wounds healed, but he got

* 'Lancet,' August 20th, 1904, and ' International Clinics,' 1905, vol. ii, 15th series, pp. 154-171.

thrombosis of his right femoral vein on the eighteenth day. He then disappeared and was not seen until seven months after the operation. He could not walk as well as he used to, his leg getting stiff. He had given up his chance of going to India; he had given up all interests in life to become the admiring centre of a group of sympathising ladies. He had many subjective symptoms. On examining him there was no evidence whatsoever of anything abnormal. Unfortunately a medical man had told him that he could feel the obliterated femoral vein like a cord! When the condition had been explained the patient refused to begin with gentle treatment, took to violent exercise, and his doctor at St. Leonard's, wrote that he was well in ten days.

These two hernia cases have been selected as examples of neurasthenia after this simple operation. They show that the medical man may have much to treat after the surgeon has gone and the wound healed. After abdominal operations neurasthenia may cause much trouble, not infrequently marring a case which has been most successful from the physical or bodily point of view. These can only be illustrated by a selection of cases.

An Irish woman was operated on for appendicitis. At the operation the right ovary was found to be surrounded by clot and infiltrated with blood. The ovary and tube were removed. For two years this woman was more or less incapacitated from earning her livelihood on account of subjective symptoms, weakness, pain, etc. Repeated examinations revealed no cause for this trouble, which finally passed off, the patient becoming vigorous and active again.

A lady of neurotic temperament had her appendix removed. For many months she remained more or less *hors de combat* from obscure abdominal symptoms, with attacks of " burning pains " in the bowels. Thirteen months after the operation she writes as follows : " The burning sensation in the bowels is still troublesome, and the heartburn is very bad. But what troubles me most is the dull pain in the back and round the loins, which has persisted ever since I left the home." How long this will go on it is difficult to prophesy.

I must relate the next case on account of its professional lesson and humour. A young lady who had been operated on for movable kidney by a distinguished surgeon was operated on later for an adherent ovarian cyst on the left side. The wound healed perfectly and the patient got well, but she remained unhappy and depressed. Two months or so later her doctor sent her up to be seen. After some preamble, she confessed the cause of her trouble. The kidney operation had suppurated extremely freely, and she had had many operations for the removal of stitches ; the abdominal wound

had healed *per primam* and she was depressed on account of the stitches not requiring removal, and felt very uneasy at their non-appearance !

Another case [*] illustrates the effect of two severe surgical operations on a patient. In 1901 she underwent a supra-vaginal hysterotomy for fibromyomata of the uterus. Some time afterwards, adhesions having formed between the small bowel and the stump of the uterus, she was operated on again for acute intestinal obstruction. She made an excellent recovery from her operations, but her doctor reports that she can do no work, is depressed, has abdominal pains, etc. In fact, though only about forty-nine years of age, her life has ceased to be of any use or enjoyment to herself or others. It is illogical to put all these ills down to the intestinal adhesions. Intestinal obstruction is but an incident, perhaps of a day or an hour, in the history of these adhesions which may have been present for years. They are often present, and cause little or no trouble. The trouble from which this patient suffers seems to be due to a form of neurasthenia consequent upon her surgical diseases and their successful treatments.

A healthy man, candidate for a commission in the Army, had to undergo an operation for varicocele in order to become physically fit. This was duly done, and it healed by first intention. After leaving the home he was seized by an inquiring turn of mind, as was also his father. They found a cord of thickening where the ligatured veins were thrombosed. From this moment, in spite of assurances, open-air exercises were discarded, his general health became depreciated, and his mind depressed. It now became time to go to Aldershot, where the regular life and heavy open-air work have restored his nervous system to the normal again. This is an example of a perfectly successful case followed by neurasthenia, which affected the parent as well as the patient.

An old lady had a bad painful hammer-toe, for which there was nothing but amputation. This was done, and the wound healed by first intention. Yet for a year she walked with a limp, and a gait like a horse with " stringhalt " or the historic " bear on hot bricks." There was much pain and tenderness in the part, yet if her attention was distracted, that self-same part could be severely handled without causing any suffering. When a year had elapsed since the operation she began to recover.

I have mentioned this last case particularly as it is an example of a class of operation which is commonly done in general practice. It is, therefore, of distinct importance to know that a perfectly successful operation may give an imperfect result. No workman, no matter how skilled, can make a fine porcelain vase out of poor clay. Neither can the most skilful surgeon attain perfect success with

* ' Practitioner,' August, 1903, pp. 160 and 161.

poor material. In an operation the surgeon supplies the means and the skill, the patient the material. The result may be due to errors on either side or on both.

Just as accidents and operations may produce neurasthenia, so can disease. At its onset a disease often produces other symptoms which mask any neurasthenia. On the other hand, the news of its presence, the suspicion of its presence, or the nature of the disease may cause the greatest depression of mind. In this connection I must give a case as an illustration.

A woman, æt. 58 years, who had been previously quite well, strong, and healthy, began to have pain in the right loin, with some abdominal symptoms. As some of her relatives had died of cancer, she was convinced that her own end was near and that she had this same disease. She was profoundly depressed and would take no assurances. As it was uncertain if the complaint was due to the right kidney or to the appendix, an exploratory operation was performed. The right kidney showed areas of septic infection and was removed, as was also the appendix, which was diseased, but not grossly. She made a perfect recovery, and it was now hoped that her mind would improve. But this was a great deal to hope for. About eighteen months after the operation the doctor in charge reported that she was very well.

As the result of a surgical disease a neurasthenic condition is not infrequently left behind. There are many examples of this, but I relate the following case because in this instance no operation was performed.

A young and healthy candidate for the Army hurt his hip slightly. Two days later he had severe pain in the hip and a high temperature. When seen it was difficult to ascertain the cause of the trouble. There certainly was acute arthritis of the hip-joint, which on the whole was thought to be "gonorrhœal." This was purely a matter of supposition. In about six weeks this arthritis quieted down, but was awakened by movements to restore function to the joint. In a few weeks it again quieted down. Practically from this time and onward for some months, although his hip was quite well, he was absolutely neurasthenic. Appropriate treatment was employed, and the doctor in charge reports that he recovered with remarkably little interference with the joint.

As this form of neurasthenia is well recognised, it will be unprofitable to recite more cases. Surgical neurasthenia which is concerned with disease is quite well known and recognised. The cases connected with railway injuries were the next to be known. Finally, with the immense advances of operative surgery it is desirable to give attention to the subject of post-operative neurasthenia.

February 5th, 1906.

THREE LECTURES

ON THE

SYMPTOMS AND TREATMENT OF GOUTINESS.*

By LEONARD WILLIAMS, M.D., M.R.C.P.,

Physician to the French Hospital; Assistant Physician to the Metropolitan Hospital.

LECTURE II.

HAVING now paved the way for the efficient action of the excretory organs by insuring for them an adequate supply of water, and having by the action of the above-mentioned drugs rendered the process of elimination more easy, let us inquire into the best means of setting these organs to work. So far as the bowels are concerned, if guaiacum is given, then the quantity in the cachet which I described in the last lecture may do all that is necessary. Where it does not some purgative salts, preferably sulphate of magnesia, in doses of thirty grains, with nux vomica (*vide* " Chronic Constipation," CLINICAL JOURNAL, August 30th, 1905), should be added to the morning dose of water, and also, perhaps, to the evening dose ; or some of the natural aperient waters which are not overburdened with NaCl† may be substituted. Either course is much to be preferred to the exhibition of chola-gogue cathartics, which are so often recommended. There is no objection to an initial dose of calomel (say two to three grains)—it is an excellent measure, especially in sthenic cases—but the practice of a sustained exhibition of hepatic stimulants is much to be deprecated. It was introduced in conformity with the theory that gout in all its forms was due to some dereliction of duty on the part of the liver, which could be counteracted by stimulation of that organ. As this theory is very far from being established, and as the continuous administration of cholagogues has well-recognised drawbacks, the practice is not to be recommended. In gouty conditions the liver, together with all the portal radicles, require un-

* Delivered at the Medical Graduates' College and Polyclinic.

† Arabella water, which contains chiefly sulphate of sodium and bicarbonate of sodium, is comparatively free from the chloride.

loading, but this may be done quite efficiently with the mixture above suggested, especially when this is occasionally reinforced with small doses of calomel (gr. j), podophyllin (gr. ss.), iridin (gr. ij), or euonymin (gr. j).

The excretory organs to whose action the greatest importance is, in this connection, universally attached are the kidneys. It is my purpose to avoid, as far as possible, expressing an opinion about any of the theories concerning the causation of gout ; but it is safe to admit that uric acid, the biurate of sodium, and the quadriurate of sodium are all, in a measure, actively engaged in producing the symptoms of the complaint, and as these substances are normally excreted by way of the kidneys, it is obvious that anything which tends to increase renal activity will materially aid the discharge of these matters and thus lessen the incidence of the manifestations. The importance of fluid, which, as already stated, is considerable in the case of all the excretory organs, is here paramount, and water must therefore be exhibited in full quantities. As aids to its discharge by the kidneys rather than by any other route, it is well to have recourse to diuretics.

There are diuretics, such as digitalis and scoparium, which act by increasing the general blood-pressure, including that in the kidneys. As will appear later on, the blood-pressure in the gouty already rules over-high, so that such drugs are carefully to be avoided. The routine prescription of digitalis, bad as it is in cardiac disorders, becomes in conditions accompanied by high arterial tension, something in the nature of a therapeutic crime. It increases the arterial tension, and acts as a diuretic only when œdema is frequent. For diuretics in the gouty state, then, we must look to those which increase the renal activity without raising the blood-pressure—such, for example, as the salts of potassium, the infusion of buchu, and theobromine. Fothergill says that buchu has upon the urinary passages the same inexplicable soothing influence which bismuth has upon the digestive apparatus. This I believe to be true, and it has often seemed strange to me that so valuable a drug should recently have fallen into disuse. It is by no means unpalatable, and it increases very conspicuously the functional activity of the kidneys. Of the salts of potassium, those which are most used are the citrate and the bicarbonate. No one, I

imagine, now gives these salts in the vain hope of increasing the alkalinity of the blood so as to obtain the solution of uratic deposits. But whatever the motive with which they are given, there can be no doubt either that they exercise a beneficent action over the symptoms or that they increase very materially the renal activity. It is probable that such merits as these and all other alkaline salts may possess are due mainly, if not entirely, to their action as diuretics, and that the salts of sodium, even though they be, as some are still found to maintain, wrong in theory, are useful in practice owing to their possessing a similar eliminative action. To insure the adequate discharge of the excreta from the kidneys, we have, then, to see, first, that enough fluids are being taken. The importance of this is so obvious that it seems absurd to dwell upon it, and in reality my only reason for so doing is to point out that the rule is liable to an exception. If there is too much fluid in the vessels, the urine is scanty because there is undue pressure in the kidneys. In such circumstances to increase the amount of fluid ingested is to decrease the amount of urine excreted. If, therefore, after a few days the urine fails to increase in quantity, the fluid should be decreased until the urine flows freely. The next thing to do is to construct a prescription which which will include such diuretic drugs as will assist in the discharge of this fluid by the renal route. If the cachet be discontinued, we can include its most important ingredient, the iodide of potassium, in this prescription, which would then be as follows :

℞ . Potass. iodide   .   .   . gr. x.
    Potass. citrat.   .   .   . ʒss.
    Inf. buchu, ad.   .   .   . ʒj.
    M. *Sig. : Ter in die.*

If, as is not altogether infrequent, the patient be anæmic, five to ten grains of the potassio tartrate of iron may suitably be added to this mixture, which should be taken immediately after the three principal meals of the day.

There is another time-honoured drug which is not used as frequently in these conditions as it might be ; this is spts. æth. nitrosi. When combined with citrate of potassium and acetate of ammonia, as in the following formula, it makes a useful and agreeable mixture, increasing notably the flow of urine and acting to some extent as a diaphoretic :

℞. Potass. citrat.   .   .   .   ʒss.
Spts æth. nitros. .   .   ʒj.
Liq. ammon. acetat. . : ʒss.
Aquam, ad.   .   .   . ʒij.

      M. *Sig.* : In a tumblerful of water three
      times a day.

In connection with spts. æth. nitros. it is important to remember that it must *not* be combined with iodide of potassium, as the result is an explosive mixture.

A diuretic of which Professor Huchard speaks in the highest terms is theobromine. He prefers it to diuretin, in which it is combined with salicylate of soda, because he believes that the latter is very liable to irritate the kidneys. Of theobromine (which he prescribes in ten to fifteen-grain cachets, three times daily) he says : " It is one of the most powerful and reliable diuretics with which I am acquainted ; it is by far the best medicament in all cases where we desire to increase the secretory activity of the kidneys, and I prescribe it all the more confidently because it does not increase arterial tension, nor has it any effect upon the strength or frequency of the cardiac contractions. It acts solely upon the renal secretory elements."

The natural mineral waters of Contrexéville, Vittel, and Evian have very powerful diuretic properties and may be prescribed with great confidence for all gouty patients. These waters can be obtained in bottles in this country, but it is infinitely preferable to send the patient to the spring itself, as there is reason to believe that a measure of their efficacy is lost either in the bottling process or in transit. Of these three places, Evian, situated on the Lake of Geneva, is infinitely the most agreeable. It has a very fine bathing establishment, and its waters act very markedly in increasing the renal output.

The next most important excretory organ is the skin. There are several drugs which increase cutaneous activity, chief among which is pilocarpine. This is a useful drug in many contingencies and may occasionally be helpful in the gouty state, but the condition in which it is most generally recommended is precisely that in which it ought never to be employed—I mean uræmic poisoning. Pilocarpine induces not only a free flow of perspiration, but it induces also a great increase of bronchial, laryngeal, and tracheal secretion, and if the patient is partly insensible these secretions may

very easily choke him. If you have a fancy for pilocarpine, therefore, let me urge upon you to reserve its use for patients who are conscious, and to avoid it carefully in uræmia and other subconscious states.

In ordinary goutiness, however, the skin is best stimulated by means other than drugs. Pre-eminent among them stands muscular exercise in the open air. This should be sufficient but not excessive—sufficient, that is, to induce free perspiration without at the same time giving rise to more waste products than the organs can coveniently deal with. When we are trying to dispose of an excess of a material we must be careful not to pursue a policy which may have for one of its results the production of that material, or a similar one, in increased measure. The nitrogenous waste which is produced by muscular exercise has to be excreted for the most part by the kidneys, and it is well that those organs, which already stand in need of stimulation, should have no more work cast upon them than is absolutely necessary.

A good substitute for muscular exercise is to be found in baths of various kinds combined with massage. These are undoubtedly best administered at a health resort, under the guidance of an experienced physician who is accustomed so to graduate them as to obtain the maximum benefit with the minimum of fatigue. Hot baths followed by massage may be administered at the patient's own house, but when this is done careful instructions should be given as to temperature and duration. The temperature of the first few baths should not exceed 100° F. and their duration should be limited to ten minutes. Both may be cautiously increased until the one reaches 105° F. and the other twenty minutes. Each bath should be followed by massage or shampooing, and thereafter the patient should be swathed in flannels and encouraged to perspire by the administration of hot water. Such baths are, however, inferior to the hot wet pack which I shall presently describe. Turkish baths, though excellent in many respects, have this against them, that very few, if any, of the establishments in which they are administered are adequately ventilated, so that the bather, especially when he is in the hot rooms, is breathing an atmosphere which is loaded with the cutaneous and pulmonary excreta of others. The home Turkish baths, of which there are now many on the market, are not open to this objection ; but then, they are lacking in those agreeable elements of shampooing, douching, coffee, cigarettes, and gossip, which reconcile people to the discipline when administered in well-conducted establishments. Of all the forms of bath obtainable under ordinary circumstances in large towns that which I have learned to value most highly is the radiant heat bath. The addition of light to the hot air certainly seems to confer upon the latter properties which, in the absence of light, it does not possess. At the Dowsing Institutes, of which there are now a great number all over the country, these baths are well and carefully administered. They may be followed by massage if so desired, but even without this addition I know of nothing so well calculated to stimulate cutaneous activity and to bring about reabsorption of gouty deposits in properly selected cases.

Of routine household procedures nothing can compare with the hot wet pack. This is an old method which has become unduly neglected. It is useful in a great variety of conditions, and as it is practically always available, I shall describe it in detail. All that is required is a mackintosh sheet, two ordinary blankets, a cotton sheet, a hot water bottle, a pail of boiling water, and a wringer, all of which, except the last named, can be obtained in an ordinary household. The wringer can be manufactured at short notice by hemming in enough of the two ends of a towel to allow of a walking-stick to be passed through each end easily. The mackintosh is placed on the bed, and on top of it the two blankets, fully spread out. The sheet, having been wrung out of the boiling water, is then laid on the upper blanket. The patient is then placed on the sheet so that his occipital prominence is on the upper margin of the sheet. With the patient's arm raised the upper corner of the sheet on his right side is carried across and tucked under his left scapula. Each blanket is then carried across in a similar manner, the hot water bottle is placed near the feet and the free ends of all the coverings are tucked under the heels. In a period varying from twenty to forty minutes perspiration will be found on the forehead and that is the signal of sufficiency. The temperature, taken in the mouth, generally shows a rise of one or two degrees. After a tepid or cold sponging the patient is removed to bed, on which the coverings should not be too heavy. Two or even three of these packs may be given in a week. Patients, especially children, for whom they are very useful in many conditions, always enjoy them, and an intelligent nursery nurse can be taught to administer them quite satisfactorily.

The use of such means as are above indicated for stimulating the skin derives its importance, not only from the point of view of excretion, but also from the view of vascular dilatation. One of the effects of the gouty poison (whatever it may be) is to irritate the blood-vessels, especially the arterioles and capillaries, causing their contraction, and thus giving rise to heightened arterial tension. Now, high arterial tension, if long continued, leaves its mark upon the vessel walls in the form of arteriosclerosis, and ultimately, in the form of dilatation and relative insufficiency, upon the heart itself. The involvement of the coronary arteries in the sclerotic $_{pr}o_c$ess may give rise to anginal attacks and the inclusion of the renal arteries to cirrhosis, but we need not multiply examples in order to realise the necessity for taking early steps to overcome the chronic contraction of the blood-vessels which is the direct cause of the increased blood-pressure. The general measures, dietetic and medicinal, already indicated, especially the avoidance of meat foods and alcoholic drinks, together with the exhibition of mercury and potassium iodide, will in the long run do much in this direction, but cutaneous stimulation by means of baths and massage causes prompt dilatation of the vessels over an enormous area which lasts a considerable time and may be repeated frequently ; and the assistance in combating the condition which is to be obtained by such dilatation is the secret of a large portion of the success which attends the balneological treatment of these cases.

So much, then, for the management of the gouty state in general. Let us now consider how we are to treat the various symptoms of this state as they arise in different parts of the body. The most important of these are those which affect the joints causing a subacute or chronic arthritis. When this arthritis is a legacy from an acute attack, its treatment, in so far as it differs from what has above been indicated, resolves itself into that which is laid down in all the text-books as proper to the attack itself. Into the details of this it is not necessary to enter here but I should like to say that where pain is at all obtrusive colchicum is the best palliative, and that it is desirable to withdraw the remedy as soon as the pain has subsided. There are, however, a great many varieties of gouty arthritis which are truly chronic from the beginning, attacking various joints, notably the small joints of the hands and the metatarso phalangeal joints in the feet, giving rise to enlargement and deformity rather than to pain. This is the so-called chronic deforming gout, so frequently labelled chronic rheumatism, which is by no means easily distinguished from rheumatoid arthritis, especially if we make the mistake of concentrating our attention upon the local manifestations of the disease to the exclusion of the general state of the patient. For in the gouty condition there is as a rule no difficulty in discovering the existence of sthenic manifestations in other organs or tissues, whereas in rheumatoid arthritis not only are such manifestations absent, but the clinical picture is essentially one of asthenia, demanding, not an eliminative, but a generous régime. The arthritis of chronic gout is probably more amenable to electric light baths than to any other therapeutic measure. The baths, especially when combined with massage, bring about the absorption of the deposits with a rapidity and completeness which is astonishing to those who have never tried them. Hot air baths, douches, and the various measures of a similar kind which are employed at health resorts stand next in order of efficacy, and where the patient's means permit it is always well to advise a visit to a suitable spa.* For the rest it is important to insist that chronic gouty joints should not be allowed to become fixed and deformed for want of exercise and movement. Massage is an excellent measure, so is electricity; so, in fact, is anything which will insure regular stimulation. In this direction much can be done by the patient himself, and there is generally no difficulty in inducing him to do it if it is brought home to him that ultimate recovery of a crippled joint depends more upon his willing and intelligent co-operation than upon the assistance

* Vichy and Royat are two places which may be recommended with confidence. Aix-les-Bains has deservedly a world-wide reputation. Buxton, Bath, Harrogate, Woodhall Spa, and Llandrindod Wells offer exceptional advantages to people who prefer to stay at home. It should be remembered that the ingestion of sulphur waters seldom suits the gouty; their external application does.

of others. Stimulating liniments are very useful adjuncts, especially when applied after the part has been steeped in hot water. Poultices and compresses containing bicarbonate of sodium or citrate of lithium are also very helpful in reducing swelling and restoring movement.

A method of treating stiff and painful joints which is very highly spoken of by some is cataphoresis, by which medicinal substances are transferred to the joint through the unbroken skin by means of the constant electric current. Theoretically, the positive pole should be that to be placed in contact with the drug, but clinically it is found that some drugs penetrate better with the negative pole, and amongst these are iodide of potassium and salicylate of sodium. A procedure which has seemed to me to give good results is to paint the part with iodine, and then place upon it a pad of lint which has been steeped in a solution of lithium citrate. The positive pole is then placed on the pad and a current of about ten cells is allowed to flow. When the pad is removed the colour of the iodine will be found to have disappeared. Whether this fact has any "suggestive" effect in bringing about the result I am unable to say.

I feel I ought not to leave this question of gouty or rheumatic arthritis without saying a word in connection with the reprehensible practice of lightly dismissing joint troubles in children as due to this cause. Such troubles, it is true, are seldom labelled gout, but they are labelled rheumatism with a frequency which is far from creditable. The truly rheumatic state in children so rarely takes the form of an arthritis that, apart from the disease closely resembling rheumatoid arthritis and associated with the name of Dr. Still, such a condition may almost be said not to exist. Rheumatism in children shows itself as chorea, tonsillitis, subcutaneous nodules, erythema, purpura, and the like, but seldom or never as an arthritis. An enlarged or stiff and painful joint in a child, therefore, especially if only one joint be involved, is exceedingly unlikely to be rheumatic or gouty in origin, and great care should be taken in so describing it. Such conditions are more often due to tubercle than to anything else, their progress is fraught with considerable anxiety, and their treatment demands the utmost care and watchfulness. Numberless limbs have been sacrificed and lives lost owing to the loss of precious time due to the otiose diagnosis of "a little rheumatism" where arthritis in a child has been present.

Of a barticular gout there are a great many forms. Chronic pharyngitis is by no means uncommon, chronic laryngitis is common, and chronic bronchitis is not rare. The gouty poisons as they affect the lower air-passages seem, however, to void themselves in acute explosions rather than in chronic irritation. Thus, an acute bronchitis of gouty origin is an exceedingly common event. It is important to remember this because bronchitis is invariably attributed to chill; and if we allow ourselves to be beguiled by such etiological suggestions we shall fail to treat the case as it should be treated, namely by mercurial purges and the addition of iodide of potassium and perhaps some colchicum to the drugs intended to combat the bronchial irritation. Asthma is another very common form of gouty ebullition. Inasmuch as iodide of potassium is one of the most useful remedies in ordinary spasmodic asthma, failure to recognise the gouty origin is, so far as the attack itself is concerned, not of much consequence ; the recognition becomes of importance only when we are considering the best means of providing against further attacks, and if we do not realise their true origin, our precautionary measures are likely to prove singularly ineffectual. One of the commonest associations of asthma, which is a symptom and not a disease, is with high arterial tension. As we shall consider this important question in some detail later, I content myself now with reminding you of the fact, and with urging you to remember to treat the high tension by appropriate means rather than relieve the asthma by habit-provoking sedatives.

The gouty affections of the nervous system consist in myalgia, neuralgia, neuritis, insomnia, mental irritability, mental depression, migraine, and epileptiform attacks.

In the skin the diathesis may show itself as an eczema, a psoriasis, an erythema, and, contrary to what is generally believed, as furunculosis. Boils are commonly regarded as a symptom of asthenia ; they are, especially when occurring in successive crops, in my experience much more often due to the gouty poison. Why this poison should favour the activity of staphylococci in the hair-follicles I am unable to say, but that it does so is to my mind abundantly clear. An excellent treatment

for boils consists in the administration by the mouth of pills of calcium sulphide (gr. j), three or four times daily (small doses are useless), and the local application of ichthyol ointment (about 15 per cent.) This does a great deal of good where the boil is a "singleton," relieving very considerably the local pain and hastening resolution. Where, however, the boils, as they often do, tend to appear in successive crops, the patient should be injected with anti-staphylococcic serum. This treatment, introduced by Professor Wright, late of Netley, is practically painless, there is no constitutional disturbance, and the result is uniformly satisfactory. It does not, of course, in any degree influence the underlying gouty condition, which should be treated on the lines already suggested.

Gouty men tend to become bald early, probably owing to vaso-constriction of the arteries in the scalp, and their nails assume a reedy appearance from longitudinal striation.

So far as the other skin manifestations are concerned, such as gouty eczema, in the existence of which some dermatologists affect to disbelieve, they are to be treated locally according to dermatological rule, but if their recurrence is to be prevented, their underlying gouty cause must receive adequate attention on the lines already laid down.

In the eye gouty iritis and gouty conjunctivitis are common. These conditions, when of gouty origin, are less liable to be acute than when they own some other cause, and consequently the local treatment need not be so vigorous. A blister and a few hot fomentations, and perhaps a little atropine are all that is required. If the blood state is properly treated the condition will quickly yield.

In the intestinal tract dyspepsia is very common. The indigestion of gouty people is usually, but not invariably, of the sthenic variety, demanding alkalies and bismuth, but it may, on the other hand, be asthenic and require hydrochloric acid and pepsin for its relief. Another form of indigestion, namely intestinal indigestion, is much more common in gouty people than is generally supposed, more especially in such as take large quantities of alcohol. It takes the form of diarrhœa, often accompanied by flatulence : it is generally painless and is usually confined to the morning. If it can be managed it is well to refrain from interfering with this discharge ; it should, indeed, be encouraged by mercurial cathartics, for the process is entirely beneficial in that it rids the system of effete matters without irritating the kidneys. Tannigen (gr. x in cachet) is an excellent simple astringent ; catechu (3j of the tincture) is another. Whatever is used it is important to remember that neither lead nor opium should ever be prescribed.

February 5th, 1906.

THE CLINICAL JOURNAL,

CLINICAL RECORD, CLINICAL NEWS, CLINICAL GAZETTE, CLINICAL REPORTER, CLINICAL CHRONICLE AND CLINICAL REVIEW.

EDITED BY L. ELIOT CREASY.

No. 694. | WEDNESDAY, FEBRUARY 14, 1906. | Vol. XXVII. No. 18.

CONTENTS.

NOTICE.

Editorial correspondence, books for review, &c., should be addressed to the Editor, 51, New Cavendish Street, W., Telephone No. 904, Paddington; but all business communications should be addressed to the Publishers, 22½, Bartholomew Close, London, E.C. Telephone 927, Holborn.

All inquiries respecting Advertisements should be sent to MESSRS. ADLARD & SON, *Bartholomew Close, E.C. Telephone 927, Holborn.*

Terms of Subscription, including postage, payable by cheque, postal or banker's order (in advance) : for the United Kingdom, 15s. 6d. per annum : Abroad 17s. 6d.

Cheques, &c., should be made payable to THE PROPRIETORS OF THE CLINICAL JOURNAL, *crossed "The London, City, and Midland Bank, Ltd., Newgate Street Branch, E.C. Account of the Medical Publishing Company, Ltd."*

Reading Cases to hold Twenty-six Numbers of THE CLINICAL JOURNAL *can be supplied at 2s. 3d. each, or will be forwarded post free on receipt of 2s. 6d. ; and also Cases for Binding Volumes at 1s. each, or post free on receipt of 1s. 3d., from the Publishers, 22½, Bartholomew Close, London, E.C.*

THREE LECTURES

ON

DISEASES OF THE BREAST.

Delivered at St. Bartholomew's Hospital.

By ANTHONY A. BOWLBY, C.M.G., F.R.C.S.,

Lecturer on Surgery and Surgeon to the Hospital.

LECTURE I.

GENTLEMEN,—I propose to-day to speak to you upon diseases of the breast. And in the first place one must consider a little the normal anatomy of the breast, and very briefly also its development. The breast is developed from epiblast, and in the fœtus it consists of columns of epithelium which pass but a very little distance from the surface. As development progresses, these columns become hollowed out into tubes, so that before puberty the breast consists of a fibrous stroma with hollow tubes which branch very slightly. But towards puberty the breast begins to grow, and at that time the tubes shoot out branches, which are the slowly developing acini. As these acini develop they also become hollowed out, so that there is now a parent stem or trunk at the nipple, containing tubes which pass down into the subcutaneous tissue. This gland, like other glands, grows as the person grows, and together with the growth of the gland there is a growth of a good deal of fat. The size of the breasts is indeed to a great extent dependent on the amount of fat which surrounds them. So that there are many cases where a woman seems to have large breasts but really has very little glandular tissue. This is often evident at operations, and when you dissect the breast out, the size of the gland itself is often found to be quite small compared with the quantity of fat in which it lies. During pregnancy of course the gland still further increases in size and becomes much more vascular ; and if you examine the gland during pregnancy, you will find that there is a great proliferation of epithelium in every part of it, and towards the end of pregnancy this results in the formation of milk.   After parturition, when the child ceases to be nourished, the breast undergoes atrophic or retrogressive changes. But these retrogressive changes even then leave it somewhat altered compared with what it was before it was ever used for lactation.   It usually becomes more pendulous and loses to some extent its original globular shape.   And it does so, of course, because the skin has been greatly stretched and the fibrous tissue which forms the septa of the breast becomes stretched also by the weight of the gland.   The more frequently a woman suckles children the more alteration takes place in the size of the nipples and in the pendulous state of the breast.   But when menstruation ceases there comes a time when the breast begins to undergo a permanent atrophy, in the same way that the uterus and ovaries also atrophy after the period of the menopause.   The changes which take place in the breast at this time are of some importance. There is now a gradual shrinkage of the glandular tissue, and slowly the acini shrivel and shed their epithelium, so that in old age there is very little of the breast left except the ducts, the fibrous tissue in which they lie, and innumerable small cysts, which are found in all parts of the breast, in the places which once were filled with acini.   So you see that in old age there are profound degenerative changes which alter the whole of the breast structure.

INTERSTITIAL MASTITIS.

Let us now turn to the condition known by the name of "interstitial mastitis"; and I want to point out to you in the first place that this, in spite of its name, is not generally an inflammatory lesion at all.   What I said just now about the breast was that as age advances the breast-tissue proper shrinks and atrophies, and the breast becomes more fibrous.   There is not only a diminution of the mammary glandular tissue, but there is also an alteration in the fibrous tissue of the breast, which becomes more dense and hard.   If you took a section of an old breast and examined it microscopically, you would find the fibrous tissue of it was more dense than that of the breast of a young woman, less cellular and more fibrous.   In any one lobule of the breast this condition may be more

advanced, and instead of the breast growing old as a whole, portions only of it may undergo degenerative changes, and an individual lobule in the breast or more than one lobule may undergo these senile changes, which may result in that part of the breast becoming harder and more fibrous and more evident to the feel than the rest of the gland. We often call that interstitial mastitis, and I want you to realise that many of the cases which you see as interstitial mastitis and are so called are really cases in which part of the breast has undergone a premature senile change.   And a notable thing in many of these cases is, that more than one of these hardenings in the breast can be found, and in characteristic cases they are to be found in both breasts.   I mentioned to you that in old age the breast not only undergoes these changes, but that its acini become altered, that they shed their epithelium, and that minute cysts form.   Now, I want you to realise that that is a normal process.   If you were to examine breasts from the post-mortem room of people between fifty-five and seventy years of age, you would find in every single breast which you examined tiny microscopic cysts, and many of these cysts you would find had lost their epithelium, and you would be inclined to think at first sight that these cysts which were not lined by epithelium were not glandular cysts at all.   But I want you to remember that cysts in the breast may either be lined by breast epithelium, or they may be lined only by a flattened layer of endothelium-like cells.   If that is the condition of the breast normally, you can easily understand how it is that in the degenerative processes which take place late in life not only may fibrous tissue form, causing interstitial mastitis, or hardening of a portion of the breast, but in these same lobules, or in other lobules, cysts may form which are only exaggerations of the normal cystic condition of the aged breast.   So that it is a common thing to find a cyst as large as a walnut, containing clear fluid, in elderly people, and these conditions very often simulate carcinoma, for a hardening of the breast in one lobule suggests the hardness of carcinoma.   A few tense, hard cysts, or a single cyst situated in a hardened piece of breast, will feel more like carcinoma than anything else, and you must remember that a certain number of hardenings in the breasts late in life may be either due to this fibrous change of a degenerative nature in a lobule, or that they may be due to this change plus the formation of a cyst, or cysts—these cysts which form late in life and which, because they occur in degenerating breast tissue, are often called "degeneration cysts." And whilst I here explain to you their origin I must now remind you that until recent years the cysts of the breast used to be described as being either serous or glandular, and it was believed that cysts might form in the connective tissue of the breast, the fluid collecting in the lymphatic spaces and the cellular tissue, which would be thereby distended. Those were called "serous cysts." The other form of cyst of the breast tissue was called "glandular." The reason of that differentiation was that some of these "serous cysts" were found to be lined by a layer of flattened endothelial-like cells. But if you take cysts of the breast at every stage during the active period of the breast's life, you will find that whilst in all small cysts the breast's epithelium can easily be demonstrated, yet the larger the cysts become the more tense they are, and the more the fluid presses upon the epithelial lining the more flattened do the lining cells become, until ultimately you get a condition in which the cells are absolutely flattened. You cannot, then, tell that the lining membrane of the cyst is composed of epithelium at all, for it looks rather like endothelium. But it is by observing these cysts in their different stages that we are able to say that all these serous breast cysts originate in the gland-tissue.

FIBRO-ADENOMA WITH CYSTS.

In the young woman's breast also there may be a growth of cysts and a growth of fibrous tissue, but it differs from that which I have been describing as occurring in the more aged. In the young woman's breast, when you examine a fibro-adenoma you find that there is a much more definite growth of glandular tissue and a new formation of a much more rapidly growing fibrous tissue, both these conditions resulting in the young woman because of the activity and normal condition of the glandular elements at the time when these growths appear. So that in a young woman there may be fibro-adenomata with cysts, which you may compare with the fibrous degeneration and the degeneration cysts of old age. But if you examine the two sections under the microscope you would find that in the young woman the fibrous tissue was evi-

dently the fibrous tissue of active growth, in the old woman it would be dense and more like the fibrous tissue of atrophy and shrinkage. You would find in the young woman that the glandular tissue was like the glandular tissue of the healthy breast, except that some of the acini were distended, and that the gland-tissue did not present that regularity of outline which you notice in the normal gland. In itself the gland-tissue in the young woman's fibro-adenoma is normal gland-tissue, and it only differs from the remaining gland-tissue by its irregularity of conformation. But in the case of the breast of the young woman also the formation of a fibroma is often associated with a distension of the acini so as to form cysts. So you may have, you see, cysts in a degenerating breast, or you may have cysts in the breast of a young woman as a part of a fibro-adenoma. What is the next development? In many cases the cysts throughout are microscopical. But any of these cysts may become large, and in the case of a young woman who has fibro-adenoma, as the cysts get larger and become distended, their walls meet with the resistance of the surrounding fibrous tissue which is also growing at the same time. The result is that as the breast tumour grows both the fibrous tissue and the cysts increase, so that you get a condition where there is no longer any gland-tissue shaped like an acinus, but each acinus has become converted into a tiny cystic cavity. And the next thing you may find is that the wall of this cavity is pushed inwards by the growing tissue which surrounds it, and you talk of this now as an "intra-cystic growth," and the cyst will be called a "pro-liferous cyst." If you look at this diagram, you will see that I have drawn the lining membrane of the cyst as being pushed in front of the advancing growth, and that is what happens. Now, between such a growth as this, the so-called fibro-adenoma with cysts, and the development of what is called "sero-cystic disease" of the breast, there is every possible gradation.

SERO-CYSTIC DISEASE.

Sero-cystic disease of the breasts is the name which was given by Sir Benjamin Brodie to a form of tumour which attained a considerable size, but which until he wrote about it had not been differentiated at all from cancer. In his day there were no such names as carcinoma and sarcoma; tumours were talked of as cancerous or otherwise. Brodie pointed out that some of the tumours which hitherto had been described as cancerous were really rather different, that they did not run the course of ordinary cancer—that, in fact, there was a class of tumour which had hitherto been merged in the cancers, but which really did not belong to them. And his description of these sero-cystic tumours is perfectly accurate, as far as it goes, to the present day. He said that there were certain tumours which grew in the female breast which had these characteristics.: they often grew for years, they caused a great enlargement of the breast, the skin over them was much more often stretched than ulcerated, the surface of the breast was bossed like the bosses of a shield, that many of these bosses were the results of cysts containing fluid underneath the skin. He said that when you opened these tumours you found that they consisted partly of cysts containing fluid and partly of cysts which were more or less completely filled up by a solid growth which had grown into them. But Brodie was also astute enough to point out that really these solid growths were not inside the cysts, but had the lining membrane of the cyst still over them, and he talked of these as " proliferous cysts," and he described this disease as "sero-cystic disease" of the breast.

So you see there are all these gradations of cysts with or without solid growth. There is in the old woman the fibrous tissue of the breast in the shrinking and the atrophying stage, without active growth, and the cysts which are only an exaggeration of the normal cystic condition of the acini in an old woman. There is the fibro-adenoma of the young woman, in which there is growing fibrous tissue and healthy gland-tissue, except that it is irregular. There is much the same condition with cystic development of some part of the glandular tissue. And then we pass on directly to the last stage, the sero-cystic disease of Brodie. As far as Brodie had taken it, all he had described was accurate, and does not require to be in any way altered at the present day. It only requires to be added to. In Brodie's day there was nothing to differentiate the nature of the solid ingrowth which he had noticed protruded into these cysts : he had not known himself what it was made of, but he said it was fibrous-looking in many cases. And so you come to this, that in the sero-cystic disease of

the breast you have this condition which Brodie described, but the solid tissue is not the same in all the cases. In what respect, then, do these tumours differ from the fibro-adenomata of young women with cysts? They differ chiefly in being on a larger scale, for many of the large tumours to which this name is given after all are only exaggerations of the fibro-adenomatous growths with cysts. But it is to be noticed that the solid ingrowth is often more cellular than the growth of fibrous tissue in the fibro-adenoma ; it is more vascular, it is less densely fibrous, it contains many more growing oval cells. Now you are getting to a stage of tissue ultimately recognised under the name of "fibro-sarcoma," and these sero-cystic tumours frequently have a fibro-sarcomatous growth. In some of them it is more myxomatous, and these fibro-sarcomatous and myxo-sarcomatous tissues are often present in the same tumour. We then come to the stage in which the solid tissue is either all myxo-sarcomatous or definitely sarcomatous, but yet grows in connection with cysts. So you will thus see that the solid growth in sero-cystic disease is very different in different cases. And is not there necessarily a corresponding difference clinically? Of course there is. The more fibrous the growth in these sero-cystic tumours of Brodie, the slower growing it is, so that some of them persist for many years.

This drawing illustrates such a condition. In this picture there is shown a tumour which had been growing for thirteen years, and you may be sure that it was fibrous. If the growth is fibro-sarcomatous, it will grow rather more quickly, and the more the sarcomatous elements predominate the more quickly will the tumour grow. In one of these pictures which I have shown you you will see that the skin has given way and that the growth has ulcerated. That is a late development of sero-cystic disease, and the skin rather gives way as a result of pressure and stretching than as a result of infiltration. Of course it is perfectly true that in all sarcomatous tumours there is some infiltration of tissues, but it is not to be supposed that in these cases the infiltration is an early event or that it is characteristic. For these tumours may go on for many years without causing any adhesion or infiltration of the skin at all, and it is only when the tumour has attained a great size or when the solid growth is much more sarcomatous than it usually is that the skin becomes involved.

Solid sarcoma of the breast without cysts is comparatively rare. You may be in the wards of the hospital for a year or two without seeing a single case of solid sarcoma of the breast. They are nothing like so common as carcinomata. As to their local conditions, they ordinarily occur as a definite lump in the breast, which protrudes the skin in front of it and is irregularly globular in shape. In some cases these growths increase with great rapidity, so that a tumour of a sarcomatous nature may grow more quickly than an ordinary carcinoma. They are tense and elastic, they do not usually cause retraction of the nipple, and they do often cause an affection of the lymphatic glands. They are very like sarcomata everywhere else in the body. On section they are fleshy tumours, mottled more or less by hæmorrhages, and infiltrating, though not so markedly as carcinoma, the neighbouring tissues of the skin, the fat and breast. These sarcomatous tumours of the breast may be, and often are, much more malignant than many carcinomata.

Like sarcomata elsewhere, these growths appear in the breast in their most malignant and in their comparatively less malignant forms. If you were to ask what else happens in sarcoma of the breast, as far as the patient is concerned I should say that in many cases the tumour proves malignant, not only by affecting the glands but by disseminating in the viscera. The rapidly growing round or oval-celled sarcoma of the breast is a thoroughly malignant tumour in every way.

VILLOUS CARCINOMA.

I have to-day been speaking chiefly of the development of cysts, and I want to deal with one form of carcinoma in which there occurs characteristically the development of cysts. It is called "villous carcinoma." Between these villous carcinomata and the development of papillomata in the ducts there is every gradation. Here is a picture of a duct papilloma of the mammary gland of a boy, though I do not want you to think that duct papillomata are common in boys, for this is the only one I have ever seen. Well, in this case there was a slight hæmorrhage from the nipple, and it was on account of this bleeding that the boy was brought to the hospital. It could then be felt that inside the nipple there was a tiny lump which felt as large as a pea, and when it was squeezed it bled, so that the blood oozed out through the ducts of the nipple. It was excised, and the specimen is in the museum. The description says : "There was a tiny raspberry-like growth growing into the cavity of one of the ducts, and this growth when examined under the microscope was found to be a compound papilloma of the villous type." Now, here for comparison is a drawing of a villous carcinoma of the female breast after removal. The breast and ducts are laid open from the nipple. One of the gland ducts is much dilated, and lying in it and adherent to its walls is a small papillary growth. That is the early stage of villous carcinoma of the breast, and I think the name "villous carcinoma" had better be applied only to a very limited class. In these cases the breast ducts are occupied by a growth which is papillary in its appearance, which is villous under the microscope, but which instead of merely growing on the surface, as does a papilloma, infiltrates the base on which it grows, extends into the tissues around, and in that way becomes a malignant tumour. There is all the difference between a villous carcinoma and a papilloma that there is between an epithelioma and a wart. You know that a wart is an excrescence or outgrowth of epithelium, and that an epithelioma is an ingrowth or infiltration of the epithelium. Papilloma of the breast is comparable to the wart, and the villous carcinoma of the breast is comparable to epithelioma. When these latter tumours grow in the ducts and block them, the ducts are liable to be distended, and so are the acini which lead into them. The result is that there is the development of many small cysts. Now, inasmuch as these tumours grow from the ducts they grow mainly in the neighbourhood of the nipple, and one of the chief characteristics of villous carcinoma of the breast is that it forms a tumour of very moderate size in the immediate neighbourhood of the areola and is associated with the formation of numerous shot-like or pea-like small cysts. In many of these cases there is hæmorrhage from the nipple. Another thing which is noticeable, and which it is most important to notice, is that though these tumours are situated immediately beneath or near to the nipple, yet the nipple is not retracted, but, on the other hand, is protruded. In most cases of ordinary scirrhous cancer near the nipple the growth causes the nipple to be drawn in and to be adherent. But these villous tumours, though they are near the nipple practically always, do not cause retraction but rather protrusion. Villous carcinoma deserves to be separated from the other carcinomata also because it runs a different clinical course, and it is mainly for that reason that it is desirable to keep it separate. It is a slowly growing tumour ; it does not usually infiltrate the skin, even though it is so near to it. It ordinarily extends slowly into the breast-tissue and the subcutaneous tissue, but it very rarely fungates. It scarcely ever affects the lymphatic glands, and I am not sure that a pure villous carcinoma ever does that. I know cases are recorded of it, but of the cases I have seen, now some fifteen or sixteen in number, in not one of them have the glands been affected, either early or late. In none of the patients that I have followed up, in whom operation has been performed and the tumour or the breast removed, have they suffered from internal dissemination of the disease, and none of them have, so long as I knew them, died of it. So you see that this is a very different clinical history to the usual one of scirrhous cancer of the breast. The cysts in this form of disease are very unlike the serous cysts of old age or the sero-cystic tumours and this tumour has a clinical history and clinical conditions of its own.

February 12th, 1906.

The Serum Treatment of Scarlatina.—

Schick strongly urges a more extended application of Moser's anti-streptococcic serum treatment in scarlatina. This has already been made the subject of extensive trial with satisfactory results in Russia, where epidemics of scarlatina of severe type are especially frequent. Schick reports sixty cases in which the serum was used, with a mortality of 16·6 per cent. ; these were, however, the sixty severest and least hopeful cases out of 660 instances of the disease. In other words, the serum was used only in cases in which there was no hope from other methods of treatment, and in which there seemed nothing to lose and everything to gain. The usual dose was that first recommended by Moser— 200 c.c.—though in two instances double that amount was injected. A serum reaction was noted in about three quarters of the cases, but it was nearly always slight, and never interfered with con-valescence.—*Medical Record*, vol. lxix, No. 3.

WITH DR. GUTHRIE RANKIN AT THE SEAMEN'S HOSPITAL, GREENWICH.

[By the courtesy of Dr. Guthrie Rankin and Dr. James, his house-physician, we were favoured with a visit of inspection over this venerable institution, with its numerous small wards and general air of homely comfort. Perhaps in no hospital with which we are acquainted is the clean orderliness and absence of hurry and bustle more pronounced than here ; indeed, the whole atmosphere of the place seems to be in harmony with the calm placidity of those old veterans of the sea who are to be found within its walls. A notable feature of the institution is the valiant effort which has been made to deal effectively with phthisis ; on the roof is a large liegehalle, absolutely open in fine weather and partially closed in bad weather, furnished with deck chairs ; the sleeping apartments are also open to the air throughout the night. Male patients, and only those connected with the sea, are re-ceived.]

The following are points of interest in connec-tion with some of the cases commented upon at Dr. Rankin's visit :

Here is a man, J. J—, æt. 43 years, the subject of locomotor ataxy. He was admitted on October 1st, last year, and was so bad that he practically had to be carried in. About twenty years ago he had syphilis, and fifteen years ago he commenced to have sensory disturbances ; then there followed giddiness, headache, and sharp darting pains all over his body. The pains have ceased during the last twelve months, but he still complains of a tight band round his waist. His gait became unsteady, and gradually that disability increased. There seems to have been no disturbance of digestion. He now has the following well-marked evidences of locomotor ataxy : absence of knee-jerks, ataxia, sensory disturbances, Argyll-Robertson pupils, de-generation in his discs, and marked impairment of muscular sense. The feature of interest in his case is that he has been carrying out Fraenkel's movements by means of the apparatus which we have here, and this exercise or re-education of his muscles has resulted in his having partially regained his power of walking. He is taking his food well, and is not manifestly losing weight. He has had many varieties of drugs, and we are now giving him occasional courses of quinine, strychnine and iron, with cod-liver oil constantly as a supplement to generous feeding. There being a specific history in the case, as there usually is in connection with this disease, we gave a trial to anti-syphilitic remedies, but found them of no use. We also gave him chloride of aluminium over a long period, but without any apparent effect : our efforts are now solely directed towards keeping his general health up to the best standard possible. We hope shortly to send him back to his home in Scotland. He has had no complications and none of the crises.

The next patient, H—, æt. 32 years, is a sick-berth steward. He was in the Navy eight years, and has never done any really hard manual labour. There is no history of rheumatic fever, and he has not had syphilis. It is over three years since he first came in. The first thing of which he complained was pain in the back, and afterwards in the stomach. He was in Charing Cross Hospital for four months last year, and was told he had aneurysm. During his stay there the pains became somewhat better. He tells us that when he came here he was practically broken up in health ; he could not sleep at night nor take his food ; the pain in the abdomen had again increased ; and he was breathless on exertion. Since his admission on April 25th he has been having injections of gelatin, and you will notice he is very positive about the improvement which has taken place in his condition. He has entirely lost the pain, is now able to sleep at night, is no longer conscious of pulsation, and takes his food well. The case is one of undoubted abdominal aneurysm. On admission there was an extensive tumour in the epigastrium over which there was expansile pulsation and a systolic bruit. Under the influence of gelatin injections the sac of this aneurysm has gradually contracted and got firmer, until now the tumour can be felt as a well-defined mass the size of a cricket-ball, which heaves with each throb of the aorta, but is no longer expansile and is painless on manipulation. Unfortunately, he is also the subject of double aortic disease, but his history does not enlighten us as to the cause. This circumstance obviously militates against the achievement of such a good result as might otherwise be looked for. A course of twenty injections were given first,

then there was an interval for three months, and he is now undergoing a second course of twenty. The gelatin is administered twice a week, alternately on the inner side of each thigh. The quantity used on each occasion is 100 c.c. of a 2 per. cent. saline solution. He has only had one disturbance of temperature, and there have been no nauseating after-effects. The swelling is now so quiescent that it might almost be taken for a solid tumour ; this is doubtless directly due to deposition of clot inside the aneurysmal sac. The site of puncture is painful on the day following each injection, but no other discomfort has been experienced.

This man is 34 years of age, and he is a fireman. He admits having consumed a large quantity of beer in his time. He was first taken ill nine months ago, when he felt sick and dizzy, and then the legs began to swell. His urine got less in quantity. Previously to that he had never had a doctor in his life. Coming up from Hartlepool he felt sick and short-winded, had headache and a constant sense of faintness. When he came in his daily average secretion of urine was thirty-five ounces, and in it were fourteen parts per thousand of albumen. It also contained granular and hyaline casts, and some renal epithelium. His present output of urine is sixty to seventy ounces, and the albumen is down to two to three parts per thousand. There is now 1·75 per cent. of urea. He has a hard pulse and a loudly accentuated second aortic sound. Hot air baths, and pilocarpine hypodermically, have been of much service to him. Within the last few weeks he has complained of deficiency in his eyesight. Mr. Cargill has made the following note of the condition of his eyes : " Congenital subluxation of each lens and consequent deepening of the anterior chambers, with very tremulous irides. There is papillitis on the right side and about three D. of œdema. On the left side the papillitis is more marked and there are four D. of œdema. The vessels of the left disc are very fibrous. The left disc shows signs of commencing atrophy, being rather pale." He has no evidence of albuminuric retinitis in the ordinary sense of the term. He has had double optic neuritis, which is beginning to clear up, leaving behind the usual evidences of wasting. Though this is an unusual condition in nephritis, Mr. Cargill informs me that it is sometimes the forerunner of the ordinary changes in the retina which are associated with albuminuria. There is no reason to suspect intra-cranial disease.

He is now taking iron and digitalis, with a hot air bath every alternate day. He is kept on a milk dietary. The swelling in the legs has wholly disappeared ; he has no longer shortness of breath ; and, apart from the defective vision, his only complaint now is that his food is monotonous, and, as he thinks, insufficient.

The next patient is the subject of enteric fever, and he is now convalescent. But although this is the sixth week of his illness his temperature still keeps up in the evening. I cannot find anything to account for this. On the forty-first day his temperature was almost normal, but since then there has been a recrudescence of pyrexia. In the cases of enteric fever which come to this hospital relapses are of common occurrence. Very often in cases of prolonged fever such as this we can improve the condition by allowing more food. This patient is still on a milk diet, but we will now give him, in addition, six ounces of chicken-broth twice a day, and a drachm of Valentine's meat essence every six hours. His temperature will be watched, and if it rises at all, the diet must be brought back to one of milk only. Our routine medicinal method for enteric fever in these wards is to give salol, in the hope that it may keep the bowel at least partially clean. A tonic may help this man's powers of resistance to the bacillus, so we will give him, instead of salol, liquor strychninæ, 5 min., salicylate of quinine 5 gr., spiritus chloroformi ⅓ dr., aquam ad. ½ oz., three times a day. His bowel will be washed out by a simple enema every morning, assisted by one grain of calomel every alternate night. The general appearance of the patient is excellent, and it is a noteworthy point of favourable prognostic significance that he is passing from sixty to eighty ounces of urine daily.

Here is a young man whose case presents some features of interest. He is nineteen years of age, and was admitted six weeks ago. He had been in China, and came directly home from there. He caught a chill at home and was ill for a month before coming to hospital. His ship was not delayed in the Mediterranean. I learn from Dr. Hewlett, whose patient this is, that clinically the symptoms have been characteristic of enteric fever, but that the blood, though giving a positive reaction to Widal's agglutination test, also yields a very marked Malta fever reaction. We have evidently to deal with a mixed infection, to which may fairly be ascribed the persistence of the fever.

He is getting well, and seems to be passing through the ordinary course of his enteric without unusual trouble. A confirmatory point in this case in regard to enteric has been the onset of pronounced deafness. He has recently complained of rheumatic pains. Now, muscular pains do not form part of enteric fever, whereas they are common in Malta fever. Patients such as this, who are the victims of a double infection, present many difficulties, both diagnostic and prognostic.

This is an ordinary seaman, æt. 20 years, who tells us he was ill for a fortnight before coming to hospital. When he was admitted he complained of a succession of shivering fits, with cough, shortness of breath, and headache ; his temperature was 102·6°, the pulse and respiration corresponding. With regard to physical signs, the left side of the chest moved much less than the right, and the apex beat could not, at first, be located. On percussion, the left chest was dull behind up to the level of the middle of the scapula, but hyper-resonant below the clavicle in front. On auscultation there was harsh breathing under the left clavicle, but the breath sounds were absent over the lower lobe, the normal tactile and vocal resonance had disappeared and ægophony could be heard at the upper limit of dulness. The heart was so displaced that the apex beat was ultimately found to the right of the sternum. These constituted the classical signs of effusion, and when the chest was tapped Dr. James withdrew over three pints of turbid, greenish-yellow fluid of a specific gravity of 1020, containing large flakes, and tending to coagulation. He centrifugalised the exudate and on examination it was found to contain large cells with indistinct nuclei which were probably squamous, and polymorphonuclear cells in bundles. The prognosis is therefore favourable from one point of view. Probably the shivering fits of which he tells us may be taken as evidence that the fluid was on the point of becoming purulent, so that he has only just escaped an empyema, if indeed he has escaped it. We must wait to see whether he gets any refilling. There is no history of tubercular disease, and the absence of mononuclear cells in the exudate makes us hope it is a simple pleurisy from chill and not one arising from underlying tubercular conditions. He experienced very bad weather indeed on board ship, so that the circumstances were favourable for the operation of such a cause. He declares he has felt quite well since the tapping, and his temperature has been normal for three days. He is now taking an iodide mixture and there has been no re-accumulation of the fluid so far. He is on a dry diet and will be kept at rest in bed for at least another week.

This man, K—, is 24 years of age. On September 26th he came to us with an indefinite history of pain in his abdomen, diarrhœa, and blood-stained stools. The pain was exceedingly severe, and the stools were those of an ordinary dysenteric diarrhœa, such as we are accustomed to associate with a catarrhal condition of the colon. The interesting point in the case is that, after coming here, he developed a tongue so characteristically "beefy," that we recognised in it evidence of gastritis. This was speedily confirmed by the onset of epigastric tenderness and vomiting. Treatment by bismuth and β-naphthol for his colitis had not relieved him, but the condition of his tongue gave us the cue, and we put him upon arsenic. From the first day he took this drug he improved, and he is now to all intents and purposes well. His sickness has ceased, the abdomen is no longer tender, the stools are normal, and he is able to digest ordinary food.

Here is an old pensioner, who has been here seven years. His trouble is right hemiplegia. Periodically he has a typical Jacksonian epileptic attack, but he has not had one now for several months. The attacks are always of the same type and begin in the same way, starting probably in his cerebrum from some irritation at the site of his old lesion. He is very contented, and has not had a bed-sore, which I think speaks well for the nursing.

Four or five months ago he developed a left-sided pleurisy, which gravitated into empyema. It was drained in the ordinary way, but he did not get well, and his temperature continued high in the evening. Mr. Turner again operated upon him, increasing the previous opening, but with a comparatively negative result. Subsequently matters mended somewhat, but a long sinus was left. We thought this sinus might be the cause of his temperature, but it would not heal, and we looked upon the future with some anxiety. Eventually it was treated with peroxide of hydrogen, under the influence of which it closed in a fortnight, and the cicatrix has remained hard ever since. The temperature became normal *pari passu* with the healing of the sinus. He is completely aphasic and manifests in a remarkable degree the curious emotional instability so often met with in old hemiplegics.

This case is a pleuro-pneumonia, and he has been seriously ill. He is a sailor, æt. 45 years. A week ago to-day he came in with all the evidences of left pleuro-pneumonia. Within three days of his admission his upper lobe became involved as well, and contemporaneously he developed delirium. Nervous symptoms have been a marked feature in this case ever since. He is an admitted alcoholic, and he had been drinking heavily immediately prior to his admission. This is the tenth day of his disease, and no crisis has yet taken place. You will notice that his breathing is hampered, the tongue is dry and coated, and he is considerably cyanosed. At times he is restless, and his mind wanders continually. There are no signs in the other lung, and the heart is normal. He has been treated with ice-poultices and antimony, replaced recently by ammonia and ether, alcohol and oxygen inhalations. The prognosis is not favourable.

The next patient is a man, æt. 46 years, who came in nine months ago. He complained when admitted of a pain situated in the region of his left nipple, but nothing was found to account for it. He ascribed his illness to bad food on the voyage home from Colombo, and believed this to be the explanation of the excessive thirst and abnormal hunger from which he suffered, and of the progressive loss of flesh which had taken place.

We found he was passing in the twenty-four hours 200–250 oz. of urine, which contained sugar varying in amount from seven to twelve grains per ounce. In addition to his diabetes he has double aortic disease and mitral regurgitation. He is still steadily losing weight, in spite of all that we have done, and the amount of water passed, though less, continues large. The quantity now is from 100 to 110 oz. The sugar has diminished, and since October 18th we have not, on any occasion, found it to exceed seven grains to the ounce, and it has several times been as low as four grains.   He has been put upon careful dietetic treatment, but every time we have relaxed the rule a little and given farinaceous food the sugar has promptly increased.   He has had practically every drug reputed to control the excretion of sugar, but they have all failed.   Eventually we fell back upon morphia, the dose of which has been gradually increased, until he is now taking six grains a day.   Since these large doses of morphia have been administered he has been infinitely more comfortable ; he has lost his thirst, he does not feel his weakness so much, and his general sense of well-being is greatly improved. The morphia has not disagreed with him in any way, nor made him feel heavy and sleepy. Recently his loss of weight has not been progressive. He is also taking cod-liver oil.   His food is as strictly diabetic as we can make it short of giving him gluten bread. You will notice that he has very widely dilated pupils, yet there has not been any mydriatic given.   His knee-jerks are still normal.

This next patient, E. R—, is 25 years of age, He looks remarkably old for his years, with grey hair and a general appearance of senility.   He has been ship's fireman, and has drunk a good deal in his day, mostly beer, he says.   He never has consumed much whisky.   He came in on August 13th with a swelling in his abdomen, and with a history of having been lately short of breath, and unable to button his clothes because of increasing girth. We tapped him, and withdrew 290 oz. of fluid— that is to say, nearly fifteen pints—and he continued to drain after that.   His abdomen was so full when he first came in that we did not attempt medicinal treatment, but after draining we put hint upon large doses of resin of copaiba.   He had fifteen grains three times a day for a considerable time. The effect was so good that he left hospital under the impression that he was cured.   The quantity of water he passed was considerable, and he did not fill up to any extent before going out.   But he had not left the hospital long before he came back again practically as ill as ever.   Since his re-admission he has been tapped three times.   On September 12th thirty-three pints of fluid were withdrawn, on October 16th twenty-five and a half pints, and on November 1st thirty-one pints.   And now, as you see, his abdomen is again full, with dulness up to two inches above his umbilicus, so that he is in a condition which will immediately demand another tapping.   The area of liver dulness is, as in all these cases, difficult to make out, but it may be assumed that the cirrhosis which is responsible for such extreme ascites is of the " hob-nail " variety. There is no jaundice and no history of hæmatemesis or melæna. A remarkable feature about this case is that—if his story is true that he has drunk beer, and not the more potent forms of alcohol—he should have contracted an atrophic cirrhosis, and not the hypertrophic type of the disease which is generally supposed to be associated with beer-drinking. The man who gets an enlarged liver from cirrhosis is usually fat and over-fed, purple in the face from the circulation being impeded, frequently jaundiced, and free from extreme distension of the abdomen such as this man has.   On November 6th he was put upon digitalis, squills, and blue pill, and since then the average daily excretion of urine has increased from an average of twenty-seven ounces to an average of fifty-five ounces. If that continues he will escape his tapping.   He has not increased in girth during the last week. In a case which fills up rapidly and repeatedly, as this one has done, the prognosis is unfavourable. Mr. Turner has been asked to see him to consider whether the plan of suturing the omentum to the parietes, so as to get increased anastomotic circulation through the adhesions, is advisable, but it is not unlikely that he will consider the condition too advanced to offer much hope of relief from this method of treatment.

This is a man, æt. 28 years, a Russian Finn. He was admitted two days ago. He can speak very little English, but his story practically amounts to one of starvation for a period of many weeks. He was on a badly found ship. He has no physical signs, but his temperature is subnormal, and his pulse is of poor quality : it does not exceed forty-five per minute. His gums are so swollen and tender that it is doubtful whether he is not on the verge of scurvy. This suspicion is strengthened by the improvement which has already taken place under the influence of full diet combined with a suitable quantity of lemon-juice. We have recently had seven sailors of one crew in the wards suffering from undoubted scurvy. At one time this hospital was rarely without such cases, but we seldom see them nowadays.

We now come to the open-air ward, which has been in use five years. It contains twelve beds, with a corresponding number of shelters out of doors on the roof.

Various forms of medicinal treatment have been tried, but all have been disappointing. Our present routine treatment is to give guaiacol night and morning, and heröin as a linctus for the cough. The diet is generous and varied. Fats are given abundantly, with two ounces of raw-meat pulp twice a day and half an ounce of cod-liver oil at bedtime. The windows of the rooms where the patients sleep are pinned open, so that life is passed in the open air practically continuously. The roof shelters are occupied during the day, the wards being only used to sleep in. During a period of a year we pursued treatment by formalin injections, which were pushed to the utmost limits of toleration and safety. One man had no fewer than fifty intravenous injections, beginning at 1 in 2000 and working up gradually to a strength of 1 in 500. From 50 to 100 c.c. were administered twice a week. We convinced ourselves that this mode of treatment had no beneficial effect, and therefore relinquished it. We have also tried Dr. Wright's method of tuberculin injections, but we have given them up likewise, chiefly because we have not the necessary laboratory facilities for testing the opsonic condition of the blood which Wright insists upon as necessary to the proper carrying out and control of his system. All our present cases have put on weight, one man having gained one and a half stones in three months. No patient is admitted into this ward unless tubercle bacilli are found in the sputum. The charts used in this ward contain headings for weight, microscopic characteristics of sputum, urine analysis, average weekly, morning and evening temperatures, pulse rates, respiration rates, chest-girth on expiration and inspiration, etc. The physical signs are recorded once a month.

We are in no doubt that our attempt at open-air treatment has been attended with considerable success, and we are hopeful that before long the Board of Governors may be induced to permit us to segregate the whole of our tuberculosis cases on this floor, so that they may all have the benefit of the advantages which even a limited open-air method provides. Under such an arrangement, moreover, the inmates of the wards elsewhere throughout the hospital will be freed from the possibility of infection from tuberculous patients being placed in neighbouring beds to theirs.

February 12th, 1906.

THREE LECTURES

ON THE

SYMPTOMS AND TREATMENT OF GOUTINESS.*

By LEONARD WILLIAMS, M.D., M.R.C.P.,
Physician to the French Hospital; Assistant Physician to the Metropolitan Hospital.

LECTURE III.

THE connection between gout and kidney-disease is one which has long been recognised. There exist, however, very decided differences of opinion as to the exact nature of this connection. And yet the matter does not seem to present any very great difficulties. Luff expresses the balance of modern opinion on the subject of gout generally when he says † that the disease is due to faulty metabolism giving rise to an auto-intoxication. He goes on to say: "This auto-intoxication coincides with or is followed by, in the majority of cases, a deposition of sodium biurate in certain of the joints or tissues, which constitutes the climax of the gouty attack. I cannot but think that, with our increasing knowledge and experience of the disease, uric acid and its salts will in all probability have to be relegated to a position of subsidiary importance in the pathogenesis of gout. The joint manifestations are probably dependent upon much more general and much larger conditions than a mere excess of uric acid in the blood. The deposition of sodium biurate is possibly merely the sign of the disease, not the essence of it."

Now, if we admit the auto-intoxication—and there is no escaping it—the connection between gout and kidney-disease seems simple enough. And not only the connection between gout and kidney disease, but the connection between gout, kidney-disease and arteriosclerosis, and this is how the matter would seem to stand. The toxin circulating in the blood has as one of its results the irritation, possibly of the vasomotor centres, but almost certainly of the blood-vessels along which it passes. The effect upon these blood-vessels is to cause their contraction and when the contraction is continued for a long period of time, the vessels

* Delivered at the Medical Graduates' College and Polyclinic.

† 'Practitioner' July 1903, p. 91.

become sclerosed. Now, this poison is normally excreted by the kidneys, so that it is projected on to these organs not only in a concentrated form but with " nozzle velocity." If the initial power of resistance in these organs is weak, its vessels quickly sclerose and the sclerotic process spreads, as it were, all over the organ. Then arise the phenomena with which all are familiar, the increased blood-pressure, the enlarged left ventricle, and the consequent progressive arteriosclerosis all over the body.

This is easy enough to understand and is very generally realised. What seems to me to require insisting upon is that this process is frequently reversed, in the sense that the arteriosclerosis, instead of beginning in the kidneys, may originate elsewhere and spread to these organs, so that the granular nephritis, instead of being the first stage, figures either as an accident or as the final event in the morbid process. For the process, like all other morbid processes, will begin at the site of least resistance, and this site will vary with the individual, so that if the renal vessels are not primarily below par there is no special reason why they should be first affected. And as a matter of fact they very seldom are, and I am convinced that a great number of the cases of granular kidney and general arteriosclerosis might be checked if sufficient regard were paid to the detection of the earlier manifestations of arteriosclerosis in other parts.

Now, although we are for the moment dealing with the gouty poison, I must not be understood to suggest that this is the only form of toxin which may give rise to the phenomena we are about to consider. I believe, on the contrary, that the reverse is the case and that the poisons of lead, tobacco, syphilis, typhoid, acute rheumatism, scarlatina, and other acute specifics frequently carry arteriosclerosis in their train ; and that worry, anxiety, and concentrated brain work are very likely to produce it. But this I am prepared to affirm, namely that by far the commonest cause is to be found in those dietetic and other errors, such as excess of flesh foods, alcoholic drinks, and insufficient exercise, which all agree in associating with the production of the gouty state.

The French have an aphorism to the effect that " gout is to the arteries what rheumatism is to the heart," which means, of course, that arteriosclerosis is as common an accompaniment of gout as endocarditis is of true rheumatism. The idea would, however, be better expressed in English by saying that " goutiness " is to the arteries what rheumatism is to the heart ; for in acute gout the poison usually exhausts its virulence during the attacks, which consequently protect the sufferer from the symptoms of goutiness. Now, if we bear this aphorism in mind it helps us in a great measure to understand that otherwise baffling element of ubiquity which characterises the symptoms of goutiness, by teaching us to regard these symptoms as due primarily to some dereliction of duty on the part of the arteries in the immediate neighbourhood. Such an explanation does not, perhaps, cover all the facts ; it serves, at any rate, to remind us of what in our search after the exact nature of the gouty poison we are sometimes in danger of forgetting, namely that this poison has a particular affection for the arterial vascular system.

Let us now consider its *modus operandi.* We have already seen that the gouty poison causes contraction of the arteries. Now, it is important to remember that this contraction is at first functional and therefore curable, but that if it goes undetected and unremedied, it becomes organic and therefore incurable. It becomes incurable in the ordinary acceptation of the term, but its effects may nevertheless be mitigated and in the earlier stages even nullified by suitable treatment. The functional, the curable, stage is called by the French the stage of pre-sclerosis, and it is, of course, in this stage that it is desirable to recognise the condition and to set about its treatment. For once the stage of pre-sclerosis is past and the stage of organic sclerosis is entered upon, the disease, though much easier to detect, is infinitely more difficult to treat. Now, how are we to recognise this first stage, the stage of pre-sclerosis ? Well, it is by no means easy, and as I have already said, in connection with goutiness generally, the first thing to remember in connection with it is not to forget it. For it must always be sought for; it never calls attention to itself by any very obtrusive symptom, and the indications of its presence are very variable. The first effect of a general contraction of the branches of the arterial tree will be increased vigour of the heart's action. The cardiac muscle is stimulated by the resistance which it seeks to overcome by slower and more forcible contractions. Now, if we keep these two facts in mind, the contraction of the vessels and the increased vigour of the heart's action, the phenomena to which they give rise, individually and collectively, are not difficult to follow.

First of all, then, with the contracted arterioles we find pallor of the surface, more especially of the face, cramps and numbness, together with coldness of the legs and feet, and fingers that "go dead"; slight giddiness and momentary mental confusion, which are very liable to be mistaken for attacks of petit mal, which may indeed degenerate into such attacks unless their true origin is recognised and treated. Further, there may be mental lethargy, and although the patient sleeps badly he is always drowsy. There is also disinclination for work, especially pronounced in the morning. Another effect referable to the nervous system is the production of neuralgias of various sorts; persistent or recurrent neuralgia or headache is very suggestive of high arterial tension. Someone has said that neuralgia is the cry of a nerve for healthy blood, so that if the arterioles which supply a particular nerve contain impure blood, and by reason of their contraction are able to deliver such blood in reduced quantities only, it is not surprising that the nerve should become painful. The facial and sciatic are those most frequently affected.

The effect of the vascular contraction in the bowels is, as one would suppose, the production of constipation, and in the kidneys, polyuria. These symptoms are fairly constant, more especially the polyuria. The vaso-constriction not being confined to the systemic vessels, but invading also those of the pulmonary area, dyspnœa is a prominent, an important, and a highly characteristic symptom. This dyspnœa, the dyspnœa of slight effort, must not be confused with the asthma which is so liable to supervene in the later stages of the affection. This dyspnœa, even when extreme, never has the characteristic laborious expiration of asthma, but resembles far more closely the panting of renal air-hunger which one so often sees in the last stages of a chronic nephritis. It is provoked by very slight exertion, it is often accompanied by a vague feeling of uneasiness in the chest, or by palpitation, and is liable to occur at night without obvious cause. This symptom derives its importance partly from the fact that it is the one which usually brings the patient under observation and largely from its liability to be confused with the dyspnœa and palpitation of ordinary dyspepsia. So again I say that the most important thing to remember about the stage of pre-sclerosis is not to forget it. The complaint of dyspnœa would naturally lead every conscientious practitioner to an examination of the cardio-vascular system, and here he will find two objective facts of an unmistakable character to help him. The first is the character of the pulse, and the second is an accentuated second sound at the aortic cartilage.

Now, in connection with the pulse there are three points which deserve the closest scrutiny.

The first is the state of what is called the tension of the radial artery. The term is not a very correct one, but it has become stereotyped and we must, therefore, use it. This tension is dependent upon three factors—the amount of blood in the vascular system, the force of the heart's action, and the tonicity of the arterial walls—and it is influenced in health by various conditions, some of which it is well to recall. Thus, it is raised by muscular effort, by coughing, sneezing, and the like, but it is lessened by passive movements and by massage. Contrary to what one would expect, it is raised during sleep and the recumbent posture, and depressed by the waking state and the upright posture. It is raised by cold baths and very hot baths, but lessened by baths which are merely warm. It is also raised at the menopause and during digestion. A condition of high tension which is persistent is always pathological. Now, how are we to determine when the tension of a pulse is unduly high? Well, I admit that it is by no means an easy matter. Most of the mechanical appliances hitherto introduced are unsatisfactory, but Rolleston * speaks well of Stanton's modification of Riva Rocci's instrument, and Dr. George Oliver is, I understand, at work upon one which will, he hopes, overcome all existing difficulties. The educated finger is undoubtedly the best guide, but this in reality is a counsel of perfection because, as Dr. C. J. Martin points out, the finger is in this matter so immensely difficult to educate, so far at any rate as slight degrees are concerned.

Nevertheless, definite high arterial tension may

* CLINICAL JOURNAL, June 21st, 1905. See also 'The Clinical Study of Blood-Pressure' by T. C. Janeway, M.D. (D. Appleton, New York).

be detected if we pay attention to the following points. Having regard to the fact that the artery is contracted, we expect to find it small and hard. And so it usually is, but—and this is important and may appear paradoxical—it is not necessarily incompressible. The smallness is generally very pronounced and when the hardness is equally so, the term "wiry" which has been applied to it is very appropriate. The beats are sometimes difficult to feel, but each one seems to tarry unduly under the finger and one is conscious of the fact that the vessel is full even between the beats.

The next point, which is closely connected with the state of tension, which we have to investigate is the pulse-rate. In ordinary cases this is slow in accordance with Marey's law that the pulse-rate is in inverse ratio to the arterial tension, and when it is slow the beats seem to have a dragging quality as if each one were prolonged. But although the pulse is slow in the earlier stages, while the heart is still capable of overcoming the peripheral resistance, there comes a time when the central organ tires, its expulsive force lessens, and instead of bradycardia we have tachycardia. When, therefore, we find a small, hard, contracted artery in association with tachycardia, we know that unless energetic measures are adopted trouble will very shortly ensue. And here let me once more emphasize the fact that such trouble does not always emanate from the kidney. High arterial tension is, in the minds of far too many, so indissolubly connected with renal disease that if, by an examination of the urine, they can persuade themselves that the kidneys are healthy, they are unable to realise that the high tension can be doing any harm. As a matter of fact the danger under these circumstances is not with the kidneys but with the heart, which, exhausted by the unequal combat against the peripheral resistance, dilates, giving rise to valvular insufficiency and pseudo-anginal attacks.

But there is another means of determining the state of the pulse-tension which, though very simple and effectual, I have never seen described in any English text-book. It is very commonly employed in France, where Huchard was the first to call attention to its value. Dr. Graves, of Dublin, many years ago noted that the number of pulsations was normally fewer by six or eight in the recumbent as compared to the upright posture.

It was reserved for Huchard and his school to deduce any practical lesson from this fact, and they have shown that in states of high arterial tension this ratio is always reduced, it may be abolished or even reversed. Thus, if the pulsations counted while the patient is standing reach eighty-eight, they ought after a few minutes in the recumbent posture to fall to eighty-two or eighty. If they do not, then the arterial tension is unduly high and this fact becomes very much emphasized if, instead of falling to eighty-two or eighty on lying down, they become increased to 100 or 102. This method, then, not only enables us to establish the existence of high arterial tension, but it enables us to some extent to gauge its degree. It is thus at once a simple and accurate means of arriving at a correct estimate of the state of the arterial tension, and he who would make an early diagnosis of the conditions which lead to arteriosclerosis will do well to remind himself that the two positions are as important in examining the pulse as they admittedly are in searching for murmurs in the cardiac area.

So much, then, for the pulse. When we come to examine the heart, as we should do, to determine the exact site of the apex beat and map out the area of relative dulness (the amount of absolute dulness affords no information of any value), if we are seeing the case in the very early stage we shall probably discover nothing abnormal. For it is, as a rule, not until the later stages, where definite arteriosclerosis is already in full swing, that the heart breaks down and dilatation ensues. When you come to use your stethoscope (never trust the man who commences an examination of the heart by listening !) there will probably be no murmur, most of the sounds may have a muffled quality, but the second sound at the aortic cartilage will be unduly loud. Under normal conditions, as I need hardly remind you, it is the pulmonary second sound which is the louder, but where arterial tension is unduly high, the aortic second sound becomes much more pronounced, and this accentuation is very properly regarded as one of the most important signs of the condition. The degree of accentuation will vary, of course, with the amount of increased tension, but it is often very loud and has even been compared to the popping of a cork when drawn from a bottle. When it assumes a ringing, metallic, or clicking note it is certain that the stage of pre-sclerosis is past and that of definite arteriosclerosis is well established.

Although there are other signs of high arterial tension, it is not necessary to enumerate them. The multiplication of symptoms tends only to confusion, and the nature of those which are liable to arise in a state of pre-sclerosis can easily be imagined if we remember the essential conditions of this state, namely a toxicity of blood, contracted arteries, and reduced blood-supply, with their logical accompaniments of high arterial tension and an underfed, overworked heart. Among the signs and symptoms to which attention has already been called three are so important as to deserve special emphasis. One symptom, that of undue breathlessness on slight exertion, is of all others the most constant and the most important. It is rarely, if ever, absent and its suggestiveness should never be lost sight of. If this breathlessness or, indeed, any other symptom, should give rise to a suspicion that the arterial tension is unduly high, there are two physical signs which, when both are present, will establish the fact beyond the shadow of a doubt. The one is the abnormally accentuated second sound at the aortic cartilage, especially if it be "booming" or "popping," the other is the abolition or reversal of the normal difference of the pulse rate in the erect and recumbent postures.

I may perhaps be charged with dwelling unduly on the nature of this condition and its symptoms, but my excuse must be that it is important from every point of view. Little is thought or written about it in this country, and yet its recognition and treatment is of the gravest possible moment to all concerned. We hear a good deal about arteriosclerosis as a clinical entity, but the text-books are silent as to how we should proceed so as to detect its early stages and as to how we should act so as to check its further development. I beg you, then to remember that the gouty poison is a powerful vaso-constrictor, that if this vaso-constriction is maintained it gives rise to high arterial tension, and that if persistent high arterial tension be not lessened, definite arteriosclerosis, leading, among other things, to apoplexy, granular kidneys, and angina pectoris, will certainly ensue. Now, how is this high arterial tension to be lessened? Obviously, by removing the gouty poison and by taking such steps as will insure the permanent re-duction of its manufacture in the system. Into the general principles which should guide us in these matters I have already entered in some considerable detail, but I may briefly recapitulate those which have a special bearing upon the question under consideration. First, then, as to diet, without careful attention to which it is quite hopeless to attempt the treatment of high arterial tension of gouty origin. The embargo upon meat foods must be absolute; and under meat foods let it be clearly understood are included fish, poultry, and game. Alcoholic drinks, tea, and coffee must also be absolutely forbidden. The patient must be encouraged to drink plenty of milk and to take fruits and vegetables freely. What I have said above about the great importance of taking plenty of fluid in the gouty state generally must be accepted with considerable reservation in the case of high arterial tension. If the passage outside the body of the extra fluid taken can be insured, then the extra fluid can do nothing but good. If, on the other hand, an appreciable portion of it remains, then, by increasing the actual quantity of blood in the vessels, and by thus adding to the state of tension, it is liable to do an infinity of harm. For this reason a flushing policy, though excellent when it succeeds, should, in the first instance at any rate, be undertaken with caution. The emunctories must, nevertheless, all be urged to do their part in ridding the system of the gouty poison, and the purgatives, diuretics, and sudorifics already referred to must be made to do their part. So far as purgatives are concerned nothing can compare with mercury, and for a diuretic it is as well to try that which has been so highly spoken of by Professor Huchard, to whose teaching we owe almost all our knowledge of the pre-sclerotic state, namely theobromine (see Lecture II). The waters of Evian, Contrexeville, and Vittel are admirable aids to all diuretic drugs, and would seem, especially the first named, to possess a special value in the condition we are discussing. The best means of stimulating the skin—that is, by warm baths and electric light baths—have already been referred to. Another excellent general measure, namely massage, is capable of rendering yeoman service in states of high arterial tension, especially when applied to the abdomen; for it helps to dispel "abdominal venosity" and to pass the blood rapidly through the organs which are credited with being actively concerned in the manufacture of the gouty poison.

This, which is mere recapitulation, refers to general measures the importance of which should never be lost sight of. We now come to the question of our ability to act directly upon the high blood-pressure and reduce it by means medicinal or otherwise. Do such means exist? Well, they do, but none of them are satisfactory, for the reason that their action is very transient and their continued employment is by no means unattended with danger. First among them stands blood-letting. Where we find ourselves in an emergency face to face with a threatening of cerebral hæmorrhage or an anginal attack, no one would, I presume, hesitate to abstract blood from the arm to the extent of half a pint or more. But it is obvious that this is a process which cannot be often repeated, and as the high arterial tension depends less upon the quantity of the blood than upon the state of the vessel-wall, it is useless to reduce the one (especially as the reduction cannot be maintained) without influencing the other. And a similar objection applies to the drugs hitherto introduced for this purpose. Nitrite of amyl, though entirely trustworthy in emergencies, is incapable of prolonged action. Trinitrine is in reality only a degree better. It takes longer to act than nitrite of amyl and its effect is maintained for a longer period, but the relief it gives is ill-sustained and it cannot be frequently repeated. Thyroid extract seems to act beneficially in a good many cases, and where tachycardia is not yet present it may be tried with considerable confidence. In the high arterial tension which is so common with women at the menopause, some observers claim to have had good results with ovarian extract. The physiological basis for its employment is certainly sound, and if it does no good, it can do no harm. Aconite has been recommended by some people and chloral extolled by others. The employment of both these drugs is, however, fraught with such obvious drawbacks that it is scarcely necessary to consider them.

In the way of drugs, then, there is nothing upon which we can in the present state of our knowledge depend for a definite and sustained action of a specific nature without incurring risks which it does not seem to me that we are justified in taking. And this is perhaps all to the good. For if we had such a drug we might be tempted to use it to the exclusion of those general principles of diet and hygiene on which the successful management of the gouty diathesis is known to depend and on which, especially when combined with the judicious employment of mercury and iodide of potassium, full reliance may always be placed.

I have already pointed out that the danger in the state of pre-sclerosis is not so much with the kidneys as with the heart, which, being overworked and underfed, is in imminent danger of dilatation. I now revert to the question in order to consider its bearings upon treatment. Where arterial tension is high, the heart is always endeavouring to force the blood through the constricted vessels. Among the vessels which become constricted are those of the heart itself, the coronary arteries. Now, it is obvious that if the heart is forced to undertake an increased amount of work, and if at the same time it is supplied with blood which is insufficient in quantity and poor in quality, among the earliest and most frequent of the complications which we must expect are those which are to be referred to the cardiac area. We have already seen that the bradycardia which is normal to a condition of uncomplicated high tension is liable to be replaced by tachycardia as soon as the heart begins to flag. At this stage and a little later it will be found that the apex beat becomes displaced, and is visible over a much larger area than it ought to be. The shock of the ventricle against the finger becomes exaggerated and the percussion dulness is increased. On listening, the first sound is generally prolonged at the apex and the aortic second sound very much accentuated at the base. There may be bruits, that suggestive of mitral regurgitation (that is, a systolic murmur at the apex) being especially common.

Now, let us ask ourselves what is likely to happen to a patient who presents himself with this cardiac condition to a physician who fails to test for, and therefore to discover, the real cause, namely the high arterial tension. He will almost certainly be given digitalis (in small doses, let us hope) with a view of toning up the heart and curing the dilatation. Now, such a line of treatment is fore-doomed to disastrous failure. The high blood-pressure has caused cardiac exhaustion. Digitalis increases the blood-pressure and consequently adds to the cardiac distress. But some one may object, "Digitalis is a cardiac tonic." It is indeed, but what good can a tonic effect if the cause of the distress be not first removed? One would not give a quinine pill to a man staggering under a heavy burden—at any rate, until the burden has been removed. And so it must be with the heart. The important, the paramount, necessity is to relieve the high arterial tension, and when this is effectually done it will usually be found that no heart tonics are required. An enormous amount of permanent harm is wrought by the exhibition of digitalis in these cases. The bruit at the mitral valve is in reality the indication, not of danger, but of a most salutary and truly conservative process. The pressure in the left ventricle becomes so high that the mitral valve leaks, as it were ; but the leak is a safety-valve process, and its occurrence, by lowering the tension in the systemic periphery, prevents hæmorrhage into the brain and other organs. It is essential, then, before giving digitalis in a case of cardiac dilatation to ascertain that the dilatation is not due to high arterial tension. If it is, digitalis will do harm, and the only proper treatment is provided by the dietetic and other measures which have already been explained.

February 12th, 1906.

THE CLINICAL JOURNAL,

CLINICAL RECORD, CLINICAL NEWS, CLINICAL GAZETTE, CLINICAL REPORTER, CLINICAL CHRONICLE AND CLINICAL REVIEW.

EDITED BY L. ELIOT CREASY.

| No. 695. | WEDNESDAY, FEBRUARY 21, 1906. | Vol. XXVII. No. 19. |

CONTENTS.

* *Specially reported for the Clinical Journal. Revised by the Author.*

ALL RIGHTS RESERVED.

NOTICE.

Editorial correspondence, books for review, &c., should be addressed to the Editor, 51, New Cavendish Street, W., Telephone No. 904, Paddington; but all business communications should be addressed to the Publishers, 22½, Bartholomew Close, London, E.C. Telephone 927, Holborn.

All inquiries respecting Advertisements should be sent to MESSRS. ADLARD & SON, Bartholomew Close, E.C. Telephone 927, Holborn.

Terms of Subscription, including postage, payable by cheque, postal or banker's order (in advance) : for the United Kingdom, 15s. 6d. per annum ; Abroad 17s. 6d.

Cheques, &c., should be made payable to THE PROPRIETORS OF THE CLINICAL JOURNAL, *crossed "The London, City, and Midland Bank, Ltd., Newgate Street Branch, E.C. Account of the Medical Publishing Company, Ltd."*

Reading Cases to hold Twenty-six Numbers of THE CLINICAL JOURNAL *can be supplied at 2s. 3d. each, or will be forwarded post free on receipt of 2s. 6d. ; and also Cases for Binding Volumes at 1s. each, or post free on receipt of 1s. 3d., from the Publishers, 22½, Bartholomew Close, London, E.C.*

THREE LECTURES

ON

DISEASES OF THE BREAST.

Delivered at St. Bartholomew's Hospital.

By ANTHONY A. BOWLBY, C.M.G., F.R.C.S.
Surgeon to the Hospital, Lecturer on Surgery.

LECTURE II.

GENTLEMEN,—Last week I spoke to you of villous carcinoma when I was lecturing on cysts, because villous carcinoma is essentially associated with the development of cysts. And that form of carcinoma really stands by itself and cannot be held to compare closely either structurally or clinically with the other carcinomata. In speaking of cancer of the breast, then, to day I am alluding to cancer in any form except in the form of villous carcinoma. And the first thing one has to consider is—Under what conditions do carcinomata occur? When and under what circumstances is this disease most common? I think we must accept at once the statement that it is so much more common in the female breast that unless one makes an exception and specifically mentions the male, one refers always to cancer of the female breast. In women it is most common between the ages of forty and sixty. But it may occur at any time from twenty-five to the latest years of life. I have seen it at the age of twenty-six, I have seen a good many cases of it between twenty-six and thirty and between thirty and forty, so it is not to be supposed that it is limited to old age or that it is uncommon before forty. Next we have to ask, Is it more common in married or unmarried women? Now, as a large proportion of women are married before the age of forty it is evident that a majority of the cases will be likely to occur in women who are or have been married. That does not mean that it is because they are married, for it may occur in either the married or the unmarried. Is there anything which predisposes to it? Is there any definite cause for cancer? There certainly is not a definite cause for cancer which we know. I myself doubt very much whether anything we know of predisposes to it except one condition, that which was recognised many years ago by Sir James Paget and to which we constantly apply the name " Paget's disease " of the nipple. But you will frequently find it stated that it is liable to follow a blow, or that it occurs more frequently in breasts that have given trouble during suckling. Neither of these is within my experience. I know there is often a history of a blow, but in the majority of cases women can think of some slight knock which they consider might account for the disease. On the other hand, I am sure, from what I have seen, that a breast that has happened to have had suppuration in it in past years is no more likely to have cancer in later years than a breast which has never had that trouble. Is it predisposed to by any of the forms of innocent tumour of the breast ? Is a person who has fibro-adenoma of the breast more likely to have cancer than a person who has not ? I do not think so. There is a specimen in the museum in which cancer appears to have originated in connection with fibro-adenoma of the breast, but that is only the exception which proves the general rule. It is one case among very many, and no one would dream of saying that fibro-adenoma is an ordinary precursor of cancer. It would not be right to say to a woman that one reason why she should have a fibro-adenoma removed is because it may become cancerous. I do not think that practically it ever does. It may become larger and may become the seat of sarcomatous growth, but not, I think, of carcinoma.

What about the other condition which I mentioned last lecture—mastitis ? You know that chronic interstitial mastitis is said commonly to go on to cancer of the breast. I do not believe that either. I do not think that the affection of a lobule by interstitial mastitis is of itself likely to lead to cancer of the breast. But, on the other hand, considering that cancer occurs between forty and sixty years of age, at the time when women very often do have some induration of a lobule of the breast which merits the term " mastitis," the two often occur together, although it is not to be said that because they occur together therefore one causes the other. You will find histories of the following kind. A patient has been examined and has been found to have what the surgeon believes to be interstitial mastitis. She is or is not treated, and four, five, or six months afterwards she is again seen. She now has cancer of the breast, and the tendency naturally is to say, " This is a case in which there was interstitial mastitis and now there is cancer, and this mastitis has led to the cancer." But the real question in such a case as that is, Was the original diagnosis correct ? Is it possible that this originally was a case of cancer, and that when it was a very small nodule deep in the breast it simulated interstitial mastitis and was mistaken for it ? Is it necessarily a fact that because the diagnosis of interstitial mastitis was made at one time and that of cancer six months later that there was, therefore, first interstitial mastitis and afterwards cancer ? The answer to all that is, of course, that it is possible that originally this condition which was thought to be interstitial mastitis was cancer; and it is because there is not a tendency to revise one's diagnosis, but rather to hold to it after it has once been made, that people are somewhat liable to say, " My diagnosis originally was right and now the condition has changed its character." You must remember it is possible that in many of these cases the original diagnosis may have been wrong. And I believe that is the proper explanation of most of these cases ; consequently I do not think that even interstitial mastitis is a frequent precursor of cancer, though I do think that it is essential to keep such cases under close observation lest the condition is more serious than it appears to be. Now, all that leads to the statement finally, that there is no definite condition which predisposes to cancer of the breast, with the exception of Paget's disease.

What is Paget's disease ? This is an entity in itself which has been studied and which is to some extent understood. Paget's disease is a form of destructive dermatitis, which, originally limited to the neighbourhood of the nipple and areola, results in ulceration and destruction of the nipple and of the skin of the areola. And this dermatitis and consequent destruction may spread, so that after a time other areas than those originally involved may be affected. This condition is liable to be mistaken for eczema, and it is indeed very like eczema in its earliest stages. You will see in this picture a characteristic drawing of one of these cases in its comparatively early stage. You will notice the redness of the areola, that there is no ulceration, no destruction of the nipple, but that there is extensive scaling and destruction of the epidermis and a raw weeping surface. This is a picture of the same condition affecting both breasts, and it represents a later stage in which the disease is more advanced on the left side than on the right. Here you see an extensive raw surface in which there is much destruction of skin, and in the third picture there is actual destruction of the nipple. This is another illustration of the same thing. Here are depicted the breasts of a woman, one of them normal, the other occupied by a red, velvety surface of ulceration, which shows no trace whatever of the nipple, for it has been completely destroyed, and in the areola the skin is destroyed in its whole depth. These pictures, then, illustrate Paget's disease of the nipple, and as in every case there was cancer they show that Paget's disease is a definite precursor of carcinoma. It is very peculiar in this respect, that if treated, even in its earlier stages, it is incurable by any means at our disposal ; no applications of ointments or lotions stops its extension ; no scraping or curetting, as we treat lupus, makes any impression upon it. It is an inveterate ulceration and inflammation which goes on regardless of treatment and extends and destroys in spite of whatever you may do for it. Yet under the microscope it is only seen as an inflammatory lesion. For how long does this condition last before the breast may become the seat of cancer? That is a question which does not admit of a definite answer, but the condition generally lasts for little more than a year, and sometimes, though rarely, for five or six years, before cancer begins. So you may say that within a time varying from about a year to six years, and generally in the earlier than in the later of those years, the patient will develop carcinoma. What sort of carcinoma will she develop? It has been said that she will develop a duct carcinoma, due to the extension of inflammation along the ducts, but this is not a fact, it is a theory. The actual fact is that the patient develops an ordinary, scirrhous, glandular carcinoma, which is generally situated deep in the breast, and is not directly connected with the condition which we have described in the skin of the areola. So you see that the relation-

ship between Paget's disease and the development of cancer of the breast is not clear. It is known that the one will almost infallibly result in the production of the other, but exactly how that occurs we do not understand. You must not think that it is the result of a direct extension of this peculiar inflammatory process from the skin to the adjacent breast. It is not. It is not an extension at all, because ordinarily in these cases there is to be found a lump of cancer separated by a considerable mass of apparently normal breast tissue from this condition of the areola. As regards its practical importance I will only say this, that knowing that Paget's disease infallibly results in cancer of the breast, it is evidently the right thing to do to remove the whole of the affected area of skin by operation. You may do more: you may remove the whole breast ; and if the disease had been going on for a long time it would be wise to remove the whole breast, because it would be inherently probable that there was in the breast already the commencement of cancerous disease which could not yet be detected by any physical examination.

So much, then, for the only condition which certainly can be shown to have a direct relationship with the development of cancer of the breast. I put all the other alleged causes aside, because I do not think that any one of them admits of definite proof.

Now, to pass on. What are the clinical conditions under which cancer of the breast first of all makes its appearance to the patient? How does the patient first find out that she has cancer? In the minds of the public the idea of cancer is inseparably connected with the idea of pain. People can hardly appreciate the fact that cancer can arise without causing pain, and because of this belief there is a tendency to overlook cancer in its early stages, for in its earliest stages it is absolutely painless. In a very large number of cases it is certain that a woman has had a cancer in her breast for months or even for longer without knowing of its presence. In a large number of the cases when the patient comes to see you for the first time she tells you that she has found a lump in her breast only " last week," and when you examine it you know from your knowledge of such growths that such a lump would take months to grow. In other cases the patient tells you she has known of a swelling in the breast for quite a long time, a year perhaps, but she paid no attention to it because it caused her no pain. These two conditions you must remember, the finding of a lump the existence of which has not been known, and the watching of a lump which causes no pain. The first thing for you to appreciate—and I wish the public could appreciate it as well—is that cancer in its early stages is to a great extent unnoticed by the patient, and as a rule causes no pain. I think the majority of women will tell you that the way they came to notice it was in washing. A woman washing with the flat of her hand across the breast feels that there is a lump there, and it may have been there for months before it is thus discovered. In one case a lady brought her daughter to one of the surgeons of this hospital because she had a lump in her breast. And thinking that the girl might be alarmed, she told her that she herself was also going to consult the surgeon, and that she wanted him to have a look at the girl's breast and her own. And the surgeon examined the girl and found she had a fibro-adenoma, and for the sake of appearances, as it were, he examined the mother's breast, and found she had a cancer, of which she had had no knowledge whatever. Yet the mother's tumour was by far the larger of the two. That will serve to illustrate to you how these tumours may grow without attracting the attention or the notice of the patient. Next, supposing you yourself see one of these cases of cancer of the breast quite early, you may often find that it has very little that is characteristic of cancer about it, for there- is a stage in every cancer of the breast which is at all circumscribed in which it has not the characteristics of cancer. What are the characteristics of cancer? The characteristics of cancer are that it is a tumour which is irregular and hard, lumpy and nodular. It is also more or less fixed. Without going any further, I would like to remind you that none of these conditions may be noticed in an early stage of cancer of the breast. A patient may have a cancer in which there is no nodular lump to be felt at all, but rather an induration of a portion of the breast in which there is not any definite tumour to be felt, in which there is no fixation but absolutely free mobility. Yet that may be cancer. Surely yes, because cancer must have its beginnings ; and if it begins deep down in the breast, buried in a nodule which is surrounded by fat, it is evident that so long as the cancer has not spread to a larger size than that of half a hazel-nut or so, it has not spread through the breast enough to be adherent or fixed to anything around it ; and consequently cancer in its earliest stages may not only be painless, but it may have none of the characteristics which cancer acquires as it becomes a larger thing and more marked.

I have said nothing yet about the extension of cancer when it passes through the breast-tissue ; but when it passes through towards the surface, it, of course, invades the subcutaneous tissue. When it does that it at first produces no alteration in the appearance of the breast until you try to draw the skin up. Then you may find there is a very slight dimpling of the skin. This very slight dimpling of the skin is the first indication that the growth is beginning to come through the capsule of the breast and to pull down the small fibrous strands which pass from the fascia to the skin, and by pulling upon these it draws the skin down. The skin itself as yet is not affected. This dimpling means that it has been drawn down from underneath, not that it is involved in the cancerous process, but the dimpling is of the greatest importance, for it is a condition practically limited to cases of cancer. Similarly the nipple may be drawn down by the growth getting hold of and pulling upon its ducts, and this dragging downwards is the result of the process of contraction inherent in the growth. For these tumours not only grow, but at the same time that they grow they contract, they draw in and pucker and draw towards themselves the parts around them, and they cause dimpling of skin and retraction of the nipple when they are near enough to influence them. But when the growth is at the margin of the breast it does not affect the nipple, because the nipple is then not within the area of its contraction, and therefore the nipple may be a perfectly normal one although the person may have a cancer at the margin of the breast. And as the growth extends to the skin, the skin becomes also altered in colour and reddened. Here is a drawing of a breast showing at some distance from the nipple a large raised hard plaque in the skin at a place where a cancerous growth has come to the surface. And this skin is not only altered in colour, but also in texture ; it is now definitely adherent, it is infiltrated, it is not like the puckered and lightly drawn in skin which is dragged upon by the subjacent bands of fascia. This skin is infected ; the growth is in it, and is spreading in its network of lymphatics, and in spreading and extending the infection may involve the skin over a great part of the chest-wall, so that you often can both feel and see tiny nodules of growth, and sometimes you can feel them when you cannot see them. In other cases, however, you can feel nothing, but can see a discoloration which looks like an erythematous rash, and this also may indicate the spread of cancer in the skin. But if you wait until the disease has advanced to this stage you have waited for a diagnosis until, of course, the disease is absolutely and hopelessly irremovable. More rarely this widespread affection of the skin may spread as extensively as these pictures show you, so that' practically the whole chest-wall, front and back, up to the clavicle and all over the scapula, may be 'involved in the infiltration of the cancerous growth. And this also may take the form of either tiny nodules in the skin or of an erythematous-like eruption. Always be very suspicious of these reddened erythematous areas of skin in cancer of the breast. There may be no induration to tell you it is carcinoma, for in these cases where there is this infiltration of the skin there may be only reddening, and nothing may be felt at all.

The last step is that the tumour may fungate. The extent to which it fungates will vary immensely in different cases, because in some classes of cancer the amount of growth is very considerable, in other cases the amount of growth is but small. In some of the cases large masses of tumour growth extend through the skin, in others the reverse is the condition. Look at these two pictures. Here is one showing a mass of cancer five or six inches across, which has completely destroyed the skin, and which is growing out as a large fungating, bleeding, foul-smelling tumour. Here is another picture. In those two pictures there is shown the same disease, cancer, but it has occurred under very different conditions. For in the second picture, instead of a fungating tumour, there is an irregular contracted ulcer with very little growth at all. Here, again, is a picture of a male breast showing quite a small growth outside the skin, quite a little area of fungating tumour, but a large area of infiltration and retraction.

These are the last local stages of cancer, and you have next to think of what else happens beyond the

breast and its immediate neighbourhood. The first thing which is noticeable is that the lymphatic glands become enlarged at an early stage, and they become enlarged first of all in the axilla. When they become enlarged in the neck simultaneously with enlargement in the axilla it is a very bad case. The glands not only become enlarged, but in them the cancer grows in exactly the same way as in the breast. It infiltrates and destroys the glands and extends through them to neighbouring structures, becomes attached to the skin and to the ribs, passes up from gland to gland towards the apex of the axilla, and afterwards extends to the glands in the neck. That is all characteristic of carcinoma. And as these glands grow big they often cause more trouble and more pain than does the original disease. In not a few cases cancer of the breast runs its course without causing a great deal of pain or distress to the patient as far as the breast is concerned. But in a number of cases where there is not a fungating growth, where there never has been a very large tumour or much pain in the breast, there may nevertheless be a considerable growth in the axilla, which presses upon the nerves and causes great pain down the arm, obstructs the lymphatics and veins, and causes swelling and œdema ; and indeed it may render the whole limb so shapeless and useless that the patient would be glad to get rid of it rather than to keep a part which is no longer anything but an encumbrance. All this may happen merely as a result of the glandular growth of the cancer, but the cause of œdema of the arm is often more deeply seated, and may be found in growth in the mediastinum instead of in the axilla.

What else happens ? What other parts does the cancer affect ? In almost all these patients who have cancer which has been growing for a long time there is some effect on the general health, quite apart from the illness which necessarily results when there is a foul, fungating, bleeding mass. As a rule this illness, or cachexia, may be taken as a measure of the extension of the disease to other, internal, parts of the body, and you should know the parts of the body to which cancer is most likely to spread, because you must be on the look-out for it. The first part you look for it in, after its involvement of the glands, is the liver, and an enlarged liver is found in a considerable number of cases. Here, again, as in the case of cancer of the breast, it does not necessarily cause pain, and it does not necessarily attract the attention of the patient. Some years ago I was asked to operate for the removal of cancer of the breast. I was told that it was a good case for operation, but I said that before operating upon it I should like to see the patient. I did so, and found that the diagnosis was perfectly correct and that cancer of the breast was present. The cancer was extensive, the breast very much infiltrated, and there were large glands in the axilla. And when I inquired further I was told that the patient had some "dyspepsia." I therefore examined her abdomen, though rather against her wish, and as soon as I passed my hand below the margin of the ribs on the right side I felt an enlarged and nodular liver. That had not been noticed, for the patient had not complained of it, and the doctor had not examined the abdomen; but I at once declined to operate. She died in ten days from the time that I saw her, of hæmorrhage into her peritoneal cavity caused by an erosion of a branch of the hepatic artery. That, of course, is a very unusual termination, but I think you will agree that it was a very good thing that this patient was spared the anxiety and pain of having an operation done which would have been perfectly useless. So you see you must keep in mind the other parts of the body where you should look for cancer when you feel enlarged glands in the armpit and the neck. Next, remember that cancer may spread to another part which you must think of particularly in this connection, namely the inside of the thorax. Many years ago Sir Benjamin Brodie, who was a very acute observer, said that not a few patients who had had cancer died of pleurisy. Since I lectured to you here last week I have seen a patient who had her breast removed four years ago for carcinoma, and within the last six months she has developed pleurisy with effusion, which, in spite of tapping, has resulted in a refilling of the chest again and again. Together with this there is general illness and loss of health, which makes one feel sure that in this patient there is a pleural effusion consequent upon a growth of carcinoma in the pleura. Some years ago a patient was operated upon for recurrent carcinoma of the breast in this hospital, and afterwards she did badly. She had trouble in her chest and difficulty of breathing, and developed a large pleural effusion and ultimately died. On a post-mortem examina-

tion being made the whole of the pleura was found to be studded with small nodules of cancer. When you come to think of it, this is rather a place to which you might expect cancer of the breast to extend, because through the intercostal spaces lymphatics pass from the mamma to the mediastinum. Is it not therefore easy to see how the pleura may become involved? I think it is rather surprising that it is not more frequently involved than is the case. But when you have spoken of the pleura you have not exhausted the seats of extension which you may find inside the chest, for you may have both the lungs and the glands in the mediastinum infected. There may be much growth in the lung, and yet it may be very difficult in many cases to find any definite physical signs of it, even though there may be a large amount scattered in different parts of the several lobes. There may be growth in the mediastinal glands, and there also it is not easily diagnosed unless extensive enough to cause pressure. All this has to be suspected and considered in any case of cancer of the breast. Then there are more widespread conditions, some of which I have mentioned to you already in connection with diseases of bone. You will remember that last month, when I lectured upon diseases of bone I told you that amongst the other diseases of bone was secondary carcinoma. I told you that in cancer of the breast there were certain bones which were particularly liable to be involved. I mentioned the humerus, the femur, the sternum, and the spine. Any pain referred to any of these parts should at once excite your suspicions, and I told you when I was speaking on this subject that carcinoma in bone may grow without causing any apparent tumour or enlargement that can be felt. When the bone is quite near the surface, as is the case with the sternum and humerus, you can perceive enlargements which you would not feel in the spine or in the femur. But you should remember that continuous aching pain in any one of these bones or in the spine, or the oncoming of symptoms suggestive of pressure on the spinal cord should lead you to be suspicious of the development of carcinoma in a patient who has cancer of the breast, or who has had cancer of the breast which has been removed, even though it has been removed for many years. Some time ago I saw a patient who had had her breast removed a considerable time before, and I was consulted because she had what was believed to be "sciatica." But it was not the characteristic pain of sciatica. With it she was very weak on the limb and she said to me, " I feel as if this leg would hardly bear the weight of my body." I said I thought that this poor patient very likely had a cancerous growth of her femur, though there was no definite evidence of it to be ascertained, and within six weeks of that time the femur spontaneously fractured one morning as she was getting out of bed. I mention that now to remind you that tumours of the bone secondary to cancer of the breast may develop merely with symptoms of pain and weakness, without there being any definite tumour to be felt.

In conclusion, it may be said that there is no viscus that cannot be involved in the spread of carcinoma; and not only may the thoracic and abdominal viscera suffer but in not a few cases growth may affect the brain, and I can recall two or three cases where patients of my own have died from cerebral tumour consequent upon carcinoma of the breast.

February 19th, 1906.

THE FEEDING OF INFANTS.*

By T. R. C. WHIPHAM, M.D.Oxon.,
M.R.C.P.Lond.,
Physician to Out-Patients at the Evelina Hospital for Sick Children.

MR. PRESIDENT AND GENTLEMEN,—When our secretaries asked me to read a paper before this Society I naturally turned to the subject of children, the study of which, I think, is too often neglected in a general hospital.

My subject is "Infant Feeding," and I have selected it as being the fundamental principle in the treatment of infants. The ailments of by far the majority of infants are gastro-intestinal, and of these the greater number are due to improper feeding. Now, of course, everyone here knows that maternal nursing is the natural and ideal method of feeding infants during the first months of life. Unfortunately from social reasons or from the necessity for working, an artificial is often sub-

stituted for a natural diet from the very first. It should be our aim, therefore, to impress upon mothers the desirability of breast-feeding, and where this is possible four nursings should be given in the first twenty-four hours,* six during the second day and after that ten a day till the end of the fourth week. You will remember that at birth the capacity of an infant's stomach is only 1 oz., and that it increases rapidly, till at two weeks it is 2 oz., at three months 4½ oz., and at the end of a year 9 oz. You will also recollect that lactation in a mother is not fully established till about the third day. From this you will see that Nature enjoins that the amount of food to be given during the first forty-eight hours of life should be small, and this is not surprising considering the changes that are taking place in the circulation and the respiratory system. After the fourth week the breast should be given according to Table I.

TABLE I.—*Schedule for Breast Feeding.*

Age.	Number of nursings in 24 hours.	Interval during the day.	Night nursings 9 p.m. —7 a.m.
1 day . . .	4	6 hours	1
2 days . .	6	4 ,,	1
3—28 days . .	10	2 ,,	2
1—3 months .	8	2½ ,,	1
3—5 months .	7	3 ,,	1
5—12 months .	6	3 ,,	0

Now, it is absolutely essential that the details here given should be strictly carried out, and that the child should not be put to the breast whenever the mother "thinks it wants it," or whenever it cries. An infant's stomach requires periods of rest the same as an adult's, and if it is fed too often there is a gastro-intestinal upset. Children, if managed properly, can easily be trained to sleep with regularity, and a healthy child will have at least one sleep of four to five hours in the twenty-four. Hence it is advisable to wake the child during the day for his two-hourly feeds, in order that he may sleep better during the night, and only wake for his one or two nursings. In this way the mother is less disturbed and has a chance of regaining her strength.

In addition to these details of breast-feeding the

---

* Read before the Hunterian Society of St. George's Hospital.

* Some authorities advise not more than two or three nursings during the first twenty-four hours.

care of the mother's breasts must be attended to, and this is a point which is often neglected by the poor. Scrupulous cleanliness is absolutely necessary, and the whole of the breasts as well as the nipple should be carefully washed after each nursing. Plain water is perhaps sufficient, or a weak boric lotion may be employed. The health of the mother too is of the utmost importance, and must be attended to as occasion arises, for on this depends a good supply of milk. In this connection a good night's rest is perhaps of as much importance as anything else. Hence the great necessity for training the child to sleep at night, as I have just told you, and, moreover, for enjoining that night-feeding should be stopped after the fifth month (see Table 1). Then on no account should the child be allowed to sleep on the mother's breast, nor even in the same bed. The temptation to frequent feeding at night is thus largely removed, to say nothing of other dangers, such as overlying.

Next we must consider how long the child should be kept at the breast. You may take it that nine months is the proper time for solely breast-feeding. After that the child should be gradually weaned, an increasing number of bottle feeds being substituted for the breast, until at the end of eleven months or a year the child is on a purely artificial diet. This method of procedure is in the interests of both the mother and the child. The mother is saved from the necessity of the breast-pump and other artificial means of stopping the secretion, and lactation gradually ceases, while the child is saved from an abrupt change of diet, which ofttimes causes acute indigestion or is refused, until a serious condition of starvation is arrived at. The bottle feeds, I need hardly say, should consist of diluted cow's milk. The amounts of dilution I shall touch upon presently, when speaking of artificial feeding, but one point in the weaning of infants must be borne in mind, and that is, that the dilution of the milk must be greater than that required by an artificially fed child of the same age. This is especially the case in sudden weaning, when an infant weaned at the ninth or tenth month should be given to begin with bottle food appropriate for one of the third or fourth month, and similarly one weaned at six months a food appropriate for a child of one month, and so forth. When the child is accustomed to the cow's milk its strength can be gradually increased. Wean-

ing in hot weather is usually to be avoided unless one can be sure of the freshness and purity of the milk supply, but the dangers from this are scarcely so great as when lactation is unduly prolonged. The importance of weaning a child after nine months is great, for soon after that time it requires a more varied diet, and if it does not get it, dire results follow. In my experience at a children's hospital breast-feeding continued for more than a year—and often one finds it continued for eighteen months or even two years—without any other dietary is an important factor in the causation of rickets. Thus out of a series of 200 well-marked cases of rickets which have recently come up to my Out-Patient Department I find that 83, or 41·5 per cent., were kept at the breast too long.

This prolonged breast feeding is generally the fault of the mother; it may be the result of slackness—the child is going on tolerably well and she does not take the trouble to change its food—or it may be from the popular idea that as long as lactation is continued another conception will not take place.

Now, under certain circumstances artificial feeding must of necessity form part of the dietary, and this is termed *mixed-feeding*. The necessity for this generally lies with the mother: it may be that her supply of milk is naturally deficient or defective in quality, or if at any time her health begins to suffer, she should be relieved of two or more nursings a day and the bottle substituted. She may thus be enabled to continue lactation for some time longer. When, however, the nursings have been reduced to two or three a day the milk should be frequently examined, as its quality is apt to deteriorate. Retarded convalescence after parturition, again, may cause the mother's milk to be insufficient until she is well enough to be out and about, in which case two or three bottle feeds a day will tide the child over until he can receive sufficient of his natural food. In all these cases the bottle feeds should be the same as when the child is fed entirely artificially.

Other circumstances, again, render it imperative that breast feeding should not be allowed from the first. No mother who has tuberculosis in any form, whether latent or active, should nurse her child; it may hasten or re-start into activity the disease in the parent, and it exposes the infant to a danger of infection. Any serious complication connected with parturition is another reason

Among such I may mention severe hæmorrhage, nephritis, convulsions, septicæmia. Again, when the mother suffers from any chronic disease nursing will only debilitate her and not correspondingly benefit the child.

In such cases we have to choose between *wet-nursing* and artificial feeding pure and simple. As you may suppose, the difficulties attending the engagement of a good wet-nurse are many. There is, first of all, the expense, and then the difficulty in obtaining a suitable woman free from all suspicion of disease. These considerations, of course, render the employment of a wet-nurse by the poorer members of the community out of the question, but if they can be successfully overcome in the case of the well-to-do, a wet-nurse is undoubtedly of the greatest service, and this is especially the case where we have to deal with premature infants and those

to dilute the milk for young infants. The proportion of fat must be made up by adding cream, which on an average contains 20 per cent. of fat, and that of the sugar by adding lactose or ordinary cane-sugar. There is also another reason for diluting the milk, and that is the dense coagulum which forms in the stomach when feeding with cow's milk. This is considerably lessened by dilution, but does not disappear entirely even when the total proteids are made the same as in woman's milk.

The *proteids* may be modified in one of five ways : either (1) by reducing the proportion by the addition of water ; (2) by ~peptonising ; (3) by separating them after the coagulation of the casein with rennet ; (4) by diluting with gruels made of barley, oatmeal, etc., for their mechanical effect upon the coagulation of the casein ; or (5) by the

TABLE II.—*Comparison of Human with Cow's and other Milk.*

	Human milk.	Fresh cow's milk.	Condensed cow's milk.	Ass's milk.	Goat's milk.	Mare's milk.
Proteids—Total .	1·5 per cent.	3·5 per cent.	14 per cent.	2·7 per cent.	3·8 per cent.	2·2 per cent.
Lactalbumen	·8 „	·5 „	—	—	—	—
Casein	·7 „	3 „	—	—	—	—
Sugar . . .	6—7 „	4—5 „	49 „	5·3 „	4·3 „	5·8 „
Fat . . .	4 „	4 „	10 „	1 „	5·2 „	1·1 „
Salts . . .	·2 „	·75 „	2 „	·4 „	·7 „	·3 „
Water . . .	87·3 „	87·25 „	25 „	90·6 „	86 „	90·6 „

with feeble powers of assimilation, who from chronic indigestion fail to thrive on artificial food. In the majority of instances, however, we have to resort to artificial feeding.

Before giving the details of *artificial feeding*, it is necessary to compare human and cow's milk, for cow's is, practically speaking, the only milk available for common use.

From the table it will be seen that the proportions of the constituents are not the same in cow's as in human milk. You will observe that in cow's milk there is excess of proteids and salts and too little sugar, the quantity of fat being the same. The cow's milk must therefore be modified to suit the requirements of the infant as far as may be.

Now, there is more than twice as much proteid in cow's milk as in human milk, and of the total proteids casein forms by far the greater amount. Proteids, especially the casein, are the most difficult part to digest, and on this account it is necessary

addition of sodium citrate. For the healthy infant reduction of the proportion of the proteids is all that is required, but during the early months, until the stomach is accustomed to the cow's milk, a reduction beyond 1·5 per cent. is advisable, even down to 0·5 per cent. The strength can be gradually increased until at the end of the second or third month 1·5 per cent. can be given, and by the end of the fourth or fifth month 2 per cent. The full proportion of proteids in cow's milk can seldom be given before the child is a year old.

The *salts* in cow's milk are in excess in about the same proportion as the proteids, so that the necessary dilution is the same for both. This constituent, therefore, can be left out of our calculations.

The *sugar* in cow's milk is about 2 per cent. less than in human milk, so that to raise it to the proportion required is a very simple matter. Thus if lactose be added, ʒj is equivalent to 2 per cent. in

7 oz. of milk, and in artificial feeding the carbohydrate should be kept at about the normal proportion. Lactose is the best sugar to use both theoretically and practically. It should be dissolved in boiling water and filtered, if necessary, and should be prepared fresh every day, at all events in summer. Failing this, cane-sugar may be substituted, but in only little more than half the quantity, as it is sweeter and more liable to undergo fermentation in the stomach. This is especially the case with brown sugar, but, on the other hand, the brown in some cases has the advantage over white in that it is more laxative.

With regard to the *fat*, except for the first few days of life, an infant can digest 2 to 4 per cent.— 2 per cent. at the end of the first week, and 4 per cent. at four or five months. Any deficiency in the fat in diluted cow's milk must therefore be made good, and this is done by the addition of cream.

The *acidity* which occurs in cow's milk on being kept even for a short time may be overcome by the addition of either lime-water or bicarbonate of soda to the milk—of the lime-water about 1 oz. to 20 oz. of food; of the soda about 1 gr. to the ounce.

Having thus considered the composition of milk generally, I shall next deal more in detail with the preparation of the infant's food, which shall be suitable to its age. For the *first three or four months* of life it is desirable that the amount of fat should be three times that of the proteids—*i. e.* about the usual ratio in breast milk. The best way to obtain this is to get a milk containing 10 per cent. of fat and 3 per cent. of proteid, and to dilute it. Now, 10 per cent. fat and 3 per cent. proteid is found in "top-milk," as it is called. Good milk fresh from the cow is allowed to stand in a cool place for four hours, and the upper third of the milk is then siphoned or baled off. Begin at birth with 2 oz. of this top-milk, 1 oz. of lactose, and 1 oz. of lime-water, diluted with water up to 20 oz. The proportion of the milk can then be increased ounce by ounce till 4 oz. in 20 are used at the end of a week, and 6 oz. or 7 oz. in 20 at the end of three or four months.

Now, of course all this is ideal, and the mothers of hospital patients have not the time, the intelligence, or the money to carry out ideal feeding, but I hope that all of you will have patients possessing these attributes, and then the value of these things will

be apparent. Therefore, as the mothers of hospital patients cannot, or will not, carry out an ideal method, it behoves us to see how we can best make use of the materials that we have—*i. e.* a stupid mother and ordinary cow's milk—and in passing led me add that I do not believe that a rigid adherence to figures is absolutely necessary for the proper nutrition of an infant. The majority do perfectly well on the approximate proportions that I am going to give you, though of course there are instances in which one or other of the constituents of the milk must be increased or diminished. You will remember that I am still dealing with children during the first three or four months of life. The child's first feeds should consist of diluted milk, in the proportion of one of milk to three of water, and to this 60 gr. or a small teaspoonful of lactose merely should be added to every 3 oz. of food. At the end of the first week 1 teaspoonful of cream should be added as well. About the third month the child should be taking one of milk to two of water, with a teaspoonful of milk sugar, and 2½ teaspoonfuls of cream to every 4 oz. of the mixture.

For the *middle period* of infancy—*i. e.* from the end of the third or fourth month to the end of the ninth or tenth—the amount of fat in the food should be twice that of the proteids. These proportions correspond to rich breast-milk. The ideal way to obtain this is to get a milk containing 7 per cent. of fat and 3·5 per cent. of proteid, and this is found in the top *half* of the milk, which has been allowed to stand, as I described just now, that for the earlier months, you will remember, having been the top *third*. The child is now, at the end of the third or fourth month, able to take as food 7 oz. of the top half of the milk, with 1 oz. of lactose and 1 oz. of lime-water, as before, diluted to 20 oz. The milk is again to be increased ounce by ounce as time goes on, till at the end of the ninth or tenth month he takes 10 oz. of this top milk in 20 oz. of food. Translating this again for use in the case of poor patients, we begin the fourth or fifth month with ordinary milk diluted with rather more than an equal part of water, and to every 4-oz. feed we add 3 teaspoonfuls of cream and 1½ teaspoonfuls of lactose (100 to 120 gr.). The milk is increased in amount till at the end of the period the infant takes half-and-half milk and water with sugar as before, and 4 teaspoonfuls of cream to 5 oz. of the food.

During the *later part of the first year* the child should be rapidly pushed on to plain milk in 8-oz. feeds, with the added sugar, reduced to about half the former amount, as much of the carbohydrate may now be given in the form of starch. Starchy foods may, indeed, be given a little earlier than this, but at all events not before the seventh or eighth month as a rule. The starchy foods which are advisable are gruels made from barley, arrow-root, or oatmeal—the last if the child has a tendency to constipation—or some farinaceous food such as Ridge's, Neave's, or Savory and Moore's, Robinson's patent barley, or the Allen-bury malted foods—Savory and Moore's or the Allenbury being perhaps as good as any to begin with, as they both contain malt. With regard to barley-water, which is the commonest starchy food,

same time ½ to 2 oz. of fresh fruit juice—such as that of an orange—may with advantage be given in the morning.

Having now settled the constituents of the baby's food, we must consider *how often* and in *what amounts* it must be given. To merely repeat the times and quantities would be wearisome, so I have tabulated them in Table IV. Suffice it to say that an infant should not be fed oftener than every two hours, and not whenever the mother "thinks it wants it." Feeding too often is naturally a source of indigestion, and the child cries. This, the mother imagines, is from hunger; more food is given, which perhaps relieves the pain for a time, but more pain follows, and so the child goes from bad to worse. After the fifth week every two and a half hours is sufficient, and after the third month once in every three hours. With regard to the night feeds, pray remember that they are frequently given too often

TABLE III.—*Composition of Feeds.*

Age.	Cow's milk.	Water.	Additions.
1 week	1 part	3 parts	1 teaspoonful (small) of lactose to 3 oz. of food
2—12 weeks	1 ,,	3 ,,	1 do. and 1 teaspoonful of cream to 3 oz.
3—5 months	1 ,,	2 ,,	1—1½ do. and 2½—3½ do. do. 4 oz.
6—9 ,,	1 ,,	1 part	1½ do. and 4 do. do. 5 oz.
9—12 ,,	Pure	—	1 do. to 8 oz., together with starchy food.

it should be made as follows : Take 2 table-spoonfuls of barley and soak it in water for a few hours, then remove the barley and add 1 quart of *fresh* water. Set it to boil continuously for six hours, keeping up the quantity to 1 quart by the addition of water, and at the end of that time strain through coarse muslin. This sets into a thin jelly when cold, and should, therefore, be warmed before being added to the food. It is best to begin by making the food consist of one third barley-water, and as time goes on to increase the strength of the barley-water rather than to use a larger quantity. The only other things that are advisable during the first year are beef-juice and fresh fruit. Beef-juice is made by adding 8 oz. of water to 1 lb. of chopped beef, and allowing it to stand for six to twelve hours. The juice is then extracted by squeezing the meat in coarse muslin or in a lemon-squeezer. A little salt should be added, and 2 to 3 teaspoonfuls may be given daily during the tenth or eleventh month. About the

and long after they are necessary. This is, of course, bad for both the child and the mother. Two night feeds are required during the first three weeks, and after the fifth month they should be discontinued.

I next come to the important question of *sterilisa-tion.* Should the milk be sterilised or not ? It is an important question and one on which authorities differ. For my own part, I think that unless one, so to speak, knows the cow from which the milk is drawn, and the way in which the milk is handled, and unless one can be certain that it is never more than twenty-four hours old, all the baby's milk should be sterilised, and this is especially important in dealing with the poorer population of large cities. The simplest and a very efficient way of sterilising milk is to bring it up to the boil, and then set it in a cool place or on ice till it is required. This method, however, has its drawbacks. Spores are not destroyed, and at an ordinary temperature spore-bearing bacteria may soon develop and make the milk dangerous. Some of these act upon the proteids and not upon the sugar, so that such milk is not always sour, and the danger may escape detection. Again, the taste of the milk is altered, and some of the lactose is converted into caramel, causing it to become a brownish colour. These, however, are but slight drawbacks ; more important are the coagulation of part of the lactalbumen by heat (the scum on the top of boiled milk), the greater resistance to the action of pepsin and trypsin, the constipating effects of such milk, and the destruction of certain natural ferments which apparently aid digestion. As the result of one or more of these changes the milk is rendered less nutritious, and possibly is liable to give rise to scurvy when used for some time. In spite of all these drawbacks, however, I give it as my opinion

TABLE IV.—*Artificial Feeding during the first Year.*

Age.	Interval during day.	Night Feeds.	Feeds in 24 hours.	Quantity per feed.	Quantity in 24 hours.
3—7 days.	. 2 hours	2	10	1—1½ oz.	10—15 oz.
2—3 weeks	. 2 „	2	10	1½—3½ „	15—35 „
4—5 „	2 „	1	10	2½—3½ „	25—35 „
6 wks.—3 mths.	2½ „	1	8	3—5 „	25—40 „
3—5 months	. 3 „	1	7	4—6 „	28—42 „
5—9 „	. 3 „	0	6	5—7½ „	30—45 „
9—12 „	. 4 „	0	5	7—9 „	35—45 „

that in the case of hospital patients it is best to have all the milk boiled.

A better and more efficient method of sterilising is by Pasteurisation (if you will allow me to use the word), but this, of course, requires care and a special apparatus. Bottles of milk are placed in a metal receptacle and exposed to steam at a temperature of 155° F. for half an hour. In this way the bacilli of tuberculosis, diphtheria, and typhoid are destroyed, and most other bacteria, though, of course, not the spores or toxins. Various forms of such apparatus are on the market, but I cannot enter into the details of their construction now. They are, of course, only within the reach of well-to-do parents. Before leaving the subject of sterilisation I need hardly add that all the water used for diluting the milk should be thoroughly well boiled.

Now a few points concerning the *administration* of the milk. The food should be warmed to about 100° F. before feeding. This is best done by placing the bottle in a saucepan or dish containing water rather above this temperature. The milk, when dropped on to the back of the hand, should feel warm, but not hot, and this is sufficient test of the temperature. The mother should on no account be allowed to suck the nipple with her own mouth. The time allowed for a feed should not exceed twenty minutes, and the infant should not be allowed to go to sleep with the nipple in its mouth. While the feed is being given care should be taken that the neck of the bottle is always kept full, so that the child sucks milk and not air. The best kind of bottle, as you know, is the boat-shaped one with a widish mouth, over which a short nipple is slipped. These are fairly easily kept clean, and the nipple can be everted and washed. The round bottles with long tubes are to be condemned, as it is impossible to keep them clean: to this kind the French have given the very appropriate name *tue-bébé.* It is best to have two bottles for alternate use. After the feed both the nipple and the bottle should be rinsed in cold water and then washed with warm soap-suds, the bottle being well scrubbed out with a brush. They should then be allowed to stand in water, to which a little borax or boracic acid has been added, while the second bottle is in use. Before being used again they should be rinsed and the bottle placed in boiling water for ten minutes. There is one point to be remembered about the nipple, and that is, always examine its aperture ; some are too small, so that the child has a mechanical difficulty in sucking, and perhaps does not get enough food ; others, again, are too large, and the child gulps down the meal too quickly, with the result that vomiting and colic often follow. The hole should be just large enough to allow the milk to flow at the rate of one drop per second when the bottle is inverted.

Now, how are we to tell if the infant is thriving on the food that is given to it? Of course appearances are some guide, but in children, who are much wasted when first seen, it is often very difficult to tell by merely looking at them whether they are improving or not as time goes on. In these, and in fact in all cases, it is best to have the child's weight regularly taken. I do not mean by this a daily weighing, for slight variations from day to day are apt to alarm a nervous mother and mislead the physician. Once or twice a week is sufficient for us to judge the progress of a case. For this purpose we must use accurate scales weighing to half-ounces. Several patterns of these will be found in the instrument-makers' catalogues. You must remember, however, that during the first two days infants lose about 10 oz. in weight, owing partly to the discharge of meconium and urine, and partly to the small intake of food. They then, if breast-fed and thriving well, steadily increase in weight at the rate of about 1¼ oz. a day, till about the tenth day they reach the original weight at birth. With children artificially fed from the first, however, there is usually a stationary period, lasting one to two weeks after the initial drop, before the weight begins to increase. This is due to the digestive organs taking some time to become accustomed to the new food, and must not be taken as an indication to increase either the strength or the quantity of the food unduly rapidly, or indigestion will be the result. The most rapid increase in weight occurs during the first three months, and the slowest from the sixth to the ninth month. In artificially fed children, as I have said, the increase during the first month is slow, but the deficiency between such a child and a breast-fed one is usually made up by the sixth month. At the end of a year the child's weight should be nearly three times that at birth.

If, then, we find that the baby is not gaining weight, although it is digesting well, and has no untoward symptoms, it means that it is not having enough food. With all infants it must be remembered that it is best to increase the food very gradually. Rapid changes are apt to upset the digestion, and it is seldom wise to add more than ¼ oz. at a time to the feeds, or even ½ oz. in the case of young babies. It is best perhaps to alternate increase in quantity and increase in strength of the food. In this way too great an increase of bulk is avoided. Of course babies are not all exactly alike in their powers of digestion, so that you must not adhere too strictly to the tables that I have given you : they represent the average infant's powers. What you have to do is to treat your patient, and if you find he wants and can digest more food than is usually required, well, then give it to him.

Next I come to deal with *loss of weight from constitutional causes or disease*, and will begin most conveniently with *marasmus* or simple wasting. This is a failure of assimilation, " a vice of nutrition " as it has been called. The condition often occurs when weaning has been rendered necessary

at about a month or six weeks. Previously to this the child has been plump and well nourished, but with a change of diet it steadily wastes. The stools usually contain undigested food, and are large in proportion to the intake. Digestion is upset, and vomiting is easily excited. Now, these cases require very delicate and careful handling, and frequently, in spite of all one's endeavours, they eventually slip through one's fingers. Although they seem to be taking sufficient nourishment, they gradually get worse. Under the age of four months it is best to put the child to a wet-nurse ; artificial feeding frequently fails. Above the age of six months the child has a better chance, and bottle-feeding may be employed. These children have difficulty in digesting the proteids and fats, so that both these constituents must be reduced by diluting the milk, while the sugar is kept relatively high. It is a mistake to increase the fat in the hope that the child will assimilate more. In those cases where the digestion of proteids is the chief difficulty the milk may be *peptonised* either partially or completely. Partial peptonisation is brought about by mixing 1 pint of milk with ¼ pint of water and adding 5 gr. of pancreatic extract and 15 gr. of bicarbonate of soda. Fairchild's zymine powders are of this strength and are most commonly used. The vessel is then placed in hot water with a temperature of 110° F.—about as hot as the hand can bear—for a quarter to half an hour. Some of the proteids are thus converted into peptones, and to prevent the furtherance of the process the milk should then be rapidly brought to the boil. It should then be kept in a cool place till needed. To peptonise the milk completely the process is continued for two hours, by which time all the proteids will be converted. Such milk is rather bitter, but infants, as a rule, take it readily after the first bottle or so. With older children a little lemon-juice and sugar will cover the taste. The peptonised milk should be diluted according to the child's requirements, though it is perhaps better to regulate the proportions before peptonising. So also it is better to peptonise each feed separately, in which case there is no need to scald the milk, and the action of the pepsin can continue in the stomach.

Another way of helping the digestion of proteids is by the addition of some *cereal gruel*, which is often of great benefit, though it must always be remembered that for healthy infants with normal digestions such additions to the food are not only undesirable, but often harmful. The gruel apparently prevents the casein from forming such dense masses of curd in the stomach, and in this way higher percentages of proteid can be digested than would otherwise be the case. The stools become more natural and the colic and general disturbance abate. Such gruel is made from barley, oatmeal, or arrowroot, one tablespoonful of the flour being added to a pint of water and boiled from twenty to thirty minutes, the whole being again made up to a pint at the end. The gruel is used to replace either the whole or part of the water in the feeds.

If these methods fail, or as an alternative proceeding, we may remove the casein from the milk and feed the child on food made with the resultant *whey*. To make whey we proceed as follows : In 1 pint of lukewarm milk 2 teaspoonfuls of rennet are stirred, and the mixture is allowed to stand until coagulation takes place. The curd is then broken up and the whey strained off. This is an age of tabloids, so that perhaps it is not surprising to find rennet tabloids on the market. Hansen's junket tablets, one dissolved in a quart of milk, act very well, and may be used, if preferred, instead of the fluid rennet. The whey contains a little proteid in the form of lactalbumen, which is readily digestible, and practically all the sugar of milk, but very little fat—less than 10 per cent. This deficiency must, therefore, be made good by the addition of cream and a little sugar to bring the percentage up to the child's requirements. Before adding the cream the temperature of the whey should be raised to 150° F. to destroy the rennet ferment, and any further coagulation that occurs during the heating should be filtered off.

Another, more recent, method of rendering the casein less dense and so more digestible is by adding *sodium citrate* 1, 2, or 3 gr. to every ounce of food, as suggested by Dr. Poynton. A solution of sodium citrate containing the requisite number of grains to the drachm, according to the number of ounces in each feed, is prescribed with a little chloroform-water to check fungus growth, and the mother is told to add one teaspoonful to each bottle. This method is a very good one, and I have repeatedly found it of much value in cases of milk dyspepsia.

In addition to malassimilation of the food these wasters often suffer from lack of fluid and benefit greatly by enemata or subcutaneous injections of normal salt solution. They must also have a good supply of fresh air and must be kept warm.

On rare occasions it may be necessary to have recourse to *condensed milk* when other methods prove of no avail, though the period of its use must be limited as far as possible. Why this must be, and why condensed milk is at times useful, I will tell you in a minute, but first let me put in a word or two of warning concerning such milk, which I consider one of the greatest scourges of the infant poor. Why it should be such a favourite with mothers, and I regret to say with many medical men also, I am at a loss to understand, and I am not exaggerating when I say that many medical men resort straight away to condensed milk when the child shows any sign of intestinal disturbance. If you ask the mothers why they use it, you will find that they have generally no reason whatever to give. The only excuse, which is at all legitimate, is that in summer it is at times difficult or impossible to obtain cow's milk sufficiently fresh to remain sweet till the following day. This may be the case with milk bought at the average milk-shop, but with a little trouble it is possible to find dairies, even in the heart of this London of ours, where you can see the milk drawn straight from the cow, and I know of two such places in the poorer districts of South London.

Condensed milk is prepared by heating fresh cow's milk to boiling point to destroy bacteria, and then evaporating it *in vacuo* at a low temperature to one quarter of its volume. Cane-sugar is added— about six ounces to the pint—and the milk is then preserved in hermetically sealed tins. The composition of such milk is given in Table II. It is usually given diluted with 16 or 18 parts of water, but I have known infants to be fed on the plain milk from the tin with, of course, the inevitable results.

A glance at the composition will show that condensed milk contains when diluted little proteid, very little fat, and an abundance of sugar ; moreover, the natural ferments are destroyed by the heat to which it has been subjected. For these reasons it is inadequate as a permanent food, and out of my series of cases of rickets 19·5 per cent. were found to be due to its continued use. As a temporary expedient it may, as I have said, be useful on occasions when other methods fail, as after dilution the casein is reduced to a very low point, whereas there still remains an abundance of carbohydrate, which is the easiest thing for an infant to digest. But let me once more impress upon you that the occasions when it is necessary to resort to condensed milk are very few and far between, and it should never be ordered unless the case is under your constant supervision. For my own part I scarcely ever order it for hospital out-patients, as there is a great danger that, its use having been once sanctioned, the mother will continue giving it after the child has got better and ceased attending. That it is possible to do without it is further borne out by the fact that in the wards at the Evelina it is very seldom employed.

I next come to lesions of the stomach and intestinal tract. It is important to discover which of the two is at fault ; and, speaking broadly, we may take it that vomiting, eructations, and a coated tongue indicate some derangement of the stomach, and that the intestines are affected if we find colic, flatulence, distended abdomen, diarrhœa or constipation, and curds or mucus in the stools. The first thing to do is to inquire into the manner of feeding of the child and to bring home to the mother any irregularities according to the broad principles that I have already described. Then, having decided from the symptoms that we have to deal with a case, say, of *acute gastric indigestion* or *acute gastritis*, the best mode of treatment is to empty the stomach and then give it rest for a time. By far the best method of emptying the stomach is to wash it out. ¯The method of procedure you all know. A catheter with a long india-rubber tube and funnel attached is passed into the stomach. The gas is allowed to escape and the stomach contents are then siphoned off by lowering the tube. Plain boiled water at about 100° F., or water to which a little sodium bicarbonate has been added, is then introduced and allowed to escape, the process being repeated two or three times, until the water is returned clear. If this is impracticable, vomiting may be induced by giving large quantities of lukewarm water from the bottle, but this plan is not so efficacious. After this nothing should be given for the next three or four hours, when ½ to 1 oz. of whey or albumen-water should be administered every hour. Albumen-water is merely the white of a fresh egg beaten

up in half a pint of previously boiled water, with the addition of a little salt. After twenty-four hours raw beef-juice or broth may be tried, but no milk should be given for at least three days. When milk is begun again it should be peptonised and diluted with five or six parts of water. In a nursing child the breast should be withheld for twenty-four hours and then resumed for two minutes every three hours, the time of suckling being increased minute by minute as the child improves. The great mistake is to begin food too soon and to give too much, especially of cow's milk.

You will notice that up to the present I have not said a word about drugs. In the cases with which I am dealing they are really of very secondary importance. Attend to the feeding, and you will in most instances bring about a satisfactory result. If, however, the bowels do not act freely, you may give calomel in ½-gr. doses every hour until they do, or if there is persistent vomiting of very acid mucus, alkalies, such as lime-water, chalk, or bismuth, are useful. The child should be kept quite quiet, and warm applications to the abdomen are often beneficial if there is much prostration.

In cases of *chronic gastric indigestion* daily lavage of the stomach should be made with alkaline water to remove the mucus and stimulate the secretion. It is necessary, also, to determine which constituent of the milk is the chief source of the trouble ; it is most frequently the fat, next the proteids, and only rarely the sugar. A too high proportion of fat brings about a regurgitation of sour, curdled milk, or a watery fluid, one to two hours after feeding, and the passage of offensive stools, either large, dry, and greyish in colour, or loose and rather green. Excess of proteids is evidenced by colic, curds in the motions, and often constipation. The food, therefore, must be regulated as occasion requires, though where serious and long-continued trouble exists a change to a farinaceous food may for a time check the gastric fermentation. Drugs here, again, are of but little real value as compared with regulation of the diet. Pepsin and hydrochloric acid are disappointing, though where flatulence is a prominent symptom salicylate of soda in 1 to 2 gr. doses is of much value.

Associated with acute gastric symptoms, we frequently find indications of *acute intestinal derangement*, and for the intestines the same general plan should be employed as for the stomach—first evacuation and then rest. Small doses of calomel, or doses of castor oil or salines, should be given until a full effect is produced, and all food should be withheld for twenty-four hours. Thirst may be relieved by small quantities of albumen or plain water, and brandy is indicated if there is much collapse. After the bowels have been well cleared out, Dover's powder up to $\frac{1}{4}$ grain may be given after each stool to check any excessive diarrhœa. Stimulants are required in severe cases, as the prostration is often great, and ℳx of brandy may be prescribed every one or two hours, according to the age. With regard to the use of opium, you must, of course, be very careful, and it should only be used to check excessive diarrhœa. Furthermore, every care should be taken to keep the child warm. With nursing infants breast-feeding may be resumed after twenty-four hours, but only at intervals of six hours, and for five minutes at a time. In between other foods should be administered. Artificially-fed children should be kept without milk for five or six days, broths, farinaceous, or malted foods being given. Milk should be resumed very cautiously, and only for one or two feeds each day to begin with : it may with advantage be peptonised. As fat is likely to cause disturbance, cream should not be added.

In the summer-time we frequently come across cases of *acute gastro-intestinal intoxication*, gastro-enteritis, or summer diarrhœa, as it is sometimes called. This appears to be infective in origin, as it occurs for the most part in artificially-fed children, and at a time when the high temperature favours bacterial growth. During the wet summer of 1903, for instance, I noticed that these cases were remarkably few in number, and I believe that such was the case at other hospitals than my own. Curiously enough, cases of cerebro-spinal meningitis were at that time especially numerous, and among my out-patients at the Evelina I frequently had two or three cases waiting for admission into the wards. The treatment of cases of gastro-enteritis resolves itself into hygienic, dietetic, and medicinal. With regard to hygiene, fresh air is of the utmost importance. Children in towns should be sent into the country if the attack does not subside in a few days, and in any case a change is advisable to prevent the danger of a relapse. The child should be kept out of doors for the greater part of the day, and its clothing should be light but

warm. Especial care must be taken to remove immediately all soiled napkins and to keep the child clean. The dietetic treatment consists in stopping all food, and especially milk, at once. Thirst may be relieved by whey, thin barley-water, or albumen-water. After a day or two, according to the symptoms, the food may be cautiously resumed. Broths (strained, of course), farinaceous, or malted foods may be first tried, and then very small quantities of boiled milk, carefully watching its effects on the stools and temperature. Speaking generally, the quantity should be a quarter or half of that usually given in health, and sufficiently long intervals allowed between the feeds—viz. at least two hours, and often better four. Here, again, the therapeutic treatment consists in first emptying the stomach and intestines to remove all toxic substances. The stomach should be washed out, and calomel, castor oil, or salines given, and this treatment should be repeated if symptoms of fresh intoxication develop. Irrigation of the colon is also advisable, as it hastens the removal of offensive material. Such antiseptics as bismuth, preferably the subnitrate or the salicylate, in sufficiently large doses—*e.g.* 5 to 10 gr., salicylate of soda or salol 1 to 2 gr., resorcin $\frac{1}{2}$ to 1 gr., are at times useful. Alkalies and chalk are of value in the acute stages and dilute hydrochloric acid later on. Astringents often do more harm than good, but with excessive catarrhal diarrhœa they are advantageous, and sometimes it is necessary to resort to opium in minute doses. Stimulants are required in many severe cases and should be always given well diluted. When there is extreme prostration warmth is essential, and where the drain is very rapid and great subcutaneous injections of saline solution will at times confer a great and lasting benefit.

February 19th, 1906.

PROFESSOR C. S. SHERRINGTON's new work on ' The Integrative Action of the Nervous System' will be published soon by Messrs. Archibald Constable and Co. In the multicellular animal the author holds, especially for those higher re-actions which constitute its behaviour as a social unit, in the natural economy, it is nervous reaction which *par excellence* integrates it and constitutes it an animal individual. This integrative action, in virtue of which the nervous system unifies from separate organs an animal possessing solidarity, is the problem which Professor Sherrington discusses in this book in a luminous manner.

THE CLINICAL JOURNAL,

CLINICAL RECORD, CLINICAL NEWS, CLINICAL GAZETTE, CLINICAL REPORTER,
CLINICAL CHRONICLE AND CLINICAL REVIEW.

EDITED BY L. ELIOT CREASY.

No. 696. WEDNESDAY, FEBRUARY 28, 1906. Vol. XXVII. No. 20.

CONTENTS.

Specially reported for the Clinical Journal. Revised by the Author.

ALL RIGHTS RESERVED.

NOTICE.

Editorial correspondence, books for review, &c., should be addressed to the Editor, 51, *New Cavendish Street, W., Telephone No.* 904, *Paddington ; but all business communications should be addressed to the Publishers,* 22½, *Bartholomew Close, London, E.C. Telephone* 927, *Holborn.*

All inquiries respecting Advertisements should be sent to MESSRS. ADLARD & SON, *Bartholomew Close, E.C. Telephone* 927, *Holborn.*

Terms of Subscription, including postage, payable by cheque, postal or banker's order (in advance) : for the United Kingdom, 15s. 6d. *per annum ; Abroad,* 17s. 6d.

Cheques, &c., should be made payable to THE PROPRIETORS OF THE CLINICAL JOURNAL, *crossed "The London, City, and Midland Bank, Ltd., Newgate Street Branch, E.C. Account of the Medical Publishing Company, Limited."*

Reading Cases to hold Twenty-six numbers of THE CLINICAL JOURNAL *can be supplied at* 2s. 3d. *each, or will be forwarded post free on receipt of* 2s. 6d. ; *and also Cases for binding Volumes at* 1s. *each, or post free on receipt of* 1s. 3d., *from the Publishers,* 22½ *Bartholomew Close, London, E.C.*

A LECTURE

ON

A CASE OF PERNICIOUS ANÆMIA.

Delivered at Guy's Hospital.

By W. HALE WHITE, M.D., F.R.C.P.,
Physician to the Hospital.

GENTLEMEN,—The patient I had hoped to bring here for you to see this afternoon is too ill to come, so you must leave it to me to describe his illness to you. The point about him which you would have noticed if he had been here is that he is extremely anæmic, so much so that the problem for us is to try to discover what is the disease which could cause such profound anæmia. Whenever you see anyone who is profoundly anæmic the first thing you have to think about is whether the anæmia could possibly be due to hæmorrhage. When the anæmia is due to hæmorrhage the patients are usually of a dead white colour, something like the colour of a sheet of white note-paper. I do not think that in any other forms of anæmia the patients are of that dead white colour, which is especially striking when the hæmorrhage has been recent. It is a common cause of anæmia. I recently saw a most striking example. I got a message from a doctor asking me to go at once to see a patient with him, and the story was that a young man, æt. 25 years, had vaulted over a table and he had, he thought, ricked his right side. He did this at seven o'clock in the evening, and the pain was so bad that at midnight he sent for the doctor, who found him in some pain. Next morning the man was much worse, and the doctor found that he was not moving the right side of the chest at all, and he wondered whether he had ruptured his lung and had in consequence got a pneumothorax. I saw him at seven o'clock in the evening and the first thing which struck me as I went to the bed was that he was the colour of a piece of white paper,

so much so that I felt certain that he had severe
hæmorrhage somewhere. On going over his chest
.it was true the right side did not move, and we
both agreed there was considerable evidence
that he had fluid at the right base. And bearing
in mind the fact that he was so anæmic, one
ventured the suggestion that he had ruptured something or other, some aneurysm perhaps, which had
led to an effusion of blood into his right pleural
cavity. We put a needle into the cavity and drew
off pure blood. I only mention this case because
of the aid to diagnosis which the tint of the anæmia
gives when there is considerable hæmorrhage. A
very common cause of anæmia, which is constantly
being overlooked, in women especially, is piles.
Women do not like to mention it to their doctor,
and you will frequently meet with considerable
success if, when the woman is anæmic, you go
carefully into the possibility of her bleeding from
piles. Often you will find that that is the cause of
her anæmia. Some of you may remember a man,
who was in Addison Ward, two years ago, with
great pain in his back. The diagnosis lay between
malignant disease of his vertebræ and aneurysm.
He suddenly, one day, had more pain and became
considerably anæmic. We took the specific gravity
of his blood about a day after the great exacerba-
tion of pain in the back, and we found the specific
gravity was low, from which we inferred that the
trouble was probably aneurysm, because a low
specific gravity indicates severe hæmorrhage, for
the first part of the blood to be restored after
hæmorrhage is the fluid and not the solid part.
So for a few days after hæmorrhage the specific
gravity of the blood is lowered. In that case
we were able, by taking his specific gravity, to
know that the man had lost a quantity of blood,
and that therefore he probably had aneurysm,
which was causing the anæmia. That turned out
to be the correct view as shown by the post-
mortem examination. He had retro-peritoneal
hæmorrhage as the result of an aneurysm. However, we cannot find that the man in John Ward
has any hæmorrhage that could cause his anæmia.
You know that the text-books divide anæmia into
primary and secondary. I took down the first
text-book which I had handy, and it was Hare's
'Text-Book of the Practice of Medicine.' He
says : " When anæmia is due to some disorder of
blood-making or blood-destroying tissues it is called

primary, and when to some other cause secondary."
That is obviously an unscientific distinction, because no man can have anæmia unless there is
something the matter with either his blood-forming
or his blood-destroying organs, unless it be the
anæmia due to simple hæmorrhage. But it is a
practical distinction at the bedside, because what
it means is this : Is the anæmia which the patient
before us has secondary to any well-known disease,
or is it due to some disease that at the present
stage of our knowledge we have to call a blood
disease because there is no well-known obvious
cause leading to the change in the blood ? With
this patient now in John Ward we applied this
distinction, and in our minds we went through
what would be the common causes of secondary
anæmia. They are legion, but some of them it is
important to remember. You must never, when a
man is anæmic, overlook the possibility of his
trouble being due to malignant disease. That
mistake is so often made. A patient may have a
malignant growth, generally in the abdominal
cavity, and deep down, producing no symptoms
but anæmia. We can find no evidence of this in
our patient in John Ward, or of any malignant
growth anywhere. In olden days, before we knew
how to stain tubercle bacilli, phthisis was frequently
overlooked as a cause of anæmia. Nowadays I do
not think the mistake is so common ; still, you must
bear in mind that a person who is anæmic may
really be suffering from phthisis. And then syphilis
is occasionally responsible for profound anæmia,
but as far as my experience goes I do not think
the mistake of overlooking it is often made, but
you should always think of syphilis, whatever is the
matter with anybody. There are two diseases of
the thyroid gland which you are very liable to get
into trouble about, for anæmia is often the first
symptom of exophthalmic goitre, and it may be an
early symptom of myxœdema. We examine our
patient, and he has no signs of syphilis, or phthisis,
or exophthalmic goitre or myxœdema. Then certain
poisons are frequently overlooked as a cause—for instance, mercury, or, still more commonly, lead. A
man is poisoned with lead, but the doctor does not
suspect what is the cause of his anæmia, and the
poisoning goes on. We cannot find that our man in
John Ward is poisoned with lead or mercury. There
are many parasites which frequently cause anæmia
and which have often led to mistakes. For instance,

that of malaria will often give rise to anæmia. Frequent mistakes have been made in this country about ankylostomiasis. And we are especially interested in it here, because you will remember that Dr. Boycott, in the year that he held the Gordon Lectureship of Pathology, worked at the cause of the profound anæmia which is common in Cornish miners, namely that due to ankylostomiasis. And if there is any chance of your patient suffering from this parasite, look at the fæces for ova. We have not yet had an opportunity of examining the fæces of our patient. Still, we shall do so. I do not, however, think he is suffering from ankylostomiasis, because he has never followed any occupation especially liable to lead to infection, such as a tunnel-maker, or a miner, or a brick-worker, nor has he any eosinophilia. A year ago, when Dr. Boycott was here, many of you must have seen the ova of the ankylostoma because there were enormous numbers of them in the pathological laboratory, sent from the mines of Cornwall. Another parasite which causes anæmia is the bilharzia. This man has no symptoms which would lead one to suspect that he has that, nor do we suspect him to be infected with *Bothriocephalus latus*. A cause of anæmia which is frequently over-looked is chronic Bright's disease. We went into that subject two or three lectures ago, so I need not go over that ground again. And lastly, you must not forget that some cases of anæmia are due to early Addison's disease.

We have now mentioned the secondary anæmias about which there is likely to be difficulty. We considered them all with regard to our patient, and we cannot find that he is suffering from any of them. Therefore, we have come to the conclusion that he has one of the primary anæmias. They are rapidly disposed of. Two weeks ago I lectured on Hodgkins' disease, and you will remember I brought in two patients suffering from it. Our patient has not got that, he has no enlarged lymphatic glands anywhere that we can detect. We have looked at many slides of his blood, and the white corpuscles are fewer than normal, so he cannot be a case of splenic or lymphatic leukæmia. There is a rare disease called chloroma affecting lymph-glands, but he has not that, nor splenic anæmia—and there is no enlargement of the spleen. And there is that condition called status lymphaticus, which occurs in children, but he has

not got that, and he cannot be a case of chlorosis because he is a man and chlorosis is a disease which is confined to women. So we are able, very rapidly and quickly, to put out of court these various likelihoods, and there remains only one, and that is called pernicious anæmia. That is what we believe our patient to have. It is a disease which we are very interested in here, because it was discovered by that great Guy's physician Addison. And here is the first edition of his famous book called 'On the Constitutional and Local Effects of Disease of the Suprarenal Capsule,' and in it he mentions pernicious anæmia. He says : " For a long period I had from time to time met with a very remarkable form of general anæmia, occurring without any discoverable cause whatever, cases in which there had been no previous loss of blood, no existing diarrhœa, no chlorosis, no purpura, no renal or splenic, miasmic, glandular, strumous, or malignant disease." (He excludes the secondary anæmias, you see.) " Accordingly in speaking of this form of anæmia in a clinical lecture I propose, with little propriety, to apply the term " idiopathic " to distinguish it from cases in which there occurs more or less evidence of some of the usual causes or concomitants of the anæmic state." The word "idiopathic " is always, as he implies, an unsatisfactory word, and by general usage it has been replaced nowadays by the word " pernicious." Addison goes on to say : " The disease presented in every instance the same general character, pursued a similar course, and with scarcely a single accident, was followed after a period by the same fatal result. It occurs in both sexes, generally not exclusively beyond the middle period of life, and so far as I know at present chiefly in persons of a somewhat large and bulky frame, with a strongly marked tendency to the formation of fat." If you will look at the man in the ward, you will find all this is strictly true of our patient. He is beyond the middle period of life ; he, I am sorry to say is dying ; he has a large, bulky frame, and has a tendency to the formation of fat. " It makes its approach with so slow and insidious a manner " —this man has been getting ill for months—" that the patient can hardly fix a date to his earliest feeling of that languor which is shortly to become so extreme. The countenance gets pale, the whites of the eyes become pearly, the general frame flabby rather than wasted, the pulse perhaps large but remarkably soft and compressible, and occasionally with a slight jerk, especially under the slightest exertion. There is an increasing indisposition to exertion, with an uncomfortable feeling of faintness or breathlessness on attempting it. The heart is readily made to palpitate. The whole surface of the body presents a blanched, smooth, waxy appearance." " Extreme languor and faintness supervene, breathlessness and palpitations being produced by the most trifling exertion or emotion. Some slight œdema is probably perceived about the eyelids, debility becomes extreme, the patient can no longer rise from his bed, the mind occasionally wanders "—and it is so with our patient, and that is one of the reasons I could not bring him down for you to see to-day—" he falls into a prostrate and half torpid state, and at length expires. Nevertheless to the very last, after a sickness of several months' duration, the bulkiness of the general frame of the man often presents a most striking contrast to the failure and exhaustion observed in every other respect." There is nothing like going to the first description, and if you will take this book and go to the man dying in John Ward, you will see that this account, which was published as long ago as 1855—that is to say, exactly fifty years ago—applies precisely, even to the bulk of the man, to the patient now dying in John Ward. So you see we believe that this man, inasmuch as he conforms exactly to Addison's famous description, is suffering from pernicious anæmia, which is what the disease is generally called nowadays.

I want, please, before describing the case to you, to get into your minds, which many people have not got, that this disease is a distinct clinical entity. It is rare, and there are many other forms of profound anæmia ; and the result is that many cases have been recorded, especially in Germany, of people who have been profoundly anæmic as the result of some well-ascertained cause, but because the anæmia has been profound the patients have been said to have pernicious anæmia. For example, you will find some cases recorded in which it has followed severe post-partum hæmorrhage, or hæmorrhage from fibroids or various other primary causes. But pernicious anæmia is a distinct clinical entity, as was foreseen by Addison, presenting different features from the anæmia due to any other cause, and not having for its cause any common well-

known condition. And his clinical insight has proved of late years to be more correct than he knew, because we have found that this peculiar disease has a perfectly distinct condition of blood, perfectly distinct from the blood, for instance, which would be present if the patient's anæmia were due to repeated hæmorrhages.

So now we come to the blood, and I want to tell you something about that.

Supposing you go into the ward and prick the man, you will notice that the blood flows with difficulty, that it coagulates badly, and is very pale and remarkably fluid. Indeed, it is after death much more fluid than is the case with most other diseases. You then put some under the microscope, and the first thing which strikes you is the enormous diminution in the number of red cells. There is a case recorded in which the number of red-cells sank to 143,000 per cm. Our man on two occasions has shown counts of 900,000 odd ; that is to say, the red cells were reduced by more than four fifths. You then look at the white cells, and you are at once struck with the fact that there is nothing much wrong with them, except that perhaps they are a shade fewer than normal. Having noticed that, turn your attention to the hæmoglobin and estimate that, and you will find, what will surprise you, that the hæmoglobin does not decrease to the same extent as the number of red cells. In other words, each red cell has got a little more hæmoglobin than it should have. This is not quite constant in pernicious anæmia, as I shall show you, but it is very frequent, probably never constantly absent in any case, and is rarely present with any other disease. It produces what is known as a high colour index, which is very characteristic of pernicious anæmia. Then you turn your attention again to the red cells, and I looked at them only a few minutes ago. If you look at the blood-film from our patient the first thing which will strike you is the extraordinary variety of shape of the red cells ; those that I saw fifteen minutes ago are so altered that it would be quite excusable not to know them for red cells. They are all sorts of shapes. The chief thing which strikes you about them is that they are much more oval than natural, and now more so than they were the other day. That would suggest that there is a return to the embryonic type of cell. They stain badly, and have undergone some granular degeneration which enables them to take the ordinary basic stains which are used for staining micro-organisms, and which reveal a granular change in the red cells. Especially they stain badly in the centre of the cell, and the centre is often pale. So they undergo granular degeneration, and stain peculiarly, with a pale centre. Next, you notice that very often they are larger than normal. We were looking at a slide the other afternoon in which that was very striking.

Those are the chief changes that you will notice when you are looking at these red cells under the microscope. But you look still more carefully, and then—though it will often take a long time to find them—some of the red cells are found to be nucleated. I did not see one in the slide this afternoon, but I saw some a few days ago in the blood from the same patient. Then, what is of very great importance, some of the large cells are nucleated cells as well as some of the ordinary sized ones ; that is to say, there are erythroblasts and megaloblasts present. If you dry the blood rapidly, sometimes crystals of hæmoglobin form very quickly, but that does not occur when the patient is taking arsenic. Our patient is having arsenic. Then it is said— although we have not had an opportunity of examining that point—that the red cells of this disease contain a large amount of nitrogen. So much for the red cells. There is a slight increase in the number of the eosinophile cells, and it is said that sometimes the total amount of blood in the body is increased and sometimes slightly diminished. Probably it is not very much altered.

That completes the description of the main changes in the blood, and they are perfectly striking and characteristic. It used to be thought that they were absolutely characteristic—that is to say, that they occurred in no other disease than pernicious anæmia. But that is found to be not quite true, but such a degree of change as is present in this man now I think could only occur in pernicious anæmia. The most characteristic features of the blood are probably the increased colour index, the presence of nucleated red cells and the presence of large red cells. Conditions of blood something like this have been rarely met with in syphilis, and not quite so rarely in cancer, especially cancer of the stomach and uterus, and in gastric ulcer, myxœdema, and ankylostomiasis. But in none of these conditions does the unusual state of the blood approach anything like the extreme degree that it shows in this man who is now lying in Addison Ward.

We have thus learnt that there are great changes in the blood, and I have taken them in such an order as to try to make the subject interesting.

Next, I want to draw your attention to the liver in trying to understand the disease. The present Lecturer on Physiological Chemistry at Cambridge, Mr. F. G. Hopkins, who was my ward clerk and clinical assistant, when he was Gull research student, worked on this subject, and found that while the normal percentage of iron in the liver is ·09, in one of my patients suffering from pernicious anæmia it was 1·038, in the next one ·204, and in the next one ·4, and in the next ·19. He found a considerable increase also in the spleen and kidneys, but the main thing he detected in these four patients of mine—who, fortunately for me, all happened to be under my care at the time that I had such an expert chemist for a clinical clerk— was that in every one of them the iron in the liver was very greatly increased. And you know that iron in the liver is demonstrated by forming Prussian blue in it. And I will pass round some chromo-lithographs which illustrate Mr. Hopkins' paper. You will see the Prussian blue iron in the top figure, which represents the liver and in the two lower ones the spleen and kidney. There is therefore an excess of iron in the liver and spleen and kidney in pernicious anæmia. Here is the liver itself from one of my cases at which Mr. Hopkins worked, and here is the Prussian blue reaction shown in the liver itself. The intensity of the Prussian blue reaction is, unfortunately, no accurate guide to the amount of iron in the liver, because, as Mr. Hopkins points out, the reaction depends on the chemical condition of the iron in the liver. But no healthy liver will give such a Prussian blue reaction as that has done. This excess of iron in the liver, and to a less extent in the spleen and kidney, suggests that there is a considerable blood destruction in pernicious anæmia. The obvious explanation is that the blood has been broken up and some of the resulting iron is deposited in the liver. The suggestion of blood-destruction is supported by the fact that the quantity of urobilin in the urine is increased. It is not increased, as far as we can make out by examining with the spectroscope in our patient now in Clinical, but generally speaking it is increased, and you will find that subject very fully discussed by Mr. Hopkins if you read his article. He concludes that there is no doubt that the amount of urobilin in the urine is often increased in pernicious anæmia. The suggestion is that the red cells undergo destruction, that as the result of that iron is deposited in the liver and other organs, and some other pigmentary part of the hæmoglobin leads to the increase of urobilin in the urine and some other part of it leads to the patient being of the yellow lemon colour which is so characteristic of pernicious anæmia. I do not want to push this suggestion too far, because the origin of urobilin is not certain. But I am supported by the well-known fact that there is an increase of urobilin in the urine in people who have been the subjects of hæmorrhage in which the blood is not discharged outside the body. If you were to get a large hæmatoma in your muscles, as the colouring matter was absorbed from it you would become of a yellow tint, and the amount of urobilin in your urine would be increased, which would suggest that some of the blood-colouring matter was being absorbed from the hæmatoma and being excreted into the urine and colouring the skin. That very liver which is going round, which was the object of Dr. Hopkins' research, excited Dr. Cleveland, when he was registrar here, to look carefully for the Prussian blue reaction in the liver of other diseases. He found it was not peculiar to pernicious anæmia, and he obtained it in various cases; I think four of them under me showed it very well. The percentages of iron which he got were ·136, ·25, ·134, ·222. One was a case of fatal hæmorrhage from gastric ulcer, the other a fatal hæmorrhage from typhoid, and in both of these the absorbed blood might very well have led to a deposition of iron in the liver. The third was a fatal pancreatitis, and there we are justified, from the general condition of the patient, in supposing that the amount of blood-destruction must be considerable The other was a case of fatal erysipelas, which is practically the same thing as fatal septicæmia, in which probably the amount of blood destruction is also great. So I have tried to bring home to you that there is no disease in which the deposition of iron in the liver and other organs is more marked than in pernicious anæmia, but it is not peculiar to pernicious anæmia. It suggests there is great destruction of red blood

cells in pernicious anæmia, and that it is somewhat supported by the yellow tint and with the passage of urobilin in the urine. We have thus evidence that in this disease there is an increased destruction of blood. We have also evidence that there is increased formation of blood. For example, we have the nucleated reds and the megaloblasts, which are especially found in the red marrow, and probably they are manufactured there and in pernicious anæmia are poured into the blood before their time, so to speak, and hence we find them. We have got a high colour index, which might be interpreted as an attempt to repair; that is to say, each corpuscle is carrying more hæmoglobin than it should, so as to make up for the general deficiency. And it is probable, judging from other cases, that in this case we shall find post mortem that the red marrow of the bones is considerably increased, again an attempt on the part of the body to lead to an excessive formation of red blood cells. Therefore, pernicious anæmia is a disease in which there is undoubtedly an increased destruction of blood, and there is strong evidence that it tries to get itself well by an increased formation of red blood-corpuscles. But we do not know the cause of this increased destruction of blood. Still, there are one or two suggestive facts pointing to the cause lying in the periphery of the portal vein. The facts are these: Pernicious anæmia has interested all the physicians here since the time of Addison, and from time to time various members of the staff have tabulated the cases which have been in since Addison's time. And in 'Guy's Hospital Reports' vol. xlvii, I investigated the subject and found that there were thirty-one of them from 1855 to 1899, and 41 per cent. of them gave a history of vomiting before admission, 34·5 per cent. a history of diarrhœa, 55 per cent. vomiting after admission, and 41 per cent. had diarrhœa after admission. Many had these symptoms who took no arsenic, some of them had the symptoms before the arsenic was given, and some after the arsenic had been left off. So we cannot attribute the symptoms to the arsenic which the patient took. Therefore you see a large proportion of the cases have considerable gastro-intestinal disturbance, and that is true of our patient, and it is merely a suggestion I throw out to you that the destruction of blood takes place in the periphery of the portal area, and this view is supported by the large amount of iron in the liver. What the cause of the destruction is I do not know.

Now a few words about the symptoms. One point which the books do not bring out with sufficient emphasis, I think, is that the state of the blood varies from day to day. If you look at the appendix of cases at the end of the article by Dr. Hopkins, you will see a blood chart of one of my patients, and you will notice how much the blood varied from day to day in the number of reds and the quantity of hæmoglobin. The same is true of our patient in the ward. Mr. Edridge has done many counts, and here are some of them. In the first one he gives us there were 905,000 reds and hæmoglobin 20 per cent. In the next count he gives us there were 1,105,000 reds and hæmoglobin 30 per cent., the next, 910,000 reds and the hæmoglobin percentage 25. Not only that, but the shape of the corpuscles varies from day to day. The slides which Mr. Edridge has prepared show that a few days ago the preponderating corpuscle was a large, oval, red corpuscle, and to-day the preponderating corpuscle is an extraordinarily distorted red cor-puscle, so much so that you can hardly recognise it as a red corpuscle at all. I put on the board before you the figures from a case that Mr. Allen, when he was my ward clerk, worked out for me, and you will see that the number of red corpuscles and the amount of hæmoglobin show considerable variations from day to day. I have here the record of the blood of a patient of Dr. Hingston Fox's that I saw only last Saturday, and Dr. Fox kindly supplied me with various countings of the reds—in February last 1,290,000, in March 3,406,000, in April 4,500,000, in May 5,000,000, in July 3,000,000, in August 2,500,000, in October 2,500,000, and then in November 3,000,000. There again you see a very good illustration of the great variations in the number of reds. The variations in this patient's colour index are as follows : In February it was 1·46, in May ·92, in July 1·35. Going back to March, I see it is 1·9. Now, at the present moment, it is 1·37, and last month it was 1·86. So I want to bring to your notice how much the blood varies from time to time. If you look at it in this disease, so much does it vary that sometimes, even in a bad case, you may hardly be able to tell from looking at it that the man had pernicious anæmia at all. You may find no nucleated reds, you may have a normal colour index, and perhaps you can only ascertain a little poikilocytosis, and that is not distinctive. Before you can deny that a case is pernicious anæmia several blood examinations must be made.

The next clinical point I want to direct your attention to is the fact that these patients have a raised temperature. Here is the temperature chart of our man in John Ward, and you can see how his temperature has remained pretty constantly up. I show you the charts of the cases which Mr. Hopkins analysed, and you can see that the tem-perature was always ranging about the figure 100°. It is very interesting that these patients should so frequently have a temperature somewhere about 100°, because you would have thought that as they had so little hæmoglobin, oxidation would be very low with them. But be the cause what it may, there is, no doubt, often a moderate degree of pyrexia in pernicious anæmia, and it is one of the characteristic symptoms of the disease. I have already mentioned the tint of the skin and the colour of the urine.

I now come to a very interesting point, and that is the condition of the eyes. When we looked at our patient's eyes in the ward, we found this state of affairs. There was over the whole retina a haziness, a mild degree of general retinitis. On looking at the disc it was found to be swollen and œdematous, and at the edge of the disc and scattered over the retina were innumerable small hæmorrhages. Some of them were flame-shaped, some were not. There is no variety of anæmia but pernicious anæmia which could possibly produce such a severe degree of this change as you can see if you look at the man in John Ward. So striking is it that it would be, even apart from the examina-tion of the blood, a very good help to diagnosis. Other forms of anæmia will produce a few hæmor-rhages. But such countless hæmorrhages as we have here, together with œdema of the disc and retinitis, could hardly be produced by any other similar disease. Unfortunately, I have no book which gives chromo-lithographs of this condition. But here is a very good photograph from Gowers' 'Medical Ophthalmoscopy.' The hæmorrhages in our case are very much smaller than you see in the photograph, and more numerous. So please bear in mind the ocular changes of pernicious anæmia.

Our man presents another symptom of this disease which is very striking, namely dyspnœa.

Our patient illustrates that these patients do not waste. And the other symptoms of anæmia, such as hæmic murmurs, palpitation, cardiac dilatation, hæmorrhages in various parts of the body, œdema of the ankles, are not more common in pernicious anæmia than other forms of anæmia, so we need not consider them now. You will remember that Addison, in his account of the disease, pointed out that it was fatal. Some years ago I wrote to a number of cases which had been in the hospital and tried from the replies to estimate the prognosis. It came out that the prognosis was, as one knew already, very bad. I was only able, after tabulating a number of cases that had been in the hospital, to find two who had not died, either in the hospital or not very long after leaving. But one patient was alive eleven years after being first seen here. Another was alive four years afterwards. The common thing is for them to come in here, to get a trifle better, to go out again, to come in again and get better, and then finally to come in and die. Remember, it is a disease which is characterised very strikingly by relapses. Probably some day we shall learn to estimate the prognosis somewhat from the condition of the blood. Of course, if the hæmoglobin is very low, the prognosis is probably bad. It is said that a high colour index indicates a bad prognosis, showing that the patient is very ill, and there is a desperate attempt at cure. On the other hand, some have thought that a high colour index would show a good prognosis, indicating a successful attempt at repair, but probably that is not right. All observers are agreed that a large number of nucleated reds, especially of large nucleated reds, is of bad prognostic import.

The only remaining thing I have to tell you about it is the treatment. And as far as we know, the only treatment which benefits these patients is to give them arsenic. We push the arsenic as far as we can; it has no curative effect, it only improves the patient for a time. That reminds me of the last thing I want to draw your attention to, and that is this : So very often mistakes are made from not remembering that the administration of arsenic will lead to pigmentation. I have known people with arsenic pigmentation called subjects of Addison's disease, pernicious anæmia, and all sorts of diseases. Our patient has a few brown spots upon him ; they are not sufficiently marked for me to be sure that they are due to arsenical pigmentation, but at any rate they are sufficiently interesting to raise the question. The patient of Dr. Fox's whom I mentioned to you, and whom I saw last Saturday, had well-marked arsenical pigmentation. Here are plates from Dr. Crocker's 'Atlas of Diseases of the Skin'; I brought them down to show you the condition. This picture illustrates strikingly the kind of pigmentation. It is due to the actual deposit of some arsenical compound in the skin. The hair-follicles are spared at first, but any parts or spots which were originally dark are more darkly pigmented by arsenic than other parts. If there is any inflammation of the skin, such as a patch of psoriasis, this gets pigmented to a brown colour. You will find this brown arsenical pigmentation is better marked on the trunk than on the limbs. It very slowly disappears. It lasts a very long time and in some cases perhaps it never disappears. You will remember the patient upstairs whose blood was counted by Mr. Allen, whose case I mentioned to you. He raised a very interesting point, as to whether arsenical pigmentation can occur on the mucous membrane of the mouth. You know that in Addison's disease the mucous membrane of the mouth does get pigmented. This man, who was in last year, got brown pigment patches on the mucous membrane of the mouth. He certainly had pernicious anæmia, was taking a large quantity of arsenic, and I cannot help thinking that the brown patches inside the mouth were due to the arsenic. Future experience only can tell us whether there can be pigment inside the mouth from this cause.

(The patient died the day after the lecture was given. The diagnosis of pernicious anæmia proved correct. The liver, spleen, and kidneys contained a great excess of iron.)

February 26th, 1906.

THREE LECTURES

ON

DISEASES OF THE BREAST.

Delivered at St. Bartholomew's Hospital.

By ANTHONY A. BOWLBY, C.M.G., F.R.C.S.,

Surgeon to the Hospital, Lecturer on Surgery.

———

LECTURE III.

GENTLEMEN,—Before discussing the differential diagnosis of cancer of the breast, I think it will be useful to turn first of all to the various forms in which cancer shows itself and the appearances which are seen upon section. You are all familiar with the common descriptions of scirrhous carcinoma of the breast, and it is rather taken for granted that all cases of spheroidal-celled carcinoma conform more or less to this type. I want you to realise that there is every gradation between the typical scirrhous carcinoma and the so-called encephaloid cancer. Let us begin with this picture. Here is a section of an exceedingly dense fibrous carcinoma of the breast, a very hard growth, to which the name "scirrhous" is quite well applied. And if you were to examine that specimen in a recent section you would find everything that is described as being characteristic of cancer. You would find that it would cut like a piece of cartilage, or like a raw potato. The section of it would at once be concave, as a result of the contraction which is inherent in the growth. Its edge would be ill defined, its cut surface would be fibrous almost throughout, but here and there in it there would be small yellowish dots or streaks. Those dots or streaks represent the only cellular element in a section which is mainly fibrous or scar-like. That would be a quite typical scirrhous cancer of the breast. Now look at these next two pictures. Each of them shows a dense dirty white growth. But neither tumour is nearly as fibrous on section or as scar-like as the first one I showed you, and there is not the same tendency to the formation of a concave surface on section. Let us take these other two specimens next. Each of them is from a patient who had carcinoma of the breast, and one of them, instead of being dense and white, is distinctly of a pinkish or reddish hue. It is evidently of a softer consistency, it is more vascular, it is less scar-like, it is more succulent.

Now take the next specimen. Here is a section of a breast in which there are scattered throughout the substance of the growth numerous minute cavities. Each one of these cavities contains a quantity of thick, almost cream-like, fluid. The section of this tumour is a section which is very rich in cells, and if you come to compare it with the first picture I showed you, you will see it looks like a completely different disease. There is here none of the dense scar-like tissue ; it is not a thing which cuts like a piece of cartilage ; there is not in such a section of this any concavity of the cut surface ; and yet this is a carcinoma. And there is every gradation between the dense form and this form, which is rich in cells and contains very little fibrous tissue. Those are all examples of spheroidal-celled carcinoma of the breast. Think how unlike they must feel from each other when in the breast. Here is a picture which shows on section a colloid carcinoma of the breast. This is the more rare form of cancer and is one of the slowly growing forms. You will see there is to the naked eye the appearance of a gelatinous tissue due to the presence of colloid fluid in the cavities or spaces. This tumour contains cavities which are comparable with the cavities found in a normal thyroid gland. Here is one more picture to illustrate an unusual variety, but still another variety, of carcinoma of the breast. This is a section of a breast which contains a considerable cavity filled with blood. It is a rapidly growing, rather soft, but still spheroidal-celled carcinoma, and there has been hæmorrhage into it. And this form of carcinoma, which is rich in vessels with cavities which are sometimes filled with blood is sometimes talked of as "hæmorrhagic carcinoma." Now, all these pictures suggest, of course, that when growths differ so much in structure the one from the other it is evident they must present different clinical aspects too ; and when you come to consider the differential diagnosis of cancer of the breast, the first thing you have to realise is that cancer of the breast presents itself to you in many different forms. I alluded in my former lecture to the more usual form of cancer of the breast, the hard, slowly growing form, which is deep seated and not very definite, afterwards becoming more nodular, and ultimately causing some dimpling of the skin or retraction of the nipple, all this, perhaps, taking a year or more to come about. But there are other forms of carcinoma of the breast which are not in the least like this. In a certain number of the more rapidly growing and vascular carcinomata of the mamma the whole breast is infiltrated from the beginning, so that it is all swollen, and there is no one lump in it which can be distinguished. In these cases the breast may be so vascular and so turgid as to suggest at once inflammation. And this form of infiltrating carcinoma, where the whole gland is occupied by growth, is a condition which simulates inflammation of the breast, and not only simulates it but is perhaps particularly liable to occur under circumstances in which inflammation occurs, namely in suckling women ; for it is well known that when cancer of the breast occurs in young women, especially in women in whom the breast is very active and vascular, as it is during lactation, it grows with surprising rapidity, and infiltrates the whole breast. A cancer such as that is as unlike the common typical scirrhous carcinoma as any tumour could well be. So when you come to think of the differential diagnosis of cancer of the breast you must definitely have in your mind the fact that cancer appears under very different circumstances, and that whereas one form of cancer may simulate an inflamed breast which is threatening suppuration, another form, and a much more common form, of cancer, the typical scirrhus, does not in the least suggest anything of the kind. With that proviso, and remembering that cancer according to the nature of the individual variety, necessarily presents very different physical conditions, you must next turn to what other things most often simulate cancer of the breast.

One of the commonest conditions to simulate cancer of the breast is the cystic tumour of old age, and especially cysts with mastitis. There is no question about it that no surgeon, however experienced, is so wise as to be able to say in every case that an individual tumour is or is not a cancer. You must realise for yourselves that not only is it impossible for you, sometimes, to be able to tell whether a tumour is carcinoma or not, but it is impossible for anybody to be positive about it. You must realise that cancer of the breast may be so closely simulated by those conditions which I mentioned to you in my former lecture, in which there is hardening of a lobule of the breast and the formation of cysts, that no one could possibly tell for certain until an operation exposed the swelling

what its nature was. That does not mean to say you will not be able to diagnose a great many cases ; but one thing you should always remember is that a tumour may feel exceedingly hard, and may at once suggest to you on feeling it that it is probably a cancer, and yet this hardness may be due to the extreme tension of the fluid in one or more cysts. Therefore you ought to have always in your minds, when you come to examine the breast of a woman between forty and sixty years of age that very hard tumours may be cysts. Whenever a cyst is situated deep in the breast and when there lies over it breast-tissue, the latter is often indurated from the pressure of the cyst beneath and the pressure of the clothes and corsets above. So in feeling such a growth as this you are feeling two things, an indurated piece of breast-tissue, and underneath it a cyst. If you suspect a cyst you will often diagnose it, because when you suspect it you can feel some elasticity about it, or perhaps definite fluctuation. When you fix the tumour and press upon it firmly with your finger you will derive a sensation of springiness which carcinoma never affords. And therefore in many cases, although at first you may think a tumour feels so hard that it almost certainly must be a carcinoma, if you remember that a hard tumour may be a cyst, and direct your examination specially to the point of finding out whether there is this springy feeling, you will often be able to correct your diagnosis and establish the more hopeful one, showing that second thoughts in this case are the best. So much for cysts which simulate cancer, but I do not want you to think that they only occur late in life. Cysts may simulate tumours of the breast of a more dangerous nature earlier than forty to sixty years of age. But I reminded you before that degeneration cysts are extremely common, and therefore it is these for which you should especially always be on the look-out.

Next to cysts, interstitial mastitis without cysts is the thing which is most likely to simulate the beginning of carcinoma. Let me advise you of one thing ; if you suspect that an individual hardening of the breast is probably interstitial mastitis, examine very carefully both breasts to see whether there are several hardened areas, for this is one of the conditions in which there is great safety in numbers. No woman ever grows two or three carcinomata in her breasts at the same time. If there are two separate lumps in one breast, thoroughly apart from each other, one on the lower and outer margin, and the other on the inner side near the sternum, for example, it is very likely that neither of them is cancer. And therefore where there is not a typical growth, where it is uncertain in nature, if you find there are several such areas of induration of the breast, remember that the mere multiplicity makes it much more probable that each is simply an inflammatory condition than that any of them is cancerous. Naturally there is a tendency on the part of the patient to feel that if there are several lumps so much the worse for her. But you must remember that cancer of the breast practically always occurs as a single lump and not as multiple tumours separated by a considerable area of healthy tissue from one another.

Chronic abscesses are the next thing which you have to keep in mind, and you must remember that an abscess may be very chronic indeed. A woman after suckling a child and having had some mastitis during lactation may subsequently have a lump form in her breast which remains hard for a long time. In many cases after lactation troubles the breast remains irregular and nodular. But sometimes, even after many months, one of these lumpy areas may gradually increase in size, and you may be inclined to think there is necessarily something growing, because of the length of time which has elapsed since the completion of lactation. And thus a part of the breast which has evidently at one time retained milk will slowly form pus without any of the ordinary signs of inflammation, without pain or redness, without heat or fever. And these very chronic abscesses which form in that way do cause a very hard lump in the breast. So that wherever there is a history that a woman has had lactation troubles, or even has had a confinement or a miscarriage within recent months, you must always suspect the possibility of a hard tumour turning out to be abscess and not cancer at all.

The other form of chronic abscess in the breast is that which is due to tubercle, and this is the thing which of all others is least often diagnosed. When tubercle has extended through the breast so as to become quite typical, it is easy to diagnose; but when tubercle is in its earlier stages inside the breast, and has not come near the skin, it is not diagnosed in the large majority of cases, and if you look up the records of cases you will find that tubercle of the breast has been removed over and over again under the impression that it was cancer. That means that you must take care to learn all you can about what it looks like in its early stage. In such cases the breast at one part is hard and presents an irregular, knotty, nodular tumour, which is liable to be fixed. It may be adherent to the skin or even to the deeper parts beneath the breast. That is all very like cancer, and, making it more like it still, it is quite common, and indeed the usual thing, to find enlargement of the glands of the axilla. You know that tubercle very often affects the lymphatic glands, and that if a person has a tubercular lesion in any one part of the body, the neighbouring lymphatic glands are very liable to be involved. In the breast it is the same. So that there is this irregular lumpy tumour in a part of the breast, more or less fixed, and there are enlarged and very hard glands in the axilla, and as these glands increase in size they also often become fixed. What more, then, is necessary to make this lump like cancer? It is exactly like it, or so much so that nobody could definitely tell the difference, unless there is something to lead him to it; but in many of these cases there is something to lead you to it if you are on the look-out. You may never notice it if you are not on the look-out for it, but if you have tubercle in your minds as one of the things which you have to diagnose from cancer you will search for the evidences of tubercle elsewhere. For example, you will ascertain whether the patient has ever had tubercular glands in the neck. Many of these patients have had them. Is she a person who has had some other tubercular lesion—for example, phthisis? Is there a family history of tubercle? If so, a tumour in the breast becomes an object of suspicion so far as its possible tubercular nature is concerned. But if this breast with tubercle in it is left alone and the tubercle spreads, what will happen? As the tubercle spreads in the breast the whole breast will become irregular and hard. The recent tubercle in the breast will be the hardest, but the old parts which once were hard will soften and break down, just as tubercular glands break down elsewhere. So if you see one of these breasts at a little later stage the diagnosis becomes easier, because there is now not a single hard tumour, but the breast is occupied by irregular lumps of different consistency. Some of them are quite hard, others of them are quite soft. A woman was admitted to the Stanley Ward last year with what was believed to be carcinoma of her breast, for she was sent to the hospital with that diagnosis. When I came to examine her my first diagnosis also was carcinoma ; but when I came to proceed with the examination more carefully I found that there was an infiltration of the whole breast, that parts of it were hard, and that there were other parts which were soft and definitely breaking down. I knew that cancer did not break down in half a dozen different places. Carcinoma of the breast may disintegrate at one place and may undergo cystic degeneration, or there may be hæmorrhage into it ; but carcinoma of the breast does not have three or four more areas of softening and other areas of irregular hardening. Moreover, in this patient the skin was bluish and otherwise discoloured at one or two places, very much like the skin is discoloured over tubercular glands in the neck. In the axilla was a mass of hard and fixed glands, which nobody could have distinguished from those of carcinoma, but on account of the condition I have described we made the diagnosis of tubercle, and removed the breast, and we then found that the condition was tubercular. A stage later the diagnosis becomes more easy still. Here is the picture of the chest-wall of a woman æt. 62 years, in whom there is a growth just like lupus. The tubercle in the breast has spread right through to the skin, and there is now, to make the diagnosis plain, a tubercular lupoid lesion of the skin of the whole breast. Under those circumstances the diagnosis becomes easy. But when you are talking of the differential diagnosis of cancer you must remember that tubercle is a condition which, though rare, is comparatively seldom diagnosed in its early stages, and that no doubt in past years a great many breasts have been removed which were tuberculous under the belief that they were the seat of scirrhous cancer, and have been included in hospital records as scirrhus.

When cancer involves the skin it appears in different cases under very different conditions and I showed you yesterday a picture illustrating a cancerous growth which was fungating. At the same time, you should know that in many cases there is no fungation of the tumour although the skin is destroyed, but rather an open cancerous ulcer.

And I want you particularly to appreciate what is illustrated by some of these pictures, that there are some cases of cancer in which there is not only no tumour or swelling, but rather a shrinkage or diminution in the size of the breast, and this condition is spoken of as "atrophic scirrhus," or atrophic cancer. Here are three pictures which show it exceedingly well. Here, first of all, is a picture of the breasts of a woman æt. 48 years. For six years there had been growing in each breast a dense scirrhous growth, and you will see that it has caused the breasts to shrivel up, so that there is practically no mammary prominence left. Here is a drawing of the breasts of a woman æt. 48 years. On one side the breast is represented by a shrunken area of skin with some nodules around it ; all prominence, such as you see in the other breast, is absolutely gone, and when such tumours as these come to the surface and ulcerate, instead of there being a fungating mass there is only a retracted ulcer and a depression or depressions on the surface.

Atrophic cancer is diagnosed generally at first sight, for the hardness is very marked, and the retraction and shrivelling and puckering of the skin are all very easily seen and felt. In cases of this class the disease may last for as long as ten or even twenty years.

Now let me turn for a short time to the question of the treatment of cancer. Operation at the present time is practically the only treatment that is considered to be wise to adopt, so long as the operator can hope to remove the whole of the disease. If you are asked if there is anything that can be done to arrest the growth of cancer, if there is any treatment that can be adopted in cases where an operation cannot be performed, either because the growth is too extensive or because the patient will not submit to operation, you must say that as far as small growths of the skin are concerned treatment by the X rays will undoubtedly in very many cases either diminish or arrest their progress, and that in a certain number of cases where the growth is superficial a cure seems to result. But there is no reason whatever to believe that electricity in any form cures cancer in the breast. It may cure certain small recurrences in the skin, it may perhaps help to prevent recurrences in cases where the main tumour has been removed by operation, and it may help a cancerous ulcer to cicatrise ; it does in some cases also relieve the patient of pain. But when we have said this we must acknowledge further that there is not the least reason to believe that cancer of the breast can be treated so as to cure it by any form of electricity. Is there any drug or drugs upon which any reliance can be placed ? There are a great many that have been tried. Twenty years ago Chian turpentine was believed by many people to be a cure for cancer. It was first of all tried in connection with cancerous tumours of the uterus, and was believed to have cured some of them. Afterwards it was tried for cancer in almost every part of the body. But there is, unfortunately, no reason to rely on it as a cure for this disease, although whether it has any influence in preventing rapid extension is a much more difficult matter to decide. Many other drugs have been tried lately, amongst them thyroid extract, but I am not aware of any drug that has been proved to be useful in any consecutive number of cases. Isolated cases account for very little, though you may naturally think that if a person has been given a drug and the tumour has disappeared to a great extent, surely it is fair to put its disappearance down to the drug. Well, that introduces a difficulty which one must allude to, namely that all cases of cancer do not run a definite course, and that there are cases where, although the tumour may not be removed, its progress may be to a great extent spontaneously arrested. Three and a half years ago I had a patient in the hospital who was admitted on account of a very advanced cancer of the breast, which had destroyed the skin, which was bleeding, and which threatened her life, both from bleeding and from sepsis. It was quite evident that she had so extensive a disease as to prevent it being removed completely with any hope of success. There were large masses of glands in the axilla and in the neck, but I operated for the removal of her breast, not with the expectation of a cure of her disease, but to stop the bleeding and with the view of saving her from sepsis. I took away also the most easily removable glands in her axilla, and I found that at the apex of the axilla were glands so involved and so attached to the large vessels and nerves, that they could not all be removed—a very unsatisfactory sort of operation. I saw no more of the patient for three years, and I supposed that she had died, but when she came back to see me at the end of that time, not only was she alive and well, but she had no enlarged glands which could be felt in her axilla, or in her neck, although she had a recurrence of carcinoma in the skin and pectoral muscle. I removed that, and at the present time she is very well. I know that I left a considerable mass of cancer in this patient more than three years ago, and I know that that mass of cancer which I left has almost entirely disappeared. Now, is it not evident that if I had been giving this woman medicine I should have been inclined to attribute the improvement to the drugs I had given. So you must realise that cancer may remain stationary or may even retrogress. In a few very rare cases it has actually spontaneously become cured.

February 26th, 1906.

WITH DR. MONTAGUE MURRAY IN THE WARDS OF CHARING CROSS HOSPITAL.

GENTLEMEN,—There is one thing about this child to which I wish particularly to direct your attention—the size and shape of his head. He is ten months old, and was sent into the hospital because he had had convulsions and was thought to have hydrocephalus. He was quite well when he was born, was weaned when four months old, and was then fed on milk and barley-water and Robb's biscuits. We know nothing about the hygienic conditions under which he lived. Certainly, however, his diet lacked fat and contained an excess of carbohydrates. It is only during the last few weeks that he has suffered from convulsions. The first two or three were simply "screaming fits," as the mother described them, but later on the visitations were definite convulsions. With the onset of these attacks the head began to get larger, and he was sent here, as I have said, because he was supposed to be a true case of chronic hydrocephalus. The first thing one noticed on seeing him was that, as you can see now, he has definite rickets. There can be no question about that ; there is the beading of the ribs and the enlargement of the wrist ; moreover he has no teeth and you will remember that he is ten months old. Not only has he had convulsions, but, as you heard for yourselves when we first came to his bedside, he has laryngismus. When he first came in, it took very little to set up an attack, and it was very pronounced in character ; it was not the single "crow" such as you heard just now, but it went on, inspiration after inspiration, for perhaps a dozen times consecutively. He has not had any tetany, which is commonly associated with this condition, neither has he had any of those "nodding spasms" which you sometimes find in association with this affection.

All these points I mention as preliminaries to what I want to point out to you in connection with the head. It is generally stated that the enlargement of the head in rickets is absolutely and easily distinguishable from the enlarged head in chronic hydrocephalus ; and, of course, in a characteristic and advanced case it is. But a difficulty in recognition does sometimes occur when the cranial enlargement first sets in. In a typical case, of course, the hydrocephalic head is globular in shape ; whereas the rickety head has a flat top, with the frontal bosses more marked, and the head is on the whole rather a long than a broad one. Then, again, with hydrocephalus you may find defects of vision. Not infrequently these children are blind, and you will make out a little rigidity and increased deep reflexes in the lower limbs and possibly be able to obtain a history of a meningococcus meningitis. As the head gets larger and larger the sutures separate and the globular character of the head is pronounced. Still, before the sutures separate the difficulty of diagnosis may be considerable. If you feel this child's head you will appreciate the point. The head in this case is distinctly flat-topped, though the fontanelle runs much farther forward than is usually the case, and suggests a "started" suture ; yet in the absence of anything like rigidity or secondary changes, and of any increase of the deep reflexes in the lower limbs, and in view of the fact that the child is distinctly observant and intelligent, I think we must not accept the diagnosis of chronic hydrocephalus. The evidence points to the condition being one of rickets, and of course the prognosis is proportionately good.

This next patient is a characteristic case of a comparatively rare disease, namely *syringomyelia*. The facts of his history are briefly as follows : He was sent to the hospital with the complaint of loss of power in the right arm. Three months ago he first noticed weakness in his right shoulder when doing his work, and this weakness gradually extended to the wrist and arm. No wasting was noticed, but for about a month he has been unable to use or extend the fingers of his right hand. On walking he had noticed some stiffness in the right leg, which has been present for about three months. He has not become aware of any numbness, tingling, or pain, or any sensation of "pins and needles," nor has there been any difficulty in micturition or defæcation. His special senses are normal. Neither personal nor family history gives any suggestion of disease.

Viewed by daylight, he is seen to be distinctly anæmic. His right pupil is smaller than the left, and it is said to have always been so. There is marked scoliosis, with the convexity to the right. If

you look at his arms and legs, you will see that the right side is more wasted than the left ; and the wasting affects the muscles of the shoulder, as well as those of the arm, and some of the muscles of the trunk. It is unnecessary to describe each different muscle, because the exact localisation does not bear very much upon the diagnosis. Still, you will observe that the muscles involved are very much those which you find affected in progressive muscular atrophy. The hand muscles are weak, especially the extensors ; and if you look at the thenar and hypothenar eminences, you will notice flattening, particularly of the thenar. The first dorsal interosseous muscle has practically lost all its power. The furrows at the back of the hands are unduly marked, pointing to wasting of the interossei, and his grip is feeble. It appeared to us when he came in that his hands were large, but there is no marked increase in the size of the bones of the face. Cases have been reported in which acromegaly has been combined with syringomyelia. The general supposition is that when the conditions are found together their combination is accidental, but there is no doubt that this patient's hands are larger than normal.

Beyond a slight sluggishness in response to the constant current, the reactions in his case are practically normal. There is no acute lower segment lesion. He has weakness and wasting, but not degeneration, as tested by the electric current.

When we look at his lower extremites we find that he has evidences rather of an upper segment lesion ; that is to say, there is some stiffness and difficulty in walking, but no marked wasting. His reflexes are exaggerated, and there is almost knee-clonus. Ankle-clonus is well marked. There is also a pronounced extensor response in the great toe, or, as it is often termed, a "Babinski" reflex. On testing sensation it is found that the following condition of things obtains : tactile sensation is fairly normal throughout, but sensation to temperature and pain is almost lost in the right upper limb, and is definitely limited in other parts of the body. He is unable to distinguish between heat and cold at all in that limb ; everything seems equally hot to him. He can just distinguish between an ordinary touch and a prick with a needle. There are no definite nutritive changes in the joints or in the skin, unless you regard his large hands as evidence of nutritive change, which I think one is fairly entitled to do.

The diagnosis depends, then, chiefly upon these two points : (1) that the paralysis resembles that of progressive muscular atrophy so far as the distribution of the affected muscles goes, and in the fact that the upper extremities are affected more than the lower ; (2) that there is loss of sensation to heat and cold and to pain, while tactile sense persists. Additional evidence is seen in the scoliosis or lateral bending of the spine, which is also characteristic of this disease ; and then you also find in the lower limbs, not a wasting and paralysis as in the upper, but evidence of a lesion in the upper motor segment, so that the parts below overact, and you get increased deep reflexes and rigidity. All that, of course, apart from the sensory defect, might be accounted for by a degeneration of the motor tract. The degeneration of the anterior cornual cells and their prolongation in the peripheral nerves would account for the wasting in the upper extremity ; and the degeneration of the upper segment of the pyramidal tract would account for the over-action of the lower part. But when we come to test sensation and to consider the additional evidence afforded by the changes in the hands and in the spine, there can be no doubt that it all forms part of the condition known as syringomyelia. Exactly how syringomyelia arises nobody knows. Post mortem there is found a cavity in the spinal cord. It is generally most marked in the lower cervical and upper dorsal regions. As a rule the condition comes on in early adult life and develops very, very gradually ; indeed, it practically always takes that course. There are many theories as to how this cavity is produced, but I will not detain you with a discussion of them now.

Our next case is an instance of a more familiar disease. He is 56 years of age. Twenty years ago he had syphilis, which was treated for six weeks ; and for the last five or six years he has been in the habit of taking six pints of beer daily, but very little spirits. Four years ago he had an attack of gastric catarrh ; and though he says he got over it, his appetite has been poor for years—at any rate, for two years—and he apparently has had slight recurrences of his catarrh. Three weeks ago he had an undoubted attack of gastric catarrh, and he says that the abdomen then swelled up almost to its present size and that this took place all in a day. The enlargement of the abdomen, as you will readily ascertain, is due to the presence of ascitic fluid, evidence being afforded by the usual signs, namely movable dulness on percussion and uniform enlargement of the abdomen. This case illustrates the point that you may get resonance in one flank and dulness in the other ; if you find one flank resonant, it is well to percuss the other before you say there is no fluid. On the whole, the right side is more likely to be distended with air than the left. When this patient sits up, you get a dull area up to within about an inch of the umbilicus, and that gives a better notion of how much fluid there is than -can be gained while he is lying on his back. I have no doubt there are some gallons of fluid here.

There can be no question that the ascites is due to local disease. He has no disease of his heart or lungs, and the urine is free from albumen. He is neither cyanosed nor pallid. Moreover the dropsy is not uniformly distributed. Although there is very little œdema of the legs, there is much ascitic fluid, and therefore the two are unlikely to be due to a common cause.

Then we come to the question of the diagnosis of this ascitic fluid. Is it inflammatory or is it simply dropsical ? Partly with the view of settling that, we drew a little off for the purpose of examination, and we found it had a specific gravity of 1011, and that it contained 2·4 per cent. of albumen. As a good working distinction, you may say that if ascitic fluid is inflammatory in origin it will have a specific gravity of 1014 or over, while if it is dropsical in origin, it will have a specific gravity under 1014. Again, if it is inflammatory in origin, it will have a proteid percentage of something over 2·5, and if it is dropsical its percentage of proteid will be under that figure. The specific gravity of the fluid here is well under the margin, and although the proteid percentage is almost up to the margin 2·4, yet the specific gravity is enough to make it clear that the fluid is purely dropsical. What can it be due to ? Since the effusion is apparently not inflammatory, it is not likely to be due to malignant disease of the peritoneum, for the result of this is a malignant peritonitis ; and it equally is not a tubercular peritonitis. Therefore it must be due to something pressing on the portal vein or its branches. The fact, if it be a fact—and the man is an intelligent observer—that this ascites came on very rapidly suggests that the pressure on the portal vein became suddenly increased, or that portal thrombosis occurred. You may get a good deal of pressure on the vein, lasting for considerable periods of time, and then suddenly, towards the end, there may be a thrombosis. But it is quite clear—and I think his temperature and the absence of other signs show it—that the thrombosis is of the simple kind and is not suppurative or infective in character. I do not say that one can definitely affirm that thrombosis did occur—that the sudden onset of the ascites may be regarded as sufficient evidence of the sudden occurrence of thrombosis—but it is suggestive of it.

We must, however, take into consideration another view. Some teach that whenever you get marked ascites independently of dropsy in other parts of the body, and independently of toxic symptoms, it is due to perihepatitis—to the thickening of the capsule and the ensuing constriction of the liver and portal vein—and not to the cirrhotic change in the liver, and that when there is very little perihepatitis and a good deal of cirrhosis the dropsy only comes on at a late stage, very likely after several attacks of hæmorrhage. I do not profess to decide between the two views. One does sometimes see a liver which is practically enclosed in a thick envelope of fibrous tissue, a typical case of perihepatitis, often due to alcoholism. On the other hand, the ordinary cirrhotic liver is a very much commoner thing, and in these cases it is common to get a good deal of ascites and very little evidence of dropsy elsewhere. You find that the patient, as in this case, is only a little dropsical.

I do not think that the cause of pressure on the portal vein in this man is likely to be malignant disease, because ascites due to the pressure of a growth under the liver does not often occur without jaundice. This man has had no preliminary wasting, no pain and no jaundice, and there is no suggestion of any primary seat of disease. Nor is the condition likely to be tubercular, because the fluid would be of an inflammatory character and there would be a different type of temperature. Again, there might be some primary focus of infection, and this we have been unable to discover. The whole history points to alcohol as the principal cause, and the suggestion is that by its interference

with the digestive processes certain toxic substances have been formed, and that these have been carried by the portal system to the liver and have produced the changes characteristic of cirrhosis. In all probability it is not alcohol directly which produces cirrhosis, because experimentally it has been found that alcohol produces degeneration and not fibrosis. It is rather that the gradual changes which are produced in the alimentary tract, and the absorption of the products of those changes, cause, on the one hand, atrophy of the cells, and on the other sufficient irritation to produce the formation of new fibrous tissue. I think the view that the atrophy and degeneration of the cells and the formation of fibrous tissue are the contemporaneous results of the same process is a more likely one than the older statement that the fibrous tissue comes first and causes degeneration of the true liver-cells by strangling them and cutting off their supply of nourishment. A piece of important evidence which we should like to have, but which we cannot get, is a knowledge of the physical signs of the liver. But it is impossible to feel the liver or the spleen on account of the quantity of fluid in his abdomen. He will be tapped in the course of a day or two and then the liver will probably be palpable.

February 26th, 1906.

LONDON AND SOUTH WESTERN HOLIDAY GUIDE. —'The London and South Western Railway Company's Official Illustrated Guide and List,' now being prepared for publication in May next, is the most comprehensive book of the kind issued gratuitously by any British railway company. In addition to about seventy pages of descriptive matter relating to popular holiday and health resorts, it will contain a complete list of golf-links, together with about one hundred illustrations, and maps of the Company's regular system, the Channel Islands, the French coast, and ocean routes in connection with the railway. Full particulars are also given of hotel and other accommodation required by visitors, and 50,000 copies of the 'Guide' are annually distributed at home and abroad. Entries and all information intended for publication this year must be forwarded before March 31st to the Editor and Manager, at 33, Dulwich Road, Herne Hill, London.

THE CLINICAL JOURNAL,

CLINICAL RECORD, CLINICAL NEWS, CLINICAL GAZETTE, CLINICAL REPORTER, CLINICAL CHRONICLE AND CLINICAL REVIEW.

EDITED BY L. ELIOT CREASY.

No. 697.　　　WEDNESDAY, MARCH 7, 1906.　　　Vol. XXVII. No. 21.

NOTICE.

Editorial correspondence, books for review, &c., should be addressed to the Editor, 51, New Cavendish Street, W., Telephone No. 904, Paddington; but all business communications should be addressed to the Publishers, 22½, Bartholomew Close, London, E.C. Telephone 927, Holborn.

All inquiries respecting Advertisements should be sent to MESSRS. ADLARD & SON, Bartholomew Close, E.C. Telephone 927, Holborn.

Terms of Subscription, including postage, payable by cheque, postal or banker's order (in advance) : for the United Kingdom, 15s. 6d. per annum : Abroad 17s. 6d.

Cheques, &c., should be made payable to THE PROPRIETORS OF THE CLINICAL JOURNAL, crossed "The London, City, and Midland Bank, Ltd., Newgate Street Branch, E.C. Account of the Medical Publishing Company, Ltd."

Reading Cases to hold Twenty-six Numbers of THE CLINICAL JOURNAL can be supplied at 2s. 3d. each, or will be forwarded post free on receipt of 2s. 6d.; and also Cases for Binding Volumes at 1s. each, or post free on receipt of 1s. 3d., from the Publishers, 22½, Bartholomew Close, London, E.C.

A CLINICAL LECTURE

ON

INTUSSUSCEPTION.

Delivered at St. Bartholomew's Hospital.

By D'ARCY POWER, F.R.C.S.,
Surgeon to the Hospital.

GENTLEMEN,—To day I thought I would discuss intussusception, and for that purpose I have inquired concerning the children upon whom I operated in this hospital during the year 1901. There were four cases of intussusception, and of those, three survived the operation. Mr. Foster Moore, my house surgeon, has been round to see the three cases which survived, and he finds that one died of tuberculous meningitis some months afterwards, and another of whooping-cough, but their mothers say that neither of them had any subsequent abdominal trouble. The third and surviving case is the most interesting of the three, and I show him to you to-day as a fine, sturdy boy of nearly five years. The record of his case is that he was a male child of seven months, who was admitted to the hospital on April 23rd, 1901, having been suddenly seized with cramp in the stomach on April 21st. The pain had made him cry out continually; he vomited every time he was put to the breast, and had sometimes passed blood by the rectum. The child had been already in the hospital from January 16th to February 16th, under the care of Mr. Walsham, who had performed abdominal section for an ileo-cæcal intussusception. So by the time he was seven months old he had been twice cured of an intussusception. The patient was collapsed and apathetic when I first saw him, the abdomen was distended, and a distinct tumour could be felt in the region of the hepatic flexure and colon. He was brought straight to the theatre as I happened to be operating at the time of his admission, and I performed abdominal section, making the incision immediately to the right of the scar of the former wound. There was a distinct tumour beneath the liver, and as I passed my finger into the abdominal cavity I could feel it. It was an ileo-cæcal tumour, which could be felt below the liver. There was enlargement and thickening at the ileo-colic angle, which had been drawn up above the level of the umbilicus, but it was impossible to bring the swelling into the wound. I felt along the colon to ascertain how the swelling could best be reduced, and in doing so found an invagination at the centre of the transverse colon. This intussusception was easily reduced by pressure applied to the distal end, without bringing the bowel outside the abdominal cavity. The ileo-colic angle came out of the wound as soon as the intussusception had been reduced, and what I thought in the first place was an intussusception proved to be the cæcum thickened by chronic inflammation, whilst the end of the ileum lay parallel to the ascending colon, to which it was adherent for some distance. The vermiform appendix was healthy and unusually long, with no ileo-cæcal or ileo-colic intussusception. The adhesions were gently broken down, and it was noticed that portions of small intestine were adherent to the peritoneal surface of the former wound. The edges of the abdominal wound were brought together by sutures of silk-worm gut, the operation being completed in twenty-two minutes. After the operation the child did not vomit the food which was given by the mouth a few minutes after recovery from the anæsthetic. The bowels were opened on the following day, and the child made an uneventful recovery, being discharged cured on May 5th. Here is the boy, and you can see the scars where the two incisions were made, one to the left of the umbilicus and the other on the right. His mother tells us he is now perfectly healthy; he has no trouble or difficulty with his bowels. He has grown up to be a fine and sturdy lad. His abdominal wall seems to be perfectly sound and free from the least trace of hernia.

I want this boy's case to serve as a text for what I have to say about intussusception to-day. It is, of course, extremely unusual for a child to have two intussusceptions, but when two intussusceptions do occur, the intussusception does not recur at the same place ; there is not an actual recurrence, it is a new intussusception. The reason is obvious. The first intussusception causes some amount of

inflammation, stiffening, and adhesion at the ileo-cæcal angle. If a second intussusception occurs therefore, it is either in the small intestine—that is to say, a true enteric intussusception—or, as in this boy, it is an intussusception in the large intestine, colo-colic intussusception. There was another interesting point about him, and that is that the tumour which we thought to be the intussusception was really due to adhesions and inflamed peritoneum, the intussusception itself being some little distance away.

Intussusception occurs at all ages in children, in adults during the active period of life, and in old people. In children and in adults it is generally acute ; in old people it is much more often chronic. In children it occurs in perfectly healthy individuals without any apparent cause. In adults there is a traceable cause in the vast majority of cases, and that cause is often a polypus, which is usually pedunculated, whilst in children I have only once seen a polypus in an intussusception. In old people the condition is chronic, because it is nearly always associated with carcinoma, or some chronic obstruction of the bowel which causes a certain amount of straining and allows one piece of intestine to be turned into another. The seat of chronic obstruction in old people is usually the large intestine, and in them therefore the intussusception is generally close to the rectum.

Chronic intussusception in adults and in children is so rare that I do not think you need be concerned about them, though some of you here remember a very interesting example that Mr. Rawling had in the summer. He diagnosed the chronic intussusception and after making an artificial anus, left it for me to treat, as he was going away for his holiday. I considered the boy to be so bad that I did not know what to do with him, and I left him alone until he died, and that is the common ending of these chronic cases of intussusception. But you need not worry about this, for they are so rare I do not expect to see another, and I doubt very much whether you will see one at all.

The acute intussusception as it occurs in children is the one which most concerns you. The onset of such an intussusception is very sudden, and it occurs in a child who is apparently perfectly healthy. Indeed, one often thinks that it is the strongest children who are most liable to the condition. It seems to pick out one child in a family, and it comes on without any warning at all. We are in ignorance as to the exact cause, but we know that during the first few months of life very active changes are taking place in connection with the growth of the intestine. You probably know that in the newly-born child the small intestine and the large intestine have much the same calibre, but in a child of six or seven months the large intestine has grown enormously in size compared with the small one. The large intestine at that age may be four or five times as big as at birth. And it is while these active changes take place that children are most liable to acute intussusception. The change in growth affects all the constituent parts of the intestine. It takes place in the mucous membrane, in the submucous coat, in the muscle, and also in the serous coat. And going with that, it must necessarily take place in the nerve plexuses of the intestine. I think that one of the causes of intussusception is errors or irregularities in the growth of the nervous and of the muscular system of the alimentary canal, which leads to constrictions of various kinds in different parts of the intestine, perhaps at the ileo-cæcal angle more often than anywhere else, for here the physiological changes are most complicated as one wave of peristalsis ends and another commences in this region.

The intussusception must be well-developed before it comes under observation, for I have no doubt that many children have attacks of colic which are really associated with a small intussusception, which unravels itself. We had an excellent instance of this about two years ago, and I wanted to show you the patient, but we have not been able to find him, and my emissary, Mr. Moore, tells me that he was attended to his original address by a couple of friendly policemen who said it was dangerous to go down the street unattended.

The boy, æt. 6 months, was suddenly seized with abdominal pain at mid-day on February 20th, 1903. The pain continued and he passed blood-stained mucus on February 21st. He was admitted into the hospital late at night on February 22nd, and was brought to the operating theatre at 1 a.m. on February 23rd. The abdomen was then somewhat distended and a tumour could be felt in the right hypochondriac region, which I diagnosed as an intussusception. The child took the anæsthetic fairly well, but struggled a good deal whilst it was

being given. The abdomen was opened in the middle line above the umbilicus and an examination of the small intestine at once revealed a piece of deeply congested small intestine thickened throughout by exudation to the consistence of thin parchment. The inflamed portion of the intestine measured about two inches in length and was marked near its middle by a more constricted portion. The inflammation was strictly limited above and below and there was no peritonitis. The rest of the intestine seemed healthy and there was no swelling in the ileo-cæcal region, but this portion of the bowel could not be drawn up to the wound. The wound was sewn up and the patient was sent back to the ward in less than a quarter of an hour from the time the operation was commenced. He made an uninterrupted recovery. In this case the intussusception reduced itself, and probably during the few minutes when we were looking at it or waiting to treat it. I am sure that is what happens in a certain number of cases, and that it is a method by which some of the smaller intussusceptions may terminate.

Intussusception is commonly associated with symptoms of shock coming on suddenly ; and children, like adults, show shock in very different ways. The mother may tell you that the child was perfectly well, until it had a fit of intense screaming and drew its legs up, or that it fainted. Children as a rule do not faint, and this history should put you on your guard. In another case the mother will perhaps say that the child became very pale for a time, aud that it then had an attack of diarrhœa. In other cases, again, it has obvious colic, and lies curled up, its stomach is tender and the tenderness is relieved by pressure. The child lies with its knees against its stomach, and it has violent attacks of crying. The attacks of crying are intermittent. The child will cry for some time, and then it will settle down and later on will have another attack of crying. These screaming fits are obviously due to great pain, and in the majority of cases they indicate something more than ordinary colic. So there is evidence pointing to abdominal trouble.

Diarrhœa is quite common in the first stage ; that is to say, the result of the sudden shock to the intestine is to empty the large intestine. But you must not be misled into thinking it is ordinary diarrhœa due to gastro-intestinal catarrh, for if you do you will give castor oil and wait until the most favourable time for an operation is past. As soon as the large intestine has emptied itself you get the characteristic symptom, the passage of blood, and the blood is found to be mixed with slime. There is no more fæcal discharge and no flatus is passed, because nothing can come through the obstruction. You ought to be able to diagnose the condition of the child before it reaches this stage, and you have no business at all to wait for a discharge of blood and mucus before you do anything or before you make up your mind that the patient has intussusception. It is this improvement in your diagnosis which has led to our improvement in the treatment of intussusception. You ought to examine the abdomen carefully. In a young child you will often not make very much out of such a case. You will see a child who is screaming and in constant pain, with tense abdominal walls, or a child who lies pale and apathetic with nothing but the history to lead to the supposition that it has any abdominal mischief. In both cases a careful examination of the abdomen is of the first importance, and if the abdominal walls are rigid you should not hesitate to put the child under an anæsthetic. It is worth while doing this in every case of painful diarrhœa associated with screaming fits in which the onset has been sudden. Do not simply give a dose of castor oil, as I fear is usually done, and trust that the trouble will pass off. Make a thorough examination of the abdomen before you give any aperient, and do it under an anæsthetic, with the child flat on the table. Pass your hand all over the surface of the abdomen, and if there is an intussusception you will discover a lump. I do not think there is any case of actual intussusception in which careful examination with relaxed abdominal walls fails to reveal the presence of a tumour. The tumour is felt differently at different times in the same patient. Sometimes it is almost imperceptible, at other times it is felt quite easily. And if you keep your hand upon it when you have once felt it you will find it undergoes a change in shape and consistency due to the rhythmical contractions of the intestinal muscle. Examination, therefore, must not be hurried. Sit by the child's cot and keep your hand upon the abdomen for a short time ; if you do not feel a tumour at once you will probably feel it in a minute or two. Palpate carefully

from the place where the intussusception is most common—that is to say, the ileo-cæcal angle—and carry your hand upwards in the course of the colon. Enteric intussusceptions—that is to say, intussusception in the small intestine—are comparatively rare, but they are very acute. So you had better look for the common forms before you think of the rarer ones.·

Then with regard to the character of the lump. You are very often misled by being told that the lump will be found to be oblong or sausage-shaped. But very often in the early stage it is nothing of the kind ; it is a small round swelling situated in the upper part of the abdomen on the right side. It is only after a time, when the intussusception has attained some considerable size, that you get a swelling of a sausage shape and it is then situated most often on the left side of the abdomen. In the most troublesome forms you find nothing but a small round tumour, which is often movable from side to side of the abdomen and is an invagination of the small intestine.

The abdominal examination should always be supplemented by a rectal examination. In some cases—and I often think they are the easiest cases of all to treat—as soon as you put your finger into the rectum you find you are dealing with an intussusception, because you can feel the end of the intussuscepted intestine. These are either invaginations of the colon into the colon or they are large intussusceptions which come down readily and easily. Both forms are easily reduced, and the prognosis is consequently better than in the ileo-cæcal varieties. In other cases where the intussusception is not so large and has not come right down into the sigmoid flexure, or to the rectum, you may be able to feel a lump on the right side through the abdominal wall. In any case when you withdraw your finger you will find the bowel is empty of fæces, and that some blood, and very often some mucus, comes away on your finger. This enables you, I think, to make up your mind as to the diagnosis.

The pulse in the majority of cases gives you no clue at all. The temperature also remains normal. The appearance of the child does not give you any information, and there is often no characteristic aspect, as there is in other serious abdominal cases. The abdomen gives you no information if you fail to find the lump. The abdomen is not necessarily rigid ; it is moving fairly well, it is certainly not distended, neither is it unduly contracted. So you learn practically nothing from the pulse, from the appearance of the patient, from the temperature, or from the general aspect of the abdomen. For these reasons many cases of intussusception are overlooked, and the progress of an intussusception is from bad to worse if it be not treated. · I have told you that in some cases, and where there is only a small intussusception, the intussusception may cure itself.　In a few of the cases treated by the older surgeons, where children were left, and for the matter of that adults too, for an indefinite time without any treatment, sloughing occasionally took place, the intestine joined itself together at the neck of the intussusception, and the patients recovered after they had passed many inches or even feet of sloughing bowel.　But these cases are so rare that they hardly ever occur, and you must not get into a habit of thinking that intussusceptions cure themselves spontaneously, any more than you can say that a strangulated hernia will cure itself.　You have no business to depend on such a course of events occurring and leave the case to Nature.　On the other hand, the intussusception very rarely becomes gangrenous in children.　In adults gangrene is not uncommon.　The tissues of children are so elastic that although great congestion and œdema is the rule in intussusception, gangrene is so infrequent that there have not been more than one or two cases of gangrene in all the cases of intussusception which I have seen.　So even in the later stages of intussusception you are justified in advocating an operation, in the hope that you will be able to unravel the whole intussusception.

If you leave the case untreated the usual ending is death from exhaustion and toxæmia.　In the first place there is complete constipation ; nothing passes, either flatus or fæces, and the child becomes more and more apathetic.　There is not very much peritonitis, but the intestine becomes paralysed and distended in the later stages. I think apathetic children, those who allow you to examine the abdominal walls without resenting it, are in a much more dangerous condition than are those who object strenuously to your interference.　I would much rather treat a child who is kicking and struggling during the examination than one which did not seem to care much what you did to it, and in

whom it was not necessary to give an anæsthetic to enable you to make the examination.　The reason is that those apathetic children are already in a condition of toxæmia, and are likely to die from exhaustion in a comparatively short period, even though they do not look very ill.

The treatment of intussusception resolves itself into opening the abdomen at the earliest possible moment after the diagnosis has been made.　There was a time, not very long ago, when nothing surgical was done for these cases.　The child was sent to the medical ward and treated by an enema, but even then a few cases recovered.　Next came a time when cases were treated by abdominal section ; it was before our asepsis was as good as it is now and the majority of the patients died.　Abdominal section, therefore, fell into disrepute and irrigation was recommended.　Irrigation proved to be dangerous and ineffective—dangerous because too much force was used and the bowel was ruptured, ineffective because it was applied too late and it was expected that the whole intussusception could be reduced without operation.　Then there came a much more satisfactory time, a time in which we find ourselves at present, when in hospital and in private houses, if you can trust the surrounding conditions, the abdomen is opened at the earliest possible moment and intussusception is reduced. In places and circumstances where it is impossible to operate at once, or when for some reason or other the practitioner does not feel that he can open the abdomen, irrigation can be used as a temporary measure until he can obtain further help and advice.　By irrigation I mean putting into the rectum eight to fifteen ounces of hot saline solution for a child three months old, and letting the fluid run in by little more than its own weight.　For this purpose have a tube not more than eighteen inches long ; for there is danger of injuring the colon with a greater head of water than this.　The tube should end in a glass nozzle, which is introduced into the rectum whilst the thighs are held together to prevent the fluid running out again, and by that means you will often get the intussusception very materially reduced.　A large intussusception in the early stages may thus be reduced to a small one and in a few instances irrigation may result in an absolute cure of the intussusception.　But we know that it is not justifiable to rely entirely upon irrigation, so the advice I would give to those who have an acute intussusception to deal with in general practice is first to make up your mind as to the diagnosis, and then to irrigate the intestine with salt solution, allowing the solution to stop in for five minutes, the child being lightly under an anæsthetic if necessary. The tube should then be detached from the nozzle, which is left in the rectum that the fluid may the more easily run out. If you take away the nozzle and expect the fluid to be expelled through the anus, you will often find that the sphincter prevents it all coming out, and then it is not easy to say whether or not the intussusception has been reduced. When the fluid has escaped make a careful examination to ascertain whether the tumour has disappeared. If it has not gone you must, at all risks, operate. If it is no longer to be felt, you may safely wait for six or eight hours until you are able to obtain the services of a competent operator to explore the abdomen. Here, in hospital, where everything is ready, there is no need to wait. I think we get far better results by immediate operation than by wasting time or trusting to such an imperfect measure as irrigation to relieve an acute intussusception. If you have a cottage hospital, you can operate for yourselves ; and remember the great importance of operating as early as possible after the onset of the symptoms. Do not wait to see whether there is going to be blood and mucus passed ; as soon as you feel the lump cut down upon it.

With regard to the operation itself, you saw the scars marking the situation of the incision in the case of the little boy. You had better incise on the right of the middle line, taking the umbilicus as the middle of your incision. Open the abdominal cavity, put in your finger, and feel towards the rectum first of all, because in the case of a large intussusception you often find the end of it actually in the rectum, and very often you may be able to reduce the intussusception without pulling the bowel out of the abdomen, but in many cases this is impossible. Push up the intussusception from the distal end in the direction of the large intestine. As you do so there are two places where there is some difficulty in getting reduction. One is at the splenic flexure of the intestine, the other is at the hepatic flexure. But with a little manipulation you can easily get past both those critical points. Then comes the really difficult part of the operation in the ileo-cæcal form, the separation of the last bit

of the intussusception. Do not be in too great a hurry. If you press gently for some time you reduce the congested and œdematous tissues and so far empty them of blood that complete reduction occurs. If you hurry or get impatient and pull, you will almost certainly tear the intestine, and you will then prolong your operation and very likely kill the child, for you must then suture. So be gentle in your manipulations, and remember that the obstruction is chiefly the result of œdema and not of adhesions. Adhesions do form, but with nothing like the readiness which you find stated in books. When the difficult point is overcome make certain that you have produced complete reduction. If you look at the cæcum you will find very often that there is a little bit of it inverted, and it is in those cases that recurrence has taken place after operation. Look carefully at the cæcum therefore to see that you have completely freed the caput cæci.

The best guide that you have brought about complete reduction is that the appendix is free, and you can see exactly where it was inserted into the cæcum. When you have got that clear look at the point where the ileum joins the large intestine. In a few cases it happens that the intussusception has not begun at the ileo-colic angle, but in the ileum, so that an inch or two of ileum may be invaginated into the cæcum, which is then continued onwards as the ordinary ileo-cæcal form. At one time I was very much afraid of the possibility of recurrence in these cases, and it was my custom, therefore, to suture the mesentery and do all sorts of things to the ileum to insure against recurrence. But with more experience I have found that this is unnecessary, and if the bowel be thoroughly unravelled there is no need to fear a return of the condition. After the operation suture the abdominal wound, and as it is important to get over the operation as quickly as possible, I prefer to put sutures through the whole thickness of the abdominal wall. I do not waste time in suturing the abdominal wall in layers. Having got your sutures in, put on a dressing. This dressing ought to be a very complete and thorough one. Small children wriggle about a good deal, and they are accustomed to a binder round the abdomen. Put a layer of gauze and a good firm layer of cotton-wool all round the body from the sternum down to the pubes, and keep it in place with a broad roller bandage of flannel. The child should be put to the breast as soon as possible after the operation, and I have no hesitation in having the mother into hospital and putting her to feed the child within an hour of the operation. It makes no difference as regards recurrence, but feeding relieves children from the extreme shock into which they often pass after an operation.

In the after-treatment you can safely give some strychnia if the patient is collapsed, $\frac{1}{100}$ grain hypodermically, and there is no reason why they should not have a little morphia, to keep them quiet. There is one thing I want to say about the sutures. You should leave the sutures in for a very much longer period than the ordinary time. The usual time for removing sutures after an operation is on the eighth day, but in intussusception I always leave them in for a fortnight or three weeks, and for this reason. A girl æt. 6 months was admitted to the hospital with an intussusception of five hours' duration. The invagination was very large, but it was successfully reduced and the patient made a very satisfactory progress until the ninth day, when two sutures were removed because the surrounding skin looked rather inflamed. The skin stitches had no sooner been taken out than the child coughed, the wound gaped, and about a foot of the small intestine shot out. The house surgeon had the child immediately anæsthetised, the protruding intestine was returned to the abdominal cavity, and the rest of the wound was brought together by sutures of silkworm gut. No further accident resulted and the child made an uneventful recovery. It was discharged about ten days later. Such an accident may be a source of very great trouble if one is working single-handed in an isolated place. So my advice to you is to keep the stitches in for a longer period than usual in these cases.

The prognosis is good in cases which are operated upon within twenty-four hours of the onset of symptoms. The children recover in almost the same proportion as I mentioned to you in these four cases ; that is to say, three out of four recover, or 75 per cent. At one time there were no recoveries ; every child with an intussusception died as a matter of course. I am speaking now of some twenty years ago. These very greatly improved figures are in consequence first of all of a better diagnosis, and secondly because the cases are dealt with surgically at a very much earlier period than was formerly the case.

* *March 5th, 1906.*

A LECTURE ON TRANSFUSION.

Delivered at the Medical Graduates' College and Polyclinic.

By A. P. BEDDARD, M.A., M.D.,

Assistant Physician to Guy's Hospital; Physician to the West London Hospital.

GENTLEMEN,—I have undertaken to say something to you to-day on the subject of transfusion. We have all seen the great good which may be done by transfusion, but every one is not equally aware that it may be by no means a harmless procedure in unsuitable cases. It is from this last point of view especially that I want to deal with it to-day. We shall consider the three following points : (1) the cases which are suitable for treatment by transfusion, (2) the materials which may be injected, and (3) the methods of introducing the fluid.

Let us take the first point, and consider broadly what are the cases which may be benefited by transfusion. They fall into two groups, namely (a) cases of collapse, and (b) certain toxæmias, such as diabetic coma, uræmia, and cholæmia. It is necessary to consider these two groups of cases separately.

"Collapse" is the term applied to the condition where symptoms are due to loss of fluid from the vascular system. The most obvious cause of collapse is loss of blood by hæmorrhage. The fluid so lost from the vascular system has to be made good somehow, and if you can artificially provide the patient with the fluid he needs, that is clearly a suitable case in which to practise transfusion. But, with the exception of great loss of blood at a surgical operation, collapse due to hæmorrhage can rarely be treated by transfusion, for it is not wise to transfuse for hæmorrhage until the bleeding point has been secured. There may be rare exceptions to this statement, but one has to deal here with general statements, and to this one the exceptions are very few and far between ; consequently in hæmoptysis, however dangerous, transfusion is absolutely contra-indicated. In the same way no case of bleeding from the stomach or intestines should be transfused until the artery has been secured by operation or the bleeding has spontaneously stopped for at least twenty-four hours. Much the most frequent cause of collapse is loss of water and salts from the vascular system as opposed to loss of blood as a whole. An obvious example of this condition is a case of severe vomiting and diarrhœa. One has only got to consider a case of summer diarrhœa and vomiting in a child to see that a large quantity of fluid is leaving the body which is not being made good by fluid absorbed from the alimentary canal. Cases of cholera and of uræmic diarrhœa and vomiting are other instances of the same condition. In all the cases mentioned so far it is clear that fluid, whether blood or water, has been lost from the body. The next point we have to consider is this, that in order to produce collapse it is not necessary for fluid actually to leave the body, provided only that it leaves the vascular system in sufficient quantity. Whenever tissues are damaged, whether by inflammation or by mechanical injury, the tissues so injured abstract fluid from the vascular system. The fluid does not leave the body, but it is lost to the circulating blood. For instance, in a burn there is damage to tissues ; and, as everybody knows, the more extensive the area burned, quite apart from its degree, the more dangerous is the condition. One of the reasons for this is that the greater the area of tissue, damaged by the burn, the greater will be the loss of fluid from the blood-vessels and the more is the patient in danger of dying of collapse. In the same way in acute peritonitis and many other such extensive inflammatory conditions pints of fluid may be transferred from the blood to the damaged tissues and unless this fluid is made good to the vascular system collapse will set in. If it is true that patients may thus lose large quantities of fluid from their vascular system although they may be receiving none by the mouth, we may wonder how they can go on as long as they do untreated. The answer is that the body contains large quantities of fluid stored in the muscles and subcutaneous tissues, and that when fluid begins to pass from the blood into the inflamed area the blood-vessels at once begin to take up water and salts from this reservoir. We can recognise clinically three well-marked stages in collapse due, for instance, to acute peritonitis. In the first stage the patient looks in fair general condition, his pulse and blood-pressure may be good ; of course he is losing fluid rapidly into his damaged peritoneum, but as fast as fluid leaves the blood-vessels it is made good to the blood by the vessels taking up water

from the muscles, etc. In the second stage there is an obvious clinical change in the patient ; his features become sharp, his face shrunken, and his skin slack. This shows that the drain of fluid into the inflamed tissues is still going on, and that the reservoir is running dry. The pulse and blood-pressure may still be satisfactory because, although the vascular system is underfilled with fluid, the vaso-motor centre by great activity so increases the peripheral resistance as to keep up for the time being the arterial blood-pressure. Patients will often continue for hours in this condition untreated, then they become suddenly worse and often die before anything can be done for them. The reason for this is that their vaso-motor centre has become tired out and has suddenly struck work, the blood-pressure rapidly falls, and death from collapse takes place. Whenever you see a patient with shrunken features due to loss of fluid you know that he is within measurable distance of death from collapse, and whatever other treatment he may require, at least he needs transfusion unless he is suffering from uncontrolled hæmorrhage.

In the case of the toxæmias already mentioned there has been no loss of fluid from the vascular system. In them transfusion is performed with the object chiefly of diluting or neutralising a poison circulating in the blood. The results obtained are certainly not very striking, and from the nature of the cases it could not be expected that transfusion would do the good which it does in cases of collapse. We shall come back to these cases when considering the methods of transfusion and the material to be injected.

We have briefly dealt with the conditions which may be benefited by transfusion, and we must now consider for a moment the important condition of shock, for which transfusion is an unsuitable and useless method of treatment. The terms "shock" and "collapse" are frequently used as if they were synonymous ; but they are not. They denote two conditions which resemble each other to some extent clinically but differ wholly both in their cause and the treatment which they require. Shock, like collapse, is associated with a rapid, feeble pulse, rapid, shallow respiration, pallor of the face, cold extremities, and a subnormal temperature. But the resemblance is entirely superficial. In shock the blood-pressure is low from the beginning, and as the patient loses no fluid from his vascular system his features do not become shrunken. Shock is due essentially to partial inhibition or paresis of the vasomotor centre, which is caused by an excess of afferent impulses reaching the centre. The impulses may start in the brain or the body generally. But mental shock produces a much less acute and severe disturbance of the vascular system, and does not necessitate the same immediate treatment which cases of bodily injury may demand. It is not difficult to picture the vascular condition of a patient whose peripheral resistance, especially in the splanchnic areas, has been reduced by partial inhibition of the vasomotor centre. The blood-pressure falls considerably, because, as everyone knows, no increased action of the heart can make good the fall of blood-pressure due to loss of peripheral resistance, and hence the futility of treating shock by cardiac stimulants. The blood, which ought to be in the arteries, runs round through the open peripheral resistance and stagnates in the splanchnic veins; and there is no adequate mechanism for emptying the blood in these veins back into the arteries. It is this stagnation of blood in the splanchnic veins which has to be treated and the question is how. Transfusion is shown both by theory and experiment to be a useless treatment, for the obvious reason that it does not treat the condition. The transfused fluid, like the blood already in circulation, runs round and stagnates in the splanchnic veins. A patient in shock is suffering, not from there being too little fluid in his vascular system as a whole, but to his blood being improperly distributed. Therefore the treatment of shock is to re-arrange the blood distribution—in other words, to get the blood out of the splanchnic veins into the arteries, and then to keep a proper proportion there. In order to empty the splanchnic veins it is necessary only to compress the abdomen digitally and keep the pressure up by pad and bandage. If this is done carefully, remembering, of course, that in emptying the abdominal veins we are driving blood into the right side of the heart, the blood cannot run round and stagnate in the abdominal veins, for it would occupy space in the abdomen and such space is no longer available. In the second place, it is obvious that in shock you must treat the fundamental defect—the absence of peripheral resistance. And with this object there are certain things not to do, and

the most important of these is not to give strychnine. The injection of a large dose of strychnine will raise the blood-pressure even in profound shock, but the rise is of short duration and the subsequent fall reaches a level lower than before the injection. It is easy to see why this happens. Strychnine acts, not upon the peripheral arteries, but upon the vasomotor centre. A large dose will stir up even an exhausted centre to give another kick, but after the stimulation is over the centre is even more exhausted than before and the blood-pressure lower.

Nobody, I imagine, at this time of day would dream of using injections of alcohol or ether as a treatment of shock. They used to be given in the belief that they were cardiac stimulants. It is now known that they are not. And further, we have already seen that a cardiac stimulant could be of no real value in the treatment of shock, because no increase in the heart's action can counteract the fall in arterial-blood pressure caused by loss of peripheral resistance. We may, therefore, conclude that alcohol and ether are useless, and it is probably true that they are therapeutically harmless in the doses usually administered. But their use is not harmless from the point of view that they may be given to the neglect of a useful drug. The pathology of shock makes it clear that the only useful drug would be one which raised the blood-pressure by increasing the peripheral resistance, not through the vasomotor centre, but by acting direct upon the peripheral arterioles; and in adrenalin we possess such a drug. I need scarcely remind you that adrenalin given by the mouth to patients other than those suffering from Addison's disease has practically no effect upon blood-pressure because it is not absorbed from the alimentary canal. And when one reads in the medical papers of hæmoptysis being treated by adrenalin given by the mouth one knows that a valuable and costly drug is being wasted, quite apart from the consideration that the action of adrenalin on the circulation would be the worst possible treatment for hæmoptysis. In shock adrenalin must be given either subcutaneously or intravenously. I am sure that it is a good general rule never to put a drug into a vein if it can be given as well in any other way. Adrenalin given subcutaneously in therapeutic doses produces a temporary glycosuria, but is otherwise harmless. A safe dose for an adult is from 20 to 30 ℔ of a 1 in 1000 solution, or, of course, a corresponding dose of any similar preparation.   Its effect upon the blood-pressure comes on within a very few minutes and has gone in about an hour, therefore the injection has to be repeated about every hour until the shock has passed off.   Given intravenously, the effect of adrenalin is instantaneous and it does not last more than ten minutes.   It is, therefore, necessary to infuse continuously a weak solution such as 1 in 20,000.   In passing it may be pointed out that there is such a thing as preventive treatment of shock, by seeing that patients are properly under the anæsthetic before an operation begins or by giving an injection of morphia soon after a severe bodily injury.

The next point we have to deal with is the material to be used for transfusion.   Any solution to be used for this purpose must have the following two properties : (1) it should be of such a strength as to be approximately isotonic with human blood-plasma, and (2) the solution must be more or less non-toxic or physiologically indifferent to the body. The matter of strength is easily arranged, but the second point is much more difficult.   In order to get a solution of the required osmotic pressure it is necessary to use a solution of a crystalloid, and these, as you know, may be divided into electrolytes and non-electrolytes.   Of the non-conductors dextrose is eminently suitable for transfusion ; it is a normal constituent of the blood and sufficiently non-poisonous to be injected in large quantities. A 5·8 per cent. solution of dextrose in distilled water is theoretically isotonic with human blood-plasma.   As a matter of fact what one buys as pure dextrose contains a small percentage of dextrin, which gives the solution a slightly opalescent appearance.   The presence of dextrin is immaterial, and in practice a 6 per cent. solution of so-called pure dextrose may be used.   Electrolytes, such as salts, on the other hand, are a very different story. Their solutions contain ions—that is, electrically charged particles—which endow these solutions with powerful physiological actions in addition to the purely chemical action of the salt in question.   You cannot, therefore, treat a solution of salts as if it were physiologically indifferent to the body in the way that a solution of dextrose is.   You know from physiology that sodium and potassium salts may be poisonous, and that their toxic action is to some

extent neutralised by calcium.   Ringer's solution as used by physiologists is an attempt to compound a solution of various salts which shall neutralise each other's toxic actions and so be indifferent to the body.   There can be little doubt that such a solution of crystalloids is the right one to use if salts are used for transfusion.   But the trouble of making it is prohibitive.   There are many ready-made tablets of mixtures of salts on the market, but none so far as I know which exactly corresponds to Ringer's solution.   The solution most frequently used is one of sodium chloride in sterilised tap water.   The strength should be one and a half drachm to the pint, and not one drachm to the pint as generally stated.   Such a solution is far from being non-toxic, and if you keep your eyes open you will see plenty of cases of poisoning by it. What are the symptoms of poisoning by sodium chloride—or, in fact, by any sodium salt ?   They are—stimulation of the nerves and muscles, from slight twitchings up to severe convulsions ; pyrexia up to hyperpyrexia ; rigors ; feeble, rapid pulse.   I do not mean to suggest for a moment that this solution is too poisonous ever to use, but I wish to emphasize the fact that the solution is poisonous, and much more so than a solution of dextrose. I further want to point out to you that certain cases are much more liable to poisoning by sodium chloride than others.   All the serious cases of sodium chloride poisoning which I have seen have been cases of uræmia, diabetic coma, or cholæmia, and it is easy to understand why.   In these toxæmias the patient has lost no salts from his vascular system ; he has all he ought to have, and you by treatment make a considerable addition to this amount ; therefore he is comparatively easily poisoned.   But in cases of collapse, such as peritonitis, diarrhœa, and vomiting, etc., the patient besides water has lost large quantities of salts as well, and therefore you would have to inject very large quantities of sodium chloride to poison him severely.

Another substance used for a particular case is sodium bicarbonate.   The special case is diabetic coma and the object is to neutralise the acid intoxication by the alkali, as well as to dilute the poison in the blood.   The strength to use is 4 drachms to a pint.   But—and it is a large "but "—you have to remember that sodium bicarbonate is much more poisonous than the chloride.

that in most cases you have no means of measuring the degree of acid intoxication—in other words, the dose of bicarbonate necessary to neutralise it— and that any bicarbonate in the circulation beyond this dose will exert its poisonous effect.

The last point I have to deal with is the method of performing transfusion, and I shall confine my remarks to the question of the choice of route by which fluid is to be introduced. And before doing so I should like to say a word about the extent to which patients are often most unnecessarily starved of fluid by the mouth. It is or used to be the custom before a surgical operation to starve the patient of food for hours ; this one can understand. But why they should be starved of water too, which is so rapidly absorbed from the alimentary canal, it is difficult to see. And again, after operations many patients are for most insufficient reasons not allowed to have any fluid by the mouth for hours. I am not suggesting for a moment that all patients should be given drink, but that no patient should be prevented from having as much to drink as he likes simply because it is the routine treatment. The three possible routes other than the mouth by which fluid can be introduced are the bowel, the skin, and a vein. The alimentary canal is often impossible for obvious reasons. There can be little doubt that fluid is absorbed from the subcutaneous tissues with considerable rapidity provided that the circulation is moderately good. The vein is the most certain and rapid way of getting fluid into circulation, but it undoubtedly has disadvantages and dangers. The choice of route in any given case depends upon two considerations—(1) the nature of the case to be treated, and (2) the kind of solution to be used ; for all solutions cannot be given by any or all of the three routes. If you adopt the attitude of not putting anything direct into a vein unless you are driven to do it, then the only thing which will drive you to transfuse a patient intravenously is the extreme urgency of the case—that is, the necessity of getting fluid into the circulation with the least possible delay. Cases of such urgency are of considerable rarity; they are cases either of severe hæmorrhage or of other less urgent conditions in which the circulation has already become so bad that it is doubtful whether fluid would be absorbed with sufficient rapidity from the subcutaneous tissues or alimentary canal. In all other cases transfusion by

the subcutaneous or alimentary route is certainly preferable, and for these reasons : Intravenous transfusion is open to real dangers which do not exist in the other cases ; they are as follows : (a) It is much more serious if the solution is not of the right strength ; (b) if there is any danger of the solution causing toxic symptoms in the dose it is deemed necessary to give, then the intravenous method is much the most dangerous. And for this latter reason it is always preferable to use a dextrose than any salt solution when intravenous transfusion has to be performed ; (c) there is a very real danger of over-distending the right heart. I have certainly seen cases where intravenous transfusion has caused death in this way. It is difficult to say at what rate fluid can be run into a vein without this danger to the heart. Modern methods have shown that the intake of the human heart in each diastole is very much less than was previously supposed. The most likely figure is 60 c.c., or a little over two ounces. That an apparently small difference in the blood-flow along the veins may make a great difference to the right heart is clearly shown by venesection. Here in the course of several minutes· we abstract at most a pint of blood from the arm and produce a very real effect upon the condition of the right ventricle. Conversely it is easy to understand that the injection of fluid into a vein may be serious to the heart. There can be no doubt that the more slowly the fluid is run in the better, and as a maximal rate I would suggest a pint in ten minutes. The rate may appear to err greatly on the side of safety, but I do not think it does. It is necessary to remember that often when intravenous transfusion is used the right heart is far from normal, and it is just in uræmic convulsions that I have seen the worst results to the heart. From what has been said as to the limited application of intravenous and alimentary transfusion it follows that the best route in the vast majority of cases is the subcutaneous one, and in some cases it is the only one. For instance, in cases of acute gastro-enteritis in children the bowel is useless for transfusion, and no one who has once been foolish enough to try to transfuse a young child intravenously will be likely to repeat the attempt. Subcutaneous transfusion may be performed in two ways, either continuously or intermittently. Personally I do not see that the continuous method possesses a single advantage to outweigh the disadvantage it certainly possesses, namely liability to sepsis. It is one thing to inject fluid under the skin at intervals and quite another to keep a passage between the skin and subcutaneous tissues open continuously for many hours. It may be said with truth that many instances of continuous transfusion show no sepsis, and that it would not matter very much if they did. But, on the other hand, it must be admitted that continuous transfusion of diabetics frequently leads to suppuration and if it does it will take you all your time to stamp it out. And again, in uræmic patients at any rate it is of supreme importance that suppuration, however slight, should not take place. Liability to sepsis is also shared by any patient whose vitality is very low, and this is certainly true of many cases which need transfusion.

I have still to say a word about the choice of route as determined by the solution to be used. A solution of dextrose is not suitable for any but intravenous injection. Large quantities given by the bowel may set up diarrhœa, and when injected by the skin they may lead to sloughing. But for intravenous transfusion for uræmia and for loss of fluid from the vascular system it is the best solution to use. A solution of sodium chloride in tap water may be given in any of the three ways. The objections to its use intravenously have already been discussed. It is the best solution to use for subcutaneous or rectal transfusion. A solution of sodium bicarbonate should not be given subcutaneously because of its liability to produce sloughing. In most cases of diabetic coma there is plenty of time to give alkali by the mouth or rectum. Strong solutions may then be used. Thus six drachms in six ounces of milk or water may be introduced several times a day into the stomach or rectum. If you wish to give it intravenously, give a pint of fluid containing four drachms of sodium bicarbonate and test the reaction of the urine and repeat at intervals of a few hours until the urine becomes neutral or slightly alkaline to litmus-paper. When this point has been reached you may be certain that the patient is no longer suffering from an acid intoxication, and nothing but harm can follow the introduction into a vein of further quantities of alkali.

In the short time that remains I will say a word about the treatment of combined shock and col-lapse. So far we have spoken of these two conditions as occurring separately, and so they may But more often perhaps they occur together in the same patient either simultaneously or successively. Every patient when put back to bed after a severe operation, and especially one on the abdomen, is to some extent in a condition of both shock and collapse, which will vary in degree according to a large number of circumstances. Considerable shock is necessarily present in cases of perforation of the stomach or intestine, of strangulation of bowel or torsion of a pedicle, and is also produced at the time of the operation where much handling of the viscera or traction on the mesentery is unavoidable. The degree of collapse will depend upon the quantity of blood lost at the operation and the amount of damage done to the tissues, not only by inflammation, but also by the amount of handling and exposure to the air that the tissues undergo. It hardly seems to be appreciated how much damage exposure, for instance, of the intestines to the air really does. It has been found that the exposure of a healthy dog's intestines to the air for one hour without doing anything else to them leads to damage which will cause an appreciable amount of subsequent collapse. And there is no reason to believe that this is not equally true of human intestines. For this reason above all operations should be performed with the greatest rapidity that is possible. And there is another consideration that points to the same conclusion, namely that of the anæsthetic. A certain depth of anæsthesia is essential to the safety of the patient and the convenience of the surgeon ; but there is no excuse, excepting possibly want of manipulative skill, for the absolutely poisonous depth of anæsthesia upon which some surgeons seem to insist. Every minute of such anæsthesia injures the patient's power of recuperation and of recovering from a condition of shock and collapse, and the same is true to a less extent of all anæsthesia to the surgical degree. Another condition in which shock and collapse occur simultaneously is in burns. The collapse has been explained and the shock is caused by the injury and stimulation of the sensory nerves in the skin. In many other conditions shock is followed by collapse. Thus in perforation of the stomach or intestine, in gun-shot wounds of the bowel, in abdominal injury with rupture of a viscus, in strangulation of the gut, all the initial symptoms are due to shock ; these may pass off or continue on until the one due to collapse sets in. There can be no doubt that uncomplicated shock is rarely fatal ; but shock none the less requires treatment for the reason that it frequently adds a serious complication to collapse. The treatment of both conditions occurring simultaneously must be a combination of the treatment of the two. That is to say, the patient is transfused, by whatever method is most suitable to the case, and this will generally be by subcutaneous transfusion, and at the same time adrenalin is injected. It has been suggested that the best method of treating such cases is by continuous intravenous transfusion of a fluid containing adrenalin in extremely dilute solution, about 1 in 20,000. This method, however, is practically more difficult to carry out and certainly more dangerous, and is only to be recommended in cases of such urgency that the subcutaneous method would appear to be too slow, and such cases are very few and far between.

March 5th, 1906.

Preparation of an Antigonococcus Serum effective in the Treatment of Gonorrhœal Rheumatism.—Dr. John C. Tarrey says there are several reasons why an antigonococcus serum has not been used heretofore in the treatment of gonorrhœal rheumatism. It has been found to be impossible to bring about an infection in animals by the gonococcus. Again, there is not the slightest indication of an acquired immunity in man to gonorrhœal infection. Finally, the consensus of opinion seems to be that animals cannot be immunised to the toxin of gonococcus as it is contained within the cell. It is, in other words, an endotoxin, a bacterial protein. Although there was apparently slight chance of success, at the suggestion of Dr. Rogers he prepared a serum for a case of gonorrhœal rheumatism of some fifteen years' standing, which had been treated in every other way without result. He was agreeably surprised to find the serum effective not only in that case but also in a high percentage of others in which it had been tried. The culture which was originally employed in producing the serum was isolated from an acute case of gonorrhœa in a male. It conforms in every respect with the characteristics of the gonococcus. The diplococci are negative to Gram's stain, will not grow on ordinary peptone agar or broth, and die on acetic sugar in a short time. For purposes of inoculation a very satisfactory medium is a mixture of rich acetic fluid and slightly acid beef infusion peptone broth.— *Medical Record*, vol. lxix, No. 6.

WITH DR. MONTAGUE MURRAY IN THE WARDS OF CHARING CROSS HOSPITAL.

THIS patient, a woman, had an intestinal hæmorrhage just before we came down, and I want you to look at the abdomen without making any further examination. I will also ask you to look at the temperature-charts, as it is a case of unusual interest. The facts are roughly these. She is 24 years of age, and was sent up for slight hæmatemesis, which was assumed to be due to gastric ulcer. The physical signs on admission were perfectly normal, and her progress for twenty-five days was uninterrupted. Then, suddenly, on Friday, the 8th, her temperature rose—the rise is sharply marked on the chart. On that day she complained of marked headache. On the 9th—that is to say, the following day—there was definite pain and tenderness and gurgling in the right iliac fossa and near the umbilicus : there was no rigidity, and the abdominal movements were good. Her bowels had not been opened since the 6th, so an enema was given. On the 12th, four days after the onset, the temperature and headache still continued, the temperature being somewhat remittent. There was no abdominal tenderness, no pain, no swelling, no limitation of movement. All the other signs were the same as before. On the 14th—six days after the onset of the fever—at 2 o'clock in the morning, she had an attack of acute epigastric pain and vomited half a pint of green watery fluid. The temperature then dropped to 97·4° and the pulse to 60. In a quarter of an hour the pain passed off and the abdomen was observed to move quite freely. There was no distension and no rigidity, and only very slight epigastric tenderness. There were no physical signs in the chest. On this day three rose-coloured spots, disappearing on pressure, were observed on the abdomen, intermingled with others which were redder and which were not affected by pressure. On the next day, the 15th, three more spots were observed. On the 16th the headache disappeared. Early in the morning, at 1.50 a.m. on the 17th, she had a rigor which lasted thirty minutes, and vomited four ounces of yellow matter, and her temperature rose to 106·4° F. At 12.15 p.m. she had another rigor, which lasted twenty minutes ; she was somewhat cyanosed, but still there were no physical signs. Widal's reaction was obtained on this day for the first time ; but there was not, and had not been, any enlargement of the spleen. The bowels were still confined, she complained of feeling somewhat stupid, and her face was flushed much as it is now. On the 19th, at 5 o'clock, she had another rigor, lasting twenty minutes, and her temperature rose to 107°. She was cyanosed for some minutes before the rigor, and passed a large constipated stool after an enema. On the 20th—that is to say, on the next day— diarrhœa began ; the stools were dark-brown and watery. There was still no abdominal distension whatever. The blood-count showed no leucocytosis, and that the polymorphonuclear leucocytes were somewhat diminished. There were no streptococci discoverable in the blood. On the 21st there was a little epistaxis, and also vomiting of an alkaline greenish fluid containing bile. On the 22nd she had her first hæmorrhage from the bowel, a clot about one inch by one and a half inch being found in the stool. The stools were frequent, and brown and watery in character. On the same day, the 22nd, the left parotid gland was found to be swollen and tender. On the 23rd, at 5 p.m , the abdomen became rapidly distended, but there was no pain or rigidity. At 7 o'clock there was more distension, considerable rigidity, and only very slight abdominal movement, while the liver dulness was almost obliterated. Next day, at 11.30 a.m., she passed a large quantity of blackish-red stool, grumous in character, not tarry, and containing no clots. The temperature dropped to 99·6° and the pulse rose to 140. Two or three hours after she passed this stool the abdominal distension almost disappeared, the liver dulness reappeared, and the abdomen was only slightly rigid. The patient was not in the least pallid, but the parotid was getting larger and more tender. On the 25th there were clots in the stools. The fifth stool on that day was the first which was at all light, and that was definitely of pea-soup colour and free from clots. The liver-dulness was normal. On the 26th she passed two large stools containing dark red blood. The parotid, although very large and tender, is not thought by Mr. Waterhouse, who has seen her every day, to contain any pus.

There is now very little abdominal fulness— rather more, perhaps, than there has been during the majority of the attacks. There are no spots, no pain, and no rigidity. She was sick yesterday, and the stools contained recent blood-clots. This afternoon she has had still further hæmorrhage.

Now that you have the whole of the facts before you, it is easier to form an opinion than it has been from day to day. To begin with, it seems perfectly clear that it is a case of intestinal ulceration. The hæmorrhages during the last week and the diarrhœa show that. The point we want to decide is, Is it a case of enteric fever or not ? If it is, is it an uncomplicated case, or is there some secondary or independent lesion ? If we consider that it is enteric fever, and that it began with the onset of the fever, we must date her illness from the first rise of temperature, on the 8th of the month : then the headache is characteristic, being severe and lasting just nine days. The fact that the headache was not in the usual position does not go for much. The diagnostic importance of the spots must also be considered. They were not uniform in size, they were not really characteristic spots, and they were mixed up with spots which were certainly not those of typhoid fever. There was, however—and this is an important observation—a positive Widal reaction. Some authorities would regard this as decisive ; I do not. There is no observation which is not open to some fallacy, and the bacteriologist and radiographer can assist, but not replace, the clinical observer. I have had re ports of a positive Widal's reaction when the case was not one of typhoid fever. In this case there was no leucocytosis, which again is in favour of typhoid fever, because it is unusual in enteric fever to get any ; while in suppuration we are likely to get some definite leucocytosis, though not if due to the B. typhosus or the B. coli communis. During the last three days her stools have been very characteristic. Again, the hæmorrhage is suggestive of typhoid, as is her general appearance and progress.

Is it an uncomplicated case ? Against this view is the difficulty, first of all, of explaining the rigors. Why should she have had these rigors ? They have been described in other cases, but are rare and unexplained. One can only assume that they were due to some secondary foci of infection, occurring, for instance, in the parotid, for we know that her parotid is inflamed ; or there may be an inflammatory focus somewhere else that we have not been able to find out. The chief objection to the secondary focus theory is that with those very marked rigors one would have expected suppuration to have set in earlier. Nor must one forget the complete absence of any persistent tenderness or any abnormal physical signs in the neighbourhood of the stomach or colon.

With regard to the abdomen, I have never seen a case of typhoid fever, with repeated hæmorrhages, in themselves evidence of its intensity, with so little abdominal distension. The only time she had abdominal distension, it came up rapidly, and disappeared rapidly after the passage of the dark watery stool of which I have spoken ; the character of this stool suggested hæmorrhage into the intestine, which distended it; and when it was got rid of, the abdomen reverted to its normal size. In cases of typhoid fever you do not get that absolute relief. There is also the fact that no enlargement of the spleen has ever been found. Still, although it is a very unusual case, our " working diagnosis " is enteric fever, and with that idea we are treating her. It is now the twentieth day of the illness. It is possible that one ought to antedate the onset of the disease. One does not generally get hæmorrhage all through the third week, which is practically what we have seen here. We are on the watch for abscesses, especially in some remote part of the upper abdomen. *

The following case, in my opinion, is one of neuritis of a toxic character, probably due to alcohol, or rather perhaps to an undue susceptibility to alcohol, for reasons which I will mention. She is a married woman, æt. 52 years. She has had four children, but no miscarriages. There are three important facts in her past history : (1) She has had a winter cough, bronchitis, and asthma for twenty years. (2) She says she has never taken alcohol in excess, but only a moderate quantity of spirits daily. (3) Some few years ago she began to suffer from morning retching and occasional vomiting, bringing up slimy mucus.

Some few months ago she noticed that her feet were swollen, and that she had pricking pains in her

---

* The patient subsequently passed a considerable quantity of pus *per rectum* and suffered from suppuration of the parotid gland. Six subcutaneous abscesses were also opened. These contained the Staphylococcus aureus in pure culture. Anti-staphylococcic serum was given. The patient ultimately recovered.

calves and over the tibiæ. After that she took to her bed, and the condition improved. Six weeks from the onset she found that her left foot had dropped ; the right foot also dropped slightly, but that has since recovered, and the left foot is better than it was a few weeks back. She has had pains in her arms and hands, with weakness and wrist-drop. When we examined her, we found first of all that her teeth are very bad, and next that her thorax is rigid, and somewhat barrel-shaped. On inspiration it moves as a whole, and does not expand. The physical signs are as follows : The limits of resonance are practically normal ; they are not increased behind, and the heart's dulness is not covered over by the lung. The air-entry is fair, and the expiration is only slightly prolonged. The adventitious sounds consist in bronchitic râles at the bases ; they have now almost disappeared. The heart practically shows no change nor does the urine. Then we come to the nervous system. There is partial anæsthesia to all stimuli —tactile, thermal, and painful—most marked in the left foot and in the right hand and arm. Sensation is normal elsewhere. There is weakness, most marked in the same regions as the anæsthesia. She has much the same wasting of muscles as the man whom we have been looking at upstairs—that is to say, flattening of the eminences and marked furrows between the bones of the hands. She has some difficulty with the first dorsal interosseous ; such muscle as there is is flabby. There is some slight spasm in the flexors of the wrist and of the knee. There has been no tremor. The skin over the fingers is glossy. There is complete R.D. in the exors of the right forearm and in the small muscles of the hand, and in the tibiales of the left leg. The R.D. is partial in the other weak and wasted muscles. Of course all these points will at once suggest that the case is one of neuritis. She has motor and sensory symptoms which, are most marked in the extremities, and which have the usual distribution of multiple neuritis. The deep reflexes in such a case are usually abolished, but you will find that the knee-jerk on her right side is increased, and it has been increased all through. You may get the knee-jerk persisting in neuritis for some time, and there are cases in which it has been increased right through the attack until the patient began to improve, but that is certainly unusual. There is no ankle-clonus. In the plantar regions there is a flexor response in the right side and none in the left. The question arises, therefore, How are we going to explain the rigidity and the increased knee-jerk? Shall we simply note them as being unusual signs and leave them, or shall we attempt to explain them? I think the most obvious explanation is this : The lesion is not quite so local in its distribution as that which you usually get in toxic multiple neuritis. The grouping of the nervous changes point to degenerative changes in the upper as well as the lower "segment," and in the anterior cornua as well as in the peripheral nerves. This may be to some extent explained by the rigid thorax without much emphysema, which suggests that the costal cartilages became calcified at a comparatively early stage. That necessarily led to a generally defective state of nutrition and possibly predisposed to degenerative changes later on. Then the toxic effects of a poison especially involving the nerve tissues produced the wasting and the sensory changes which we have noted. It is important to recognise this condition, because, while she is recovering generally from the neuritis and has rather more power than she had, still, the likelihood of complete recovery is less than it would be if the condition were clearly limited to the peripheral nerves, since there is little power of repair in the motor tracts of the spinal cord. She is having a simple, nutritious diet, strong beef-tea and strychnine, the beef-tea being given more from the point of view of acting as a stimulant than as a nutritive substance.

March 5th, 1906.

Cancer and its Treatment. Mayo Robson.

Cancer is a disease that has attracted much attention of late, not only on account of the extreme gravity of the malady, but also because of the determined efforts now being made by scientific men in all parts of the world to solve the mystery of its causation. Mr. Mayo Robson's excellent work on 'Cancer and its Treatment' has therefore appeared at an opportune moment, and the publishers, Messrs. Baillière, Tindall, and Cox, have done their part well by printing it on good paper and in legible type. The object of the author is "to convince those who have the chance of seeing patients in the early stages of their illness that in many cases cancer can be prevented by treatment in the precancerous stage ; that even when cancer has developed, if it be seen early and thoroughly removed, it is frequently a curable disease ; and, lastly, that even in the later stages much may be done by surgical treatment to give real relief." Mr. Mayo Robson asks if it is too much to hope that some of the views he has enunciated may filter through the profession to the public and serve to convince them that until a true prophylactic for cancer is discovered they will be consulting their own interests best by seeking medical advice earlier. To trifle with their ailments in the early stages is to lose the favourable moment, and ultimately to hear the verdict, alas ! too often pronounced, "Too late." The very fact that cancer is often only submitted to the surgeon when it has either ceased to be a local disease or, if still local, when it has invaded the tissues to so large an extent that its complete removal is difficult or impossible, has not only misled the public, but has even biassed many members of our profession as to the true facts of what surgery can do for this fatal disease. "Too late" has yet to be said in one half or three fourths of the cancer cases when seen by the operating surgeon. Many even intelligent persons, having abandoned all hope of permanent benefit from surgical treatment, throw themselves into the arms of so-called cancer specialists, who fatten on the credulity and ignorance of their victims, and only when all hope of benefit by recognised methods has passed are they allowed to escape from their clutches. Mr. Mayo Robson says that "although cancer is not infectious in the ordinarily accepted sense of infection, there is a very large accumulation of facts which seem to prove that it is locally infective and capable of distribution by contact and inoculation," and his conclusion is that "it seems highly probable that cancer is both contagious and inoculable among human beings, as it undoubtedly is among the lower animals. These facts are so suggestive that, although it may not be necessary to advise segregation of cancer patients, it would seem most desirable that all dressings taken from cancer patients should be burnt ; that linen soiled by cancerous sores should be destroyed or disinfected by boiling ; that contact with cancerous ulcers, whether of the lip, tongue, breast, uterus, or other parts, should be avoided ; and that common use of beds and utensils with cancerous patients should not occur."

THE CLINICAL JOURNAL,

CLINICAL RECORD, CLINICAL NEWS, CLINICAL GAZETTE, CLINICAL REPORTER,
CLINICAL CHRONICLE AND CLINICAL REVIEW.

EDITED BY L. ELIOT CREASY.

| No. 698. | WEDNESDAY, MARCH 14, 1906. | Vol. XXVII. No. 22. |

CONTENTS.

* *Specially reported for the Clinical Journal. Revised
by the Author.*

ALL RIGHTS RESERVED.

NOTICE.

*Editorial correspondence, books for review, &c.,
should be addressed to the Editor, 51, New Cavendish
Street, W., Telephone No. 904, Paddington ; but
all business communications should be addressed to
the Publishers, 22½, Bartholomew Close, London,
E.C. Telephone 927, Holborn.*

*All inquiries respecting Advertisements should be
sent to MESSRS. ADLARD & SON, Bartholomew
Close, E.C. Telephone 927, Holborn.*

*Terms of Subscription, including postage, payable
by cheque, postal or banker's order (in advance) : for
the United Kingdom, 15s. 6d. per annum ; Abroad,
17s. 6d.*

Cheques, &c., should be made payable to THE
PROPRIETORS OF THE CLINICAL JOURNAL, *crossed
" The London, City, and Midland Bank, Ltd., New-
gate Street Branch, E.C. Account of the Medical
Publishing Company, Limited."*

Reading Cases to hold Twenty-six numbers of
THE CLINICAL JOURNAL *can be supplied at 2s. 3d.
each, or will be forwarded post free on receipt of
2s. 6d. ; and also Cases for binding Volumes at 1s.
each, or post free on receipt of 1s. 3d., from the
Publishers, 22½ Bartholomew Close, London, E.C.*

A LECTURE

ON

HÆMATEMESIS.

Delivered at St. Bartholomew's Hospital.

By W. P. HERRINGHAM, M.D., F.R.C.P.,
Physician to the Hospital.

GENTLEMEN,—There are a considerable number
of cases of hæmatemesis admitted into this hospital every year, and their diagnosis and their
treatment are matters both of difficulty and of
importance. If you turn to text-books on
medicine and look up the subject of hæmatemesis,
you will find such cases are divided, very logically
and beautifully, first of all into those in which the
blood is not effused directly into the stomach
cavity but is swallowed, having been originally produced either in the nose, as in epistaxis, or in the
lungs, as in hæmoptysis, or in the œsophagus, as
in the case of cancer of that part, or of aneurysm,
or even at the base of the skull in a case of fracture. Secondly, there are the cases in which
the blood is effused directly into the stomach.
And these, again, are subdivided, first of all into
those in which the stomach-wall itself is diseased ;
secondly, those in which hæmorrhage occurs from
some neighbouring tumour bursting into the
stomach ; and thirdly, those in which the hæmorrhage is due to some general disease, and is not a
local affair at all.

Such divisions and classifications are excellent,
I think, for text-books, and are to be recommended
to you when you are writing examination papers.
But clinical instruction and clinical experience
take a different view of things, and tend to make
you recollect first of all those things which are
most common, and only after those the things
which seldom occur. I have no hesitation in saying that, when you come to practise medicine, in
99 out of every 100 cases of hæmatemesis you will

not refer to any such classification at all. Very few cases of hæmatemesis are due to swallowed blood, and of those which are due to effusion of blood into the stomach cavity nearly all are due to disease of the stomach-wall. I have seen—and I suppose everybody who has seen many cases has observed —hæmorrhage due to general diseases. For instance, I have seen it at the end of a fatal case of typhoid fever, and I have seen it in pernicious anæmia. It also occurs in other hæmorrhagic fevers. And I have seen aneurysms bursting into the stomach. But those rare cases are usually of no particular difficulty in the matter of diagnosis. The disease is pretty obvious in those cases, and they are of no importance with regard to treatment.

Again, if you will refer to your books you will find that cases of hæmorrhage due to disease of the stomach-wall are divided into cases of congestion, cases of inflammation (those are generally said to be very slight), cases of erosion, cases of ulcer, and cases of cancer. But here, again, you find that clinical experience does not leave you with that sort of classification in your mind. When you come to recall the cases you have seen you will find that they group themselves, curiously enough, not according to their cause but according to their ages. You will remember, first of all, that the largest number of all cases of hæmatemesis occur in young women between twenty and thirty years of age, and you will very likely recall that in not a single one of them did you feel quite sure what was the matter. Take a typical case. A young girl, æt 19 years, was admitted under us in 1902. Three years before she had been treated for gastric ulcer in another hospital. She had been having indigestion again for some time, and the week before admission she brought up half a pint of blood, and passed the usual black stools containing blood. Again on the day before admission she did the same thing, and this time we saw the melæna in the hospital. After she was admitted she went on for a month under ordinary medical treatment, and improved somewhat. Then she again had a slight hæmatemesis—that is to say only about a couple of ounces—and a month after that again she had a return, again of a small amount. She had no sign of disease except slight abdominal tenderness. After a time she improved and was discharged. She came in again the next year—that is to say eighteen months after her discharge—because

she had again had hæmatemesis, up to half a pint of blood. She had this vomiting of blood three times during the first few days in the hospital, and always to about the same amount. She seemed to be perfectly natural in every other respect. Then she improved again and went out, after a month's stay here. What has been the matter with her? Is it to be supposed that she had a gastric ulcer? That is the question which always arises in one's mind. I should say most probably not. In the first place, there are plenty of such girls, and if they all had gastric ulcer one would think there would be some corresponding frequency either of ulcer or of the sequelæ of ulcer—scars, contractions, and so forth—to be found in the female post-mortem examinations which are made; but this certainly is not the case, and in the second place the symptoms of these patients do not as a rule give the impression of a grave disease. Of course we must not push that sort of evidence too far. We know very well that some cases of definite gastric ulcer are quite latent until the last moment, when they perforate or the patient dies by a sudden hæmorrhage. Still, when you see a number of such cases in which the symptoms are all very slight, it certainly has a share in the formation of your conclusion as to their nature.

And yet this patient certainly had gastric hæmorrhage. And what else could she have had besides gastric ulcer? Of late years some stress has been laid on the existence of bleeding points in the stomach, merely little capillary oozings in the mucous membrane. Surgeons have operated on cases of repeated hæmatemesis, and they have found such points and ligatured them, and sewn the patient up, and the bleeding has stopped for a time. Again, other surgeons have found oozing in the stomach, but no definite ulcer, only an erosion. Such a case as that occurred to us. A young woman, æt. 31 years, was admitted here. She was a servant of a medical man, one of ourselves, and she had therefore been under skilled observation for a considerable time. Nothing had been noticed in her health until a fortnight before she came in, when she began to complain of slight indigestion. Two days before coming in she had some headache and some vomiting. The day before coming in she had slight hæmatemesis to about two ounces. She was admitted into the hospital and certainly looked very ill, much more ill than such a slight hæmatemesis would account for. On the day of her admission she had a hæmatemesis of considerably larger quantity, between half a pint and a pint of blood. She looked so much worse after that, that after a consultation we decided that although the hæmatemesis was slight, it was evidently having so severe an effect upon her general condition that it was dangerous to leave her without doing anything further. We thought it was one of those cases with bleeding points, or at any rate that operation would enable us to discover some slight injury which could be relieved. Therefore she was operated upon. When the stomach was opened and turned more or less inside out, it was seen to be of a very deep red all over and many bleeding points appeared. In fact, the stomach seemed to bleed wherever it was touched. That was the impression left on my mind when I saw the operation done. Many such bleeding points were ligatured and the patient was returned to bed. But she died the next morning, not, however, from hæmorrhage, but entirely from the shock of the operation. At the post-mortem examination we found that at the cardiac end, as far as possible removed from the wound, so that it would have been very difficult for the surgeon to see or reach it, was a slight erosion, in the middle of which was a small thrombosed vein which had been opened; a thrombus was formed in its lumen; and that, I suppose, was the source of her hæmorrhage.

But another case occurred which is also of interest in this connection, that of a young woman æt. 27 years, who was admitted with the history that for eight years she had had indigestion and pain after taking her food. She had been in another hospital a year before for this set of symptoms. For the last two months the pain had been continuous, although much worse recently, and she had had occasional hæmatemesis to a small amount. On the day of her admission she brought up half a pint of blood. On the day following there was another hæmatemesis, and four days later she had another attack of hæmatemesis. Next day she had an attack of violent pain. She improved up to about a month from the time she came in, but not very much, and then she had a return of her symptoms, followed in a fortnight by a return of the hæmatemesis. She had another attack of hæmatemesis a month later. So that she had three attacks at intervals under our actual eyes.

She improved so little in her general appearance and symptoms that I thought it would be wise for an operation to be done, and this was carried out. Her stomach was turned practically inside out, but nothing was found to be the matter with it. So that in cases even of repeated hæmatemesis there may obviously be no serious disease of the stomach whatever.

And that is borne out by the course of the disease in these patients. I am speaking entirely of this class of young women. I have not seen a single case in the last four years which was let alone and which proved fatal, and all of them, even the obstinate one which I mentioned last, improved eventually under medical treatment. It could not be said that surgical operation had anything to do with it, because nothing was done in that way. I do not mean to say that the improvement remains for ever. It does not; the symptoms recur. A great many of our patients have been treated in previous years at other hospitals; some have returned to us because of a second attack after being treated here. But they improve in the second attack, just as they did in the first.

Moreover, the same recurrence takes place, even after operation. We had a girl here who was a school teacher, æt. 26 years, who had been eight years ago an in-patient here for gastric pain and vomiting. Evidently she was thought to have gastric ulcer. She remained well two years. Two years ago she was again ill in the same way and came to our out-patients. Six months later she went into another hospital, where gastrotomy was performed. She had considerable hæmatemesis. The bleeding points were ligatured; she knew all about it, and told us the whole history of her case. She kept well until eight weeks after the operation and then began again with the same train of symptoms, and subsequently had the biggest hæmatemesis in her life, amounting to one and a half pints. That was after the operation had been performed. She came in to us six months afterwards with a precisely similar attack to those which she had had before. So you see that operation had had no lasting effect. Under such circumstances it seems to me that, except in the very rarest cases, it is highly inadvisable to operate for simple hæmatemesis in young women.

There are similar cases occurring in young men, but they are very rare. There is only one such case in a male to about twenty females in these four years, and he was a young man, æt. 26 years, who gave the same sort of history that the girls do. Twelve months ago he had painful indigestion, which lasted two months. And the day before he came in he had a sudden hæmatemesis amounting to about two pints. He began to improve from the time he was taken in and put under proper treatment.

That is the sort of case which occurs in young men and young women under thirty years of age.

When you come to the ages past thirty, you will find the cases of hæmatemesis are more frequent in men than in women. Between thirty and forty years of age I have had five or six in men during the last four years, and at this time of life the effects of alcohol are beginning to tell. You have then not only to consider the idiopathic disease of the stomach, but also that secondary congestion which occurs from cirrhosis of the liver. Such was probably the condition at the bottom of the trouble in the case of a young man æt. 33 years. He was a tremendous drinker of alcohol, and for four months he had had morning sickness and vomiting. The day before he came in he had a large hæmatemesis, and on the day of his admission another. We took him in ; he looked a very good colour ; his lungs, heart, and urine were all natural. But his liver extended to one inch below the ribs, pointing to some enlargement of it, probably cirrhotic, such as one gets in patients who have a history of intemperance. He died within a week, having had two severe hæmatemeses, which we saw. Apparently also he had a severe internal hæmorrhage which was not vomited. But no post-mortem examination was allowed.

You also get cases of true gastric ulcer in these men. A man, æt. 38 years, was admitted with a history of gastric pain. There was a rapid onset of severe symptoms, hæmatemesis to a pint, repeated again within a few days, and symptoms of internal hæmorrhage, which were followed by death. We found in his stomach a small ulcer, sharply cut, deeply punched out, typical of gastric ulcer such as are described and such as you see in museums, with a tuft in the centre, containing blood-vessels which had been eroded, and from them the hæmorrhage had come. To one case of this age great interest was attached by the fact that gastro-enterostomy was performed, and here again no permanent good effect

followed. The man was 33 years of age, a healthy, muscular labourer. He was not at all intemperate and had never had syphilis. He was a healthy-looking fellow. He had several attacks of hæmatemesis. In the last one he came to me in the out-patient department and looked so bad that I took him into the hospital. And on his having another attack of bleeding I felt that if that was to go on he would probably die, and I advised him to undergo an operation, thinking that if we did a gastro-enterostomy, short-circuiting the food as it were, the irritation of the food passing over the gastric ulcer which I felt sure he had at the bottom of his disease would be relieved, and the ulcer would be allowed to heal up. Operation was performed. He went to the convalescent home at Swanley, and while he was there he had a return of the vomiting and a slight hæmatemesis, but on the whole he was considerably better than before, and he remained so for eight months. He still had occasional vomiting, but he had no hæmatemesis. Eight months after the operation he began again to have slight hæmatemesis. I admitted him because I was afraid of what might happen. The day afterwards he had a hæmatemesis amounting to one and a half pints and he looked very ill. He had had nothing to eat by the mouth since admission, but yet he had severe hæmatemesis. He remained in the hospital with us for two months, slowly improving, but very slowly, and still remaining exceedingly anæmic. I never saw a man in whom the loss of blood produced such a lasting effect. He was discharged at his own request as he was very impatient and wanted to get out, but the anæmia was not anything like cured.

After forty years of age cases of cirrhosis of the liver increase, and they are more common than gastric ulcer, although genuine gastric ulcer still occurs. I need not instance cases of that ; the hæmorrhage is generally caused by a distended or varicose gastric or œsophageal vein in the terminals of the portal system, which get obstructed by contraction of the liver. But sometimes you cannot see any such vein ; you cannot see any real source of the hæmorrhage into the stomach. And in those cases a second possibility arises. We had a man, æt 60 years, who had had, I think, no illness at all until three weeks before admission, when he had pain in the abdomen. The day before admission he had hæmatemesis of a pint, and he died eight days afterwards with constant repetition of the hæmate-mesis. There was no symptom of disease that we could find in life to show what was the cause of the hæmatemesis from which he died. He had no tenderness, and his liver was not enlarged. There was nothing to show that he had gastric ulcer or cir-rhosis of the liver, and when he came to be ex-amined in the post-mortem room we found that his liver was slightly cirrhotic, but only slightly. It weighed fifty ounces, which is almost the natural weight for a man of his age, and in the stomach there were no distended veins and nothing to show where the blood came from. There was a general staining of the mucous membrane, which was very likely derived from the clot itself, nothing more. But he had in addition to this cirrhosis of the liver very marked interstitial nephritis, and that happens in a certain small proportion of cases of hæmate-mesis. We have had another patient, who has been in the hospital several times with attacks of hæmatemesis to a large amount, and he has obvious signs of chronic interstitial nephritis. You know that interstitial nephritis and cirrhosis of the liver are both of them well-known causes of severe epistaxis, and we know that chronic interstitial nephritis has a very marked effect on the lumen of the arteries. Cirrhosis of the liver we know dilates the veins; you can see these dilated veins on the face, and sometimes on other parts of the body, but how it occurs I do not think any of us quite know. So after forty years of age you have not only to consider cirrhosis of the liver and gastric ulcer, but also interstitial nephritis.

It is curious that cancer, which you would think would complicate the diagnosis, very seldom does, for the bleeding of cancer is not usually as profuse as that which leads to sudden hæmatemesis of red blood. The bleeding of cancer is a slow and gradual oozing, so that the blood is extravasated little by little into the stomach, and it does not irritate the stomach enough to produce vomiting. In consequence the blood lies for a long time in it, and is subjected to digestion by the gastric juice, thus producing the coffee-grounds stuff which is vomited in these cases. This material is generally held to be significant of malignant disease.

You may have gathered from what I have said that I am not at all in favour, except in the very rarest cases, of operation for hæmatemesis alone, And if you do not operate, how else shall you treat the patient? Such cases are treated here in the first place by rest of the whole body. Rest—that is to say, making the patient lie in bed and keep there—is the best of all treatments for hæmor-rhage anywhere. Next there should be rest of the part which is bleeding. Those who have been in the wards know that we do that by depriving the patient of food by the mouth for as long as they can bear it, the period varying up to a fortnight. Some, of course, cannot stand it for so long as that. But during that time nothing whatever is allowed them by the mouth, unless it be sips of water, a teaspoonful at a time. These people are fed entirely by means of nutrient enemata, generally one every three hours, the enema consisting of meat, milk, and egg, which is usually pancreatised and alkalised. The thirst is very well relieved by injection of a pint of saline fluid once or twice in the day. If you are feeding patients by nutrient enemata, remember you have to wash out the rectum thoroughly with a large soap-and-water enema at least once a day, otherwise there will be a mass of decomposing stuff in the rectum which will not only prevent absorption of other food, but cannot possibly do the patient any good. After a fortnight we give these patients whey and then whey mixed with milk, gradually reducing the quantity of whey, until eventually pure milk is given, and then the ordinary milk diet of the hos-pital. For severe hæmatemesis the immediate treatment is in the first place the giving of ice to suck, secondly the injection of morphia, which has a wonderful effect, and thirdly the administration by the mouth of adrenalin. I have no doubt that that is a valuable styptic in cases of bleeding of the stomach. It has been said, in objection to adre-nalin, that by increasing the general blood-pressure throughout the body it might tend to produce a recurrence of the hæmatemesis, pressure being brought to bear upon the bleeding point. But the observations of Dr. Hadfield made in my wards in cases of administration of adrenalin proved fairly conclusively that no such general rise of blood-pressure could be traced. It may happen experi-mentally in animals, but it does not appear to happen in man, and as a result no such danger of recurrence of hæmatemesis is to be feared. I always employ it in cases where there seems danger of there being hæmatemesis. For the pain which generally accompanies gastric inflammation there is not a drug in the whole Pharmacopœia which is to be compared with bismuth. People give it in fifteen-grain doses generally, but sometimes very large doses are administered. In the smaller doses in which I give it, it has had a most wonderful effect in relieving pain ; and it is well to remember in employing bismuth, first of all that it colours the stools a dark brown, which may be mistaken for melæna, and in the second place that physicians are widely at variance as to how the drug acts. Some say that it acts simply mechanically, making a sort of covering over the sore place. On the other hand, some say it acts physiologically, as an astringent. There is no clear evidence either way, and in consequence, as you will generally find to be the case, the opinions expressed are extremely dogmatic. And as some physicians are also examiners, it is well to remember that point.

March 12th, 1906.

A LECTURE ON DIET.

Delivered at the Medical Graduates' College and Polyclinic.

By HARRY CAMPBELL, M.D., F.R.C.P.

GENTLEMEN,—I will begin this lecture by a question: How far is man to be regarded as a vegetable feeder, and how far as an animal feeder? We doctors ought to be in a position to answer it authoritatively.

That branch of vertebrates known as the mammalia falls, in respect of diet, into three classes : (1) the purely flesh feeders, or carnivora ; (2) the purely vegetable feeders, which include the herbivora and many of the frugivora ; and (3) the mixed feeders. (2) The herbivora, of which the horse, the ox, and the rabbit may be cited as examples, subsist on bulky, unconcentrated vegetable food, such as grasses, leaves, and the like, and have a correspondingly bulky digestive system. The frugivora, which include such animals as the squirrel and the monkey, consume, on the other hand, a more concentrated vegetable food, such as they find in seeds and nuts ; being more intelligent than the herbivora, and gifted with no inconsiderable prehensile powers, they are able to pick and choose their food, and, as might be expected, their digestive system is much less bulky than that of the

herbivora. (3) Lastly, there are the mixed feeders, including, it should be observed, many of the frugivora, their intelligence and ability to grasp objects enabling them to procure a certain amount of animal food, which of all foods is the most nutritious. Thus we find squirrels consuming eggs as well as nuts, and many of the monkeys supplementing their vegetable diet by small birds, lizards, grubs, and the like.

We have now to ask, To which of these three great classes does man belong? Is he by nature purely carnivorous, or purely vegetarian, or is he a mixed feeder? In other words, which kind of diet best satisfies his digestive and nutritive requirements? There can be no doubt as to the answer. Man is naturally a mixed feeder, and that I may convince you of this fact I will ask you to cast your minds back to the anthropoid stage of his evolution—the stage, *i. e.,* which corresponds to that of the existing anthropoids—the gorilla, chimpanzee, gibbon, and orang. We have beyond all doubt descended from a being closely allied to these creatures, and are therefore justified in assuming that the diet of our simian ancestors was much the same as that of the present-day anthropoids, a conclusion rendered all the more certain by the remarkably close resemblance which exists between their digestive organs and our own. You see, then, what great interest attaches to the study of the diet of the anthropoid apes. Unfortunately, we do not know exactly what their natural food is ; for, owing to their extreme shyness, it is difficult to observe them closely under natural conditions. So far, however, as I am able to form an opinion from the observations of travellers and from my own observations of anthropoids in captivity, I cannot doubt that they are essentially frugivorous—*i. e.* that they subsist chiefly upon concentrated vegetable food, nuts, seeds, and the like, supplemented, as in the case of other frugivora, by less concentrated kinds, such as young shoots and luscious fruits. But though these form the staple of their diet, there is no doubt that they also consume a certain amount of animal food, such as birds, snakes, lizards, eggs, insects, and grubs ; and from this we may safely conclude that our simian forbears, though essentially frugivorous, were to some extent carnivorous also, and must thus be classed among the mixed feeders.

It is a long leap from the highest ape to the

lowest existing man, but I am going to ask you to take that leap with me. The most primitive peoples of to-day have not yet reached the cibicultural * phase of culture ; *i. e.* they neither cultivate the plant world nor breed animals for food, but subsist on wild fruits, seeds, roots, and such animal food as they can procure by hunting and fishing. These peoples, intensely interesting by reason of the link they constitute with our long vanished progenitors, survive in parts of the world which by their remoteness and inaccessibility have afforded them protection from more advanced and powerful races, and I need hardly say that a study of their diet, preserving as it does its primeval simplicity, is of the utmost value to our present inquiry. I have, fortunately, been able to obtain, as the result of prolonged investigation, a fairly detailed account of it. It would appear, speaking generally, to be about one half animal and one half vegetable, though considerable differences obtain among different precibiculturists in the relative quantity of animal and vegetable food consumed. Thus some, such as the Esquimaux, are of necessity almost wholly carnivorous, while with others, such as certain acorn-eating Californian tribes inhabiting oak forests, the proportions are about two thirds of vegetable to one third of animal diet. But setting aside these differences, the great point of interest is that none of the existing precibiculturists are purely vegetable feeders, the fact being that the uncultivated vegetable kingdom does not by itself afford adequate sustenance for man. In the light of such facts as these it is obvious that we cannot regard him as purely vegetarian by nature. There can, indeed, be no shadow of doubt that he is naturally a mixed feeder, for the uncultivated plant world does not afford the precibiculturists a sufficiency of food, even though they all (with the exception of the Esquimaux, who in their barren, frost-bound haunts are compelled to subsist almost entirely on animal food) understand how to increase, and that considerably, the yield of vegetable food by special methods of preparation, whereby indigestible, acrid, and even poisonous substances are rendered wholesome and palatable. Thus, objectionable ingredients they remove by

* I have ventured to coin this word, inasmuch as we have need of a term signifying the artificial production of food, animal as well as vegetable. The term *agriculture* has not this wider significance.

maceration and heat, while by means of pounding and cooking they break up the indigestible cellulose framework of vegetable tissue, thus liberating and rendering digestible the contained starch and other food-stuffs. The discovery of cookery was in truth an epoch in man's history, providing as it did the master key by which were unlocked vast storehouses of nutriment up to that time inaccessible. And yet in spite of the precibiculturists being able by it and other means greatly to augment their supply of vegetable food, they are compelled to supplement their dietary from the animal kingdom ; they are, indeed, essentially hunters and fishermen ; and if such is the case with them, how much more must man have been dependent upon the animal kingdom for his food before he had learnt to increase the yield of vegetable food by artificial means.

Now, we have seen that our anthropoid ancestors were in the main frugivorous. What is the inevitable conclusion ? Surely it is this—that the evolving man must steadily have increased in carnivorism from the anthropoid stage of his philogenetic career right up to the time when he began to prepare his vegetable food in special ways. We can understand how with his ever growing intelligence he was able to procure a constantly increasing supply of animal food, and how he thus came to be a wandering hunter ; and it was not, indeed, till the period of fixed agriculture was reached, and he became rooted to the soil, that he abandoned hunting as the serious occupation of his life. Thus it came to pass that it was precisely when man was leading the active outdoor life of the hunter that he was most carnivorous, and there can be little doubt that such a mode of life is the one best suited to a highly animalised diet—far better than a life that is sedentary and confined.* All the carnivora are impelled to great activity in their search for food, and it is probable that this very activity is favourable to the digestion and assimilation of animal

* I must guard against misapprehension here. I do not mean to say that a highly animalised diet is the one best suited to an active outdoor life, but rather that a life of this kind minimises the evils which tend to result from the consumption of large quantities of animal food. Those who are called upon to expend much muscular energy demand an ample supply of carbonaceous food, and such are better able to tolerate a purely vegetarian diet, with its large percentage of starch and sugar, than the inactive and sedentary.

food. We know that many carnivorous animals, such as dogs, are made ill by much meat when kept in close captivity, whereas under a more active mode of life they are able to consume large quantities with impunity.

If, then, we are asked what kind of food is best suited to man's requirements—animal, vegetable, or mixed—we can unhesitatingly answer that a mixed diet most assuredly is, the desirable proportion of animal to vegetable in it varying with his mode of life ; and we can explain how for hundreds of thousands of years man subsisted largely on animal food, how during this, his most carnivorous, period he led a nomad life which fitted this sort of diet to him, and how—now that he has become rooted to the soil—he cannot tolerate animal food to the same amount, though still capable of coping with considerable quantities of it.

While, however, we are from the foregoing data forced to conclude that man is largely carnivorous by nature, we must not lose sight of the fact that individual humans differ considerably in their ability to cope with animal food. It is certain that much of it is bad for some, and that not a few thrive best on a diet that is entirely, or almost entirely, vegetable. Such persons are probably exceptional and may be regarded as being in respect of their digestive and metabolic capacity more nearly allied to the anthropoids than to the average individual—as constituting, in fact, reversions to a far-off ancestral type. That good can sometimes be effected, especially in the case of the gouty and headachy, by curtailing or entirely excluding animal food there is not the slightest doubt. We can sometimes cure headaches simply by restricting the allowance of butcher's meat and bird ; in other cases we may have to exclude these from the dietary altogether, allowing fish only ; sometimes, again, it may be necessary to prohibit even fish, limiting the patient to ordinary vegetable food, together with milk, butter, and cheese, always taking care, however, as we reduce the amount of animal food, to supply the necessary quantity of proteid in the form of cheese, protein, plasmon, and the like.

I have said that there are those who thrive best on a purely vegetable diet. How far, we may now ask, is it possible for mankind at large to become vegetarian ? Civilised man has learnt to obtain from the vegetable world a much richer supply of

nutriment, and this in a highly condensed form, than can man in his primitive stage. For though precibi-cultural man secures to himself a considerable proportion of his vegetable food in a compact and easily digestible form—*e. g.* when he gathers seeds and grinds them into flour—civilised man can do much more than this ; for he knows how to extract from the vegetable kingdom pure starch, sugar, albumen, and fat, and by combining these in proper proportions, together with the requisite quantity of extractives and salines, it is possible to obtain in a highly condensed form food amply sufficient for his full nutrition. It has to be remembered, however, that such a dietary is highly artificial, and the fact—which is undoubted—that some thrive on it scarcely justifies the assumption that man is by nature purely vegetarian. Nor must it be forgotten in this connection that most so-called vegetarians consume a large quantity of milk, butter, and cheese, as well as eggs, all of which are derived from the animal kingdom.

Here I may point out by the way that such cannot legitimately claim, as the few genuine vegetarians certainly can and do, that they subsist on a diet that does not involve the taking of life, inasmuch as it would be absolutely impossible for either milk, butter, cheese, or eggs to be sold at a profit without most of the young bulls and cockerels being killed for the purpose of food. It is clear, therefore, that those who include dairy products and eggs in their dietary cannot claim to be wholly guiltless of the slaughter of dumb animals, though they would doubtless repudiate the charge with horror.

I have said that we doctors ought to be in a position to speak authoritatively to our patients on this question of animal as against vegetable food. And this, I repeat, we assuredly are, for it is as certain as is the daily rising of the sun that present-day man is in his nature largely carnivorous. It may be a sad fact and a terrible that we who claim to be the "roof and crown of things" should slaughter dumb animals and eat of their flesh—of that which has once throbbed with the pulse of life ; but so it is, and for long ages so it has been : it was, in fact, on a diet drawn largely from the animal kingdom that man evolved from the ape, through the homosimian, and reached the proud position that he now occupies. I must not be thought to argue, however, that the entire human race may not one day be able to subsist on vegetable food alone ; I believe it to be possible, though at present the difficulties in the way—economic rather than physiological—seem well-nigh insurmountable.

I now propose to touch—very briefly it must be —on a subject no less important than the one we have just considered. Assuming the various food-stuffs—proteids, fats, starches, etc.—to be com-bined in due proportions, how much food ought a man to eat ? The ideal quantity—which, however, may often be exceeded without hurt—is what we may term "the minimum normal," by which I mean the smallest quantity needful to maintain a man at his normal weight and in normal health and activity. But how, it may be asked, are we to know what the normal weight is ? We may define it as the lowest weight compatible with the most perfect health and fullest activity of which he is capable. Hence the minimum normal diet is the smallest quantity of food adequate to maintain a man at the lowest weight compatible with the highest attainable level of health. Any quantity over and above this is useless, if not actually harm-ful. Young people often eat more than is necessary, and frequently, it would seem, without harm ; but note this, that with every added year the power to cope with an excess of food steadily diminishes, and after middle life even a moderate excess is necessarily harmful. There are, of course, wide personal differences in this respect. Even chil-dren may suffer from quite a small excess, as evidenced by the deposit of lithates in the urine, by irritability of temper, and such like ; while, on the other hand, some who are well on in years can tolerate with seeming impunity a large excess, even two or three times the needful amount. I say "with seeming impunity," for doubtless they all do suffer from their gluttony, in that they fail to enjoy the best attainable health. It is a fact, however, that some of them live to be very old. Quite recently I dined at the same table with a voracious old gentleman of some ninety years, who managed to dispose of at least double the amount of food which would satisfy the needs of many a younger man, and though one can hardly doubt that he would find life far more enjoyable (certainly those around him would, for he is not always in the most amiable of moods) if he reduced his food to within physiological limits, it must be confessed that he looks hale and hearty, and bids fair to

weather out many another year. People of this class have prodigious digestive capacity.

We must not, therefore, be too dogmatic in deal-ing with this question of the quantity of food. We must be prepared to judge each case on its own merits. Some there are who, in order to enjoy the fullest measure of health, need always to restrict their allowance of food to the minimum normal, and with every year after the meridian of life the more urgently necessary does such a restriction become ; but there are others who manage to live to extreme old age on a diet which greatly exceeds the actual needs of the organism.

Lastly, let us briefly consider some of the evils resulting from eating too much. The most obtru-sive of these is obesity, and this has many disad-vantages. Not the least is the mere dead weight of the superabundant fat. Take a young man of twenty in full training—i. e. without an ounce of superfluous fat, weighing, we will say, eleven stone, and now suppose him at sixty to have put on six extra stones. Imagine what an encumbrance this extra weight must be, and how severely it must tax a heart which has long lost the elasticity and vigour of youth. Why, even in the young man quite moderate exertion, such as running upstairs, is competent to induce some breathlessness and palpi-tation, and this, mark you, in spite of youth and training. How incomparably greater, then, must be the strain of such an exercise in our man of sixty who is continually weighted with six stone of un-necessary adipose tissue, and on whose heart and arteries the inexorable process of senile decay has already begun to tell. Such a hypothetical case enables us to realise the imperative need of reduc-ing the weight of elderly stout people, above all when there are indications of cardiac weakness.

Not only does obesity impose extra work upon the heart ; it also greatly hampers the movements of respiration, and it is largely for this reason that stout people are so liable to pulmonary troubles, and so apt to succumb to them. With all stout bronchitic patients we should use every endeavour to reduce the weight to the normal.

Another evil resulting from over-eating is indiges-tion. Digestion is much more likely to be good on a minimum normal than on an excessive diet : the digestive organs can deal more efficiently with, and metabolism at large proceed more economi-cally and easily on, a moderate than on an excessive diet. When a large quantity of food is eaten gastro-intestinal digestion is defective, and the liver is burdened with an excess of imperfectly digestive material which it is unable to pass on as normal plasma into the systemic blood-stream, and as a result the tissues are bathed in a plasma which is faulty both from surcharge of nutriment and perversion of composition.

What, let us now ask, becomes of the excess of absorbed nutriment? This is a question of great practical interest. You might think that the organism, after storing a sufficiency in the shape of such substances as fat and glycogen, would allow the surplus to escape unused, the excess of albumin and sugar, *e. g.*, simply draining off by the kidneys without suffering further change. But, except in cases of very great excess—as when very large quantities of sugar, or eggs, have been eaten—or in actual disease, this does not occur. What actually happens is this : after the limit of storage has been reached, *the whole of the surplus is chemically dealt with—metabolised, as we say— by the tissues*, especially by the muscles, which contribute the furnace, *par excellence*, of the organism.

Now, that the excess of food absorbed is not simply cast off unutilised, but is, on the contrary, laboriously metabolised in the laboratory of the tissues and worked off into urea, carbonic acid, water, and the like, it is to my mind one of the most remarkable facts in the physiology of nutrition, and one the clinical importance of which cannot well be exaggerated. For what does it imply? It implies, as we all know, that an excess of nitrogenous food leads to an extra production of urea and kindred products ; and it also implies— though this is not properly realised—that an excess of combustible food, whether in the shape of proteids, fats, sugars, or starches, leads both to an *increase in the output of carbonic acid and water and in the demand for oxygen*. Excessive eating, therefore, not only throws extra work upon the digestive organs and kidneys, but also upon the lungs, increasing as it does both the demand for oxygen, and the production of carbonic acid. It also puts extra work upon the heart, and indeed upon all the organs of the body.

It is of imperative importance that we should be alive to this fact in the treatment of acute dyspnœa, whether cardiac or pulmonary. Dyspnœa is due partly to the accumulation of carbonic acid in the blood, and partly, though in a less degree, to the dearth of oxygen[*] ; and inasmuch as every particle of absorbed food increases the accumulation of the one and the demand for the other, it follows that in all cases of urgent dyspnœa we should give as little food as we dare. If it has ever been my privilege to save life—and we physicians need to be chary in taking to ourselves the credit of so great an achievement—it has surely been by adopting this plan of treatment. I always prescribe a meagre diet in urgent cases of lung disease, such as pneumonia, and if called upon to treat a case of acute bronchitis in an obese individual, I am rejoiced if I can persuade the patient to remain for some days entirely without food ; nothing is so calculated to diminish the dyspnœa and relieve the over-burdened heart in these cases as complete abstinence. The same plan should be adopted in acute cardiac dyspnœa.

The plan of reducing or altogether withholding food is, again, often useful in the acute phase of the specific fevers by the relief it affords the heart and circulation. If you are dealing with a case of enteric fever in which there is coma or delirium, do not hesitate to starve your patient ; it is better that he should remain a few days without food than that his stomach should be distended with material which it is quite incapable of digesting. And here let me say that in cases of failing heart we shall get far more good by carefully attending to the patient's diet than from the administration of alcohol, on which physicians have for so long relied as a cardiac stimulant, especially in acute febrile disorders. I have long been convinced, gentlemen, that we can help the heart far better by carefully regulating the diet than by administering to it so evanescent a stimulant as alcohol. The custom has too frequently been to overburden and dislocate the heart by giving an excess of food (which not only creates the need for a more active circulation, but also distends the neighbouring stomach), and having done this to pour in alcohol so as to stimulate its flagging energies. Surely the wiser plan would be to lessen the burden and dispense with the stimulus. A tired horse can travel farther with a light weight on his back and without

---

[*] Haldane and Priestley have recently shown that this second factor has nothing to do with the excitation of dyspnœa, thus settling a question which has been debated for nearly half a century.

any stimulus whatever, than when heavily weighted and at the same time constantly urged along with whip and spur. Think over this.

We all recognise how greatly we can benefit our gouty and plethoric patients by reducing their food. Here is a case in point. A man, æt. 65 years, came complaining of giddiness, fulness in the head, and flushes ; he had had several attacks of epistaxis, which if occurring constantly after middle life suggest, as you know, granular kidney; and there was no doubt that he was suffering from this disease, for not only was his blood-pressure excessive, but he was passing a large quantity of water with some albumin. Now, by restricting the diet and giving calomel and salines, the epistaxis, giddiness, fulness of the head, and flushings rapidly disappeared, and the patient expressed himself as feeling better than he had done for years.

There is not time to give further instances of the great good that may often be done by reducing the quantity of food, but I should like to say, before leaving the subject, that you need have no fear that by pushing this plan of treatment you will starve your patient to death. People do not so easily die of starvation as is generally thought, and it is very difficult for the physician to kill his patients in this way. I have never myself seen any one die from lack of food, except when the digestive tract has been obstructed (e. g. from malignant disease) or in the all too familiar instances of neglected children among the poor, and in these cases death generally results rather from giving the wrong kind of food than too little of it. On the other hand, I am certain that many lives may be saved by a judicious reduction of the diet, even to the point of temporarily withholding it altogether.

I have spoken of the " minimum normal quantity" of food," but have said nothing as to what on an average its actual amount is. Certainly much less than most people suppose, not a few being able to maintain health and strength on so small a quantity as ten ounces a day. Some interesting experiments carried on with a view to determine the exact amount have served to show that the more thoroughly food is masticated, the less is the quantity needed ; and not only so, but it is found that on this well-masticated reduced diet there is a general levelling up in bodily and mental vigour. Whenever, therefore, you desire—and if I have succeeded in convincing you of my main thesis it will be often—to reduce the quantity of food to a minimum, insist upon thorough mastication.

March 12th. 1906.

ON LEUKÆMIA: ITS TYPES AND CHARACTERS, PATHOLOGY AND TREATMENT.

An Address to the Brighton and Sussex Medico-Chirurgical Society.

By F. G. BUSHNELL, M.D.,

Pathologist Stephen Ralli Memorial Laboratory, Sussex County Hospital, Brighton.

MR. PRESIDENT AND GENTLEMEN,—Certain recent work carried out on the pathology and treatment of this disease, and the mystery which still surrounds it, induced me to offer this subject to the Society. I can only hope I may be successful in presenting what is an admittedly involved subject with reasonable clearness, and that it will be of some interest.

I have divided the paper into certain preliminary remarks, (a) on the cells of normal blood, (b) the types, and (c) characteristics of leukæmia and its allies, (d) a brief account of its pathology and treatment.

Three cases under the care of Dr. W. Broadbent, M.R.C.P., and Dr. D. Hall, M.R.C.P., to whom I am much indebted for the loan of the notes, taken by Dr. Stephens, serve as illustrations of the disease (see appendix).

(a) I may remind you that the colourless cells of the blood are about 10,000 to the c.mm. and are classed into granular and non-granular. In the granular class, which have minute granules in the cytoplasm, we have a further division according to their affinities for acid or basic dyes. (These terms do not necessarily mean that they are acid or alkaline to test-paper, the dyes really being a compound of acid and base, but in the acid dyes the acid radicle is in the excess, as in eosin ; and in basic dyes the base, as in methylene blue. Ehrlich's so-called "neutral" stain acts really as an acid dye.) Thus we have the acidophil (or neutrophil) leucocytes (generally known as polymorphonuclears from the appearance of the nucleus), the eosinophil, the mast-cell, and the myelocyte.

In the non-granular cells are the lymphocytes, large and small, rarely with basophil granules.

In further detail, the *polymorphonuclears* form 60 to 70 per cent. of those present in normal blood. They average 13·5 μ in diameter and have a twisted, deep-staining nucleus, usually single, but when at rest and in the marrow this may be spheric.

Its cytoplasm stains diffusely with watery solutions of acid dyes, but with alcoholic solutions of acid dyes (as Jenner's eosin methylene blue in methylic alcohol) or in differential acid stains (as Ehrlich's triacid of orange G methyl green and acid fuchsin) shows granules. Thus with Ehrlich they are purple on a pink background. They have been termed "neutrophilic" because neither simple acid nor basic dyes bring them out clearly, but they are acidophil. The cells are actively amœboid and are the chief cells in fresh pus. Transitional forms between them and lymphocytes occur in leukæmia and in normal marrow. They do not occur in blood of lower animals. *Eosinophil cells* form 1 to 4 per cent. of white cells. They show a number of highly refracting, rather large, rounded granules of uniform size grouped loosely around the nucleus. They stain bright pink with eosin. The nucleus stains lightly with basic dyes and is frequently divided into two. The cell is a little smaller than the neutrophil and more irregular. It is actively amœboid. It is abundant in connective tissue, bone-marrow, and cœlomic space. *Mast-cells* ½ per cent. normal blood. The nucleus is tri-lobed and the protoplasm remains unstained with Ehrlich's fluid, but shows purple granules with basic dyes. In chronic myeloid leukæmia they may be 5 to 10 per cent. A *myelocyte* is a non-amœboid cell with pale single round or oval nucleus, often placed excentrically, usually with neutrophilic granules in body, averaging perhaps 15·5 μ in diameter. They form 20 to 40 per cent. in myelocythæmic blood.

The large and small *lymphocytes* form together about 30 to 40 per cent. of colourless cells. The large lymphocytes average 13 μ and the smaller 10 μ in diameter. The latter has a spheric nucleus, non-amœboid, which stains intensely with basic dyes. The protoplasm has an affinity for both basic and acid dyes ; thus it may be purple with eosin and methylene blue or grey with Ehrlich's. In large cells the nucleus stains less well and may be indented. They may be amœboid and phagocytic. In acute lymphocythæmia these cells may form 80, 90, or 99 per cent. of leucocytes.

As you know, erythrocytes are present about five million to c.mm. and stain readily with acid dyes. Erythroblasts or nucleated red cells occur normally in marrow and are immature forms of red cells. They are present in severe anæmias and myeloid leukæmia. Of the blood-plates and plasma it is not so necessary to give a description.

The origin of these cells is closely connected with the disease I am about to describe.

Nucleated red cells occur in embryonic life in liver, spleen, and elsewhere, in adult life in bone-marrow (but at birth are not found in circulating blood normally). From these cells the red discs are developed, but their primary origin is probably from the mesoblastic vascular cells.

One of the latest views is that of Pappenheim, who considers that leucocytes and red corpuscles have a common ancestor, a lymphoid cell.

Be that as it may, we have good grounds for believing that both granular and non-granular leucocytes are derived in the fœtus from this lymphoid cell, the indifferent cell of Wolff, the small myelocyte of Dominici. Its characters are those of the large lymphocyte.

As is well known, the femur marrow of the human fœtus from three and a half to the fifth or sixth month consists largely of colourless non-granular cells. These are the "indifferent lymphoid" cells of Wolff, Pappenheim, Dominici, Hirschfeld, and others. Eosinophil myelocytes and polymorphonuclear cells are found also at three and a half months, and neutrophils appear between fourth and sixth months in marrow, but may be found in fœtal thymus and liver.

In the normal adult the seat of the proliferation of the granular cells is practically the bone-marrow. Non-granular cells are found to multiply in the germ-centres of the lymph-nodes (and in the connective tissue throughout the body).

Curiously enough, confirmation of the common source of origin in one cell of leucocytes in the fœtus may be found in the blood of certain cases of myelocythæmia in the adult.

Dr. Broadbent's second case, H. W—, Dr. Browning's case ('Lancet,' June 19th, 1905), among others, illustrate this point. At one time enormous numbers of large mononuclear cells or lymphocytes may be present in the blood, at other times there may be the very faintest granulations in these cells, on another occasion myelocytes may be present in similar profusion. This is regarded by some as a "reversion" of the granular myelocyte to the embryonic non-granular "premyelocyte," or lymphoid cell. A further stage is seen in the "polymorphism," so-called, of myelocytic blood, where the picture is that of all transitions from the large lymphoid to the myelocyte and to the polymorphonuclear. Further support is lent to this view by recent histological findings in acute lymphocythæmia (characterised, as you know, by the presence of large lymphocytes in the blood) by Aubertin, by whom a marrow origin is given to this disease. The distinction between it and acute myelocythæmia tends to be lost.

(b) I now turn to the types and characteristic features of leukæmia and its allies. You are aware that the researches of Ehrlich separated the leukæmias into two broad classes : (1) the myeloid or myelocytic, in which the granular leucocytes are as a rule increased in the blood and the proportions vary from the normal, where the myelocyte forms find their way into the circulation. (2) The lymphoid, lymphocytic or lymphatic, in which nongranular forms predominate and are usually both absolutely as well as relatively increased, the small forms in the chronic and the large forms in the acute. (3) To these must be added *pseudo-leukæmia* (which some people label "Hodgkin's disease," but others would exclude it). Pseudo-leukæmia is an ill-defined disease and is characterised by general glandular enlargement, with a bloodpicture differing in quantity from true chronic leukæmia. Pappenheim, I may say, considers that the one differs from the other only in the involvement or not of the bone-marrow. Pinkus classifies pseudo-leukæmias into those in which the polynuclear elements are diminished with a relative, perhaps small, increase of lymphocytes and those in which there is no blood change and the growths have practically malignant characters. The first is practically leukæmia and the second lymphosarcoma, which shows the difficulties of division with our present knowledge.

By the way, I may mention that perhaps, as Salaman suggests, clinical differences in these cases arising from growth from lymph-cells may depend on the age of the latter at which the growth originates.

(4) A variety of leukæmia that needs only to be mentioned is the so-called "mixed leukæmia." It is true that a mixed blood-picture of myelocytes and lymphocytes may occur which may or may not depend on independent and concurrent affections of myeloid and lymphoid tissues. It is, however, capable of other explanations (e.g. "rever-

sion" to embryonic non-granular type or reaction of myeloid tissue to lymphoid hyperplasia, etc.).

(5) The last type of leukæmia is one of which little has been written, but which I think is illustrated in Dr. Hall's case, Harris. Von Leube (and Parkes Weber follows) gives the name "leukanæmia" to a morbid condition in which the clinical and blood-change symptoms of pernicious anæmia are combined with those of the blood and organs allied to myelocythæmia (and pseudoleukæmia). In short the features of pernicious anæmia and leukæmia are combined, the bloodpicture of the former with the enlarged liver, spleen, and prevertebral hæmolymph-glands and marrow (perhaps also lymph-gland) changes. No abnormal pigment is found in urine or viscera. There is evidence of hæmogenesis in viscera.

It is doubtless the same disease or allied to the *anémie splénique myéloide* of Vaquez and Aubertin, Weil and Clerc—in fact, a myelogenic form of splenic anæmia of adults (see also case of Scott and Telling in an infant in ' Lancet,' June, 1905, of a myeloid condition of viscera with slight myelocythæmia and marked hæmogenesis in viscera).

(c) The characters of the disease. I am unable to find a histological analysis of leukæmia based on many cases ; in fact, it does not exist. In myeloid leukæmia there are bone-marrow changes, with large increase of neutrophil myelocytes, with enlargement of spleen and often of liver. But the lymphoid tissues outside the spleen and marrow are not markedly, if at all, affected. In the blood, marrow, liver, and spleen are found marrow types of cell. The characteristic marrow-cell or mononuclear neutrophil cell may form half the cellular elements in the blood and organs (where also cells intermediate between original mother lymphocyte and adult polymorphonuclear are found). The disease may last two to five years.

In lymphatic leukæmia there is a chronic and acute form. The former may last two to four years, the last about six weeks. The lymphatic glands are usually enlarged, but not beyond the limits of the capsule as a rule ; the spleen may be greatly enlarged. (Since writing this I have examined a case of acute lymphocythæmia of Dr. E. Hobhouse, F.R.C.P., in which no enlargement of the lymph-glands was present.)

In the chronic form the blood and organs are flooded with small lymphocytes, the other types of leucocytes being hardly noticeable. Collections of lymphocytes of various sizes (described either as metastases or as " swellings of similar elements ") are scattered throughout the whole organism. The changes in the spleen and marrow are those of replacement by lymphoid cells.

(*d*) As to the etiology and pathology of the disease, the rival theories are the neoplastic and the parasitic. An impetus has been given to the neoplastic recently by Banti, who believes that the myeloid and also lymphatic leukæmia is a true tumour development, a sarcomatosis of the medullary or lymphatic tissues. Banti accounts for the presence or absence of the specific elements in the blood by erosions which he has observed of vessels of marrow- and lymph-glands, especially in the endothelium of the veins, followed by subsequent thrombosis. In support Banti quotes a case where there was myeloid infiltration of serosa of stomach and intestines, as well as the not unusual appearance of myeloid cells in liver, spleen, and glands.

In this respect I have been much impressed by the phenomenon known as metaplasia which I have observed in epithelial growths, and which Rolleston records as occurring in carcinoma and neoplasms of the stomach, breast, and uterus. Ribbert says that " there is no such thing as metaplasia in the sense that one tissue can be transformed into another totally different from it. Strictly speaking, such a change is only possible in tissues which are seemingly different, but which histogenetically are identical." This allows that innate vital tendencies to aberrant growth may exist ; they may equally play a part in the etiology of leukæmia. (Dr. H. C. Bastian has contributed a paper to the Royal Society, in March, 1905, on " Heterogenesis," and though it perhaps bears upon the " new growth " theory of leukæmia, the subject is too vexed a one to enter into here.)

If, then, Banti's theory is accepted, it may be possible to explain myeloid and lymphatic leukæmia as due to eroded vessels in marrow or lymphatic sarcoma and leukanæmia (myeloid splenic anæmia) as marrow sarcoma without such erosion. True myeloid sarcoma differs perhaps in the stage of development of the marrow-cells forming the tumours.

The second or parasitic theory regards the marrow changes as a definite defensive reaction to infection and not merely as an exuberant growth without finality or obvious purpose.

Thus there is evidence of its being epidemic in region ; it occurs in members of the same family, and is said to have been transmitted from mother to fœtus (Ahren's case, ? re-infection). There is fever, gastro-intestinal symptoms, and albuminuria. The work of C. Price-Jones and of W. Carnegie Dickson on the response of marrow to infection, and its occurrence in variola where there is a myeloid leucocytosis may be also perhaps taken as support. Then again Dominici and Hirschfeld and Wolff believe that the spleen may assist the bone-marrow in its blood-forming functions in certain cases. Acute lymphatic leukæmia, which Auburtin and Weil now ascribe to disease of marrow, is accounted an infection. Finally, Jousset, in the ' Archives de Médecine Expérimentale,' Juillet, 1905, claims to have identified in twenty-four cases of classical myeloid leukæmia a cocco-bacillus which was granular and polymorphous. The bacteriological technique there described is most thorough. The parasitic theory, however, does not explain the influence of intercurrent infections on the blood-picture of leukæmia, which act as do the X rays or arsenic sometimes.

I would conclude with a few words on treatment. Since 1903, when Senn recorded a case of myeloid leukæmia successfully treated by X rays, a large number of similar cases have been published. Among others Bryant and Crane give two, Ledingham and McKerron one, Brown one, which showed marked blood improvement, also Krone, Guilloz, Byrom Bramwell, Cooper, Capps, and many others. In fact, with few exceptions the cases of myeloid leukæmia have improved objectively and subjectively, but whether this is permanent has yet to be seen. It is said to have a specific influence on lymph-follicles. Foster, the first case treated at the Sussex County Hospital, died ; and White, the second case, improved in general and splenic conditions, but the blood-picture was unaffected practically. There may possibly be hope in the use of goat or other animal's serum immunised against marrow and therefore containing marrow antibodies, but I can find no references to such work and its *rationale* would be uncertain in the state of knowledge.

CASE I (Table I).—H. F—, Dr. W. Broadbent. M.R.C.P.

Admitted November 16th, 1904. Has been getting thinner since August and irritable, has been at work up to date.

Father æt. 48 years.

Sister æt. 22 years.

Mother æt. 43 years. First child still-born, no miscarriage, 7 alive, all healthy except one.

No previous illness.

Morning cough. Enormous swelling of spleen.

Liver enlarged.

General and slight enlargement of superficial lymph-glands, movable, discrete, painless.

January 20th, X rays commenced (see blood table).

though no improvement in the picture resulted, his general condition was better on leaving.

CASE 3 (Table III).—Dr. D. Hall.

F. H—, æt. 25 years, admitted April 28th, 1905.

Father died.

Jaundiced since three days old.

Attacks of pain in upper abdomen, motions pale grey, like baby's stool.

Always been of yellow colour, gets "rheumatism."

Frequent attacks of epistaxis, no other hæmorrhage.

Lump in abdomen ten years ago, got bigger.

No ascites present, spleen fills up left side of abdomen, liver enlarged.

TABLE I.

Case and Date, etc.	Hglbn. per cent.	Polymorph. per cent. and per c.mm.	Eosin poly. and myelocytes per cent and per c.mm	Lymphocytes per cent and per c.mm. Small.	Large.	Myelocytes per cent. and per c.mm.	Transitional percent and per c.mm.	Mast per cent.	Erythrocytes per c mm.	Leucocytes per c.m'm.	Ratio white to red.
H. F— 1904											
Nov. 21	—	32·9	2·7	24·3		40·9	—	—	3,600,000	1,160,000	—
Dec. 4	30	Absolute numbers given on this occasion 414,787 (normal 6500)	44,720 (normal 300)	37, 877 (normal 2500)	23,433 (normal 600)	639,183	—	—			
„ 19	—	516,750	23,850	47,700		166,950	31,800	Present	4,560,000	786,850	—
„ 31 1905	—		—			—	—	—			
Jan. 26	X rays on Jan. 20th					—	—	—	2,144,000	903,000	—
„ 28	—	—	—	—		—	—	—	4,720,000	1,900,000	—
Feb. 11	—	—	—	—		—	—	—	4,400,000	1,515,000	—
„ 27	—	—	—	—		—	—	—	4,500,000	660,000	—
March 14	36	49·0	3·0	9·5	9·0	23 0	5·0	—	2,400,000	861,000	1 to 3
April 8	40	—	—	—		—	—	—	2,480,000	329,000	—

CASE 2 (Table II).—Dr. Broadbent.

H. W—, æt. 41 years, painter, admitted July 10th, 1905.

Illness began in September, 1904, with pains in knees, severe, with swellings about ankles. Afterwards suffered from pain in epigastrium and vomiting. Stomach increased in size.

On examination spleen could be felt above symphisis pubis; it is smooth. Liver and lymphatic system—No abnormality detected.. Long bones—No tenderness on percussion.

Suffered from hæmaturia and sudden deafness and giddiness in hospital while under X-ray treatment. In August inguinal glands were enlarged. The blood was examined on many occasions, and

Heart enlarged. Urine 1015, acid, no bile, no albumen.

Inguinal glands slightly enlarged, no hair on pubes nor on face, testicles small.

P.-M. Notes—Marrow, spleen, liver, pancreas, gall-bladder (suppuration, calculi), examined.

Weather very hot, examined two days after death. R. M. present and signs of advanced decomposition. Body very thin, skin and conjunctivæ yellow. Subcutaneous fat small in amount and very yellow. Testes very small.

Thymus gland—No relic seen.

Thyroid gland not enlarged.

Lungs—Small calcareous nodule in substance of lung; left weighed 2 lb. ¾ oz.

Heart-muscle pale brown, no clots in cavities, mitral valve incompetent.   Pulmonary pericardium, artery gelatinous clot, excess of fluid, brownish with reddish sediment.

Stomach contained much undigested vegetable matter, no ulceration.

Liver—Uniformly enlarged, weighs 3 lb. 11 oz.

Spleen—Uniformly enlarged, weight 2 lb. 10 oz.; on section it is firm, rather red, no infarcts.

Kidneys show post mortem green colour; left 5½ oz. ; suprarenal capsules nothing noteworthy.

Testes and prostate very small.   Lymph-glands reddish but not enlarged, hæmolymph glands not enlarged.

TABLE II.

	Case and date.	Hglbn. per cent.	Poly-morph. per cent	Eosin poly-morph. per cent.	Lymphocytes per cent.		Myelocytes and transitional per cent	Mast per cent.	Erythrocytes per c mm.	Leucocytes per c mm.
					Small.	Large.				
	H. W.— 1905									
	July 18*	45	56·3	0·8	17·6	17·6	0·8 3·2	2·0	2,560,000	625,500
	„ 22	40	—	—	—	—	—	—	1,604,000	700,000
	„ 29	40	—	—	—	—	—	—	3,056,000	793,000
	„ 31	—	25·5	0·7	2·9	7·5	48·2 5·7 (eosin) 9·2 (trans.)	—	—	—
X rays omitted to Sept.	August 5	—	29·0	9·8	7·0	3·6	38·5 6·0 (eosin) 6·7 (trans.)	—	—	—
	„ 7	35	38·3	2·6	9·2	7·0	32·0 2·5 (eosin) 9·2 (trans.)	—	2,320,000	893,000
	„ 22	40	28·6	1·6	3·7	10·3	46·0 2·0 (eosin) 3·7 (trans.)	1·1	2,608,000	1,024,000
	Sept. 6	—	59·0	0·4	3·1	9·0	22·5 3·6 (eosin) 2·2 (trans.)	—	1,768,000	1,119,000
	„ 19	45	41·6	1·0	5·6		43·3 3·5 (eosin) 1·6 (trans.)	1·8	—	—

Nucleated red cells present on all occasions practically.

* On this occasion a lymphocytic type of blood was observed.   On July 31st myelocytes distinctly present in large numbers.

TABLE III.

Case and Date.	Hglbn. per cent.	Poly-morph. per cent.	Eosin morph. per cent	Lymphocytes per cent.		Myelo-cytes per cent.	Transi-tional per cent.	Erythrocytes per c.mm	Leuco-cytes per c.mm.	Remarks.
				Small.	Large					
F. H.— 1905										
May 6	15	60·8	1·2	23·1	0·5	8·6	4·6	1,120,000	11,000	Index 0·7, mast 0·6.
„ 17	—	—	—	—	—	—	—	—	6400	Poikilocytosis, poly-chromasis, nucle-ated red cells.
June 3	25	64·8	3·1	28·3		1·8	1·8	1,280,000	2400	Index 0·1, mast 0·6.
„ 10	20	—	—	—	—	—	—	1,736,000	3800	Index 0·58.
„ 26	22	—	—	—	—	—	—	1,840,000	2200	0·6.

and is green in colour ; ducts are dilated and bile-stained, but parenchyma not altered apparently. Gall-bladder is thickened, shrunken, contains branded white gall-stones, but probe passes easily into common bile-ducts; there is a collection of about one drachm of creamy pus in relation to it.

Pancreas—8 oz., nothing noteworthy.

Marrow of ribs, sternum, humerus, radius, and ulna increased in amount, of reddish colour, but not very firm.

No hæmorrhage present.   No evidences of syphilis.

March 12th, 1906.

THE CLINICAL JOURNAL,

CLINICAL RECORD, CLINICAL NEWS, CLINICAL GAZETTE, CLINICAL REPORTER,
CLINICAL CHRONICLE AND CLINICAL REVIEW.

EDITED BY L. ELIOT CREASY.

No. 699. WEDNESDAY, MARCH 21, 1906. Vol. XXVII. No. 23.

CONTENTS.

NOTICE.

Editorial correspondence, books for review, &c., should be addressed to the Editor, 51, New Cavendish Street, W., Telephone No. 904, Paddington ; but all business communications should be addressed to the Publishers, 22½, Bartholomew Close, London, E.C. Telephone 927, Holborn.

All inquiries respecting Advertisements should be sent to MESSRS. ADLARD & SON, *Bartholomew Close, E.C. Telephone 927, Holborn.*

Terms of Subscription, including postage, payable by cheque, postal or banker's order (in advance) : for the United Kingdom, 15s. 6d. per annum ; Abroad 17s. 6d.

Cheques, &c., should be made payable to THE PROPRIETORS OF THE CLINICAL JOURNAL, *crossed " The London, City, and Midland Bank, Ltd., Newgate Street Branch, E.C. Account of the Medical Publishing Company, Ltd."*

Reading Cases to hold Twenty-six Numbers of THE CLINICAL JOURNAL *can be supplied at 2s. 3d. each, or will be forwarded post free on receipt of 2s. 6d. ; and also Cases for Binding Volumes at 1s. each, or post free on receipt of 1s. 3d., from the Publishers, 22½, Bartholomew Close, London, E.C.*

THE
DIAGNOSIS OF CHRONIC ENLARGEMENT OF LYMPHATIC GLANDS.

A Clinical Lecture delivered to the Charing Cross Hospital Post-Graduate Class.

By JAMES GALLOWAY, M.D., F.R.C.P.,
Assistant Physician and Physician to Skin Department Charing Cross Hospital.

GENTLEMEN,—We have recently had under our observation in the hospital an unusual series of cases of enlargements of lymphatic glands due to various causes. In some of these the diagnosis has been difficult, and has been possible only by the combination of clinical observation with laboratory investigation. I am glad to be able to show you some of the patients themselves, and to bring before you in the case of others the evidence which established the diagnosis. I will ask you, therefore, to follow me first into the wards, then into the lecture theatre, and finally into the laboratory, where our Clinical Pathologist, Mr. Leathem, has certain specimens ready for our examination; but so that we may retain more order in our peripatetic discussion; I will first hand you this table, which will indicate some of the evidence to which I wish to draw your attention. You will see that the details are only partly filled up, and as we go along I will ask you to fill in the remainder as they are presented for our information. The headings of the columns indicate the diseases of which we will have something to say ; and I have added an additional column, under the heading of " Spleno-Medullary Leukæmia," as I hope that we may see a patient suffering from this affection, and be able to compare her condition with the others.

A CASE OF LYMPHOSARCOMA.

Our first patient is this lad, aged about 17 years. He is at present too seriously ill to admit of thorough examination, so I must ask you to listen,

Record of Blood Examination.*

	Normal average.	Lympho-sarcoma.	Lymphadenoma (Hodgkin's Disease).	Glandular tuberculosis.	Lymphatic leukæmia.	Spleno-medullary leukæmia.
		Case H.	Case F.	Case X.	Case Fl.	Case M.
Red blood cells (No. in c.mm.)	5,000,000	5,120,000	5,120,000	3,600,000	4,200,000	4,700,000
Hæmoglobin . . .	100 per cent.	80 per cent.	75 per cent.	—	82 per cent.	96 per cent.
Leucocytes (No. in c.mm.)	7500	10,500	16,000	12,000	146,000	200,000
Varieties of leucocytes (differential count).						
Polymorphonuclear neutrophiles	62–70 per cent.	64·5 per cent.	80 per cent.	81 per cent.	3·4 per cent.	53·2 per cent.
Small lymphocytes . .	20–30 ,,	13·9 ,,	13·5 ,,	15·2 ,,	1·8 ,,	4·8 ,,
Large lymphocytes . .	4–8 ,,	13 ,,			91·2 ,,	11·0 ,,
Eosinophile leucocytes .	1–4 ,,	2·6 ,,	3·5 ,,	1·3 ,,	2·4 ,,	1 ,,
" Mast-cells " . .	⅒–⅕ ,,	4·3 ,,	3 ,,	—	—	0·2 ,,
Myelocytes	—	1·7 ,,	—	1·6 ,,	0·8 ,,	29·8 ,,

* In order to facilitate reference the grouping of the leucocytes in this table is made as simple as is possible.

to the record of his case and be content to palpate gently the enlarged masses in his neck.

He was taken into the hospital first of all on the surgical side, on account of severe dyspnœa, which appeared to call for immediate tracheotomy. The rest in bed, however, was sufficient to enable him to tide over the attack of dyspnœa from which he suffered on admission. He was then transferred to this ward, under the care of Dr. Montague Murray.

On examination it was found that he presented these enlarged glandular masses which you see in various parts of his body. The largest of the visible masses are in the neck, but there is little doubt that the lymphatic glands in the mediastinum are also affected by the growth. The X-ray photograph which I show you is evidence of this, even if the clinical symptoms permitted of doubt.

The lad's general state did not alter rapidly. He lay quite comfortably while at rest in bed, but the glandular tumours gradually increased in size. Some time ago, on exertion, an attack of dyspnœa recurred, and was of such a severe character that tracheotomy was performed, with immediate relief. The wound was allowed to heal, and he continued to be comfortable for some time longer; but three nights ago he had another attack of urgent dyspnœa, rendering it imperative to perform tracheotomy again, and on this occasion the tube was introduced with difficulty, and you see that he is still wearing it. You will notice, however, that in spite of the tube he suffers from some difficulty in breathing, and is slightly cyanosed. We are told

that the enlargement of the glands commenced about six months ago, and that they gradually increased in size from his admission to the hospital, in the beginning of December. You can see for yourselves that the size of the neck is much increased, and on gentle palpation the individual glands can be made out, but only with a little difficulty. At first the separate glands were much more distinct than they are now, and an especially large one existed on the left side. This particular gland appears now to be much less prominent than before.

It is interesting to know that as it was thought possible that this large gland on the left side was exerting special pressure on the trachea and other structures in the neck, it was exposed carefully to the X-rays by Dr. Ironside Bruce, and has apparently become smaller. Enlarged glandular masses can also be felt in the axilla and in the groin; and the clinical symptoms, the appearance of the distended superficial cutaneous veins on the trunk, and the shadows of this X-ray picture, give evidence of similar enlargements in the thorax. The fact is perhaps worthy of emphasis that separate glands can be felt now with much more difficulty than in the earlier period of the disease, as if the connective tissue surrounding them had been involved in growth, the glands being masked in a more widely spread tumour.

I will now ask you to make a note in your table of the blood examination which has been made in his case. You will observe that the character of the blood does not vary much from the normal, that there is a slight degree of anæmia, that there is also slight leucocytosis, but that the varieties of leucocytes correspond closely to the normal average.

A Case of Lymphadenoma (Hodgkin's Disease).

We have recently had in the wards one or two cases which could be fairly definitely placed in the category of Hodgkin's disease.

One of these was a male patient who was sent to me by Dr. Hope Murray from Beckenham. He was a man of middle age, and up to the period about eighteen months previous to admission to hospital had been in good health, and actively engaged in an out-door occupation. The glands in the neck began to enlarge, and at the same time he suffered from some difficulty in breathing. On examination of the pharynx, a condition resembling adenoid growths was discovered, and an operation for their removal in the ordinary way was performed with much relief to the patient. His health, however, improved only temporarily. The growths in the neck increased in size, and others in the axilla, in the groin, and elsewhere became noticeable. He began to acquire a curiously pallid appearance, and apparently suffered from anæmia. On admission to the hospital the neck was much increased in size. The ovoid shape of the enlarged lymphatic glands could be readily seen, and a very characteristic clinical picture of Hodgkin's disease was presented.

Nevertheless his health was not greatly impaired. He remarked mainly upon the fact that he became breathless in the course of his work, became easily tired, that he was very pale, and was concerned about the tumours. A careful blood examination, which is noted in the table, will show you that the amount of actual anæmia was very slight, the leucocytosis was of a moderate character, and that the different varieties of leucocytes did not vary much from the normal. The relationship in number between the polymorphonuclear cells and the lymphocytes was not disturbed. Therefore, on account of the clinical history, the slow progress of the case, from the fact that the glands remained distinct and that there appeared to be no spread of growth into the ordinary connective tissues, we came to the conclusion that the patient suffered from true lymphadenoma. It is very important to observe, however, that the line of demarcation

between lymphosarcoma and lymphadenoma is occasionally very difficult to define, and in the earlier stages of this case especially the diagnosis of lymphosarcoma seemed to be more likely than that of lymphadenoma ; on the other hand, the blood examination made it possible to distinguish this case definitely from lymphatic leukæmia.

A Case of Glandular Tuberculosis simulating Lymphatic Leukæmia.

I now wish to draw your attention to the record of evidence in a third case. It is an example of a group in which accurate diagnosis is sometimes difficult, but of very great importance.

The patient is a young lady, aged about 21 years. She appeared to be in the best of health till about the beginning of October. At about that time she commenced to feel ill, and felt herself unfit for the active out-door life which was her custom. · After some time, towards the end of October, she sought medical advice, when it was found that she had a considerable degree of fever, that she was obviously anæmic and ill, and that she had marked enlargement of the cervical lymphatic glands.

After a good deal of consideration, a tentative diagnosis was made of lymphatic leukæmia, on the grounds that the lymphatic glands were enlarged without obvious cause, that the disease was evidently severe and apparently rapidly progressive, and that there was no evidence in the body elsewhere of tuberculous infection. A blood examination made at the time seemed to lend some support to the diagnosis, as a certain degree of leucocytosis was discovered in addition to simple anæmia.

Shortly after the patient was re-examined, with the result that the physical conditions mentioned were corroborated. In the interval the fever had proved to be continuous, and a dry, resounding cough occasionally occurred on movement, suggesting pressure on the bronchi. A blood examination was again made carefully, with the result noted in the table. You will see that in this case the anæmia was considerable, that leucocytosis was noticeable, that the characters of the leucocytes did not vary greatly from the normal, and especially that there was no excess whatever of lymphocytes, the polymorphonuclear cells being in their usual great preponderance. It was clear, therefore, that the diagnosis of lymphatic leukæmia could not be established, and the blood examination left little reasonable doubt that the patient was suffering from some infective condition of the glands, and of these by far the most probable was tuberculosis. The subsequent course of this case tends to establish the diagnosis. The fever has been continuous —there has been no increase of lymphocytes— some of the glands have softened, suppurated, and had to be opened, and there has been a certain remission of the general symptoms.

It is in this variety of chronic glandular enlargement — namely of glandular tuberculosis, either primary or as an early occurrence in general tuberculous infection—that diagnosis is of so much importance. The prognosis of acute lymphatic leukæmia and of acute glandular tuberculosis are, indeed, both of the utmost gravity. In the case, however, of the acute leukæmia, as a rule the progress is a rapid one towards its termination, whereas in the case of the tuberculous infection there may be remissions in the course of the disease, and it may be possible in the earliest stages to obtain a certain amount of relief by surgical interference. In such a case the early excision of a gland may be advisable from the point of view of ascertaining the diagnosis.

Syphilis causing unusual Glandular Enlargement may simulate Lymphadenoma and certain Varieties of Leukæmia.

I should like to draw your attention at this point to the fact that it is not only in tuberculosis that great enlargement of lymphatic glands may occur. It is well known to occur in the early stages of syphilis.

I recollect very well the case of a young woman being admitted to this hospital with a tentative diagnosis of lymphadenoma. The glands in her neck were greatly enlarged. There was no sign of suppuration, and enlargement of the lymphatic glands in other parts of the body rapidly became noticeable. The key to the diagnosis was found when an indurated crack was noted in the centre of the lower lip, which was the sore of inoculation, and confirmation was obtained later, when a severe framboesiform cutaneous syphilide developed.

It is in the early stage of syphilis, in all probability, that the greatest glandular enlargement may occur, but in the later stages of syphilitic disease, especially when associated with other debilitating influences, chronic glandular enlarge-

ments of considerable size may manifest themselves, giving rise to serious difficulty of diagnosis as to their causation—whether due to syphilis or to some process of the nature of lymphadenoma or leukæmia.

A Case of Leukæmia, with Enlargement of Lymphatic Glands.

The next patient to whom I wish to direct your attention is this woman, who has recently been admitted to the hospital. She is about 55 years of age, and you will see that she is thin, pallid, and debilitated. The loss of health has been gradually progressing during the last six or eight months. What she has complained of, in addition to the gradually increasing weakness, is abdominal discomfort. She herself noticed the appearance of lumps in the abdomen. On examination you will find that the lymphatic glands throughout the body are distinctly enlarged, and there is not only enlargement of the glands in the ordinary situations such as the groin, the axilla, and the neck, but there are oval masses resembling tumours about the size of hazel-nuts or smaller, in the subcutaneous tissue in many parts of the body—for instance, here in the lateral aspects of the abdomen and chest. They make their appearance in relation with the course of the lymphatic vessels. In addition to what I have described she has recently developed tumours in the abdomen. Indeed, it was on account of the recognition of the abdominal masses that she was referred to the hospital.

The diagnosis in this case is by no means easy. The character of the abdominal masses, the appearance of the subcutaneous nodules, and the general loss of health point very suggestively to the occurrence of malignant abdominal growth with glandular infection, and the appearance of secondary tumours throughout the body. Indeed, it was not possible to come to an accurate conclusion till the blood was examined. On reference to the table you will see that there is no remarkable anæmia, but the number of white blood cells is greatly increased, approximating to 150,000 per c.mm., and examining the table more closely, you will find that of the varieties of leucocytes the lymphocytes are in great preponderance. No less than ninety-three per cent. of the white blood cells are lymphocytes, and the great majority of these are large lymphocytes. The result of the blood examination is corroborated by the histological structure of one of the small subcutaneous nodules which has been removed. It cannot be distinguished from a lymphatic gland. You will agree with me, therefore, that without the blood examination the difficulty of diagnosis in this case would have been almost insuperable. The resemblance of the case to one of malignant disease is very close, whereas there can be little doubt that what we have to deal with is really an example of the ill-defined group of cases known as "lymphatic leukæmia." Fever is a usual symptom in cases of lymphatic leukæmia, but this case is remarkable in presenting hardly any rise of the body temperature.

From a consideration of this case, and of those previously mentioned, you will readily understand how difficult the clinical diagnosis of cases of lymphatic leukæmia may be, how they may be mistaken on the one hand for cases of glandular tuberculosis and on the other hand for cases of true malignant growth.

A CASE OF SPLENO-MEDULLARY LEUKÆMIA.

By way of contrast I now present to you this patient, who has been under our observation for the last two and a half years. She was admitted into this hospital when I had charge of Dr. Mitchell Bruce's wards, and was then emaciated and extremely debilitated. The abdomen, however, was large and the spleen extended downwards almost to the pubes. No enlargement, however, of the lymphatic glands was noted. The blood examination, in addition to the symptoms, clearly established the fact that the patient was suffering from spleno-medullary leukæmia.

On her admission it was found that there were of red blood cells 2,300,000 per c.mm., hæmoglobin 34 per cent., white blood cells 440,000 per c.mm., polymorphonuclear cells 52·5 per cent., eosinophiles 6 per cent., nucleated red blood cells 6 per cent., myelocytes 34·4 per cent.

On referring to the last column of your table you will see the present state of her blood, and on examining the patient you will notice that she is now in comparatively good health. She has gained flesh, and instead of being able to totter only a few paces, she walks, in connection with her occupation, four or five miles every day. It is true that the spleen is easily felt, though it is not nearly so large as it used to be. Her improvement has been most encouraging, and has been progressive ever since treatment, by means of the X-rays, which has been done with the necessary care by Dr. Ironside Bruce.*

TREATMENT—THE USE OF ARSENIC.

I have referred to treatment once or twice during the course of this demonstration. The treatment in these cases of chronic glandular enlargement must vary according to the nature of the disease. Sometimes treatment is of little service, in other cases much advantage may be gained by medical or surgical interference.

There is one drug, however, which has to be considered in almost every case, namely arsenic, and I would remind you of the beneficial results obtained by the administration of arsenic in some of the diseases to which I have drawn your attention. The drug is usually administered by the mouth, and has the very serious drawback of producing gastritis and consequent intolerance. I would therefore suggest to you the advisability of administering the drug by subcutaneous injection. The difficulties produced as the consequence of irritation of the gastric mucous membrane are much diminished by this method of administration, the effects of the drug can be better regulated, and satisfactory results are occasionally obtained. A preparation which is serviceable, and which has certainly done good in cases under my own observation, is the solution of arsenate of iron prepared for hypodermic injection by Messrs. Squire. It is made in two strengths.

The milder solution contains $\frac{1}{18}$ grain of iron with $\frac{1}{100}$ grain of arsenious acid in the cubic centimetre; the stronger solution contains $\frac{1}{6}$ grain of iron, with $\frac{1}{30}$ grain of arsenious acid in the same quantity of the injection.

It is well in commencing treatment to use the milder of the two solutions, on alternate days, proceeding to the stronger solution if found advisable. The solution is very little irritating, and can be borne even by sensitive individuals. You will note that the dose is 1 c.cm.

We will now go to the clinical laboratory, where specimens of the blood of the various cases which we have been considering are arranged for microscopic examination, but I would venture to impress upon you before leaving the theatre the great assistance which can be rendered by a careful blood examination in such cases of obscure glandular enlargement as those I have mentioned, which must come under observation not infrequently.

March 19th, 1906.

* "Two Cases of Leukæmia, treated by the Röntgen Rays," W. Ironside Bruce, 'Lancet,' January 27th, 1906, p. 211.

PULMONARY EMBOLISM AS AFFECTING PATIENT AND DOCTOR.

By ALFRED PARKIN, M.S.

I WILL first give short notes of the case on which these remarks are founded and will then proceed to discuss the various points which naturally arise.

The patient, a lady æt. 52 years, came under my care on November 1st, for an ordinary attack of lumbago with right-sided sciatica. Knowing that she was by no means easy to deal with, I persuaded her to go to bed so that the condition might be better treated. The pain subsided and I was on the point of letting her get up when she developed a sharp attack of bronchitis. This was due to her being a strong believer in the open-air treatment of everything and she had therefore slept in a room having the windows well opened, when outside there was a very thick fog—in fact, the thickest fog of the year. Two days later she developed acute pleurisy on the left side; this was followed after two days by acute pleurisy on the right side. Four days after there were indications of a small quantity of fluid on the right side of the chest, but the left-sided pleurisy had almost gone so far as physical sounds were concerned.

The patient now began to convalesce, and the temperature, which had not been above 100·5° F., came down to normal. She also began to grumble very much at being kept in bed, but fortunately for me, I was not at all satisfied with the condition of the right lung and persuaded her to remain where she was. This lung did not clear up well and there was one spot where tubular breathing and bronchophony were heard.

I saw her on the 20th, and she seemed to be rapidly getting well and quite free from all pain, no accelerated respiration and nothing to indicate that there was the least complication to be expected.

The next morning at eight o'clock I was rung up on the telephone and told that she was not quite so well; she had some pain in the chest, not much, and they thought I ought to see her again that day. I happened to ask if she was breathing quickly and was told that she was breathing in a jerky or gasping sort of way. Suspecting that something of which I was ignorant was going on, I hurried up and arrived there in twenty minutes, to find that

the patient was of a greyish colour, quite pulseless, and breathing about 45 per minute. She died about ten minutes after I got there. There were before death no physical signs in the chest which could be of use in diagnosis. There were many râles, but no cardiac sounds to be heard.

A situation such as the above is, you will all agree, one of considerable embarrassment for the medical attendant. To see a patient one day, to tell the friends that her condition is satisfactory, and to go up the next morning to find that she is dying puts the medical attendant in a very awkward position. It always seems to me that the public expects a medical man to actually prophesy what is going to happen to the patient he is attending—broadly, whether the patient is going to get better and how long that process of getting better will take; or if he is going to die they expect to be told that he is, and almost the exact day on which that interesting event will take place. One might murmur " Would that I had the gift of prophecy!"

From a medical point of view in this case the probable causes of death I would put down as follows:

(1) Angina pectoris; if so, a first and fatal attack, which is not unknown.

(2) Cardiac failure from an undiagnosed large pleuritic effusion; this is an uncomfortable suggestion for a medical attendant.

(3) A large pericardial effusion, also unsuspected. This is equally possible.

(4) Pulmonary embolism.

The last diagnosis was the one which I thought most probable.

Turning again to the point of view of the friends after the patient was dead, the question at once and without further consideration or time for reflection arose: What explanation was to be given for what was to them an unlooked for calamity? It seems to me that the medical attendant has three distinct courses open to him.

(1) He can say he does not know the cause of death, and that he can give no good explanation of it. The reply to that is obviously pertinent, viz. " You are paid to know it, and if you do not you are gravely at fault and must have treated the patient without sufficient skill."

(2) He can try to conceal everything in his ignorance by saying that the cause of death was heart

failure, which he had suspected might happen. The reply is that he, knowing this, ought to have told the friends of the possibility; this reply is difficult to answer.

(3) To my mind the third and best course is to say that the death was as much unexpected by the medical man as it was by the friends, that one of four things, given above, must have happened, and that the best course would be to have a post-mortem examination, so as to make certain that nothing had been overlooked and to prove that the death was an unfortunate but natural result of disease. To me it seems a very strong position to take up if one can say that the death was unexpected, that it could not possibly have been foreseen, and moreover, the strongest point of all if it could have been foreseen it still could not have been prevented. It need hardly be said that this position cannot be taken up unless the medical man has taken every care by watching all possible physical signs and reasoned out his diagnosis when the patient was living.

At the post mortem, at which I was assisted to a considerable extent by Dr. Daly, there was recent pleurisy on the left side, this being the side first affected. On the right side there was more extensive pleurisy and about two ounces of fluid. At the apices there was healed tubercle. There was no pericardial effusion. The coronary arteries were slightly atheromatous. The right auricle was full of ante-mortem clot, which was adherent to the wall of the auricle and was decolorised. The pulmonary artery at its division was blocked by a detached piece of this clot and the clot spread into practically all the branches of that artery. There was no evidence of disease elsewhere.

It now only remains to state what little is known of this condition. A blockage of the pulmonary artery by a clot is an almost certainly fatal condition, but is not so if only a small branch of the pulmonary artery is affected. I have seen one case in which the diagnosis seemed certain and in which recovery took place. Everything depends on the size of the embolus, as if the emboli are extremely small, as in ulcerative endocarditis, only small wedge-shaped infarcts of the lungs result, which undergo further changes.

Large emboli which may cause death instantaneously or within the hour are due to either ante-mortem clotting in the right auricle or to the detachment of a part of a clot formed in any vein. The exact cause of this clotting is not known, but it occurs after confinements, generally at the end of the second week—that is, when the patient is about to get up. Naturally when it does occur it is a cause of great inconvenience to the medical man in attendance, who cannot explain to himself why it should happen.

Thrombosis in the veins themselves, which may result in subsequent blockage of the pulmonary artery, occurs in the course of diabetes, typhoid, gout, and after operations either on the veins themselves or operations for pelvic tumours in which large veins have often been ligatured, as in the removal of large uterine myomata, where the veins in the broad ligament are often the size of one's finger.

There is no satisfactory explanation why thrombosis and detachment of clot should occur in only a small percentage of cases; but seeing that it is very likely to happen in what we call depressed states of health, it is probable that there is some blood condition necessary for its production, and there is no doubt that sepsis or septic changes lead to this blood condition. Even after parturition it is probable that embolism is due to certain slight septic changes, and as supporting this view in the case I have described I would mention that there was in this case on the right side a patch of lung substance about one inch across quite solid and obviously broncho-pneumonic. In the recorded cases of death from embolism after the excision of varicose veins, varicocele, and abdominal operations generally it is only too likely that septic changes were the ultimate cause of the thrombosis. It is curious that in septic thrombosis of the superior cava from ear disease the emboli are so minute as to cause a septic pneumonia or, possibly, an ulcerative endocarditis.

In the case I have described it is very probable, from the size of the clot in the right auricle, that the clot had been forming during the night, and that a part became dislodged as soon as she got out of bed to pass urine, for it was then that she was suddenly seized. Previous to getting out of bed she had been chatting to her husband in excellent spirits. In fact, the husband refused to believe that there was much amiss, and when I arrived at the house was calmly having his breakfast.

March 19th, 1906.

A FEW REMARKS ON THE VARIOUS METHODS OF TREATING SYPHILIS.

By CAMPBELL WILLIAMS, F.R.C.S.

WHENEVER I have occasion to speak or write upon the treatment of syphilis I always feel inclined to preface my remarks with profuse apologies to those long defunct Chinese doctors who, well nigh upon five thousand years ago, forestalled the modern syphilographer by inditing treatises upon certain phenomena which they not only ascribed to a luetic origin but also treated with mercury. It seems almost incredible that although fifty centuries have passed away since then, time still finds us with no better remedy at our command. Our dosage, preparations, and mode of administration have been elaborated or altered, but nevertheless the principle and also the fundamental drug remain the same as in the olden days of Ho-Ang-Ti in the year 2637 B.C. Most probably they administered the medicament in pilular form ; and I should conjecture from what I have seen of Chinese pills that it would require a roomy œso-phagus and a strong effort of will on the part of the patient to negotiate the bolus. One would deduce that the diurnal mercurial dose was at least a full one, according to modern views, since they dilate upon ptyalism and its appropriate treatment. But one need only go back more than a little over one hundred years to find that what was thought to be the proper treatment for syphilis was inseparable from excessive mercurialism. Some years ago when I was acting resident medical officer to the London Lock Hospital I came across some old case-sheets. I gleaned from their perusal that the amount of mercurial ointment which a patient was expected to rub in *daily* was "one ounce." A bowl or porringer was served out to each patient for the purpose of gathering and measuring the excreted saliva. Apparently the efficaciousness of the treatment was gauged by the amount expectorated. I noted that the average duration of the stay in hospital was about a month. The case-sheets had written across them "Evadit"—but there was no note as to the dental condition of the outgoer. The treatment of syphilis has gone through, so to speak, many phases of favour, albeit with good reason, in that the changes of method of administration have not been fanciful but for the purpose of more successfully combating the disease. We no longer make the cure worse than the malady. For the dosage should be regulated to the immediate and remote wants of the patient and in no case allowed to produce those disastrous results which were of such frequent occurrence in former days. The modern practice of administering mercury is either by the mouth, in the form of pills, tabloids, or fluid preparations ; by inunction and consequently lymphatic absorption from the skin ; or by means of instillation into the muscles or veins by the aid of the hypodermic syringe. Volatilisation or fumigation, though it still has some adherents, is seldom employed nowadays. It is needless for me to say that the vast majority of syphilitic cases are still treated by remedies administered through the mouth. There are many weighty reasons, most frequently the condition of the patient's finance or movements, which tend towards the continuation of a method which the present-day school of "instillers" regard as inefficient and antiquated. Personally I employ all the methods and see good points in each, and not infrequently combine or utilise two forms of administration synchronously—for specific reasons. As the result of experience I would beg to advise the young practitioner not to be too insistent upon intra-muscular injections as being the only way of curing syphilis, particularly so when his patient is either timid or neurotic and fears the momentary prick of the needle or else complains of severe after-pain at the site of a former injection. With certain soluble salts of mercury this is usually trivial, but it is not always so. What is barely discomfort to a phlegmatic person may be agony to one whose nervous system is on the border of degeneracy. If he adopts the uncompromising attitude of *Aut injectio aut nulla*, and refuses to treat his syphilitic cases by other means, he will assuredly lose a certain proportion of his practice. The patients will leave him and find some other medical man who has more *savoir faire* and will drug or rub his cases when they prefer it to injections. Every method has its advantages and drawbacks, its successes and failures. Necessarily, owing to numbers, the greatest proportion of failures are found in the mouth-treated cases. Perchance one reason for this is that the patient too often practically treats himself. For, having procured a prescription from his medical attendant, he thinks that all that is required is to keep on swallowing the daily pills regardless as to whether they are efficiently effecting their purpose or no, and frequently discontinues treatment just when it ought to be persevered with. The treatment of syphilis is not of the rule of thumb order. What is one man's dose may be insufficient for another person or too much for a third party. One patient will absorb a particular preparation which on the other hand will pass inert through some one else's intestinal tract or set up most violent diarrhœa with another individual. In each case it is necessay to find out the idiosyncrasy of the patient. One may possess a "stock pill" which usually agrees, but it is not a necessary corollary that it is acceptable to everybody's internal economy. Not only must the preparation suit, but the dosage must be such that it both removes symptoms and likewise keeps the patient free from further ebullitions of the disease until such time as one may reasonably assume, through experience, that he or she is cured. A sporadic visit does not give one the necessary opportunities for inspecting a case, which should be seen at stated and regular periods. A patient will frequently declare that all symptoms or signs of syphilis have disappeared. But an expert examination too often proves the contrary. In few diseases is the practitioner more at the mercy of his patient's obedience and perseverance than with syphilis. For by whatever system one elects to treat a case you are dependent for success or otherwise upon the mode of life and manner in which the patient seconds your efforts and carries out your instructions. Neglect to take, use, or accept the medicaments regularly will bring you, if not discredit, at least failure and ofttimes unmerited reproach. Carelessness, irregularity, and alcohol are factors which are responsible for many cases of uncured syphilis. Let us now review the advantages and disadvantages of the mouth method of treatment. Countless numbers of syphilitics have been cured by it and will continue to be so, provided that it be properly and judiciously employed. Most of the disadvantages are, or should be, preventable, either by the patient's own efforts or through the watchfulness and resource of the medical adviser. First, let us consider the point of irregularity in taking the prescribed pill. This is held out as a serious drawback, but the same applies

equally to the inunction treatment, should the patient either fail or forget to rub or be rubbed, nor is the hypodermic plan free from reproach when the case does not turn up for the appointed injection. Conversely the over-zealous patient, in his anxiety to get well, may swallow more than double the daily number of globules which one intended him to take. If they induce stomatitis and diarrhœa, he certainly should not blame either the drug or the doctor. One must admit, however, that stomatitis, dyspepsia, and diarrhœa, of varying grades of severity, occur more frequently with this method of treatment than with the inunction or hypodermic systems. It is seldom met with when the latter plan is restricted to certain salts. In certain cases it would not seem to be the mercurial preparation that is wholly to blame, but rather some article of food or drink which, though not ordinarily irritative to the individual, becomes so under a mercurial régime. Uncooked vegetables, such as lettuce, or beer may be the exciting agents ; anyhow, the logical deduction is that they are so. A patient has been getting on comfortably and well with a certain pill, when suddenly he develops most violent diarrhœa. It may be found that beer is the cause, for occasionally it seems to have a most purgative effect in the presence of mercury. You stop the beer, and the patient is able to resume taking the identical pill without any signs of intestinal upset. The effect of uncooked green food is well known, and the patient is usually warned against its ingestion. One occasionally meets with individuals who cannot tolerate the oral administration of the drug. It matters not how small the dose may be nor the nature of the preparation, the result is always the same, more or less griping and purging. In the majority of ordinary diarrhœic cases one finds that one of the following pills can be successfully taken :

    ℞. Hydrarg. tannas . . gr. 1¼.
       Pulv. opii . . . gr. ¼—½.
       Ext. hæmatoxylin. .⎱ āā gr. ¼.
       Ext. gent. . . .⎰
       T. d. s.

Or as an alternative variation in prescribing :

    ℞. Hydrarg. gallas . . gr. 1½.
       Pulv. opii . . . gr. ¼—½.
       Confect. rosæ . .⎱ āā gr. ¼.
       Ext. hæmatoxylin. .⎰
       T. d. s.

It sometimes produces indigestion, owing to the astringency of the gallate constituent.

In many instances, however, all that is necessary is to " mask " the grey powder as follows :

℞ Hydrarg. c̄ creta . . gr. 1.
Bismuthi carb. . . gr. 2.
Pulv. opii . . . gr. ¼–½.
Ext. hæmatoxylin . gr. ½.
T. d. s.

Should dyspepsia be present it may often be relieved by incorporating one grain of pepsin, papain, or ingluvin with each pill. I am of the opinion that a small dose of pepsine materially assists the digestion of the pill, and consequently favours assimilation through the chylopœtic tracts. It is not a good plan to get more than sixty or seventy pills rolled at a time, since they are apt if kept too long to become hard and indigestible. Moreover I have noted that when Pulv. hydrarg. c̄ creta has been held in stock for a considerable period it seems to gain unwonted purgative power. I am totally unable to assign any chemical reason for this phenomenon.

One of the most simple domestic remedies for combating mercurial diarrhœa is the raw egg. It presumably forms a non-irritative albuminate of mercury. Two or three eggs swallowed in the course of the twenty-four hours, together with discontinuation of the offending drug, rapidly subdues the symptoms of enteritis. Mercurial diarrhœa is most frequently met with when the more potent salts of mercury are administered. These are Hydrarg. iod. rubrum (Hyd. biniodide), Hydrarg. subchlor. (calomel), Hydrarg. iod. flavum (yellow mercurous iodide) and Hydrarg. iod. vir. (mercurous iodide). The last named salt, from being a favourite one, is often an offender, particularly because unless it contains a slight excess of mercury it is apt to be unstable, and, as was pointed out by the late William Martindale, prone to get transformed into the highly irritative Hydrarg. iod. rubrum.

The majority of patients do very well on either grey powder or blue pill, and unless there are urgent reasons for changing to the more drastic preparations it may be wise not to employ them, particularly so if the patient and doctor are not readily accessible to each other.

Mercury frequently receives the entire blame for stomatitis or gingivitis when it is only partially responsible for its intensity. The state of the teeth should demand attention as soon as or before treatment is undertaken, and an endeavour made to get the gums and dental alveoli into a healthy condition. Patients who are the subjects of pyo-alveolaris or whose gums are inflamed owing to the presence of tartar, combined with a neglect of cleanliness, have their symptoms intensified by a dose of mercury which would not give evidence of its having being administered were the mouth but in a normal condition. It must be admitted that these people do not suffer to a similar extent under either the instillation or inunction *régimes* which is a point urged in their favour by their respective champions. But if one cannot entirely prevent the state of the gums, one can at least modify the inconvenience, and as far as possible ward off dental decay which is apt to ensue in those under mercurial treatment. First, the teeth should be scaled, when carious stopped, and if rough or sharp they should be filed smooth. It is needless for me to point out that the dentist should be apprised of the syphilitic state of his patient in order that he may pay due regard to his own fingers, and also thoroughly sterilise his instruments after the interview.

One of the best methods for hardening the gums is to paint them night and morning with sp. vini. rect. 90 per cent. Mouth washes of alum or myrrh should be advocated and used four to five times daily. In the case of poor patients who cannot afford much money to buy their medicine, an admirable and cheap plan is to rub a little powdered alum into the gums by means of the forefinger. But the chief agent in keeping the mouth clean is a soft tooth brush. A hard one can easily be rendered soft by soaking it in hot water for a couple of hours. Teeth should be cleaned at least twice daily, but the nocturnal cleansing is the most important. The food which collects between the teeth is often left *in situ* if resource be not had to either a tooth-pick or a bit of thread, in addition to the brush, otherwise the food necessarily putrefies during the hours of sleep. Camphorated chalk is an excellent preparation as a dentifrice, but the patient should be advised to combine the use of ordinary soap with it. This is done by well rubbing the tooth brush on a cake of soap before laying it on to the powder.

In justice to the mouth method of treatment it

must be admitted that some of the cases of stomatitis which are alleged as being due to its action are not really such, in the ptyalitic acceptation of the term. They are mucous patches, the result of under and not over dosing. It is not the drug which should be blamed, but the diagnosis.

I append a very pleasant and efficacious mouth wash which not only hardens the gums but keeps the mouth sweet. It should be used three to four times daily and swished about the oral cavity for five minutes each time of usage.

℞.　Plumbi acetas　.　.　ʒiiss.
　　Aluminæ trisulph.　.　ʒv.
　　Aq. fervent　.　.　ʒxx—i.e. Oj.

Dissolve the salts separately, mix, filter, to the clear filtrate add Ess. menth. piper ʒss. Label the mouth-wash: To be used four or five times daily.

In an ordinary straightforward case of syphilis, where one is not confronted with chronic dyspepsia or an easily irritated intestinal mucous membrane a pill or tabloid of either Hyd. c̄ creta or Pil. hydrarg. in a total daily dosage of 4 grains or even 3 suffices. Many people do not require the addition of sedatives, such as Ext. lettuca, Ext. hyoscyamus, or Pulv. opii. In fact, the reverse may be the case when chronic constipation is troublesome, and it may be advisable to add either Ext. belladonnæ gr. $\frac{1}{10}$ or aloin gr. $\frac{1}{10}$ to each pill or perchance both may be required. Again, where the patient is run down it may be advantageous to combine iron and tonics with mercury as in the following pill.

℞.　Hydrarg. c̄ creta　.　.　gr. i.
　　Ferri redact.　.　.　.　gr. i.
　　Quin. sulph.　.　.　.　gr. $\frac{1}{2}$.
　　Ext. nucis. vom.　.　.　gr. $\frac{1}{6}$.
　　Pulv. opii　.　.　.　gr. $\frac{1}{8}$.
　　Ext. gent.　.　.　.　gr. $\frac{1}{4}$.

　　Ft. pil.　T. d. s.

This combination is particularly useful when there is anæmia, as is often seen prior to the dermal eruptions when the toxine of syphilis is exerting its baneful effects. Sometimes the inclusion of ferri arsenias, gr. $\frac{1}{10}$, is valuable, but many stomachs will not tolerate arsenic. It either makes them feel sick or irritates the bowels. Mercury in itself, apart from its germicidal powers, has a tonic effect and increases the number of red blood-corpuscles, provided that an overdose be not given. This statement can be verified by means of the hæmocytometer. In appropriate dosage the red blood-corpuscles can be seen to gain in numbers, but decrease when an excess of the drug—that is, an excess for the individual in question—is administered. Moreover when treatment is agreeing an increase of bodily weight is frequently noted. Patients will tell you that, instead of experiencing depressing sensations from its ingestion, they have not felt so well for a long time as they have done since starting their pills. This feeling may not be wholly unconnected with a more regular life, earlier hours, less alcohol, and sterilisation and systematic evacuation of the bowels. Perhaps grey powder, either alone or in combination with Pulv. ipecac. co., is the stock remedy which is most frequently prescribed. There are many who pin their faith and preference to Pil. hydrarg. One often sees the latter preparation cause a rapid disappearance of symptoms which had persisted notwithstanding the administration of hyd. c̄ creta. Grain for grain it exerts a greater and more rapid action on the system and consequently upon the disease. Many a man has scored over a rival by either intelligently or haphazardly resorting to this little juggling device. So far no reference has been made to the prescribing of mercury in fluid vehicles or to the treatment by the iodides alone. It is my firm conviction, founded on twenty-three years' experience, that the IODIDES DO NOT CURE SYPHILIS, THEY ONLY CLEAR UP SYMPTOMS, and unless mercury be employed either in conjunction with them or subsequent to their discontinuation that one may assuredly, sooner or later, expect a relapse. No one can deny that the various iodides are most wonderful adjuvants in the treatment of syphilis, but I regard their curative powers as nil. They "scotch" but do not kill. I strongly suspect that many of the cases of syphilis of the nervous system can be attributed to the fact that iodides have been employed, if not entirely, well, practically to the exclusion of mercury throughout the treatment of the case. I do not wish it to be thought that I disapprove of iodides beyond denying that they possess curative powers. For I frequently prescribe the following mixture, to be taken at bed-time, as an addition to the customary three pills per diem. The purpose in view is that of hurrying up either the healing of the initial lesion or the absorption of the indurated cicatrix and the enlarged lymphatic glands. It certainly seems to do so. If you do not believe it, try half a dozen cases with its aid and half a dozen without, and you will be convinced of its efficacy.

> ℞. Liq. hydrarg. perchlor.   .   ʒj.
> Potas. iodidi   .   .   . grs. 5–10.
> Syr. zingib.   .   .   . ʒj.
> Aq. chloroformi .   .   . ʒj.

To be taken at bed-time. Take the dose in a tumblerful of water. Extreme dilution mitigates iodism and also the irritant effect of the drug upon the stomachic mucous membrane.

Many people content themselves with some modification of the foregoing prescription as the staple treatment throughout the case. It is without doubt a most efficacious formula. It clears up symptoms which have resisted various other efforts. But it is very hard on the stomach and is apt to ruin a hitherto first class digestion in a short space of time. Moreover, and apart from the unpleasant metallic taste which the mixture gives rise to, it may not be tolerated by certain patients who are extremely susceptible to develop iodism. Another favourite preparation with the profession is the Liq. arsenii et hydrargyri iodidi (Donovan's solution). This is more frequently employed than the pill of imilar name and constitution. In certain cases it is a most valuable remedy. But it possesses those drawbacks which are inseparable from all arsenical compounds when relegated to irritable stomachs. The amount of arsenious iodide which a usual dose would contain is sufficient to produce arsenical pigmentation of the skin just as Fowler's solution will sometimes do when it is administered for any considerable length of time.

As regards the iodides. There are three forms, namely the iodide of potash, soda, and ammonia, from which one can pick and choose. Some people who cannot tolerate the potash salt can manage to struggle on with either the ammonia or the soda compound. But should none of these be acceptable, resource may be had to the Syrupus acidi hydriodici. It is claimed for this preparation that it is guiltless of producing coryza, gastritis, or other symptoms of iodism such as iodic acne. This is probably due to the small amount of iodine which it contains.

There are certain cases of syphilis which, owing to causes such as intolerance of orally administered drugs, impoverished digestive organs, failure of absorption, stomatitis, syphilo-dyspeptic glossitis, or a paralytic state due to thrombosis, demand treatment either by inunctions or injections. What might have been a preference for a different method to the mouth treatment now becomes a necessity, for rubbing and instillation are both much more rapid in action than stomachic drugging. The most speedy reaction follows on· intramuscular injections ; if the patient will only allow you to continue with them, you can fairly rapidly pump in a remedial dose. But let us assume that the treatment is objected to, or flatly refused. Then we can proceed with inunction. The advantages of the mouth method can be summed up as follows. It is a cheap, convenient, and personally applied method. Patients have not got to haunt the doctor's consulting-room, nor to give themselves, together with a considerable quantity of their time, into the hands of a rubber. They are free to conduct the affairs of life without running the risk of scamping treatment. The medicaments are easily portable, and if the urgency of business calls them away they are still able to uninterruptedly pursue treatment. Over or under dosage can be corrected at will. In the vast majority of cases an effective preparation or combination can be evolved which will suit the consumer's stomach. And lastly, and certainly not the least consideration with some patients, is the element of privacy. The medicine can be swallowed surreptitiously, and, to use a slang phrase, "the show is not given away," as so frequently happens with inunction.

Personally I am a great believer in inunction, provided that it is satisfactorily performed. A perfunctory rub will not do. Consequently to get the full and best results of this method of treatment one should employ a professional rubber. When the patient essays to rub him or herself they are apt to get tired and to scamp the process. For it takes from twenty to thirty minutes of energetic massage to efficiently dispose of one drachm of ointment. This, in addition to the preparatory steaming or hot bath which precedes the operation, means giving up of at least one hour a day to treatment. When patients are undergoing a course of inunction —a course is somewhere about forty-two baths— they not only have to be careful about their diet but they also require close watching. Sometimes rapid loss of flesh ensues, or they may become debilitated or anæmic, to say nothing of the possible occurrence of sudden ptyalism. It is for these reasons mainly why cases do well when under the supervision of rubbers and doctors who are constantly in touch with the process. Part of the secret of Aachen's success is that the patients, having got there, give themselves up completely to treatment. They get an appropiate diet, are expected to drink such alcohol as they are ordered, to take exercise that shall not overtire them, and above all receive their rubbings regularly and efficiently according to the needs of their case. But everyone cannot afford either the time or expense which a stay at either Aix, Harrogate, or Strathpeffer entails, at each and all of which places sulphurous waters may be drunk. It is claimed that the inhibition of sulphur-water plays a great part in the case. But I have never been converted to that idea. My theory is that it is entirely the *régime*, and not the "liqueur," which is responsible for the benefits obtained. When one has the necessity for advising rubbing to a young man "about town" the wisest thing one can do is to pack him off, out of it. His intentions and promises too often yield to the temptations of late, very late, hours, combined with a consumption of alcohol and a forgetfulness of treatment which is not conducive to success. But whilst I am a staunch upholder of the efficacy of inunctions in all stages and conditions of syphilis, excepting the advanced tabetic cases, I'nevertheless do not concur in the total suppression of all specific treatment during the interim of bath courses. Continuity of treatment until one can reasonably assume that a cure has been effected is the maxim I work upon. What I advise during the periods which are allowed to intervene between systematic courses is that a mild course of mercury should be administered by mouth. This keeps up the advantages already gained. When a patient is in requirement of a further course of baths, say in three months time, it is to my mind not only a tacit admission that he is still actively syphilitic, but that a relapse may be expected. It therefore stands to reason that the much debatable organism which one assumes to be the cause of syphilitic phenomena is only temporarily repressed and consequently requires but time and rest from mercury before it, so to speak, "raises its head again." My experience is that the interbath mercury prevents this. The technique of inunction is of the simplest description. The pores of the skin are opened and mild

sweating induced by means of hot-air or hot-water or vapour baths. The temperature of the usual hot water bath should be about 105° F. Some patients will even stand and relish a temperature of 110° F. Before starting on treatment the heart should be examined for obvious reasons and the state of the kidneys should be noted as to renal sufficiency for mercurial excretion. Kidney disease and faulty elimination may produce ptyalism when only a small amount of mercury has been used or given. The patient usually remains immersed in hot water for ten to fifteen minutes before being rubbed dry in preparation for inunction. The ointment is rubbed into all portions of the trunk and limbs indiscriminately. When a rubber is employed one is not tied, as in personal inunction, to the groins, axillæ, and other easily accessible sites. The usual amount of ointment which is employed at the start of a course is one drachm. It takes an experienced and energetic rubber from twenty to thirty minutes to effectively dispose of this quantity. But the amount may quickly require to be reduced if the patient shows signs of either enfeeblement or ptyalism. Many people will not stand more than five rubbings per week. Some find every other day as much as they can bear. The weight should be carefully noted from day to day. It is often necessary to administer an iron tonic, such as ferri perchlor., during the course. Scrupulous attention should be paid to the teeth, which should be cleaned at least three times daily with soap and chalk powder, whilst liberal use should be made of alum acetate mouth-wash, which I have already given the prescription of. It is often advised that it should be used every hour. In fact, at establishments where rubbing is conducted the patients walk about with a bottle of mouth-wash in their pocket and when at a loss to occupy a few minutes employ the time by rinsing out the mouth. After a rubbing the patient should keep quiet for an hour or so, taking care not to catch cold. Exercise must be regulated to the powers of the individual. It should not over-tire the body or produce symptoms of fatigue. The diet should be plain and nourishing. It is recommended that meat should form a marked element of the dietary. Uncooked vegetables and salads should be avoided and fruit consumed with caution. Light wines, such as hock or Moselle, may be taken in moderation or even beer, provided that it does not produce diarrhœa. Watchfulness as to the state of the skin must be enjoined lest mercurial erythema or suppuration of the hair-follicles eventuate. A matutinal bath with appropriate soap will materially obviate either occurrence. The following ointment will be found to be a satisfactory one. It is really nothing more than ordinary blue ointment made with lanoline instead of lard. Lanoline does not undergo degeneration like lard does with the formation of dermal irritating butyric acid. But as lanoline is sticky it requires the addition of an oil, such as olive or almond oil, to facilitate its usage and penetrative powers.

℞ Ung. hydrarg. (made with lanoline) ʒj
  Ol. amyg. vel. ol. olivæ opt.   .   ʒj

Mix. Divide into 16 or 32 packets according to the dose prescribed.

The drawback to the employment of this ointment is that it is dirty. Some people prefer the oleates because they are cleaner. But they are in my experience more prone to set up dermatitis. The chief drawback to the inunction method is the attendant expense at the time which it entails. But when a patient will undertake, not only to rub himself but to rub properly, these objections cease to exist. Another plan which has been advocated in Denmark is to wear an undershirt impregnated with mercurial ointment. It is affirmed that gradual and satisfactory absorption of the drug ensues by this means.

The treatment of syphilis by means of mercury injected into the tissues was advocated by Scarruzio of Milan as far back as 1864. Perhaps the name which is best known in connection with the earlier essays of this mode of medication is that of Ragazzoni, whose original solution contained approximately Hyd. iod. rub. gr. ½ c̄ sod. iod. gr. ⅛, ad. aq. dest. ℳ v. Formerly the various solutions, peptonised or otherwise, were instilled into the subcutaneous tissues. But as this method was not infrequently followed by abscess formation the expedient of injecting less irritating salts into the deeper or intra-muscular regions was evolved. Practically no form of mercury, soluble or insoluble, has escaped trial. The vehicles for suspension or solution have varied from water to oil or paraffin, whilst solubility, stability, sterility, and increased absorption properties have been striven after by the addition of such agents as pepsin, asparagin, formamide, chloride of sodium or ammonia, iodide

of potash or soda, and benzoic acid. Sufficient historical data have been quoted for this paper's purpose to show that the modern method is but an advance on the former régime. I often wonder how many men who use a hypodermic syringe know who invented it. Too often the real originator of a process, instrument, or even operation remains unknown, whilst the kudos and financial benefits which his brains should have reaped go elsewhere. If ever a man deserved a memorial for his services to mankind, either from the point of alleviating suffering or combating disease, then this inventor should have one.

Intra-muscular injections are usually and most easily affected upon the buttocks—the right and left sides alternately. The point chosen should be about the junction of the outer and middle thirds, a little above the level of the great trochanter. This will miss the great sciatic and small sciatic nerves. The great sciatic at first rests in the hollow between the great trochanter and the ischial tuberosity. Emerging from the pelvis below the lower border of the pyriformis muscle, it descends, with the small sciatic resting upon it, under cover of the gluteus maximus. The reason for the above piece of anatomy is that sometimes the nerve gets injected, and intense neuritis follows. I remember seeing the late Christopher Heath cut down upon a great sciatic nerve for the purpose of stretching it. The cause of the intense sciatica was a misdirected intra-muscular injection of sal alembroth owing to the patient jumping at the moment the needle should have penetrated the proper site. I had happened to have been witness to the accident at another hospital.

The technique of injection requires ordinary surgical cleanliness. The skin should first be washed with spirit soap and afterwards sterilised with sp. vini. rect. ninety per cent. or else ether. The needle is then plunged in rectangularly at the appointed spot till it is assumed to have penetrated through the subcutaneous tissues. The depth necessarily varies with the amount of fat present. In an ordinarily well nourished individual about an inch length of needle suffices to reach the muscular regions. The fluid is expelled slowly from the syringe and after the needle is withdrawn it may be gently dispersed by finger massage. The puncture should be sealed up with a minute portion of antiseptic wool saturated in collodion. An ordinary syringe and needle will do, provided that the mercurial solution is squirted in immediately the syringe is filled, and not allowed to remain more than a few seconds in contact with the metal. I have found it preferable, but not essential, to have platino-iridium needles. If you will but take the trouble to wash and boil the ordinary steel ones directly you have used them, they do not corrode or rust. It is also advisable to subsequently dip them in absolute alcohol; it thoroughly dries off any water. If extra sterilising precaution be deemed necessary, it can be obtained by passing the needle twice or thrice through a spirit flame.

The choice of an injection lies between a soluble and an insoluble preparation of mercury. In this country the soluble ones have received most favour, the reason being that the majority of them not only cause less after-pain but that all are free from the danger of causing cardiac dyspnœa of an embolic origin, pulmonary embolism, and pneumonia. They are also less liable to be followed by cellulitis or abscess troubles. In France calomel injections have been largely employed, with surprisingly good and rapid results. Dr. A. Fournier speaks very highly of them. In America the neutral mercury salicylate in liquid albolene has been strongly advocated by Dr. Gottheil of New York. But they are both attended with the slight embolic risk inseparable from the injection of all insoluble salts of mercury.

In the following list I have tabulated nearly all the numerous preparations which have from time to time been advocated by their various champions.

Soluble or else convertible into soluble preparations, administered in water:

(1) Sal alembroth (ammonio-mercuric chloride).
(2) Hyd. cyanidum or oxycyanidum.
(3) Hyd. iod. rub. c̄ sod. iod. (Ragazzoni).
(4) Hyd. lactas.
(5) Hyd. oxidium c̄ asparagin.
(6) Hyd. oxidium c̄ formamido.
(7) Hyd. perchloridum.
(8) Hyd. sozoiodol.
(9) Hyd. succinimidum.
(10) Hyd. et sod. disulphocarbolas (hermophenyl).

Insoluble preparations administered in Liq. paraffin or vegetable oils.

(1) Grey oil (inject. hyd. hypodermica).
(2) Hyd. ox. flavum.
(3) Hyd. subchlor. (calomel)
(4) Hyd. salicylas (neutral salt).
(5) Hyd. tannao.
(6) Hyd. thymolacetas.
(7) Hydriodol (cypridol).
(8) Hydrarg benzoas (practically insoluble in cold water).

Soluble salts—aqueous medium.	Insoluble salts—oleaginous medium.
℞ Hydrarg. sozoiodol . . . . . grs. 2½ Sod. iodidi . . . . . . grs. 5 Aq. dest. . . . . ♏100 Dose 10 to 15♏, containing ¼ to ⅓ gr. of the salt.	℞ Hydrarg. salicylatis neut. . . . . grs. 10 Paraffin liq. . . . . . . ♏100 Dose 3 to 10♏, containing respectively 3/10 to 1 gr. of the salt.
℞ Hydrarg. succinimid. . . . . grs. 2½ Aq. dest. . . . . ♏100 Dose 10 to 15♏, containing ¼ to ⅓ gr. of the salt.	℞ Hydrarg. . . . . grs. 10 Adipis lanæ anhyd. . . . . . grs. 30 Paraffin liq. (carbolised 2 per cent.) . ♏100 Dose 10♏, containing 1 gr. of the *base*.
℞ Hydrarg. lactatis . . . . . grs. 2½ Aq. dest. . . . . ♏100 Dose 10 to 15♏, containing ¼ to ⅓ gr. of the salt.	℞ Hydrarg. subchlor. (calomel) . . grs. 5 Ol. olivæ (sterilised) . . . . . ♏100 Dose 10 to 15 or even 20♏, containing respectively ½, ¾, or 1 gr. of the salt. NOTE.—The larger quantities must be given most cautiously. The intense pain following its injection may necessitate a local hypodermic of ¼ gr. morphia.
℞ Sal alembroth . . . . . . grs. 5 Aq. dest. . . . . ♏100 Dose 10♏, containing ½ gr. of the salt.	

Let me say at once that personally I only use the calomel, the salicylate, or the grey oil preparations from the insoluble group, and even those but very seldom, particularly calomel, whilst of soluble series I restrict my choice to Hyd. sozoiodol, Hyd. lactas, Hyd. succinimide, or Sal alembroth. The three former produce much less after-pain than any of the others. I append the strength and dosage of their respective formulæ and would advise those intending to embark upon a system of intra-muscular therapy to limit their resources to the soluble preparations of sozoiodol, lactate, succinimide, or sal alembroth. Calomel or the neutral mercury salicylate formulæ may act more quickly on the disease, but they carry an infinitesimal risk with their employment, and the after-pain which follows an injection of calomel is usually *very* severe.

Special syringes have been devised for injecting mercury. They are either entirely of glass, and can be sterilised by boiling, or they have a glass barrel with vulcanite mountings, piston rod and washer. But an ordinary hypodermic syringe will do if similar precautions to those which I advised for steel needles be adopted.

Injections are usually given about once every five days to start with. After four or five applications once a week will suffice for the next four visits and afterwards only one per fortnight will be required. But the entire length of treatment should extend over two years—or even longer should the needs of the case demand it. Patients, however, are few and far between who will submit to such prolonged repetition of a procedure which, apart from being tiresome, is expensive and time-tying. Another disadvantage is that once a dose is in the body it has to have time to work its effects off. You cannot get it out again. If a patient should be in the zone of ptyalism without showing any marked symptoms of the condition, it may just turn the balance and produce well-marked mercurialism. It is a fact which I believe is not generally known that a sudden alteration in the weather—an abrupt and marked rise in temperature—tends to precipitate the evolution of ptyalism which is hanging in the balance. One should therefore exert the closest scrutiny over the gums on every occasion before giving an injection, and if there be any doubt refrain for a few days before instilling another dose rather than run the risk of salivating the patient, even to the slightest degree.

The intravenous method of injecting mercury directly into the blood-stream was, as far as I can ascertain, first advocated and practised in 1893 by Barcelli and several other Italian syphilographers. The idea was given prominence to in this country by my friend Mr. J. Ernest Lane, Surgeon to the Lock Hospital, who wrote and spoke upon the subject as far back as 1896. Mr. Lane, though he thought most highly of this process, advised certain restrictions as to its indiscriminate use. The preparation which he employed was a 1 per cent. solution of Hydrarg. cyanide, and he injected 20 minims of the solution, or roughly ⅓ grain of the salt, into the median basilic vein. At first an injection was given every other day, but subsequently a daily instillation was employed—that is, unless there were valid reasons against doing so. The advantages claimed for this method are that it is absolutely painless, if the injection be properly administered—that is, into the vein and not into the surrounding tissues—it causes no dyspepsia, there is certainty of absorption, the dose is small and can easily be regulated. The disadvantages are that it is sometimes difficult to bring the vein into sufficient prominence, or that the patient may be much frightened by the ligature preparation on his arm, and also that after all the injection may end, not as an intravenous but as a subcutaneous one. It sometimes causes severe diarrhœa, according to the salt of mercury used, or it may set up polyuria and transient albuminuria. Occasionally thrombosis of the vein occurs, spreading from the puncture side. Thrombosis is most usually found in cases where the solutions have been used cold. They should always be warmed to a temperature of 100° F. before being thrown in. It is needless for me to point out that only soluble salts must be employed. Those insoluble in water, and which are suspended in oil as the vehicle for conveyance, would necessarily be followed by the gravest, and probably fatal, results. The technique is that, having thoroughly sterilised the area over the selected vein, it is brought into prominence by the application of either an ordinary bandage or an elastic band applied above the elbow. The needle is then inserted into the dilated vessel and the fluid injected slowly as soon as the compression of the tourniquet has been released. The fluid is immediately carried away by the blood-stream. The puncture is sealed up with wool and collodion. It is sometimes difficult to give the vein the necessary prominence ; in fact, occasionally the little operation has to be abandoned on that account. The treatment is not one that all patients will submit to—it frightens them. Moreover the fact of it having to be repeated daily is a great disadvantage. In using the needle great care must be exercised not to plunge it right through the vein, or to miss the vessel and inject the liquid into the perivenous tissues. Needles with short points have been devised with the object of preventing transfixation of the entire vein. When the injection fails to enter the vessel it comes to be practically a subcutaneous one, and is always followed by pain and not infrequently by abscess or sloughing of the skin. The action of mercury administered in this fashion—i. e. into the vein—is very rapid, but on the other hand its effects pass off with an equal celerity. It is advised that varicose veins should be shunned, as ulceration is apt to ensue at the site of the puncture owing to the nutrition of the skin being impaired. The method is not one that I can recommend for general use, in that it often requires a great deal of persuasion to get the patient to regard thrombosis of his vein in the light that one would wish it to be seen, viz. an accident that may occur with the best regulated injection.

I have not attempted in this short paper to give any local treatment ; but I would like to remark as regards primary sores that it is best to use lead lotion as a dressing and to eschew irritating preparations since they are liable to produce inflammatory induration in a simple sore which may often be mistaken for true syphilitic proliferative infiltration. In conclusion, let me urge that the administration of mercury be withheld in all cases of a doubtful nature until the diagnosis is conclusively proved.

March 19th, 1906.

THE CLINICAL JOURNAL,

CLINICAL RECORD, CLINICAL NEWS, CLINICAL GAZETTE, CLINICAL REPORTER, CLINICAL CHRONICLE AND CLINICAL REVIEW.

EDITED BY L. ELIOT CREASY.

No. 700. WEDNESDAY, MARCH 28, 1906. Vol. XXVII. No. 24.

CONTENTS.

* *Specially reported for the Clinical Journal. Revised by the Author.*
ALL RIGHTS RESERVED.

NOTICE.

Editorial correspondence, books for review, &c., should be addressed to the Editor, 51, New Cavendish Street, W., Telephone No. 904, Paddington; but all business communications should be addressed to the Publishers, 22½, Bartholomew Close, London, E.C. Telephone 927, Holborn.

All inquiries respecting Advertisements should be sent to MESSRS. ADLARD & SON, Bartholomew Close, E.C. Telephone 927, Holborn.

Terms of Subscription, including postage, payable by cheque, postal or banker's order (in advance): for the United Kingdom, 15s. 6d. per annum; Abroad, 17s. 6d.

Cheques, &c., should be made payable to THE PROPRIETORS OF THE CLINICAL JOURNAL, crossed " The London, City, and Midland Bank, Ltd., New-gate Street Branch, E.C. Account of the Medical Publishing Company, Limited."

Reading Cases to hold Twenty-six numbers of THE CLINICAL JOURNAL can be supplied at 2s. 3d. each, or will be forwarded post free on receipt of 2s. 6d.; and also Cases for binding Volumes at 1s. each, or post free on receipt of 1s. 3d., from the Publishers, 22½ Bartholomew Close, London, E.C.

A LECTURE

ON

SOME HEPATIC AFFECTIONS IN INFANCY.*

By F. J. POYNTON, M.D., F.R.C.P.Lond.,

Sub-Dean to the Medical Faculty, University College, London; Assistant Physician University College Hospital and the Hospital for Sick Children, Great Ormond Street.

IN this lecture, I wish to dwell particularly upon two unusual cases of jaundice in infancy and upon that curious condition termed by Dr. Cheadle "Acholia." No single lecture could adequately deal with jaundice in childhood, and it is for this reason that I prefer to single out cases which I have observed myself and which especially illustrate points in their practical management.

For our purpose the rough division of jaundice in infancy into slight and severe is sufficient. The type of slight jaundice is the well-known icterus neonatorum, with which both doctors and the general public are well acquainted. Though common enough the causation is obscure and the condition a very interesting one. The jaundice is, as a rule, moderate in degree, and the conjunctivæ may not be tinged. The urine, too, is generally free from bile. This jaundice makes its appearance about the second or third day and lasts three or four days or even longer. Recent investigations tend to discount the old idea that the occurrence of this jaundice is encouraged by delay in cutting the cord, and, as might be expected, more stress is laid now upon the invasion of the alimentary canal by micro-organisms. This invasion of course coincides with the change from fœtal life to infancy. Another factor put forward in explanation is the increased hæmolysis at this time, and yet another is a viscid

* Delivered at the Children's Hospital.

condition of the bile, which, should there be any biliary infection, may be unable to pass along the minute biliary passages, and thus pent up be absorbed into the circulation.

A necropsy that I made about seven years ago, when medical registrar to St. Mary's Hospital, will interest you as bearing upon the viscid nature of the bile in some cases of infantile jaundice. A child had died when six days old with intense jaundice, and I investigated the biliary apparatus with the intention of finding a malformation. I found, however, no malformation at all, but a liver gorged with bile, and in the gall-bladder bile as viscid as tar, in fact so inspissated as almost to deserve to be termed semi-solid. My colleague, Dr. Still, in a lecture given at this hospital in 1901, gave his experience, which was similar to mine upon this point, and in another important paper read before the Pathological Society of London, enlightened many of us, myself certainly, upon this condition of the bile and the occasional occurrence of gall-stones at an early age.

In his lecture he menti ons cases of jaundice of the type of icterus neonatorum which lasted as long as six weeks, and these observations of his lead me now to narrate two cases which both puzzled and interested me exceedingly.

The first was a little girl, æt. 3 months, whom I saw eighteen months ago in consultation. She had been jaundiced at birth and was still so. There was no clear evidence of the cause. The parents were healthy and well-to-do, and the child showed no signs at all of any hereditary disease. The umbilicus was natural and had never given any trouble. When I saw her she was very definitely yellow, the conjunctivæ were stained, as were also the mucous membranes and skin. The urine was dark and stained the napkins ; the motions were large, white and undigested. The liver was definitely enlarged, not unduly firm and not tender ; the spleen was not palpable, and there were no hæmorrhages. The temperature was often subnormal, although occasionally it would rise over the normal line. An important point in the history was the occasional appearance of a little bile in the stools, and at these times the jaundice became a little fainter. The child, who had never taken the breast, was thin, did not gain weight, and suffered from flatulence. It will be apparent that such a case can hardly be classified under mild jaundice,

and it will be necessary now to say a few words about severe jaundice in infancy.

Pyæmic jaundice from a septic infection of the umbilical cord is one type of severe jaundice which is terribly fatal. Such a condition could be at once excluded here, for there was not a single point in its favour. Syphilitic disease of the liver with jaundice, dating from birth, is another fatal form which could be certainly excluded.

Epidemic jaundice need not trouble us, nor need that extraordinary and fatal jaundice which Dr. Rolleston mentions in his recent monograph on diseases of the liver—a jaundice met with in some Brahmin children, whose mothers take a dry diet with a decoction of pepper, spices, curries, and such-like condiments. It was not possible to exclude that remarkable form of jaundice which may develop in several children in one family, the causation of which is most obscure, for it might well have been that this was the first victim. Yet even if this were the case, one felt that the actual cause was mysterious, and for that reason, no one, I think, would hesitate to be most cautious in condemning the case as necessarily fatal, for even in these family cases it must be remembered that though four or more children may die from the jaundice, some may develop it and yet recover.

There is, however, another form of severe jaundice which it was very difficult to exclude, and this is the jaundice associated with obliteration of the ducts. Such a condition may, as Dr. John Thomson has shown, last for months before proving fatal. In such cases there are, as a rule, deep jaundice and hæmorrhages, and enlargement of the liver and spleen.

You will understand, then, how important in our case was that observation that bile was occasionally noticed in the stools, for it made it clear that there was not a complete obliteration of the biliary passages.

The practical difficulties in this case were threefold. The first was the difficulty in diagnosis, the second in prognosis, and the third was the difficulty of treatment.

It seemed hard to believe that a child whose jaundice varied a little from time to time, who was not more jaundiced at three months than at birth, and in whose stools a little bile was occasionally noticed, was doomed to die, and we accordingly adopted the view that there was no complete or advancing obstruction, but that the fault perhaps lay with the bile, which was, we pictured, too thick to pass down ducts which might be smaller than normal.

This hypothesis had the advantage of giving us some encouragement to struggle with the difficulties of treatment, and you will admit that an essential for successful treatment in a long illness is a hopeful mind.

Such cases as these are most troublesome to manage, for, owing to the absence of bile, the motions contain undigested fat and proteid. It is the fat particularly that cannot be digested, and not only does the child as a result not gain flesh, but the undigested fats also may produce irritation in the bowel, and in this way flatulence, pain, and diarrhœa. The undigested proteid is also harmful. If the fermenting food begins to set up serious symptoms—such as diarrhœa and vomiting—these children are very soon carried off, for they are thin, their temperature often low, and their resistance to disease feeble.

On the other hand, if the hypothesis that the bile might be unduly viscid had any foundation, it was reasonable to suppose that each week the child survived the fluid might become less tenacious, and the ducts a little larger. Accordingly we tried milk and Benger's food. And a milk which is very valuable, in my experience for such cases, is asses' milk. It is easy to digest, it contains very little fat, o·9 per cent., and another point about it is that it can be given pure without boiling or dilution.

Another useful mixture that we used in association with the asses' milk, alternately or in rotation, was a mixture of chicken tea or veal tea and whey, the value of which I learnt from Dr. Cheadle. With the idea of liquefying the bile, small doses of bicarbonate of soda were administered regularly for many weeks, and a few drops of brandy were also given to stimulate the hepatic functions.

There can be no doubt that this careful dieting, this exclusion of fat, and pre-digestion of much of the proteid, improved the general health of the child, and the weight rose. There were fluctuations, but the general tendency was improvement, and after some months the jaundice gradually and slowly disappeared, the liver became smaller, and some bile appeared in the stools, although it is interesting to find that the child at one time was

not jaundiced and yet was passing white stools. The food was altered with the improvement, thus the Benger's food was replaced by pure asses' milk, and later cows' milk was again utilised. Eventually the recovery was complete, and the child is now an unusually healthy-looking little girl.

Citrate of soda, upon the value of which I devoted a lecture two years ago, has also a use in this class of case at a time when the jaundice has disappeared but the digestive processes are still imperfect. Let me remind you that about two grains of citrate of soda are added to each ounce of milk. Another useful device is to add raw meat juice in teaspoonful doses to the pure asses' milk. Lastly, in such a case the employment of cream will need much care, for the digestion of fat is very feeble for a long time, and undigested fat may cause much disturbance in small children.

The second case is another of the same type, and a few details about it will serve the purpose of a recapitulation of the salient points that I have already emphasized.

This infant was a boy, æt. 4 weeks, and a first child of healthy and well-to-do parents. This case I saw in consultation, and we could find no cause at all for the symptoms.

The child was very distinctly jaundiced, the jaundice affecting skin, mucous membranes, and conjunctivæ. The urine stained the napkins, and the motions were, when I saw them, quite white, and the milk passed undigested. The child had a ravenous appetite, but the motions were bulky; and it was clear to us that although the appetite was good very little food was absorbed.

The jaundice had been first noticed on the third day. The liver was large but not tender, the spleen could not be felt, and there was no fever or purpura. In this case the umbilicus showed still a raw surface discharging a little clear fluid. This was not satisfactory, but there did not appear the least evidence of anything like a septic infection.

The interesting feature in this case, one noticed by all who had seen the child, was the occasional appearance in the stools of a little bile with a coincident diminution in the jaundice. The rule, however, was that there was no sign of bile in the stools. The child was thin, suffered from flatulence, and had only gained three ounces since birth.

Encouraged by my former experience, I gave a

favourable prognosis, and commenced treatment on the same lines—milk and Benger's food, chicken tea and whey, some bicarbonate of soda, brandy, and an occasional dose of grey powder.

The weight improved remarkably, but the child remained jaundiced. There were slight difficulties, and some weeks were less encouraging than others, but the general result was progress.

When the child was two months older I saw it again, and found that though still yellow the colour was much less distinct, and the motions were now usually mustard coloured. Asses' milk was taken with great advantage, and I have heard recently that there is steady improvement, the jaundice has disappeared, and the stools, though still lacking in bile pigment, are very much more natural. In this case also I am in hopes that there will be complete recovery.

Now, in the description of the first of these two cases I commented upon the fact that for some time after the jaundice had disappeared the stools remained very pale, and it is this observation that leads me to consider next the curious disorder termed by Dr. Cheadle "acholia." It is to his instruction that I am mainly indebted for a knowledge of the condition, which appears to me to be less common in hospital practice than in private.

We can at once single out a very striking feature of "acholia," and that is the occurrence of putty-like, very offensive, greasy stools, without the presence of any jaundice at all. The stools may be, in fact, absolutely white, and yet there not be a trace of jaundice.

One of the most distinguished physicians of this hospital in earlier days, Dr. Gee, called attention to this peculiar condition of the stools in children in a disorder which he, in 1888, termed "cœliac disease"; and Dr. Gibbons again directed our attention to it in 1899.

The occurrence of white stools without jaundice in adults has been noticed in various diseases; for example, in some cases of pancreatic disease, as in the cases described by Dr. T. J. Walker, published in 1889. In his cases the cause was complete obstruction of the pancreatic duct by calculi. Again, in the remarkable tropical disease known as "sprue" a similar condition of the stools is met with.

Now, a most instructive correspondence has recently been published in the 'Lancet' as to the meaning of these colourless stools. This correspondence has shown that there may be plenty of bile passed, and no obstruction or fault be discoverable in the biliary apparatus, and yet the stools be quite colourless. To quote verbatim a sentence of Mr. Mayo Robson's in a letter in the 'Lancet' for December 16th, 1905:

"The characteristic white stools often seen in pancreatic disease, in the absence of jaundice, owe their pale colour entirely to the solidification of the fat when the motion cools, although there may be a normal amount of bile entering the intestines." This sentence is founded upon Mr. Robson's wide experience of pancreatic disease and upon the researches of Dr. Cammidge, who has further shown that when these colourless stools are freed of their fat the normal colour reappears.

It is clear, then, that if these investigations are accurate, and the evidence certainly appears to be quite convincing, that the passage of colourless stools without jaundice is no proof of hepatic disease.

Why, then, you may ask, do I introduce this subject into my lecture on hepatic disease and use the term "acholia"? I do so because, though we may admit that pancreatic disease is a most important cause of colourless stools, we must also admit that in the condition termed by Dr. Cheadle "acholia" there is some strong evidence in favour of the view that a disturbance of the hepatic functions may also produce white stools without jaundice. I shall bring this evidence forward in the course of a short clinical description of the condition "acholia."

The onset of the illness is usually abrupt, and sometimes this abruptness is remarkable. The age of the child is usually under five and generally under two years.

The characteristic symptom is a complete change in the character of the motions which become, as I have already emphasized, colourless, greasy, and offensive. They are often more bulky than natural and sometimes more frequent. The general health quickly suffers. At first there may be slight fever, but generally this soon passes and is replaced by a subnormal temperature. The child rapidly loses firmness, wastes, and becomes feeble, languid, and irritable. The food is badly digested and ferments, with the result that the abdomen becomes distended and tumid.

You will readily understand how difficult it is to distinguish such a condition as this from tubercular disease of the alimentary canal and peritoneum.

This point Dr. Cheadle has emphasized, and further considers that a condition of acholia may exist in tubercular disease of the bowels. Nevertheless he points out that the majority of these cases are not tubercular, and however ill and wasted the children may become, the rule is for recovery to occur under appropriate treatment even though that recovery may be very slow.

In attempting the differential diagnosis, you will lay stress upon the frequency of a sudden onset in acholia, and bear in mind that although in rare cases colourless stools are met with in tubercular disease, the sudden onset of such a change in a child who has not been suspected of tubercular disease is very suggestive of a non-tubercular condition. Examination of the abdomen may show it to be swollen, but there are no tubercular masses and there is no ascitic fluid ; it is a distension of atonic bowel by the fermenting contents.

An examination of the lungs shows no disease, and the temperature is usually subnormal, whereas in tubercular disease it is as a rule raised.

Let me in passing warn you against that most tempting assumption in the diseases of childhood over which one is very apt to fall into error —the assumption that a wasting disease, be it abdominal or thoracic, is necessarily tubercular, because at the time you can think of no other explanation. It is this mistake which makes us overlook acholia, suppurative pericarditis, empyema, and even typhoid fever. I hope I shall not be too elementary or dogmatic when I remind you how important it is to bear in mind that the first step in correct diagnosis is to find positive facts, and that if we fail to find these positive facts a diagnosis, however reasonable in our experience, is at the best an assumption, and should not blind us to receiving and accepting any positive facts that may arise later in the illness.

Turning now to the causation of acholia, there is not very much evidence to help us. Dr. Cheadle attaches considerable importance to difficult and painful dentition, for some of his more severe cases have been associated with this. He believes it probable, as did Dr. Gibbons, that the process is a nervous one and a reflex irritation from the painful teeth. To surface chill he also attaches

importance, and it has seemed to me that sudden chilling is a very possible cause of acholia. There was, in fact, an interesting observation made upon this point a year or so ago by Dr. von Praagh, who found in a child suffering from acholia, that when the feet, which were usually cold, were kept thoroughly warm, the condition promptly improved.

Is the condition of pancreatic or hepatic origin, or are both organs affected ? That is a question which is not at all an easy one to answer, and leads me to mention the evidence in favour of the view that some part at least of the disorder is due to disturbance of the hepatic functions and not the pancreatic. It is an investigation by Dr. Willcox, medical registrar to St. Mary's Hospital, upon the stools in a case of acholia under the care of Dr. Cheadle. This investigation was published in Dr. Cheadle's lecture upon acholia in the 'Lancet' of May 30th, 1903. The case was one of moderate severity in a boy, æt. 3 years and 4 months, the stools were almost colourless, and while in this condition they were analysed by Dr. Willcox and gave the following results :

19·8 per cent.⎫
24·3 ,, ⎬ of fat in four estimations.
44·9 ,, ⎪
49·65 ,, ⎭

That is, from twice to four times the normal amount.

In the specimen yielding 49·65 per cent. of fat there was no colour, and bile pigments, and bile acids were *entirely absent*. In the specimen yielding 24 per cent., there was a small amount of bile pigment and bile acids.

Unless, then, we believe that the bile was so altered in the intestine by the disorder as not to be recognisable to ordinary tests, it seems clear that the bile-forming function of the liver was in this case, and presumably in other cases of acholia, almost or entirely in abeyance. I have no doubt that this important point will be further investigated and finally settled one way or the other in the near future. For it is clearly important to know certainly whether this condition of acholia is entirely biliary, entirely pancreatic, or both biliary and pancreatic in origin.

It seems to me some indirect support of the hepatic origin is provided by the case that I first described, which passed through a stage in which, although there was no jaundice visible, the motions remained for a while colourless. The previous jaundice made it quite clear that the liver was disordered, and if the view that this was in part due to the viscidity of the bile is correct, it seems possible that a stage had been reached when that viscidity was not so considerable as to cause resistance sufficient to produce jaundice, and yet was sufficient to prevent an adequate supply of bile to the intestine to counteract the pale colour due to the excess of fat in the stools. Unfortunately, at that time I had no opportunity of having the stools analysed, and can only give you the fact that for a time the stools were white, and yet the child not obviously jaundiced. Should such a condition come again under my observation, I should make use of Dr. A. E. Wright's most interesting observation and examine the blood-serum to see if there was still a trace of jaundice to be detected, for he tells us that the serum may show the yellow tinge when none is visible in the skin.

The prognosis in these cases of acholia is good, and I am not aware that anyone has demonstrated the morbid lesions which would account for the symptoms. A series of observations of this kind would doubtless help us, for very definite lesions may be found in the liver or pancreas, although one suspects that these lesions are not as a rule striking, since recovery so often takes place.

The treatment is much on the lines already indicated in the two cases of jaundice. As Dr. Cheadle points out, fats must be greatly restricted and starches only given in small quantities. Broths, beef-tea, fish, meat food, skim milk, malted biscuit, and fresh fruit or baked apples, are indicated. In very bad cases Benger's food and milk and asses' milk are valuable. Brandy in small doses for severe cases is useful, and, should diarrhœa supervene, bismuth and opium are indicated. Dr. Cheadle also advises small doses of the three chlorides—chloride of arsenic, chloride of iron, and chloride of mercury. The gums, if needful, should be lanced, and if there is great nervous irritation, chloral and bromide are useful. The extremities must be kept warm, and rest in bed will be very helpful in maintaining an equable temperature.

In conclusion, I must ask you to look upon this lecture as one which is dealing with an obscure group of children's diseases, and so is most imperfect. I do not wish you to accept that acholia is a disease, for it may well be a symptom of various different conditions; nor do I pretend that the two cases of jaundice are examples of any new disease. The subject is, however, a useful one, for it shows that a good deal can be done for these cases, and that, although one may be battling in the dark, it is wise not to lose heart, but treat the symptoms as they arise. Above all, do not forget how difficult a matter it is to get fat digested in these cases of prolonged jaundice.

March 26th, 1906

THE TREATMENT OF RINGWORM.*

By J. M. H. MACLEOD, M.A., M.D., M.R.C.P.,

Assistant Physician for Diseases of the Skin, Charing Cross Hospital; Physician for Diseases of the Skin, Victoria Hospital for Children; Lecturer on Skin Diseases, London School of Tropical Medicine.

GENTLEMEN,—The treatment of ringworm has been chosen as the subject for consideration this afternoon for two reasons, (1) because ringworm is one of the common forms of skin disease to be met with in practice specially among children of the poorer classes, and when it involves the scalp is so intractable as to have become the opprobrium of the practitioner, and (2) because recently considerable advance has been made in its treatment.

For the sake of completeness I will refer briefly to the treatment of ringworm of the glabrous skin, nails, and beard, but will devote the time chiefly to the consideration of scalp-ringworm.

Ringworm in all its forms is a purely local affection, due to the presence in the epidermis, hairs, and nails of fungi belonging to the group of the hyphomycetes, and it is not as a rule associated with any defect of general health, so that local treatment alone is necessary. The successful treatment of the disease obviously depends, then, on the destruction of the fungus and the removal of its effects. For this purpose any of the familiar parasiticides are adequate provided they can reach the fungus, but therein lies the difficulty; for when the mould is situated in the nail-substance or deep down in the hair-follicles even the strongest parasiticides rubbed on the surface are incapable of reaching it. To illustrate this difficulty I had a patch of tinea of the scalp painted daily for several weeks with tincture of iodine and at the end of the time epilated a few stumps. On examining those microscopically I found that the spores in the bulb of the hair were not even stained by the iodine and were actively growing.

In an intractable disease such as ringworm there is naturally an almost endless variety of remedies, many of which have been put forward at first as specifics, but on further experience have invariably proved to be disappointing and been relegated to

* A Lecture delivered at the Medical Graduates' College and Polyclinic.

the long list of uncertainties. Time will not permit of my even mentioning half of them, nor would it serve any useful purpose were I to do so ; instead I will confine myself to the consideration of the few remedies which personal experience has led me to favour.

Ringworm of the glabrous skin (Tinea circinata) is comparatively easily cured. When it takes the form of pinkish, scaly circinate or solid patches situated on various parts of the smooth skin the time-honoured treatment of painting the lesions with tincture of iodine, with or without the addition of 30 per cent. of acetic acid, the application of Coster's paste (iodine ʒij, oil of Cade ʒj), or the rubbing in twice daily of a parasiticide ointment such as salicylic acid gr. xx, sulphur precipitate gr. xx, ammoniated mercury gr. xv, and lanoline ʒj, will generally suffice to destroy the ringworm in about fourteen days.

When the ringworm is of animal origin the lesions are generally more inflamed and purulent, forming raised conglomerate patches dotted over with pustules. In these cases even milder parasiticide treatment is called for than in the above case, for the inflammatory reaction itself leads to the destruction of the ringworm fungus, and all that is necessary to effect a cure is the employment of boric acid compresses alternated with the application on lint of boric acid or dilute nitrate of mercury ointment.

There is a type of ringworm of the glabrous skin, however, which calls for energetic treatment, namely the form which affects the crutch and axillæ (T. cruris or Eczema marginatum), and which is so prevalent in certain parts of India, where it is known as Dhobie itch. In the treatment of this type of ringworm mild parasiticides are valueless, and it is necessary to resort to powerful measures. One of the most serviceable remedies in such cases is chrysarobin (Kemp's goa powder). This may be employed in the form of an ointment up to 10 per cent. strength. Another plan is to wash the affected part with soap and water and then rub in by the finger the goa powder moistened in a little lemon-juice. In doing so it is of course advisable to wear a finger-stall, for not only will the chrysarobin irritate the bare finger, but if it were not carefully washed off and the eye were rubbed by it a severe conjunctivitis would be the result. Another effective treatment in such

cases is the use of compresses of a 25 per cent. solution of hyposulphite of soda in water.

Ringworm of the nails (onychomycosis) is, fortunately, a rare complaint, as it is so obstinate that it may persist for years or indefinitely in spite of more or less active treatment short of extirpation of the nail and scraping of the nail-bed.

Sabouraud recommends the following treatment : The scraping down of the nail with a piece of broken glass and the continuous application of a piece of lint soaked in an iodine solution (iodine gr. iij, iodide of potassium gr. vj, water ʒj) under oiled silk and covered by a finger-stall. Another method is to soften the nail by wearing a finger-stall containing soft soap, then to scrape it down as thoroughly as possible and apply on lint some parasiticide ointment such as salicylic acid (10 per cent). But even with the most active parasiticide treatment it may be quicker in the end to remove the affected nail or nails, scrape the nail-bed, and apply a parasiticide ointment to it to kill any fungus which may have persisted in spite of the scraping.

Ringworm of the beard (Tinea barbæ) may be roughly divided for purposes of treatment into two varieties : (1) the dry, more or less raised and scaly form, and (2) the intensely suppurative type derived from lower animals. Of the two the suppurative variety is the more easily cured, for the suppuration destroys the fungus, and all that may be necessary is the application of mild parasiticide ointments such as boric acid or the dilute nitrate of mercury ointment, with occasionally the employment of boric acid compresses. When the suppuration is slight or absent the line of treatment which is obviously indicated is to set up an acute inflammatory reaction and imitate Nature ; for, as in the case of the hairs of the scalp, even the stronger parasiticides rubbed into the part cannot penetrate sufficiently deeply to destroy the fungus in the root of the hair. One of the most valuable remedies for setting up this reaction is 5–10 per cent. of oleate of copper made up in an ointment and applied thoroughly twice daily till an acute reaction sets in. This may take place in a few days or it may be considerably delayed. After the reaction has developed it may be quieted down by boric acid ointment in the manner already indicated.

Another mode of producing the reaction which I have found to be of great value is by means of the Finsen light, and for this purpose the smaller lamps, such as the London Hospital lamp, are very serviceable. A series of short exposures of fifteen to thirty minutes are given, with as much pressure exerted on the lens as the patient can bear, till the whole affected area has been exposed and has reacted, the reactions being then controlled. I am not in favour of the employment of X rays in the treatment of Tinea barbæ as though the production of an X-ray reaction is not necessary for the curing of the disease, it seems to me unwise to risk the possibility of its occurrence when the disease can be satisfactorily dealt with by other means which, so far as after-effects are concerned, are harmless, while the X rays comparatively readily cause a reaction in the face.

Ringworm of the scalp (Tinea tonsurans).—I now come to the most important division of my subject, namely the treatment of Tinea tonsurans. Ringworm of the scalp forms a considerable proportion of the cases of this disease in children, especially in hospital practice. Out of about 700 cases of skin disease which came under my care at the Skin Department of the Victoria Hospital for Children during the year 1904 there were 130 cases of Tinea tonsurans and 18 cases of Tinea circinata, and the treatment of these cases, owing to the intractability of the affection and the length of time they were under treatment, formed at least one third of the work of the department. Ringworm of the scalp is essentially a disease of childhood, being very rare after puberty, as the scalp after puberty no longer forms a suitable soil for the fungi; when it does occur in the adult it is generally of animal origin and comparatively easily cured.

When a case of ringworm of the scalp comes up for treatment it is necessary in the first instance to examine it most carefully in order to decide upon the line of treatment which ought to be adopted. The choice of treatment in an individual case depends on various considerations, such as (1) the extent of the ringworm; (2) its distribution, whether it is definitely circumscribed or widely disseminated over the scalp; (3) its clinical characters, whether it is dry and scaly, or mixed moist and suppurating; and (4) on the age of the patient and coarseness of the hair. Ringworm is much more easily cured in the infant than later when the scalp is thicker and the hair coarser. The scalp must be examined in a good light, and the diseased

area should be marked round with an anilin pencil. If the ringworm is confined to a few definitely circumscribed patches the hair for half an inch around the patch should be clipped short; if the disease is widely disseminated the scalp should be shaved or the hair cut short with patent clippers, leaving a small fringe in front for the sake of appearance. After the hair has been cut the first thing to do before attempting active treatment is to apply a parasiticide ointment over the whole scalp to stop the spread of the disease. For this purpose an ointment containing half a drachm each of sulphur precipitate and salicylic acid in an ounce of vaseline should be rubbed in twice daily, and the scalp washed every day with soft soap or a mixture of two parts of soft soap and one part of spirit, and, after it has been dried, swabbed over with carbolic glycerine (1 in 8), or tincture of iodine in 60 per cent. spirit (1 in 8). This limiting treatment may be persisted in for a week before more active measures are adopted.

With regard to the choice of a method, it may be repeated at the outset that in ordinary cases of tinea tonsurans no parasiticide short of a caustic when applied to the scalp is capable of reaching the fungus in the hair-bulb, except in the case of infants, when the scalp is covered with fine lanugo hairs, and the sulphur and salicylic ointment mentioned above will generally effect a cure. There is another exception to this statement, and that is suppurating ringworm of the scalp or kerion, where the patches are irregularly swollen and dotted over with small pustules or patulous hair-follicles exuding pus. The treatment of such cases consists of the constant application of mild antiseptic dressings. On no account should the lesions be incised, as has been occasionally done from mistaking them for superficial abscesses, since instead of obtaining pus from them only a few drops of a sero-sanguineous fluid will ooze from the wound. The whole scalp should also be treated daily with carbolic-glycerine. For some time after the inflammation subsides the affected areas remain red and bald, but in about a couple of months the hair will be found to be growing again in the form of fine, downy hairs. These cases are easily cured, and the suppuration may be regarded as Nature's method of combating the disease.

The vast majority of cases, however, belong to the dry, scaly type associated with only slight inflammation, and it is these cases which give so much trouble in their treatment. There are two methods of dealing with such cases—namely by the production of (1) artificial kerion, and (2) by causing an artificial alopecia.

(1) *The method by artificial kerion, or, as Aldersmith calls it, " cure by Nature,"* consists in as far as possible imitating the conditions found in ordinary kerion by rubbing the irritants into the scalp. The facility with which the kerion may be produced depends on the type of scalp and its susceptibility to react to irritants. In certain children comparatively mild irritants, such as 6 per cent. to 12 per cent. oleate of copper ointment rubbed in twice daily, will set up a sufficient inflammatory reaction to loosen the diseased hairs, which should then be epilated and the reaction caused to subside by applying mild antiseptic dressings. Unless the hairs are loose and can be epilated without breaking it is useless to attempt it, for fungus will be certain to be left in the follicle. When the ringworm is very extensive, the effect of the oleates should be carefully watched in case of absorption taking place. The cases which react sufficiently to the oleate of copper or mercury are exceptional, and more powerful measures are generally required. A strong irritant which I have found most valuable in a number of resistant cases is an ointment consisting of equal parts of common salt and vaseline rubbed up with a few drops of water in a mortar. The ointment should be rubbed in twice daily, and the scalp bathed between times with hot water, and after bathing swabbed over with carbol-glycerine. This, in certain cases, is a most effective irritant, but its use is apt to be very painful, and may have to be intermitted from time to time. It has the advantage when rubbed over the scalp of having a selective action and causing an inflammatory disturbance, chiefly in the diseased patches.

Another powerful irritant in this connection is croton oil, but its successful use demands some experience and considerable care. It is to Aldersmith that we are mainly indebted for this method, and a detailed description of it is given in his text-book.

The individual patches are first marked out and then painted with croton oil, care being taken to prevent the croton from spreading beyond the patch by rubbing in a little sulphur ointment

around it. About four hours after painting the patch a sticky oatmeal poultice is applied over it, and covered with a piece of oiled silk. The poultice should be changed every four hours, and each time it is taken off the part should be bathed and carbol-glycerine applied, and it should be worn during the night and kept in position by a nightcap. Next day the patches are bathed with warm water, and after the whole scalp has been swabbed over with glycerine and carbolic, are re-painted with croton oil and subsequently poulticed. This procedure is persisted in till sufficient reaction is set up to loosen the diseased hairs. After the hairs have been successfully epilated or sponged away, boric acid compresses are applied to reduce the inflammation. After the inflammation has subsided, a red bald patch is left, but fine downy hairs grow over it in about six to eight weeks.

This is an excellent treatment for small patches of ringworm, but it requires care to prevent scabs forming, sloughing, and subsequent interference with the growth of the hair. It is apt to be painful also, and should not be employed in children under five years. It is advisable also to find out the susceptibility of the patient to the irritant by painting a small patch first and watching how it reacts.

For the destruction of isolated stumps the croton oil is applied by means of a needle impregnated with it and inserted into the follicle. To needle successfully requires considerable practice. The first essentials are to have the head steady by using a head rest or placing the patient on a couch, and to have a good light. By means of a hand lens the stump is localised and epilated by forceps, and a fine blunt-handled needle such as Aldersmith's is then dipped in croton oil or croton oil and carbolic (8 to 1), and inserted into the follicle, so as to impregnate it with the croton oil. This sets up a suppurative folliculitis which kills the fungus.

By the artificial kerion methods any case of ringworm of the scalp can be cured, but experience is required in obtaining successful results. In extensive cases the great disadvantage of the method is the tenderness and pain which the irritants cause, which is often so great that the patient cannot bear the affected part to be touched, cannot lie on it without much discomfort, feels faint and giddy, and is unable to sleep. For large areas the salt treatment is best, for smaller areas the croton oil method, and for isolated stumps the needling with croton oil is most valuable.

(2) *Artificial alopecia, or depilatory method.*— No hard and fast line of distinction can be drawn between the artificial alopecia and the artificial kerion method in so far as the loosening and falling out of the hair is concerned, but the difference lies in this, that whereas in the artificial kerion method the hairs are loosened by a process of suppuration, in the artificial alopecia the defluvium is associated with only slight inflammatory change.

The simplest method of causing artificial alopecia without preventing re-growth of the hair, if it were feasible, would be to epilate the patches by forceps, but unfortunately, the stumps are brittle and almost invariably break in the follicle.

A method of producing such an artificial alopecia which occasionally is successful is the boric-ether method also recommended by Aldersmith. The scalp is first shaved, then washed with Hebra's soap lotion and water (soft soap two parts, spirit one part), then dabbed over with the following lotion : Acidi borici, ʒj ; meth. æther, ʒiss. ; ol. rosmar, ♏xij ; methyl. spirit, ad. ʒv ; for fifteen minutes with a sponge. Every morning the scalp should be washed, and half an hour later the lotion should be dabbed on, and this procedure is repeated every two hours during the first two days. At nights the scalp is covered with a paste made of precipitated sulphur in water, but no grease applied. If the treatment is going to be successful the hair falls out rapidly, or at the latest in about four months, leaving bald patches.

The most recent method of producing artificial alopecia areata is by means of the X rays. I will not at the present time discuss the details of the technique of this method, but will describe the principles of it and will refer to some important considerations connected with it.

The action of the X rays on the scalp is simply that of a powerful depilatory agent. The X rays do not destroy the ringworm fungus, as is seen in this culture (exhibited), which was grown from a hair which had been exposed to the X rays ten times for ten minutes each time at a distance of 15 cm. from the anticathode. To produce the depilatory effect a definite dosage of the X rays is required, which varies slightly in different individuals. This dosage, with the scalp at a constant distance from the anticathode of the tube, has been

fairly satisfactorily measured by Sabouraud and Noiré of Paris, and a means has been introduced by them for estimating it.

The X-ray tube is enclosed in a protecting shield with an opening to which cylinders are fitted varying in diameter, and of a length such that, when applied to the scalp, the distance from the anticathode will be 15 cm. The affected area of the scalp is exposed through these cylinders, each exposed patch being carefully protected by lead foil to prevent overlapping when another exposure is given to an adjacent patch. This process is tedious and requires the utmost care.

It has been found to be more satisfactory and on the whole safer to give the required dose of X rays at a sitting than to run the risk of giving a series of exposures, for the effect of the X rays is cumulative, and there is a latent period of at least ten days before a reaction becomes apparent.

The hair is clipped short, the diseased areas mapped out, and the exposure given. A mild antiseptic ointment such as 10 gr. each of sulphur precipitate and salicylic acid to the ounce of vaseline is then prescribed to be rubbed into the scalp each night, and instructions are given for the scalp to be washed in the morning with soft soap and then scrubbed over with tincture of iodine in 60 per cent. spirit (1 in 8). This antiseptic treatment is to prevent the spread of the disease before the hairs come out and during the defluvium. The hair falls out about the fourteenth day, the defluvium being preceded by a slight transient itchiness and erythema of the exposed area. Occasionally this erythema is not noticed. If the exposure has been of the correct dosage, the hair begins to grow again as a fine down about eight weeks later. From the time when *all* the diseased hairs have fallen out—*i. e.* in four weeks—the case ceases to be infective, and the child may then mix freely with other children, and, so far as disease is concerned, the child is cured.

This mode of treatment, if brought off successfully, gives brilliant results, and for extensive cases is far superior to any previous method and has the great advantage of being practically painless.

But to bring it off successfully is by no means easy. The above brief outline of the method may suggest that it is perfectly simple, but this is a great fallacy. To obtain satisfactory results in the X-ray treatment of ringworm it is absolutely necessary (1) that the operator should know ringworm thoroughly and be able to recognise every diseased hair in the scalp, and (2) that he should have a sufficient knowledge of the X rays, their production, measuration, and application to enable him to use them with the minimum of risk to the patient. If his knowledge of ringworm be inadequate, unless a defluvium of the whole scalp be produced, his results are bound to be disappointing, and if his knowledge of the rays be insufficient, he is playing with fire and assuming an unwarranted responsibility.

It is impossible to exaggerate the dangers of the X rays and the serious results which may follow their use, and a comparatively slight over-exposure may result in permanent alopecia. On no account should a scalp be exposed to the X rays when it is inflamed from the previous use of strong irritants, and all the inflammation should be allowed to subside before the exposure is given. One of the most harmful irritants in this connection is tincture of iodine, and if the scalp be exposed before the effects of the iodine have worn off a dosage of the rays which would otherwise be harmless may set up a severe dermatitis.

Another accident which may have serious consequences is the inoculation of the scalp with pus-cocci and the production of impetigo and folliculitis about the time when the hair is falling out. This is generally the result of scratching the scalp, which becomes irritable just before the hairs fall out, and is in a state of diminished resistance as a result of the exposure to the rays. The impetigo and folliculitis are apt to delay the re-growth of the hair and may even result in the formation of scars.

The results may be unsatisfactory in another way, namely from the want of proper care at home in the application of the mild parasiticides already referred to, and the diseased hairs in falling out being allowed to infect areas of the scalp not previously diseased.

With regard to the question of injury that the rays might cause to the underlying brain, a question which has often been asked, there is as far as I am aware no evidence of any injurious effect resulting from the exposure. I do not think it advisable, however, to expose children under three years of age and before the fontanelles are closed. There is also the possibility of the new hair not being of such a strong type as the original hair and falling out at some remote period, causing early baldness. This also is simply an hypothesis, which is not yet as far as I know supported by definite evidence.

In view of these eventualities it behoves us, however, to walk warily, to refuse, however expert we may be, to treat any case of ringworm of the scalp by the X rays without first explaining the risks to the parents and making them understand them before giving their consent. Of course this treatment is at present in its infancy. A time may be near at hand when the measurement of the dosage of the X rays may be done with absolute accuracy and the risks minimised. Till such a time it is unwise to employ this treatment without thoroughly realising the dangers, and it is better for anyone, except the expert, to be content with the old well-tried methods, which, though slower and perhaps more painful, are not attended with the same grave responsibility.

March 26th, 1906.

A DISCUSSION ON
POST-MORTEM EXAMINATIONS WHICH DO NOT REVEAL THE CAUSE OF DEATH.

MR. JUSTICE WALTON in the Chair.

<table>
<tr><td>Dr. F. J. Smith.</td><td>Mr. George Pernet.</td></tr>
<tr><td>Dr. Wynn Westcott.</td><td>Dr. Shepley Part.</td></tr>
<tr><td>Coroner Troutbeck.</td><td>Dr. Arthur Powell.</td></tr>
<tr><td>Dr. Claude Taylor.</td><td>Mr. Schroeder.</td></tr>
</table>

Dr. F. J. Smith, in opening the discussion, said the question might be asked : Is the occurrence of an autopsy without pathological appearances to account for death an example of any large class of deaths, or is it an accident due to carelessness or an incomplete survey of the conditions found? The daily press of the evening genus and more particularly the halfpenny species would lead to the supposition that the latter is the case, when it is gravely reported that an expert specially engaged by one of His Majesty's coroners stated that a man died from "threatened apoplexy." One can imagine that the appearances were really compatible with death from natural causes, but that something more in the nature of a definite diagnosis was required from one with such expert knowledge. It is statements like this that bring expert evidence into ridicule. But there can be no question but that the first hypothesis is the correct one : one has only to think of a few of the diseases of the nervous system, epilepsy for instance, or some of the chronic scleroses, or again of some of the zymotic diseases such as whooping-cough, to realise at once that in the absence of clinical history of the case a post-mortem examination done with the most scrupulous care will fail to reveal the cause of death in the absence and even in the presence of a prolonged microscopical research. Or take, again, numberless vegetable poisons ; without something to go upon suggesting a prolonged and careful chemical analysis what chance would there be of detecting death from any alkaloid or similar substance, possibly with the exception of strychnine ? I know of none that would reveal its presence to naked-eye inspection. The argument need not, however, be laboured ; for it is only in the mind of ignorance and quasi- or pseudo-specialism, that has for its own notorious reputation to twist the indefinite appearances of natural death into some alleged definite indications of the precise cause of death, that any doubts exist. The larger one's acquaintance with natural post-mortem appearances, the greater is one's hesitation to attribute them to some fixed and definite cause acting while life was still present or even to ascribe death to some gross change found. At the London Hospital our records for a period of some nineteen months finally put a crown of proof on the argument. During these nineteen months there were 2123 post-mortem examinations performed carefully and recorded with exactitude and in no less than 102 there were found no naked-eye changes whatever to which death could be attributed. I propose to briefly analyse these 102 cases and then to consider some reasons why such need not surprise us. There were in the period covered by my Report 150 cases of death ascribed by clinical evidence to marasmus (*i. e.* wasting without obvious clinical cause) and diarrhœa and vomiting, and of these no fewer than 83 showed nothing whatever in any internal organ to which death could be ascribed, and in all these it would have been impossible from autopsy alone to explain why the thread of life had snapped when it did. The remaining 19 cases were of various denominations, the most frequently occurring being prematurity, of which there were four examples. It might be argued that immaturity can be detected by inspection, and so it can in many cases born at six, seven, or even as late as eight months; but if immaturity be taken in its physiological sense of incapability to live an extra-uterine existence, there will be found several in which by inspection alone it would be hazardous to assert positively that such was the case. I have, for instance, five such cases, æt. respectively 1 day, 8 days, 18 days, 5 weeks, and 8 weeks, the first of which was born during eclampsia of the mother. Besides these children, there were one at 7 weeks, in which a guess was made that the child might have had congenital syphilis; one at 4 months, with liver and spleen somewhat larger than usual; one at 20 months, in which there was a doubtful history of laryngismus stridulus; and two at 2 years each, in one of which there was some slight evidence of rickets, but in the other every organ in the body seemed perfectly healthy, and no reason could be ascribed why life which

had lasted for these two years should not have continued. The remaining five cases were adults. One, a girl of 22, was known to have had acute mania; another, a man of 25, was seen to faint with the heat and died at once; and the other three remained without a label from lack of clinical and post-mortem evidence, and would in former days have been described as death from the visitation of God. I maintain, if this be the experience in the post-mortem room of a hospital with a large medical school attached, a similar experience must be common in places where no critics are present to ask questions or to discuss the morbid appearances disclosed; there are no keener critics than a body of medical students.

The reasons why we do not hear of more verdicts "cause of death unknown" is, first, that when a medical man who has seen the patient during life does the autopsy, he is competent to say that what he found post mortem was quite compatible with the symptoms he had observed during life, and can label the disease accordingly; and, secondly, that when a stranger does the autopsy he magnifies natural appearances into morbid ones, and makes a statement accordingly, a statement which nobody cares to, or perhaps can, controvert.

How such cases occur is, after all, not very difficult to answer; for, if one takes a general survey of all the possible causes of death, one is immediately struck by the very few absolutely tangible and definitely certain causes of death of which the naked eye makes us at once aware. Two or three limbs torn off, or crushed and mangled, an internal organ lacerated, with the pleuræ, peritoneum, or meninges filled with blood, severe cerebral hæmorrhage or extensive softening, a few forms of extensive kidney destruction, pus deluging a serous membrane, a consolidated lung, cancer blocking a tube or causing perforation thereof, a few cases of corrosive poisoning, are nearly all in which we can positively assert that such a condition is immediately, or after a very short interval, incompatible with a continuance of life. In the great bulk of cases (probably about 95 per cent. of all cases of death) kidney, heart, lung, stomach, may any or all of them be grossly diseased, and we may say that the disease was the cause of death, but only because we have known something of the symptoms that preceded the fatal termination;

they are none of them in their nature necessarily fatal *within a given short period of time*, and our evidence before the law must run : " I found gross disease of such and such organ, and it would be sufficient to account for death sooner or later, and may have caused it now." Apart from this line of reasoning, we have well-known physiological, physical, and physico-chemical principles upon which to rely.   The basis of the first is the fact that cellular and somatic death, or the death of the individual in the ordinary sense of the word, and the death of the individual cells of the organs, by no means coincide, the interval between the two events being very variable, possibly amounting to several hours ; in physiological experiments this is well shown. The physical principle is the well-known law that fluid will, when left alone, sink down to a position of stable equilibrium ; in other words, and directly applied to our subject, blood while liquid will sink and soak into the lowest possible part of the vessels and organs of the body, filling them to the highest available point, and thus simulating ante-mortem congestion to such an extent that the microscope may be necessary to distinguish between a vital reaction to an irritant and a mere physical phenomenon.   The physico-chemical principle is the well-recognised fact that cells, both those necessary to life and those less important ones, may be slain by substances of a foreign nature gaining access to them, and stopping their vital functions without leaving any demonstrable traces behind.   This subject has been the object of many physiological researches and has been proved up to the hilt, but one might illustrate it by asking, What changes would any one expect to find after a hypodermic dose of any powerfully poisonous alkaloid, such as conine, nicotine, morphine, or strychnine ? and yet assuredly death is directly due to the physico-chemical action of these substances upon nerve-cells.

We may consider these points from a practical point of view by taking the individual organs of the body, those at least, such as the brain, heart, and lungs, which are necessary to life, and disease of which may cause death ; indeed, it is usually asserted that death only takes place through one or the other of them, an assertion which fairly well expresses the truth, though in some, such as hæmorrhage and septicæmia, it might be difficult to assert that one only was the ringleader in the catastrophe.

A dead body is invariably laid on its back, and hence the meninges at the base of the brain become full of blood, usually liquid, and unless care be taken it may be assumed that meningitis or cerebral congestion of a fatal character was present before death.   The gross organic changes, such as hæmorrhage, gross softening, tumours, abscess, pus on the meninges, tubercle, and adherent meninges are easily detectible and not likely to be overlooked, but such diseases as epilepsy, convulsions due to peripheral causes, leave no traces by which they can be recognised.   An excess of sub-meningeal fluid or excessive appearance of puncta cruenta may make one suspect that they owe their origin to ante-mortem influences acting fatally upon the brain ; but in uræmia, in bronchitis and emphysema, in pneumonia, in morbus cordis, I have frequently found the brain in a condition indistinguishable from that which might easily be caused by these troubles, and if one thinks for a moment about the actual dying of the patient—the real essential Why did he die ?—in these cases, it is very easy to see that they frequently do die in all sorts of diseased conditions actually and proximately because of the serious disturbance of the normal physiology of the brain. Meningitis itself, when early, requires a good diffuse daylight for the recognition of the simple, dry, greasy appearance presented, and I have more than once been in doubt whether it was present or not, and should have overlooked it— even when tubercular in origin—had I not had the ante-mortem symptoms to guide me.

With regard to the heart, it is an established axiom in physiology that it never stops in systole, but always in diastole, and yet post mortem it is very frequently found in a condition of apparent contraction, due to *rigor mortis*, and as *rigor mortis* is universal in muscle the following is a justifiable statement.   If the heart be found flabby, with other muscles stiff, it is probable that there is something in the condition of the heart-muscle itself to account for it—some form of degeneration, fatty, fibrous, or simple ; but to state that this was the cause of death is going much beyond anything we have justification for.

Take any disease you like, and one can undertake to say that the heart may in two consecutive cases be found, in the one contracted and in the other flabby, in the one a good colour and in the other a bad colour, and who can say without the clinical history whether the heart was the real cause of death or whether it was merely what one may call an accessory to the fact? In carcinoma brown atrophy is a very common appearance; in cirrhosis of the liver, in fatty liver, in old age with atheroma, a fatty heart is frequent, but fatty degeneration takes a long time, and who, by naked eye or even with the aid of a microscope, can say at what stage of the diseased process the organ failed from absolute incapacity, or that it has been only unequal to some unusual strain? Again, the opposite is true, and cancer, cirrhosis, etc., may kill and yet the heart be found quite healthy. Are we then in the one case to say the heart killed and in the other the independent disease? Such a position is one of pure guesswork, and only the clinical history can decide.

It is when the lungs are considered that the greatest difficulties are met with in deciding between appearances that may have been the *ultimate cause* of death and those which may be an *accidental accompaniment* of death and those which are mere post-mortem effects. There can be no question but that when somatic death takes place—death, that is, of ordinary parlance—all the cells of the body do not die at the same time, and from the mucous lining of the bronchial tubes a certain amount of mucus continues to be exuded post mortem, and it is impossible to estimate whether the mucus thus found was enough to cause death or not. Again, supposing, as is frequently the case (I believe almost universally), a little pus can be squeezed out of the medium-sized and smaller tubes, are we therefore to say that bronchitis was the cause of death? I hold very strongly we are not justified in so doing unless we have an account of the symptoms immediately preceding death, for these give just the information we require.

Hæmorrhage into the lung, tubercle, consolidation, sub-pleural ecchymoses, are all obvious and evident enough, and their indications may be translated into lethal expressions; but what about œdema of the lungs? It often kills, I have no doubt, but it is equally often found in septicæmia, uræmia, apoplexy, etc., when its indications are, to say the least, very doubtful. Supposing, then, it is the only gross change found, are we justified in saying it was the cause of death? Assuredly not without the clinical history of symptoms preceding

dissolution. And we are bound to include œdema of the lungs amongst those post-mortem appearances which leave the legal cause of death unexplained.

Again, what is known as hypostatic congestion of the lungs may be what its name implies, a pure and simple mechanical effect capable of taking place post mortem, though often enough in certain debilitated conditions of the system it is a very real ante-mortem phenomenon easily capable of killing, and it wants very great experience of clinical history combined with post-mortem findings to say how far it was the cause of death. The phenomenon, moreover, can hardly be distinguished from the very early stage of pneumonia. In both there is precisely the same dark red, almost black, condition of the bases of the lungs or of one lung, and it requires very nice discrimination and long experience to say this degree of resistance to the finger is natural and that is pathological; in fact, again, without the symptoms and the temperature that preceded death I believe the distinction to be oftentimes impossible.

One cannot pass over in silence the extreme difficulty one meets with in deciding from naked-eye anatomy whether the kidneys are or are not healthy. I admit that gross changes are common enough and easy enough to detect, and yet one often has to call the kidneys normal to the naked eye when the clinical history has shown that they at any rate allowed much abnormal material to filter through them, and that they were the clinical cause of death whatever may have been the proximate and essential cause. Even if gross changes be observed we are again face to face with the difficulty—they must at some time have led to death, but have they caused it *now*?

It follows from what I have said that these cases occur with moderate frequency, we have seen also the reasons why they occur, and we have now to consider their importance from a medico-legal point of view. This may be summarised in a sentence, though details must be discussed rather more fully. That procedure of a coroner's court by which a verdict is arrived at on the evidence of the pathologist alone is simply a farce; for no such person, even if skilled, can by naked-eye evidence alone determine the true cause of death in a completely satisfactory manner. It is absolutely essential that with him should be associated the medical man who last saw the deceased alive. Do not let me be misunderstood. I am not denying the value of expert pathological evidence, I am merely stating that it is insufficient for the needs of justice and the safety of the public and requires to be supplemented by other medical evidence ; but I do go so far as to say that if only one person can possibly give evidence at an inquest that one should be a medical man who has seen the person alive, even if it be only in his death agony. The real, genuine pathological appearances of organs as opposed to the more accidental exudations and congestions so often distorted by self-assertive would-be experts into evidence of the cause of death are not likely to be overlooked by any medical man, though I must admit that it is possible they may be ; for I have myself seen carcinoma of the sigmoid leading to perforation of the gut remain entirely unperceived by a medical man ; but this class of mistake is of infinitely less importance than that of attributing a death from morphine-poisoning to bronchitis, which is a very possible or even probable mistake which might be made by one who relied upon post-mortem evidence only.

Let us imagine a person in South-West London, for example, is taking medicine containing morphia and that some evilly disposed person gives an overdose ; the medical man in attendance, feeling that the disease should not have proved fatal, may refuse a certificate ; a post-mortem examination is made and an inquest held without any reference to or communication from the medical man. Alleged signs of bronchitis are found and a verdict in accordance is given, and a foul murder is hushed up, probably for ever. The mere possibility of such an occurrence makes one shudder, and yet the ignoring of the medical man in attendance makes such, one might say, probable. In my own experience within the last few months a case in point has occurred : Dr. Wynn Westcott asked me in September last to make a post-mortem examination on two children who had died after taking liquozone, a strong solution of sulphurous acid. On autopsy I could find no possible nor even probable cause for death ; and had one not known that repeated doses of simple irritant poison may leave no traces in the alimentary canal beyond those attributable to mere post-mortem changes, I should have been obliged to say that I could find nothing to account for death had I not had the invaluable, nay in-

dispensable—if justice was to be done—support of the evidence of Dr. T. W. Morcom Harneis, who had attended the deceased children for some three or four days, with all the symptoms of irritant poisoning. It was on his evidence combined with mine that a correct verdict was given, viz. poisoning from the effects of taking liquozone in repeated doses.

It may be urged that the mere fact of no cause being found on autopsy *primâ facie* sufficient to account for death should make the pathologist suspect some insidious form of poison ; but a reference to my analysis of cases will at once show that such a connection is by no means necessary, and common experience leads in the same direction, especially perhaps in that terrible cause of infant mortality so-called overlaying ; I believe that in the majority of such cases there are no pathological conditions found after death.

I need say nothing more ; to any unprejudiced mind the case is clearly proved that the medical man's evidence of the last hours is more important than the expert evidence of the post-mortem findings ; and if an expert be necessary he must have the medical attendant associated with him both at the autopsy and in court.

Dr. WYNN WESTCOTT (H.M.'s Coroner for North-East London) said : Having held more than 15,000 inquests, I may be allowed to say that my experience fully confirms Dr. Smith's opinion, that whenever a medical practitioner has been in attendance upon any sick or injured person in his last illness, such medical man should be called upon to give evidence at any inquest. And should there be any legal or medical reason for scientific precision as to the exact cause of death let there be a post-mortem examination of the body by all means, so that the cause of death may be registered accurately. The more learned the practitioner who makes this examination the more accurate will be the result. So let us agree to cultivate the pathological expert, for he alone can help us to discover the cause of death when no evidence of medical attendance is procurable, as, for example, when unknown persons are found dead. But to assert, as some persons have done, that post-mortem examinations, which in so considerable a proportion of cases give only negative or uncertain results, even when made by collegiate professors of pathology and forensic medicine, should alone guide the coroner's jury to a verdict, seems to me to wilfully discard clinical evidence of the utmost value, and thus to multiply enormously the chances that the cause of death will be given incorrectly.

To find by post-mortem examination that a man has grave heart disease is no proof that he has not died from poisoning, the symptoms of which may have been recognisable before death, and may have been recognised, and such evidence may be procurable for a fee. To find that a man has grave kidney disease, with calculi and cysts, is not absolute proof that he has died of those lesions, for he may still have died from one of many unnatural causes, as, for example, from the inhalation of escaped gas in his bedroom, an accident that I have known in my own experience.

Dr. Smith has referred to two deaths following the use of liquozone, in which the post-mortem appearances were very slight, and for this reason great pressure was brought to bear upon him to retract his opinion that sulphurous acid caused the death. But no impartial person who read the complete and very carefully given and undisputed evidence of the parents and of the medical attendant has since questioned the propriety of the verdict that these two healthy children sickened and died from no other discoverable cause. And although there might not have been in England lately any similar deaths, yet I can find records from Italy and Germany noted in the text-books, showing that in those countries the internal use of this dilute acid, although greatly popular for a short time, was discarded because of the gastrointestinal irritation which it so often caused. History has repeated itself.

To pass from the uncertain results occasionally afforded by post-mortem examinations, even when made by experts in hospitals, I am, of course, quite cognisant that the post-mortem examinations made by the general practitioner are often of much smaller value, either from lack of knowledge, lack of facilities, or from want of time. Pathological anatomy was not taught in a systematic manner when I was attending the medical schools, and there are still thousands of medical practitioners no older than I, who studied when I was at college, and these gentlemen cannot be regarded as likely to obtain very scientifically accurate results from post-mortem examinations, unless they have had special facilities since qualification. I believe also that there are many younger practitioners who possess but a small knowledge of pathological appearances, for which reason it will be desirable in the future to make further facilities for the employment of specialists.

I consider it necessary that County Councils should obtain for coroners full permission to pay fees higher than the ordinary fees specified by the Coroners Act of 1887 in special cases, provided always that the discretion of the coroner, who alone is responsible in his choice of a specialist, should not be hampered. Some Councils have seemed inclined to seek statutory powers to appoint physicians and surgeons themselves ; but I find that the

medical coroners object, as I should object, to be deemed unfit to choose the medical expert witness best suited to any notable case. As to whether the coroners of the legal profession might perhaps not object so much to the action of the County Councils in this matter is no business of mine.

There is, however, a reason why the performance of post-mortem examinations should be gradually separated from the life-work of the general practitioner. And this is the danger to parturient women, women who are to be confined, and some other patients, the danger which is involved in the performance of this dirty work, the work needing to be done at odd times and in the intervals of bed-side attendance. Perfectly clean and aseptic hands are difficult to secure at all times, but after making examinations of the internal organs of the dead the difficulty is greatly enhanced.

Some present-day Professors smile away the maxim of good old Bichat, that death follows failure either of the heart, the lungs, or the brain. Yet there is some great practical value remaining in the knowledge that a man has died either from heart failure, or from lack of breathing, or from coma — the absence of sense, motion, and will. The physiological factor is more vital than the anatomical, and the last hours of life do often more show forth the reason for dying than does a dissection of the stiffened or decomposing corpse.

(*To be concluded.*)

The Cornish Riviera.—We have received from Mr. J. C. Inglis a copy of the book issued by the Great Western Railway Company on the Cornish Riviera. This handy volume affords pleasant reading and imparts at the same time information of great value to those concerned with questions of health. Medical men will find in its pages useful descriptions of the various health resorts in Cornwall which will enable them to direct their patients to the places best suited to the varying conditions of particular cases. In mildness of climate the Cornish Riviera rivals the chief foreign health resorts, and in equability it certainly holds its own. It has also to be borne in mind that the chief centres of interest to the seeker after health in the Cornish Riviera can be reached at slight cost and little fatigue, thus avoiding the weariness of travelling to a foreign spa and securing the continuance of those home comforts so essential to the well-being of the convalescent and to the recovery of the invalid. We congratulate Mr. Inglis on the excellent book he has brought to our notice and recommend it as a safe guide for all desiring to know how to go to the Cornish Riviera and what to see when there.

THE CLINICAL JOURNAL,

CLINICAL RECORD, CLINICAL NEWS, CLINICAL GAZETTE, CLINICAL REPORTER, CLINICAL CHRONICLE AND CLINICAL REVIEW.

EDITED BY L. ELIOT CREASY.

| No. 701. | WEDNESDAY, APRIL 4, 1906. | Vol. XXVII. No. 25. |

CONTENTS.

* *Specially reported for the Clinical Journal. Revised by the Author.*

ALL RIGHTS RESERVED.

NOTICE.

Editorial correspondence, books for review, &c., should be addressed to the Editor, 51, *New Cavendish Street, W., Telephone No.* 904, *Paddington ; but all business communications should be addressed to the Publishers,* 22½, *Bartholomew Close, London, E.C. Telephone* 927, *Holborn.*

All inquiries respecting Advertisements should be sent to MESSRS. ADLARD & SON, *Bartholomew Close, E.C. Telephone* 927, *Holborn.*

Terms of Subscription, including postage, payable by cheque, postal or banker's order (in advance) : for the United Kingdom, 15s. 6d. *per annum : Abroad* 17s. 6d.

Cheques, &c., should be made payable to THE PROPRIETORS OF THE CLINICAL JOURNAL, *crossed "The London, City, and Midland Bank, Ltd., Newgate Street Branch, E.C. Account of the Medical Publishing Company, Ltd."*

Reading Cases to hold Twenty-six Numbers of THE CLINICAL JOURNAL *can be supplied at* 2s. 3d. *each, or will be forwarded post free on receipt of* 2s. 6d. ; *and also Cases for Binding Volumes at* 1s. *each, or post free on receipt of* 1s. 3d., *from the Publishers,* 22½, *Bartholomew Close, London, E.C.*

A CLINICAL LECTURE

ON

SYRINGOMYELIA.

Delivered at the National Hospital for the Paralysed and Epileptic, Queen Square, W.C.

By J. S. RISIEN RUSSELL, M.D., F.R.C.P.,
Physician to Out-patients at the Hospital, and
Physician to University College Hospital.

LADIES AND GENTLEMEN,—Syringomyelia, as most of you are no doubt aware, is a disease in which there is proliferation of the neuroglia in the central part of the spinal cord. The neuroglia which normally exists at the posterior part of the central canal becomes proliferated, and then in time it breaks down owing to various reasons, and thus a cavity is formed. This cavity is unlined by epithelium and varies in regard to the extent to which it affects the spinal cord both in the longitudinal and transverse directions. It so happens that the cavity most often exists in the cervical region, but it may extend throughout the cord and may thus involve the lumbar enlargement. On the other hand, it may pass upwards so as to invade the medulla, in which case it usually becomes excentric, limited to one side instead of preserving the central position which it does in the spinal cord. In the cord the cavity is, as a rule, more or less central, whereas when it invades the medulla it usually becomes limited more or less to one side. The size of the cavity varies, not only in so far as its vertical limits are concerned, but also in the amount of the transverse area of the cord that is involved. Here, again, we find great variations. The cavity may be more or less limited to the central region without invading to any extent the lateral or posterior columns of the cord. On the other hand, it may invade the posterior columns and not the lateral columns, and may thus give rise to various symptoms that are due to affection of those particular tracts. Similarly it may invade the ventral horns of the spinal cord, and destroy the grey matter of which these horns are composed.   In consequence of the invasion of the lateral and posterior columns ascending and descending degenerations result, ascending degeneration owing to involvement of the posterior columns, and descending degeneration as a consequence of the affection of the lateral columns.   This brief review of the morbid conditions which exist in the spinal cord and medulla in these cases must suffice, as time will not permit of our considering this part of the subject in greater detail.

Now let us deal with the clinical picture of the disease.   The most typical clinical picture of syringomyelia is that which results when the cavity exists in the most common position, namely the cervical region of the cord.   When the cavity occupies this region a variety of symptoms result which depend on the position of the lesion rather than on its nature.   This disease is a good example of how the clinical picture of a disease of the nervous system may vary according to the position of the lesion and according to its extent.   I shall be able to show you this afternoon a case which is in reality an example of syringomyelia, but which may cause some of you to have grave doubts as to the accuracy of the diagnosis in view of the fact that it is so different from a typical case of the disease of which you may have seen an example.   On the other hand, I am going to show you another case that is not one of syringomyelia, but in which the lesion is situated in the position usually occupied by the cavity in syringomyelia, and in which a clinical picture has resulted which very closely resembles that of syringomyelia.   What I wish to bring out clearly at this stage of my lecture is that a disease of the nervous system may have very different clinical pictures in different cases, according to the position occupied by the morbid process, and also according to its extent, and that one disease may be closely simulated by another, in virtue of the fact that the morbid process of the one happens to occupy the position most commonly selected by that of the other disease.

To begin with, let us clearly understand what the ordinary clinical picture of syringomyelia is. It is usual to find that there is atrophic paralysis in the upper limbs and a variable amount of spastic weakness in the lower limbs.   You recognise how this comes about : the atrophic paralysis in the upper limbs depends on extension of the cavity

into the ventral horns of the spinal cord, with destruction of the grey matter there, while the spastic weakness of the lower limbs depends on extension of the cavity into the lateral columns of the cord.   Instead of our finding spastic weakness in the lower limbs, which is the most common condition, we may find that the lower limbs are somewhat ataxic, owing to extension of the cavity into the posterior columns of the cord.   The most common and typical picture of the disease is, however, one in which there is atrophic paralysis in the upper limbs, and spastic weakness, which varies in degree, in the lower limbs.   In addition, it is usual to find nystagmus, notably on lateral movement of the eyeballs.   Further, we may expect to find curvature of the spine ; it may be a lateral curve (scoliosis), or it may be an antero-posterior curve (kyphosis), or the two may be combined in the same individual.   We are also justified in looking for evidences of trophic lesions in the skin, notably about the hands.   There may be whitlows which are painless, scars, it may be from whitlows, old burns, or injuries which have not caused the patient pain at the time they were inflicted.   Finally, we can determine in most cases, irrespective of the particular type of the disease that is under observation, a variety of affection of sensibility which is peculiar and characteristic.   There is loss of the power to appreciate painful and thermal impressions, so that the individual is unable to distinguish between heat and cold, and is unable to recognise a painful stimulus on various parts of the body, and yet a tactile impulse can be accurately perceived. Although there is analgesia and thermal anæsthesia we may find no anæsthesia, there being the most perfect preservation of tactile sensibility, so that the lightest touch may be perceived by the individual in the same regions of the body where painful and thermal impressions are not recognised.   These, ladies and gentlemen, are the main characteristics of an ordinary case of syringomyelia.   I want, in the next place, to bring to your notice a case that is not one of syringomyelia.   This girl is suffering from hæmatomyelia—that is to say, hæmorrhage into the spinal cord.   In September, 1902, suddenly, during the night, without any cause that can be assigned, and without any trauma, she developed the symptoms which necessitated her admission into this hospital.   The symptoms were as follows: paralysis of her lower limbs with, in addition, a certain amount of paralysis of the upper limbs. The paralysis was notably atrophic in character in the upper limbs, evidence of which I can still show you on the right side. The left upper limb is practically normal both as regards motor power and also as regards the state of nutrition of its muscles, although there was some loss of power in it at first. In the right limb there is very marked muscular atrophy, notably along the ulnar border of the forearm. The same thing obtains with regard to the small muscles of the hands. You can see that the thenar muscles are markedly atrophied, and you notice the abnormal position of the hand that has been permitted by the affection of its intrinsic muscles. There is also a certain amount of contracture. There is no spasticity, but there is definite contracture. In the lower limbs she had spastic paraplegia, from which she has largely recovered, but the remains of it are still evident, as there is a certain amount of spasticity of the limbs and the plantar reflex is of the extensor type (Babinski's sign). The ankle clonus which used to be present has disappeared; her knee-jerks, which were exaggerated, have returned practically to the normal standard, though that on the right side is still a little too active, as is that on the left also, but to a less extent. She can walk a little now, as compared to her total inability to do so at first. As regards the affection of sensibility, Dr. Gordon Holmes has very kindly had these charts made for me, which I now pass round for your inspection. The patient had complete inability to perceive pain over the dark-shaded areas and comparative blunting of this form of sensibility over the lighter shaded areas, so that the degree of shading illustrates the amount of the loss of sensibility. There was more defect of sensibility on the right hand and forearm than on the left, and you will notice a sharp line of demarcation between the æsthetic and the anæsthetic areas. With regard to heat and cold, the defect corresponded to the analgesia. Although she had so much analgesia and thermal anæsthesia, she had no defect whatever of tactile sensibility. The patient still has the analgesia and thermal anæsthesia to a great extent, but she has no loss of tactile sensibility and never had any defect of this kind. The case thus resembles one of syringomyelia in many respects, but differs from the most common type of that disease in there being no trophic disturbances of the skin, no nystagmus, and no lateral

or other form of curvature of the spine. We, however, know that all of these defects may be absent and yet the case may be one of syringomyelia, so that the absence of curvature of the spine, nystagmus, and trophic lesions of the skin cannot be regarded as sufficient to preclude the possibility of syringomyelia in such a case, although the mode of onset of the symptoms negatives a diagnosis of this disease and supports the view that the patient is suffering from the effects of a hæmorrhage into the spinal cord (hæmatomyelia).

The next patient that is now being brought in is the case to which I referred when I said that some of you might have considerable hesitation in accepting the diagnosis of syringomyelia. Nevertheless there can be no doubt that we are in the presence of a genuine case of that disease. In introducing you to the typical clinical picture of syringomyelia I commenced by calling your attention to atrophic paralysis in the upper limbs. The atrophic paralysis in syringomyelia usually affects the small muscles of the hands, and is indistinguishable from that which we meet with in progressive muscular atrophy. In this patient a search for muscular atrophy in the hands fails to discover any such defect. The left arm is somewhat wasted as a whole as compared with the other upper limb, but there is no notable atrophy limited to any groups of muscles in the hands or forearms, such as we are in the habit of finding in ordinary cases of syringomyelia. Further, I told you that trophic lesions of the skin were common in this affection, and that, like the muscular atrophy, the trophic lesions are most commonly met with in the upper limbs. In this patient, however, a careful search has failed to determine the slightest sign of any trophic disturbances of the skin. There are no evidences that he has ever had whitlows, and there are no scars on his hands the results of burns or other injuries such as may occur in these cases. He has, however, a scar on his body from a burn, which resulted many years ago, and he did not feel any pain at the time when it occurred. While examining the hands for these trophic lesions of the muscles and skin, remember that in many cases the bones are affected There may be evidences of trophic changes which destroy the terminal phalanges, or more than one phalanx may become necrosed and may drop off, and thus lead to shortening and deformity of the fingers. Furthermore, in your examination for trophic lesions remember to examine carefully the various joints, and notably the shoulder-joint, for a condition of things which may resemble Charcot's joint in tabes. The joints most commonly affected in tabes are the knee and hip, while in syringomyelia the shoulder is the joint usually selected. We have examined this patient carefully but cannot find any evidences of trophic changes in any of his joints to suggest anything like the condition known as "Charcot's joint." You recognise therefore that so far as the upper limbs are concerned we are without any of the ordinary or extraordinary evidences that would support the diagnosis of syringomyelia. When we look to the patient's lower extremities, however, we find that they conform absolutely to what I have already told you is the rule in the disease, for he has spastic paraplegia. Indeed, the spastic paraplegia is so marked that the man has lost the power of progression in consequence of this defect. The limbs are so rigid that in trying to lift the one leg in the way that I am doing I lift the whole of the patient's body and the other limb with it, a condition of things which is highly characteristic of an organic paraplegia. The spasticity is so great that I cannot get the limb sufficiently relaxed to allow the full effect of the knee-jerk to be seen. You will appreciate that I am in reality dealing with a very exaggerated knee-jerk when I tell you that the hamstrings are tightly contracted, and are in consequence preventing the full effect of the knee-jerk from being obtained. In testing for ankle clonus, I am unable to get the foot back into the position necessary to obtain a clonus with ease, but with some difficulty I have succeeded in evoking this abnormal phenomenon. Oftentimes ankle-clonus is regarded as absent because of the difficulty you have seen me experience in getting the foot into the proper position. You notice, however, that as a result of perseverance a good clonus is now becoming manifest. Let us now examine the plantar reflex. There is the extensor type of response, well marked on the right side, and also on the left (Babinski's sign). We may therefore claim that in so far as the lower limbs are concerned the patient's condition conforms to what I have told you is the rule in syringomyelia.

We must now proceed to examine the patient's cranial nerves. On searching for nystagmus we find that it is present when the man looks in either direction, but is especially well marked when he turns his eyes to the right. Apart from this the cranial nerves are perfectly normal; there is no other defect noticeable in the regions supplied by them. The most notable defect present, other than the spastic weakness and certain sensory changes to which I shall refer in a few moments, is a very pronounced lateral and kyphotic curve of the spine. Now that we are examining the trunk, I want you to notice that although we did not find any muscular atrophy in the position where we usually look for it in syringomyelia, there is very marked atrophy of the scapular muscles and of those in the neighbourhood of the shoulder-blade. These defects are, however, rendered less striking owing to the very pronounced curvature of the spine which monopolises our attention. I want you to observe one other point in connection with the patient, and that is that he presents, what is not at all common in syringomyelia, great spasticity of the left arm, so that you see that I can scarcely move it away from the side of his body. After a few passive movements I am able to manipulate it more easily, but it is still very stiff. In the same way I cannot straighten his fingers except with difficulty, and as I get one sufficiently relaxed to do so, another that was previously straightened becomes flexed again by the spasm. On the other side—that is to say, in the right arm—he is somewhat spastic, but not nearly to the same extent as on the left side. The sensory defects that are present are very striking. Let me pass the sensory charts round for your inspection. The first represents the analgesia, the loss of sensibility to pain. Notice that the areas which are darkly shaded indicate complete loss of ability to perceive pain, while those which are shaded more lightly indicate a lesser degree of analgesia. The same applies to heat. There is loss of the power of perceiving heat practically all over the body, except that it is less marked over the buttocks, the posterior part of the thighs, and on the left side over a small area on the thorax and on the inner side of the thigh. The face is, however, an exception, as he has complete preservation of the power of appreciating heat on the right side of the face. This is the only area where he has complete preservation of the power of perception of heat. Although the patient experiences similar difficulty in recognising cold he can do so in a great many more places than he can heat. Thus he can appreciate cold on nearly the whole of the face, except on a small area on each side. In regard to tactile sensibility, on the other hand, he recognises the lightest form of stimulus everywhere. We are, therefore, dealing with a case of syringomyelia in which there are no trophic disturbances in the skin, no joint changes, and no changes in connection with the bones. It is further a case of the disease in which there is no muscular atrophy in the ordinary position where you expect to find it in syringomyelia, viz. the small muscles of the hands, but in which, nevertheless, there is atrophy in a less common position, affecting the shoulder muscles. The case otherwise presents a typical picture of the disease, with one extraordinary feature added, namely the extreme amount of rigidity that . is present, and notably the degree of this in the left arm.

Before demonstrating the next case I want to call your attention to the fact that there is yet another type of syringomyelia of which I have, unfortunately, no example that I can bring before you this afternoon. There is a case of the kind among my out-patients at present, but I have been unable to get the woman to come up to-day. The variety I refer to is called Morvan's type of syringomyelia, and is sometimes known as " Morvan's disease." In that form of the affection trophic changes in the upper limbs, such as cutaneous eruptions, ulcers, painless whitlows, and changes in the bones are the most striking features. Apart from these defects there may be very little the matter with the patient except that the characteristic abnormalities of sensibility are to be found. These defects of sensibility and trophic lesions in the skin may be the only manifestations of the disease. You may thus have a case with no muscular atrophy, no spastic weakness in the limbs, and, in fact, no abnormality except trophic lesions in the skin and analgesia and thermal anæsthesia, and yet the patient may be suffering from syringomyelia.

I am also unable to show you a case in which the cavity has invaded the lumbar enlargement so as to cause atrophic paralysis in the lower limbs, abolition of the knee-jerks, and paralysis of the sphincters.

When discussing the morbid anatomy I told you that the disease might be limited to the spinal cord, or that it might extend up into the medulla. I also told you that when it passed into the medulla the cavity tended to become excentric as a rule, and unilateral in position. This patient supplies us with an example of syringomyelia in which the cavity has extended into the medulla, and we shall be able to show you how certain of the cranial nerves have become involved in consequence of this. Before doing so, however, I want to call your attention to the general features of the disease that are present in him in addition to the affection of the cranial nerves. Let us begin with these charts, which show the defects of sensibility that have been determined. You will see that he has blunting of sensibility over one side of his body. Tactile sensibility is affected here as well as thermal sensibility and sensibility to pain. Over the area shaded blue there is some tactile anæsthesia. In this other chart we have the areas of analgesia depicted, and in the green chart is represented the areas over which the patient is unable to detect heat ; while the last chart shows the parts in which he is unable to recognise cold. This gives me an opportunity of saying that although dissociation of sensibility is such a characteristic feature in syringomyelia, you must be prepared to meet with cases in which there is inability to perceive tactile impressions as well as failure to detect thermal and painful stimuli. In the late stages of syringomyelia notably it is not uncommon to find an individual with tactile anæsthesia as well as thermal anæsthesia and analgesia. This is illustrated by the charts which I am handing round in connection with this man's case. Apart from defects of sensibility what other indications has he of syringomyelia ? He certainly has no spastic paraplegia, which means that in him the cavity has not invaded his lateral columns. Furthermore there is no ataxy evident in his gait, which is an indication that the cavity has not extended into his posterior columns. When we examine the parts of his hands in which you most commonly look for muscular atrophy in syringomyelia, we find that there is absolutely no evidence of defect of this kind, but, as in the case of the patient who has just left the theatre, we find that he has atrophy of the shoulder muscles. His supra- and infraspinati are markedly atrophied, and he has a good deal of atrophy of the fibres of the lower half of the trapezius, in addition to which, if we get him to draw his shoulders back against resistance, you can see that the rhomboid stands out clearly on the one side, whereas it is practically absent on the other. The muscle stands out well on the left side, but there is very little evidence of the corresponding muscle on the right side. The other muscles about the shoulder girdle are intact. When he presses the hands forwards against resistance there is no winging of his scapula, such as results when there is paralysis of the serratus magnus. Thus, although he has some tilting of his scapula, due to atrophy of the trapezius, he has no winging, such as is seen when there is paralysis of the serratus. The latissimus dorsi and pectorals are perfectly good, as you can see when he presses his arms down towards the sides of his trunk. On examining the upper arm muscles, we find that there is a good deal of atrophy in all of them. There is weakness with atrophy of his biceps, and the same applies to the triceps. There is, however, no affection of the forearm muscles or of those of the hands. He has curvature of the spine, and the most prominent vertebra is the seat of a good deal of pain. These people often have pain, notably at the acme of the curve. He has a lateral curve (scoliosis) with its convexity to the right and accompanied by a certain degree of kyphosis, though this is not very pronounced. This is all there is to be said about the general features of the disease presented by this patient. Now as to the special features which he presents in consequence of extension of the cavity upwards into the medulla, a condition that you do not often have an opportunity of seeing. Let us begin with an examination of his eyes. You can see that he has well-marked internal strabismus on the left side, and that when he attempts to move the eyes to the left the right eye moves inwards perfectly, but the left does not move outwards beyond the mid position. There is complete paralysis of the external rectus on the left side. In addition to the inability to move the left eye out, he has nystagmus of the right eye, which is moving in, and when we make him look to the right you can see that he has marked nystagmus in both eyes. He, therefore, has the ordinary phenomenon which we meet with in syringomyelia, namely nystagmus, and, in addition to this, there is paralysis of the left external rectus muscle. Is there any other feature that these cases may present in connection with the eyes other than the nystagmus and paralysis of

ocular muscles brought about by implication of the nerves or their nuclei by the cavity in the medulla ? Another condition which may be present is independent of any lesion in the mesencephalon, and is wholly due to the cavity in the cervical cord. The cavity may implicate the cilio-spinal centre, and, in consequence of this interference with the sympathetic, the palpebral fissure may be narrowed on one or both sides, with partial ptosis, which disappears on looking up, and a pupil that is small and which does not dilate when shaded. These phenomena are not due to a lesion of the ocular nerves or their nuclei, but are the result of damage to the cilio-spinal centre in the cervical cord. Indeed, you all recognise in the partial ptosis, with narrowed palpebral fissure and small pupil, the ordinary effects of paralysis of the sympathetic. Moreover, this is a condition of things that you may meet with in syringomyelia, when there are no indications that any other cranial nerves are affected, and when, in truth, the whole of the clinical picture is due to a cavity in the spinal cord. If you next observe the facial movements, you will see that the patient has complete power of raising the eyebrow and wrinkling the forehead on the right side, whereas there is absolute inability to do so on the left side. There is complete paralysis of the upper part of the left side of the face, as revealed by this and by his failure to close the left eye. When attempting to show the teeth he can move his lips on the right side but not on the left, so that the lower part of the face is also paralysed. There is thus complete paralysis of the left seventh nerve. In spite of such complete paralysis of the seventh he has no defect of the auditory nerve ; he can hear my watch quite clearly on both sides. If we now turn our attention to the fifth nerve, you can see from the charts what defects of sensibility there are in the distribution of the nerve. The motor division of the fifth is, however, absolutely intact, for the temporals and masseters act well, and when he opens his mouth, even against resistance, the lower jaw moves down mesially. The paralysis of the face may make it appear as if the jaw did preserve the mid position, but as a matter of fact it does, which proves that he has no paralysis of his pterygoid. If he had paralysis of the external pterygoid on the same side as he has the facial paralysis, the jaw would be deflected to the left when he opened his mouth. He would thus not only have atrophic paralysis of his temporal and masseter muscles in consequence of affection of the motor division of the fifth nerve, but also paralysis of the external pterygoid, which would reveal itself by his chin deviating to the left when he opens his mouth, the jaw being as it were twisted in this way by the unopposed action of the external pterygoid on the right side. Let us next look at the patient's tongue. The left half is atrophied and puckered, and marked fibrillary tremors can be seen on the affected side, in addition to which the tongue as a whole is tremulous. His palate is also paralysed on the left side. When he says " ah " the palate moves up on the right side, but there is absolutely no movement of the left side of the palate. Testing the palate is not always an easy matter, as some experience is required to prevent your mistaking movements communicated from the normal side for independent movement of the paralysed side. The uvula, instead of going up mesially, moves up to the side which is not paralysed.

This completes the clinical picture in so far as the affection of the pons and medulla is concerned. Although the patient has been under observation a good many years, there has never been any noticeable defect pointing to affection of the opposite side of his pons and medulla. It happens that in all the cases of syringomyelia that I have seen in which the cavity has extended into the medulla and pons the rule has been observed, for the cavity has in each case been excentric and unilateral.

Let me now repeat the main points I wanted to bring out clearly this afternoon. Syringomyelia is a disease which usually presents us with a very definite clinical picture, in which are included muscular atrophy, with certain other trophic lesions in the upper limbs, spastic weakness in the lower limbs, nystagmus, lateral curvature of the spine, and certain defects of sensibility. The cavity may, however, extend down into the lumbar enlargement, when, instead of there being spastic weakness in the lower limbs, there may be an atrophic paralysis, and instead of being exaggerated the knee-jerks may be abolished. The case may be one in which, although there is a cavity in the cervical cord, it does not cause any paralysis, does not lead to muscular atrophy or to spastic weakness, but may merely occasion trophic lesions of the skin and defects of sensibility. The cavity in the cervical cord may cause very little manifestations as regards paralysis, and may give rise to no defect in regard to locomotion, but may extend up into the medulla and pons and occasion paralysis of cranial nerves. It must, however, be remembered in this connection that partial ptosis, narrowing of the palpebral fissure, and pupil defects may be due to a cavity in the spinal cord, and do not necessarily mean that the cavity has extended to the mesencephalon.

I have said little of the sphincters in this disease, for the reason that they usually escape in syringomyelia ; but, as I have incidentally mentioned, they may be affected when the cavity extends down into the lumbar enlargement and causes atrophic paralysis in the lower limbs. This class of case is, however, quite exceptional, and when, as usually happens, the cavity is mainly confined to the cervical part of the spinal cord, no notable defect of the sphincters occurs.

April 2nd, 1906.

A LECTURE

ON

THE OPERATION FOR INTERNAL HÆMORRHOIDS.

By P. LOCKHART MUMMERY, F.R.C.S.,
Surgeon King Edward VII's Hospital for Officers,
Assistant Surgeon St. Mark's Hospital for
Fistula and Other Diseases of the
Rectum.

GENTLEMEN,—There are many different methods of operating for internal hæmorrhoids and much has been written by the advocates of the different methods for their pet operations.

The operations most commonly employed at the present time for the cure of piles are the ligature operation and some form of excision of the piles, of which Whitehead's operation is perhaps the commonest.

Much has been said by some writers in favour of Whitehead's operation in contradistinction to the ligature method. The advocates of Whitehead's operation originally based their claims for this operation upon the fact that it is more radical and could not be followed by recurrence, that there is less pain and less risk of secondary hæmorrhage. None of these claims have stood the test of time, however, and they have now fallen back upon the somewhat weak argument that Whitehead's operation is more compatible with modern surgical principles.

It is wrong, however, and most unwise to lay down any rules with regard to the treatment of such a condition as piles or to insist upon the performance of one operation for all cases.

That operation is the best which gives the best results with the least risk and the least amount of discomfort to the patient, and beside this nothing else matters.

Many of those who condemn the ligature operation for piles assume that the ligature operation as performed to-day is the same as it was fifty years ago, and seem unacquainted with the modern operation by ligatures. No one operation is suitable for all cases of piles, and what may be the right operation in one case may be quite unsuitable in another. While by no means wishing to deny that there are cases to which Whitehead's operation is best suited and will give good results, I do not think it has justified its claim to the premier position in the treatment of piles.

It must not be forgotten that Whitehead's operation does not consist in excision of the piles, but in excision of the whole of the anal mucous membrane. The surgeon must assume therefore that the anal mucous membrane is a useless structure, and that the rectal mucous membrane which is brought down to take its place is capable of entirely replacing it. This is certainly not the case. The mucous membrane lining the anal canal is richly supplied with sensory nerves, as a reference to the drawing will show (Fig. 1). These nerves pass between the external and internal sphincters and are distributed to the mucous membrane covering the internal sphincter and to the muco-cutaneous junction. The mucous membrane lining the rectum itself immediately above the internal sphincter (and which in Whitehead's operation is made to replace that normally lining the anal canal) is not supplied with sensory nerves at all. Now, the object of this rich nerve-supply to the anal mucous membrane is to give immediate warning of the presence of flatus or fæces in the anal canal, and to enable the individual to effectually control the passage of flatus or fæces when they reach the lower end of the rectal canal. The

maintenance of the nerve-supply to the mucous membrane of the anal canal is almost as necessary to perfect control as the presence of the sphincters themselves. Without proper sensation in the anal canal the reflex path is broken, and leakage and the unconscious passage of flatus will occur.

In Whitehead's operation the dissection is carried up between the sphincters and the anal mucous membrane, and the whole of the nerves supplying the mucous membrane of the anal canal are divided and the sensitive mucous membrane is removed (see Fig. 1).

This in itself is a very serious objection to the operation ; as although it would seem that in some cases sensation of some sort is ultimately established in the new mucous membrane of the anal canal, this is by no means always the case, and patients who

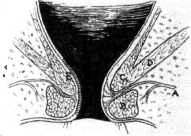

Fig. 1.—A. Sensory branch of pudic nerve, passing between external sphincter (B) and internal sphincter (C) to the mucous membrane of the anal canal. D. Levator ani. The shaded mucous membrane (E) is that part removed in Whitehead's operation.

have been operated upon by Whitehead's method often complain of inability to prevent the unconscious passage of flatus, and further, that when they get diarrhœa they have very little control over the action of the bowel.

This partial loss of control which results from lack of sensation in the anal canal causes an intense amount of distress to any sensitive person. It is also, unfortunately, a condition for which very little, if anything, can be done to afford relief.

Cases where partial loss of control from this cause results after Whitehead's operation are far from being uncommon. The following cases are instances of this condition :

A. B—, an elderly gentleman, was operated upon for piles by Whitehead's operation three and a half years ago. The operation was performed by a well-known surgeon who was thoroughly acquainted with the operation. Directly Mr. B— began to get about again after the operation he noticed that he had not the same control over his anus as formerly. He frequently could not prevent the passage of flatus, and when his fæces were at all liquid he had to seek immediate relief at the nearest lavatory or there was a disaster. He also frequently stained his linen. His condition has not improved with time, but is rather worse now than it was just after the operation. At the present time unless he has previously starved himself he is afraid of going out shooting or to any public entertainment or ceremony on account of his uncertainty as to what may happen. He has no sensation in the anal canal and but little contractile power in his sphincters.

S. A—, a middle-aged gentleman, was operated upon by a surgeon of repute for piles, by Whitehead's method. The wound healed well, but he was not comfortable after the operation. He had loss of sensation in the anus and partial loss of control over flatus and liquid fæces. Seven months after operation the wound broke down and there was severe ulceration of the anal canal, with complete loss of control and great pain. Severe contraction followed, and at present there is but little control over the anus, and he has to pass bougies to prevent further contraction.

I have gone rather fully into this result of Whitehead's operation, as it is one which is not often mentioned and is worth serious consideration.

That Whitehead's operation is more severe than the ligature operation there can be no possible doubt ; it takes longer to perform, and the time during which the patient has to be kept in bed is usually longer.

These points are perhaps not very important ones, but the greater liability to complications and increased risk of Whitehead's operation as compared with the ligature are of considerable importance. The complications which may follow the ligature operation are few and invariably unimportant, while there is practically no risk.

On the other hand, the complications which occasionally follow Whitehead's operation are often serious. Severe ulceration and delayed healing have been often seen, and cases where a serious degree of stricture has followed Whitehead's operation have been seen by most surgeons. One of the worst features of these complications is that little or nothing can be done to remedy the patient's condition.

The local excision of piles, with immediate suture of the wounds, is perhaps the ideal operation and gives good results in suitable cases. When there are only two or three isolated piles this method is excellent, but it is not a good operation when the piles are very large or there are more than two or three. It takes longer than the ligature method, and I have been unable to persuade myself that the period required for healing is any shorter.

At St. Mark's Hospital nearly every operation for piles has been tried at one time or another, but the operation which is performed in the great majority of cases is the ligature operation. This is not for any sentimental reasons or because the surgeons are conservative, and like adhering to the older method, but because it is found that the ligature operation gives the best results. At St. Mark's Hospital the results of an enormous number of operations for piles by ligature show that this operation is almost without an equal in surgery for good results and freedom from risk.

The method of performing the ligature operation which I have adopted is as follows :

The patient, having been previously prepared for operation by thorough evacuation of the bowels and cleansing of the skin, is placed in the semi-prone position on the right side.

The sphincters are then well dilated. The lower bowel for about three or four inches is then thoroughly cleansed with spirit soap and then well irrigated with a weak solution of lysol and cleansed with sterile swabs soaked in the same solution. I pay a good deal of attention to this preparatory cleansing of the mucous membrane and believe it to be of much importance.

All the piles are now seized in artery forceps and drawn down outside the anus. Each pile is now treated in turn, starting with the lower ones. The pile is first cut away from the submucous tissue with scissors until only the upper portion is left, which consists of the mucous membrane above and the vesssels passing into the piles which lie immediately below the mucous membrane at the upper end. This narrow pedicle is now firmly ligatured with stout silk in one piece and without transfixing it. If the pile is very large part of it is cut away, otherwise it is left. Any bleeding points left by cutting the pile are ligatured with fine silk. When a large pile has been removed the wound is brought together with catgut sutures so as to hasten the healing process. The whole of the anal canal and wounds are next smeared over with sterilised iodoform ointment so as to seal up the lymphatics and cover the wounds with a protective coat.

A piece of drainage-tube about three inches long and to which a loop of silk is attached is placed in the rectum to allow the passage of flatus. Sterilised pads of wool are then placed round the tube and over the anus. This operation takes less than ten minutes to perform. The incisions are made through clean tissues, and the wounds are protected from infection for some considerable time after the operation. No morphia suppository is used and no morphia given unless the patient complains of pain, when a hypodermic injection is given. The anus

tight enough to cut through practically everything but the vessels—and upon carefully cleansing the anal canal before making the incisions and keeping the parts as clean as possible afterwards.

Severe pain after operation is generally due to one of two causes, the most common being inflammation and consequent swelling of the parts. This, I am persuaded, can be to a very large extent prevented by careful cleansing of the mucous membrane before commencing the operation and by keeping the wounds protected with sterile ointment afterwards. The other cause of pain is the inclusion of some portion of the skin at the anal margin in one of the ligatures; this cannot occur if the operation is properly done.

The results of the operation by ligature leave little to be desired. The risk is almost nothing, complications are scarce, and when they do occur of very little importance, and recurrence is hardly

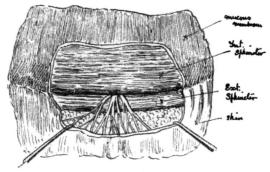

Fig. 2.—Drawing of a dissection of the anal canal laid open. The mucous membrane and skin have been removed to show the sensory branch of the pudic nerve passing between the sphincters to reach the mucous membrane and skin of the anal canal. (After Hilton.)

is douched with 1 : 60 carbolic and the dressings changed twice daily. The bowels are opened with castor oil on the third or fourth day and the parts afterwards carefully cleaned. The remains of the piles shrivel up and disappear, and the ligatures usually come away about the eighth or ninth day, and the patient is allowed up about the tenth day.

There is little or no pain after this operation and in quite half the cases no morphia is needed. In a few cases the patient complains of a sudden jumping pain occasionally, which is due to the sudden contraction of the sphincters and is the result of their having been stretched; it is quickly relieved by morphia.

The absence of pain after this operation depends mainly upon tying the ligatures very tight and their proper application—the ligature should be tied

ever seen. During the last two years at St. Mark's Hospital I have met with only two cases of recurrence after the ligature operation. In one of these cases recurrence did not occur until sixteen years after the operation and in the other twenty-three years, and this is in a large out-patient department, nearly half of which consists of cases of piles. Most of what is frequently said against the ligature operation for piles is absolutely untrue of the operation as it is described here. There is no more pain than after most other operations and in many cases far less.

The patient is not confined to bed for more than ten days to a fortnight and can return to his or her ordinary occupations in less than three weeks.

April 2nd, 1906.

A DISCUSSION ON POST-MORTEM EXAMINATIONS WHICH DO NOT REVEAL THE CAUSE OF DEATH.

MR. JUSTICE WALTON in the Chair.

Dr. F. J. Smith.
Dr. Wynn Westcott.
Coroner Troutbeck.
Dr. Claude Taylor.

Mr. George Pernet.
Dr. Shepley Part.
Dr. Arthur Powell.
Mr. Schroeder.

(*Concluded from p. 384.*)

Mr. Coroner Troutbeck said : I should like to associate myself strongly with the opinions already expressed on the importance of having, if possible, clinical evidence in a case when it is available. Now, I notice that both Dr. Smith and Dr. Westcott agree with what I think is the universal opinion amongst coroners, and that is, that to have post-mortem examinations performed by general medical practitioners who are not generally employed in that work is not the most satisfactory way of dealing with such examinations. But general medical practitioners, when they have clinical evidence to give, obviously ought to be called to give it. That is, I think, so clear that it hardly requires arguing. But the difficulty is that in many cases there is no clinical history, except the clinical history which is given entirely by laymen. This is a difficult thing to state without going into the particulars of each case, but I have looked out the numbers of inquests for the last five years in London—and they are contained in the published Reports of the London County Council, and can be purchased by anybody for ninepence a copy—and I see that during the last five years ending December, 1904, there were 38,324 inquests. There is an average in those inquests of about 48 per cent. of cases which are stated to be due to natural causes. Now, with reference to the first point raised by Dr. Smith, there is in the return a column for cases where death is stated to be due to causes unascertainable. During the five years, with over 38,000 inquests, there are only 116 of such cases returned. In the face of so skilled an opinion as that of Dr. Smith it seems to me excessively strong criticism on the manner in which at least some causes of death were ascertained. I personally have a district which I suppose is different from

most districts in London, in that in it there happen to be five of the great general hospitals of London, with medical schools attached, and that circumstance makes the percentage of hospital cases in my district considerably larger (I should say twice as large) than that in other parts of London. And looking back, I calculate that I must have held in my time inquests on at least 2300 persons who have died in hospitals. The practice in the district is that there shall be, almost invariably, a post-mortem examination, and in these hospital cases it is made by the pathologist of the hospital, in the presence of the house-surgeon or the house-physician, as the case may be, who has attended the case, and very often, if the hospital is a keen one, in the presence also of the physician or the surgeon. And therefore there is every advantage in such cases. You have the highest skill in pathology, and many generations of pathologists, and you have the highest skill in the clinical attendance, and you have the very great advantage of method in the observations made clinically. These are all there and they are all in writing, and the result has been that, rightly or wrongly, evidence has been given to prove that, with two or three exceptions only, the cause of death has been ascertained. I do not profess myself in the least qualified to criticise those pathologists who came to that conclusion ; I assume that they were the highest in their profession in England ; they were attached to some of the greatest hospitals and schools, and they are St. Thomas's, St. George's, Westminster, Charing Cross, and King's College. I have only to mention their names to show the class of evidence which it must have been. But it is, of course, obvious that the same apparent result has been obtained with evidence of very widely different character, evidence which I need not dwell upon, but which has been sufficiently described by Dr. Westcott, who has told us what he thinks of it. Now, one has to observe this. The coroner has no business whatever to take an inquest when the cause of death is not supposed to be violent, unless the cause of death is unknown. And in practice that practically means where there is no clinical history. And that means that in a large proportion of cases—I do not think I am overstating it if I say 40 per cent.—in 40 per cent. out of the 38,000 there was no clinical history. And yet you have this in the face of what Dr.

Smith's very weighty criticism is, you have this result, that general practitioners, who cannot have a tithe of his experience, or of the experience of these other pathologists, are prepared to go and say they have found a cause of death, and they apparently state it without the slightest qualification or doubt. That is not very satisfactory, and I think it is shown that some great authorities do not regard it as satisfactory. You find that in one district in London during that time 54 per cent. of the cases are stated to be due to natural causes ascertained, but only 19 per cent. of the whole of the cases are cases where a post-mortem examination was made. That means that in no less than 35 per cent. of the whole of the cases in that district a verdict was returned where, *primâ facie*, there was no clinical history at all, and (the absence of a history being the only justification for an inquest) where there was no post-mortem examination; the result could only have been guesswork, and the absence of the post mortem must have been due to the fact that the coroner had come to the conclusion that a post-mortem examination by a general practitioner was of little or no value and not worth paying for. It cannot be regarded as satisfactory. I admit that one must take into consideration the grave reasons that Dr. Smith has given us for doubting that in all cases the cause of death can be ascertained by post-mortem examination, but it is a reason for only entrusting these examinations to people of he highest skill and experience; at the present time there are obvious practical difficulties in the way of our doing that, and it seems to me that a reform in that direction is more than ripe for dealing with.

Dr. CLAUDE TAYLOR said : Of course one has heard criticism on the action of coroners recently, and on that question I may say that it seems to me that if the coroner feels that he must take only the highest evidence that he can obtain the same principle might apply all round. To a certain extent it is the right principle. But where are the rest to come in other than those who are of the highest position in their profession? Is a medical man never to be trusted unless he has very high qualifications and holds very high positions? One might say that it is unsatisfactory to think that the poor in London depend for their health, or when their health is impaired that they should be de-

pendent for the recovery of it upon those whom certain of the community feel are not of the highest position. It seems to be the general impression that only the highest are suitable for these inquest cases. It is an ideal, but it seems to me that it is hardly practical unless there is, as has been suggested, some radical change in the present legal arrangements to obtain and pay for these services. As regards the question of ordinary practitioners making the post-mortem examination, it seems to me that there is advantage in such men making examinations provided they have had instruction in the subject, and are competent to make an ordinary examination that does not require special examination of certain organs or microscopical examinations which sometimes are necessary in order to discover the probable cause of death. There is an advantage in practitioners from time to time making these examinations, and having the opportunity of making them, and being rewarded for making them, because it keeps them more in touch with the internal facts of disease which they have to gather from indirect evidence when they see the patient in life. It is of advantage to them in their practice, and it seems to me that it is their due when they have attended the person who is the subject of the inquiry, and it is, using the medical phrase, their case. It does seem to me only right that they should be entrusted with the further duty of carrying the case to completion and making the examination which is necessary, on the understanding that if they are unable to find a satisfactory cause there may be an appeal to a higher authority. Of course we recognise that a preliminary examination may to a certain extent spoil the condition of affairs for the higher authority; but in most cases that would not be so, and I think it is only right and fair to the medical practitioner who has had to do with the case, and who has done his best, that he should be the first one, other things being equal, to be consulted as to the post-mortem facts also.

Mr. GEORGE PERNET said : I agree as to the importance of having the clinical history of a case. It is really an important point in an investigation as to the cause of death. And in that connection I may mention the fact that even from a histological standpoint, unless you know the whole facts, clinical data and history—that is, the whole story—you may go wrong even after making a careful microscopical examination. With regard to the examination of bodies after death, it has long struck me, especially after studying in Paris at the Morgue, where bodies are examined in a very thorough manner, that in London we might get a great deal of medico-legal education out of these cases which we do not get at the present time. Now, whenever a case is to be examined the medical man who attended the case during life should be present at the post-mortem examination, which he should either make himself or else see done, if it is a complicated case, by a man engaged in teaching medico-legal medicine. Again, these post-mortem examinations should be made public to all medical men, and students too who have reached the fourth year of their studies. These should be allowed to attend these examinations just as they are in Paris. If that were done in London, we should derive a great deal of benefit and knowledge out of the enormous material that a city like London supplies which at present is to a large extent wasted. If we had Morgues in convenient centres as regards the hospitals, the fourth-year students and medical men in the district could attend the post mortems.

Dr. SHEPLEY PART said : There are points in favour, I think, of the general practitioner being allowed to do post-mortem examinations. The salient point is one which has been laboured almost, and that is that he is already acquainted, and in a way which nobody else can be, with the clinical symptoms which had gone on before. But there is a point which has not been touched upon ; and as my work has led, in various parts of the world, to a considerable amount of medico-legal work coming into my hands, it is one which appeals to me rather strongly, and that is the question from the medical witness's point of view, and the variety of treatment that he receives from coroners, more especially lay coroners. And it is more especially on the lines of some such case as this. Some years ago I was practising for a short time in the West of England, and I was called out one night about eleven o'clock, and found when I got to the house that the girl was dead. I had seen her in the afternoon perfectly well and spoken to her. She was quite well then and had not been ill for some considerable time. The history that I got was that she had been seized with pain in the abdomen, and as far as I could on hearsay evidence I went into the case. But there was no justification for me to go before the court and say I knew the cause of death. I had not seen her in her trouble during life ; she was dead when I got there. She presented no appearance which could be called characteristic of anything. The coroner sent a policeman first and wrote to me, and the policeman tried to cross-question me as to what conditions I was informed of in the house. The coroner wrote and asked if I could give an opinion as to the cause of death, and I said no, that it was impossible without a post-mortem examination to say and I had no evidence to give. I did not receive any further communication from the coroner, but two days afterwards I heard that the inquest had been held, and a verdict of death from natural causes had been returned by a bucolic jury. No medical witness had been called whatever. My opinion in that case was given to the coroner in a private communication ; and as at that time I was in practice there I can look upon it as a considerable hardship that my opinion should have been obtained and not paid for. I grant that it was not worth much as evidence ; still, it had put me to more or less trouble. Then, again, with regard to the question of speaking somewhat dogmatically. I would put it to you, sir, that when you are called before a jury of laymen to give evidence on technical questions they do expect that you will give a definite answer, and if you do not make a more or less dogmatic statement they will ask you for it, and they will press you for it. It is not always easy to say " I do not know." Most of us will admit it is a most difficult thing to ask a man who is supposed by his very position to be an expert to say " I do not know." He does say so at times. I have frequently heard it said that there was nothing definite. And then the question is put repeatedly, in form after form, by jurymen : " What do you think was the cause of death ? " Or it may be put from the Bench in that way. I have had it done to myself : " Cannot you give me something more definite than that ? " One is very strongly tempted to say, " I think probably so-and-so." But it is not returned as that ; and we get it in the Council reports, sir, as a definite verdict. But please do not credit the medical man with having given it in that definite form. The object of an inquiry is to get a dogmatic statement of the cause of death, and with lay or legal coroners it is very often, I think, looked upon as a *sine quâ non*—at least, judging from personal experience in various parts of this country and several of our Crown colonies—to give such a statement. It has been my lot to be pressed into a very tight corner over and over again for a definite and dogmatic statement or opinion, when, as Dr. Smith truly says, it is utterly impossible to give one.

There is a class of case which, in the East, we come across very frequently, cases found dead, probably from beri-beri. Beri-beri is one of those hopeless causes of death which Dr. Smith referred to, which in a very large number of cases will give you absolutely no sign of anything abnormal, and you can only depend upon collateral evidence for a presumption of death from beri-beri. The person may be very much emaciated, but many things cause emaciation. But I would plead for a little more charity for the general practitioner, because the practical difficulties which confront him in saying " I do not know," especially if he is in practice in the district, are very great, and I can speak with the more freedom because I am not in practice in London at the present time. And I do not think that the remuneration in this country— one guinea for a post-mortem examination—will ever get a thorough examination done with any satisfaction, and until the public is prepared to pay expert fees for expert work they will get their money's worth, but no more. Medical men are more or less business men, and neither the hospital expert nor the expert who happens through force of circumstances to be in general practice will give twenty-five guineas' worth of work for one guinea. It is not to be expected.

Dr. ARTHUR POWELL said : I have to do about a thousand medico-legal post-mortem examinations each year, and in a very large number of them, I am ashamed to say, my evidence is that I do not know what the deceased died of. Among the causes of death which Dr. Smith did not mention was that from beri-beri, which was particularly before my mind. Of course in this country you do not get it so frequently, but tetanus is another disease which I thought he might have mentioned, and also drowning as a cause of death. And in a large number of cases in which I have had no

reason to doubt the person has been drowned I cannot give, from the appearances of the body itself, any evidence that the death was due to drowning. I should like the coroners present to let us know if their experience has been the same as mine. In probably five thousand inquests which I have attended I have never yet known a case in which the general practitioner, when called in, has not been able to give a cause of death. And that is in contrast to the expert, who has sometimes been unable to give a cause. The death may have been attributed to syncope or something of that sort, and that seems to satisfy the jury in our part of the world, which is very much behind the times. I have many dozen times had experts who alleged that they could not find any cause of death, but that has never been the case with the general practitioner.

Mr. CORONER TROUTBECK said : I have heard evidence given by some leading police-surgeons on the point. They are not pathologists, but they have considerable experience of post-mortem examinations in the case of bodies taken out of the Thames ; and I do not remember a single case, unless the body was so decomposed that nothing could be ascertained, where the police-surgeon has not been able to find when death was due to drowning.

Mr. SCHROEDER said : In regard to the point about general practitioners not finding a cause of death, a great many inquests come under my notice—perhaps the records of 50,000 inquests have come under my notice—and I can only recall two in which the general practitioner was not able to find the cause of death. But I agree that probably had post-mortem examinations been made by a pathologist they might have hesitated. There is another remark, and that is with reference to the last speaker but one. In the country districts it is certainly very common for the coroner not to call any medical witness, or, if he calls one, to wait for the jury to ask for a post-mortem examination to be made. That is simply keeping to the old practice of hundreds of years ago, when the coroner went down to the place at which the death took place with his jury and examined the body himself and did not call in a medical man, and I believe in some districts it is done in deference to the County Council. One hopes that the provincial County Councils will follow the better lead of cities which call for medical evidence in every case. But

I have had a long correspondence with many coroners, and that is the answer they gave me, that they defer to the wishes of the County Council to keep the expenses down, and hence they do not call the medical man. It is open for a jury to require the coroner to call the medical witness, not only to call him, but to ask for a post-mortem examination, and if he does not do so on being requested by them he is liable to certain penalties. You have only, in your district, to let the twelve men and true know of that, and if the coroner does not do his duty he can be called to account for it. With regard to calling for his opinion in advance, in the district for which I am deputy-coroner in London that is done, and I have held this year over 700 inquests and never had any difficulty in connection with medical men giving an opinion in advance. In some districts it used to be paid for; it is not so now because coroners have no legal power to pay a medical practitioner for his opinion. I do not know that they are bound to give it; it may be a common law duty, but there is no statutory enforcement.

Mr. JUSTICE WALTON said: Although I speak with some reluctance and some diffidence upon a question of this kind, still, I may say how it strikes an outsider who, after all, has to spend a good deal of his time in dealing with questions of evidence and investigating facts. What struck me whilst I was listening with great interest to this discussion was, first, that after all you must distinguish very much between cases and cases. I do not know, but it appears to me there must be a considerable number of cases in which the cause of death can be ascertained without any reasonable doubt by the facts quite independently of any medical evidence at all; there must be a considerable number of cases where the facts speak for themselves, and I should think, on the other hand, that there must be cases—and I speak with all diffidence—in which the cause of death is reasonably and fairly disclosed by what I may call the condition of the dead body. But putting these cases on one side, I suppose you then come to a large class of more obscure cases, and I suppose it is that class, which may be very large—it may be a large percentage of the cases which have to be investigated, I do not know—it is that class about which we have been talking. Now, dealing with that class, it seems to me that everybody agrees with Dr. Smith first of all in this proposition that a post-mortem may afford no evidence at all of the cause of death. There are cases of that kind, and then, of course, a post-mortem is simply useless. It may be negatively useful, from the fact that it does not disclose anything, but it is not positively and affirmatively useful in affording evidence beyond that. Therefore it is only in certain cases that the post-mortem examination gives any evidence at all and throws

light on the cause of death, except in the negative way I have mentioned. It is then useful, as I understand it, in disclosing a morbid condition which is or may be sufficient to account for death. But in a large proportion even of such cases, as I gather the post-mortem—I am speaking of cases where a diseased condition which may account for death has been disclosed—the post-mortem examination cannot be treated as in itself proof of the cause of death. That, I gather, we are all agreed about, and therefore even in those cases—I am speaking of the obscurer cases, leaving out of consideration others—where the post-mortem examination does afford some evidence of a diseased condition which may be the cause of death it is, after all, only a link in the chain, it is not a complete proof by itself. Of course, if there was no other evidence at all, I suppose it might be such a strong link and such a large link as to be almost a chain of itself. But, speaking broadly and generally, it is only a link. And what is behind it? What is the rest of the chain? If there is a clinical history, again, I think everybody seems to be agreed that the clinical history is an all-important link also in the chain. You must have your post-mortem examination, and if there is a clinical history it would be rash to act on the post-mortem examination, in the best of cases even, without the clinical history. Where there is no clinical history, which is the fact in the vast number of cases in which there is an inquest, because there is no inquest where there is a satisfactory clinical history, where there is no clinical history you cannot have evidence of it. But looking at it as a matter of evidence, it must still be remembered that although there is no clinical history, there may be, and there usually are, not always perhaps but very often, material facts, the non-medical facts, of the case. Of course if there are such facts you must consider them. You must take all the facts of the case which are relevant and material—the clinical history, which is only part of the facts of the case, the non-medical facts which may be equally important, and it may be that in a certain number of cases the post-mortem examination will add a very important link. It will be in some cases, I should think, an all-important link, an essential link in the way of testimony. That is what strikes me, looking at it merely from my point of view, my non-medical point of view. As regards the other question as to who should make the post-mortem, it seems obvious that the post-mortems should be made by a competent man. A man may be a very good and useful general practitioner and yet possibly not be very competent to make a post-mortem, at any rate in cases of difficulty, but I do not venture to speak upon that, or as to how the post-mortem should be made. These are matters of considerable public interest, and matters in which the public interest might very well be served by the advice and suggestions of the medical profession. But let me say this : I protest against the notion that the man who says "I do not know" is the less to be respected for saying that. Quite the contrary. I am always delighted to find a man who says "I do not know." The difficulty is that most people are so unwilling to say it ; they say that they do know when they do not and when they ought to say so. Much time would often be saved and progress made by such a simple admission. I ought almost to apologise for intervening, but that is how the matter strikes me.

Dr. SMITH, in closing the discussion, said : I am very pleased to find that we are practically unanimous. As a matter of actual fact, I fully recognised the difficulties that have arisen through the position which I have dealt with, and I did not really venture to offer a full solution of those difficulties. I have heard a very excellent suggestion, and that is that the medical man should be paid for his written evidence, whether he gives it in court or whether he does not. But that leads me rather far from my present point, which amounts to this, that expert evidence from the post-mortem room only is quite insufficient for arriving at the correct verdict. I think Mr. Troutbeck has a little misunderstood my position in connection with the enormous percentage of verdicts which are returned, definite verdicts, which are not verdicts of "found dead and nothing to show for it." That is due to the fact that the medical evidence is attended to in a very large number of cases. As I illustrated it, here is a child with laryngismus stridulus. The doctor sees it in the attack, or he has seen it in a previous attack, or he has diagnosed laryngismus stridulus from the previous attack. The child dies. No post-mortem evidence of disease is forthcoming, he certifies it as laryngismus stridulus, and it goes down as such. Therefore, no wonder we get an enormous percentage of verdicts which are perfectly correct, and that I have not controverted. What I do controvert is that those verdicts are correct *because* scientific post-mortem evidence is used in the place of or as a substitute for the clinical evidence, and I venture to go one step further—that is, to say that this medical evidence is not so frequently forthcoming as it should be. I believe it would be forthcoming in a very much larger proportion of cases if efforts were made to procure it, and efforts in the right direction. How is it we refuse certificates? It is that the death did not quite accord with what we believe to be the natural procedure of a person's life, or of his disease, etc., and, if a post-mortem examination is made disease may or may not be found. But the medical evidence would still be forthcoming. I understand a coroner's business is to find out by what means this person came by his death ; and I say unhesitatingly it is absolute nonsense to view the dead body without making an internal examination. In the case of the girl referred to by one speaker, who died after he had seen her, I have a strong suspicion of the cause of her death even now, because there is practically only one cause of acute abdominal pain fatal in half an hour or so, and that is ruptured ectopic gestation. That could have been proved or disproved in five minutes by a post-mortem examination. There is another little criticism, and that is with regard to "found drowned." That is an exceedingly wrong verdict, absolutely wrong, and should never be permitted by a coroner. "Found in the river" if you like. "Found drowned" is an absolutely different matter, and the verdict should be, if there is no evidence of drowning—and that is fairly conclusive, water in the stomach and in the lungs, and so on (froth in the passages means nothing)—but if there is no evidence of anything of that sort "found in the river" would be the proper verdict to return. Then there is your own case, sir, which you suggested. I will present a little problem to you, which you can think over at your leisure. A man is cleaning a window thirty feet from the ground. He is seen to fall to the ground. He is picked up with his skull battered in, having fallen on to the hard pavement. What is the cause of death? Is it possibly epilepsy which caused him to fall? Is it hæmorrhage into his brain which likewise caused him to fall? Was it a person who tipped the ladder and caused him to fall, either maliciously or by accident? Or was it the fractured skull which formed the final stage? There is where our trouble comes in—of deciding why he fell. The cause of death might, or might not, be obvious. However, I can only say I am very much obliged for the interest you have all taken, and I hope this discussion may at some future time be useful when the question of the reconsideration of the Coroners Act comes more to the front. I feel certain that the time is distinctly ripe for a radical change in coroners' inquests altogether—a very radical change. An inquest, to my mind, is an exceedingly cumbrous mode of inquiring into what is, as most coroners admit, in 50 per cent. of the cases natural death. I say that in those 50 per cent. of cases an inquest in the ordinary sense of the word as now carried out was totally unnecessary. Whether a post-mortem examination was necessary or not is another matter, but an inquest certainly not.

Mr. JUSTICE WALTON said : As to the case you put, Dr. Smith, I had to argue a case of that kind some time ago, and I should say it is a very doubtful case. If the man was on the scaffold and was knocked off the scaffold by the tumbling down of Charing Cross Station, and he fell and broke his skull, I should not think a post-mortem examination would scarcely be necessary. There are certain cases in which the facts speak for themselves.

THE CLINICAL JOURNAL,

CLINICAL RECORD, CLINICAL NEWS, CLINICAL GAZETTE, CLINICAL REPORTER, CLINICAL CHRONICLE AND CLINICAL REVIEW.

EDITED BY L. ELIOT CREASY.

No. 702. **WEDNESDAY, APRIL 11, 1906.** **Vol. XXVII. No. 26.**

CONTENTS.

NOTICE.

Editorial correspondence, books for review, &c., should be addressed to the Editor, 51, *New Cavendish Street, W., Telephone No.* 904, *Paddington ; but all business communications should be addressed to the Publishers,* 22½, *Bartholomew Close, London, E.C. Telephone* 927, *Holborn.*

All inquiries respecting Advertisements should be sent to MESSRS. ADLARD & SON, *Bartholomew Close, E.C. Telephone* 927, *Holborn.*

Terms of Subscription, including postage, payable by cheque, postal or banker's order (in advance) : for the United Kingdom, 15s. 6d. *per annum ; Abroad,* 17s. 6d.

Cheques, &c., should be made payable to THE PROPRIETORS OF THE CLINICAL JOURNAL, *crossed " The London, City, and Midland Bank, Ltd., Newgate Street Branch, E.C. Account of the Medical Publishing Company, Limited."*

Reading Cases to hold Twenty-six numbers of THE CLINICAL JOURNAL *can be supplied at* 2s. 3d. *each, or will be forwarded post free on receipt of* 2s. 6d. ; *and also Cases for binding Volumes at* 1s. *each, or post free on receipt of* 1s. 3d., *from the Publishers,* 22½ *Bartholomew Close, London, E.C.*

The Index and Title-page for Vol. XXVII will be published with the next issue of THE CLINICAL JOURNAL.

A CLINICAL LECTURE

ON

GONORRHŒA IN WOMEN.

Delivered at Charing Cross Hospital.

By AMAND ROUTH, M.D., F.R.C.P.,

Obstetric Physican and Lecturer on Midwifery to the Hospital.

GENTLEMEN,—Gonorrhœa is a disease caused by specific infection by the gonococcus discovered in 1879 by Neisser. In 1885 Baum succeeded in growing it and separating it from other diplococci. I shall refer later to the difficulties in the scientific identification of this organism.

In males gonorrhœa is relatively trifling, though, of course, there are many exceptions. In women it is one of the most serious diseases, especially as regards the danger, during or at some time subsequent to the acute attack, of the internal pelvic organs becoming involved. The more remote risks and complications are also very serious, and may render a woman a permanent invalid, or, if married, may cause her to be sterile. Gonorrhœa is far more serious in a woman than syphilis, especially when it is remembered that if the husband has a neglected chronic gonorrhœal urethritis, euphemistically called " gleet," he may reinfect his wife after she is apparently cured, for, unlike syphilis, an attack of gonorrhœa does not render the patient immune. A woman too may have her endometrium reinfected after being cured, by discharges from a gonorrhœal salpingitis.

With regard to the symptoms of gonorrhœa in women, it is better, I think, for the sake of making things plain, to divide cases of the disease into two main groups, those which begin in a sudden acute manner, and those which come on insidiously. There are, of course, a large number of cases which do not come into either of those groups, cases which really are between the two, but, speaking generally, those are the two chief types of gonorrhœa in the female sex.

Let us take first the *acute form*, that which comes on quite suddenly. We can take the case of a woman who is perfectly healthy, newly married we will say. Her husband has not quite got over an acute gonorrhœa. He infects his wife and after the incubation stage she develops the acute disease. The incubation period of gonorrhœa is not like that of measles or scarlatina, lasting a definite time ; it varies with the severity of the attack. If it is going to be a very sharp, acute attack the incubation period is short, perhaps two or three days. If it is going to be a mild attack, the incubation is longer, perhaps five days. You see that question of incubation exemplified best in cases of ophthalmia neonatorum. A woman with this disease is confined, say, on Monday, and if it is going to be a sharp attack, almost certainly by Wednesday night or Thursday morning the child will have a smart attack of conjunctivitis. If it is going to be a mild attack, it will perhaps be another day or two before anything is seen. So the disease runs an incubation period of varying length. The first thing a woman notices when she has this acute attack coming on is that the parts are very hot and dry, and that passing water causes her pain. So one of the first symptoms is painful micturition. The parts are swollen and very tender, as well as hot and dry. In about two or three days the patient gets a profuse discharge, the swelling goes down a little, and the soreness is perhaps a little less marked. But the painful micturition continues, and she has this irritating, thick, purulent discharge. Sometimes the swelling is so great, especially in women who have not had children, that the pus in the vagina cannot get away properly, owing to the swelling of the hymen and introitus vaginæ, and therefore remains pent up and sometimes decomposes, so that it may become very offensive. If you saw the patient under those circumstances you would find it very difficult to examine her because of the great tenderness. It is a good plan, before anything is done in the way of a thorough examination of the parts, to foment them, or to let the patient sit in a hip bath and to have the vagina douched, either with warm water or some sedative such as warm borax solution (ʒij. to Oiij). After two or three days of rest and douching and other treatment you are able to find

out exactly what is amiss, and you can, perhaps, pass a speculum and see the extent of the mischief caused. You will find that the vagina is bright red—intensely red—and that the vaginal portion of the mucous membrane is also bright red, and very likely pus is coming out of the cervix too. If the vagina is primarily involved the cervix follows within a few days, and you will sometimes find the vulva, vagina, endocervix, and urethra all inflamed in a week. If that acute stage is untreated it will go on for another ten days or a fortnight, and then the discharge will get less, and it might pass on into the chronic form without anything happening. On the other hand, it may lead to endometritis, salpingitis, and perimetritis, together with other complications of which we shall speak presently.

I will relate to you a case which I saw not very long ago—that is to say, during last year—because it bears out most of these points. The patient had been married nine years and had had two children. Her husband, who was apparently a respectable man, took too much to drink one night and had connection with a strange woman. Two days after that impure connection he went with his wife and the following day he had a severe urethritis—that is to say, the incubation period was three days. Two days after he had had connection with his wife she developed great vulvar pain and painful micturition. A day or two later she had a profuse leucorrhœa, and the doctor found that pus was coming from the urethra, showing that there was definite urethritis. Her period came on ten days after this, with severe dysmenorrhœa, showing that the endometrium had become inflamed. A few days after that she had severe bilateral pain in the ovarian regions, probably pointing to the occurrence of salpingitis. A few days afterwards she had a rigor with acute pain in those regions, and abdominal swelling. No doubt she had an attack of perimetritis, spreading from the tubes. I saw her about a month after this with her doctor, and the abdomen was then distended with a hypogastric tumour due to matted bowel roofing over the inflamed pelvis. The tumour was tender, resonant, and elastic. *Per vaginam* I found the uterus was absolutely fixed by a large exudation in Douglas's pouch and behind the broad ligaments, and *per rectum* a distinct swelling of the tubes could be felt on each side. The swelling reached down two inches along the posterior wall of the vagina. In a few days she was very much better. I changed an alternating morphia and purgative treatment which the doctor had been giving her, and put her upon sulphate of magnesia, a drachm every three hours. Although for twenty-four hours she was in a good deal of pain the changed treatment made a lot of difference, and she soon got well. I saw her a fortnight ago—that is to say, after four or five months—and the uterus was movable to a great extent, but there was pus still coming away from the endometrium, showing that the gonorrhœal infection of the endometrium is not yet well, and it will probably require some local treatment before she is cured. She still has profuse menstruation, lasting fourteen days, followed by leucorrhœa for ten days.

Now, with regard to the *insidious form.* That form comes on as a rule in a newly married woman whose husband has had a gleet for many years, which, for some time, had been supposed to be cured. He has very likely gone to a doctor, perhaps the doctor who treated him for his gonorrhœa, and asked if he may marry. The doctor makes a superficial examination, does not find any evidence of the disease, and says "yes." Or perhaps he does not realise the danger of a gleety husband, and says he may marry. Great care should be taken in recommending marriage to a man who has had gonorrhœa. The patient should be told to notice the urethral orifice the first thing in the morning to see if there is any sticking together of the lips, or if any flaky urine is passed in the morning. If there is, you may be sure there is some chronic urethritis still, and he should see a surgeon and have the discharge examined bacteriologically for gonococci, because it is well to recognise that there is such a thing as latent gonorrhœa. You must realise that a man or woman—the man as a rule in the glands of the urethra and the woman in her cervix and endocervix—may have a few lurking gonococci, which produce apparently no symptoms in the individual, but when passed into the genital passages of another will set up active mischief by direct infection. In such a case you find, for instance, that if the woman has a catarrh in the cervix of gonorrhœal origin, she may infect a man pretty smartly, and he, if he resumes connection with her, will re-infect her, and light up the old mischief. Although one attack of syphilis renders a patient immune one

attack of gonorrhœa does not do so. Some people think the contrary is the case.

I will now read you the notes of a case of what one would call latent gonorrhœa. Mrs. J. G—, married, no children. The patient consulted me in 1888 for inflamed glands in the groin. I found she had vulvitis and vaginitis, urethritis, and some swelling of Bartholin's glands. In a subsequent interview with the husband I found he had had connection with a woman several times and had had some balanitis and urethritis and had also inflamed inguinal glands, which eventually suppurated and were treated by Mr. Stanley Boyd. He was so certain (and so was the woman in question) that she was healthy, that she consulted me to prove it. I found, however, that she had had an inflammatory attack after coitus four years previously and had had leucorrhœa and occasionally dysuria since. There was a chronic endometritis, and I have no doubt that this was a case of latent gonorrhœa and that gonococci, present in the cervical glands, had infected the husband and that he had subsequently infected his wife, the gonococci becoming more virulent in the new environment. There was no evidence of syphilis in either husband or wife.

Next, I want to speak about *treatment.* As soon as the acute stage is a little lessened an attempt should be made to stop the further progress of the disease. After douching the vagina pass a duck-bill speculum and draw down the cervix, the patient being by preference under anæsthesia. Then apply strong iodine solution, the liquor (1 in 9), or better still a stronger solution (1 in 4), to the endocervix as far as the internal os. This can be done through a Fergusson's speculum if preferred.

Having in that way purified the cervix, the object being to kill the gonococci, you then apply nitrate of silver solution, about a drachm to the ounce, to the whole of the vagina. There are not many glands in the vagina, but there are some. I prefer to apply nitrate of silver because it has such good results. When applying this nitrate of silver through a Fergusson's speculum and drawing the speculum slowly, out, the nitrate of silver colours the whole of the vagina a milky white, and that whiteness enables you to judge whether you have applied it to every part. After seeing that every part has been touched by this solution, withdraw the speculum gradually, and paint the whole of the vulva in exactly the same way. Then there is nothing left but the urethra to do. That is a very painful organ, and I generally apply pure carbolic acid along it on a Playfair's probe. Carbolic acid ceases to hurt the patient after a few minutes—it is its own sedative, as it were—and one application rarely fails to cure. This method of treatment will often cure a patient at the one sitting. Sometimes the procedure has to be repeated in five or six days, as there is a tendency for it to come back again. Although it is sometimes rather scoffed at, you will find it is an excellent way of cutting short these attacks of gonorrhœa in women. This can be done in the acute or the subacute stage, as well as in chronic cases where the gonococci are lingering. If the catarrh is very bad it is a good plan to give oil of yellow sandalwood in capsules, 15 drops three times a day. It does not produce a rash, as is the case with copaiba or cubebs, and the capsule can be easily taken. I have, however, now given that up in favour of salol. Some prefer urotropine, 7 grains. But salol in 5-grain doses three times a day in cachets is an excellent urinary antiseptic. This substance divides up in the stomach into salicylic acid and carbolic acid, and comes away as both in the urine, so that it disinfects the whole urinary tract and soon cures any persistent urethritis which is not of a specific character. Of course the patient must be douched every day, and the best plan is to use plain water first, or boric acid in water, and then use lead or sulphate of zinc solution, a drachm to the pint, so as to get into every nook and cranny of the vagina. In chronic cases this sort of treatment is usually enough, but if it has spread on into the uterus other treatment is required, as we shall see presently.

With regard to the *diagnosis*, if you can get a definite history of gonorrhœa you can be fairly sure what you are dealing with. But histories in these matters are notoriously unreliable, so it is better to proceed apart from such history. There is first of all the sudden onset, and the presence of thick pus in the meatus. Of course, if the gonococcus could be distinguished with scientific certainty that would be an end of the matter ; we should have far less trouble in being absolutely certain than we have now. But I have often been disappointed by failure to get the gonococcus discovered in secretions from cases which have been almost certainly

of specific origin. In chronic cases gonococci persist in the cervix longer, but are often absent from the urethra and the vagina fourteen days after the acute stage has passed. Even in prostitutes with leucorrhœa gonococci were only found in three per cent., though Kapytowski found that eight per cent. of healthy prostitutes had gonococci in their vaginal secretion. Klein states that women may become accustomed to the presence of gonococci, but that the organism will infect a healthy male with virulence, and that he in turn can cause reinfection of the same woman. Apparently the conjunctiva and urethra and vagina of animals are immune to this infection. You will see at once that the scientific discovery of gonococci becomes extremely important in many medico-legal cases, because you know that if a woman is infected by her husband with gonorrhœa or syphilis it is called legal cruelty, and the husband can be divorced for this cruelty *plus* desertion. In the absence of cruelty desertion is not a sufficient cause for divorce, neither is adultery of itself. I need scarcely say that in the absence of certainty as regards either history or clinical course or where gonococci are absent, it would never do for a doctor to definitely state that a woman had gonorrhœa from her husband. You must get the facts before you state them, and it is much better merely to state the strong probability rather than the certainty under such circumstances.

I will give you the following memoranda as regards the *bacteriological tests* for gonococci. You will doubtless notice that new tests are being sought for to prove the presence of gonococci. As a matter of fact I find bacteriologists are very reluctant to swear in a medico-legal case that gonococci were certainly present, and you will see that a skilled cross-examination could throw much doubt upon the scientific certainty of most of the tests.

Mr. A. N. Leathem, our bacteriologist, believes that the gonococcus can in some cases be distinguished with scientific accuracy, and gives four points which are essential for the scientific identification of the organism.

These are :

(1) The shape and arrangement of the diplococcus.

(2) The occurrence of groups of cocci within the pus-cells.

(3) The staining reaction. Gonococci stain

well with the ordinary aniline stains but are decolorised by Gram's method.

The number of known pathogenic cocci which do not retain the stain by Gram's method is very small, and, excepting the gonococcus, they are not very likely to be found in the urethra. Of these non-Gram-staining cocci the *Diplococcus intracellularis meningitidis* resembles gonococcus also in shape and in occurring within the pus-cells. But culturally the difference between the two is distinct. *M. melitensis* is non-Gram-staining and is excreted in the urine, but is not likely to lead to difficulties in diagnosis.

(4) *Cultivation.*—Gonococcus is not grown easily in artificial culture media. A simple one that Mr. Leathem finds very satisfactory is human blood agar—that is, ordinary nutrient agar with a drop or two of human blood smeared over the surface. Gonococcus will not grow on ordinary agar. If a very small quantity of the suspected pus is planted on this blood agar and incubated at 37°C., gonoccocus if present will appear as small, almost transparent, greyish colonies in from twenty-four to forty-eight hours. From these colonies films are made and found to be decolorised by Gram's method. Subcultures are then made on blood agar and on ordinary agar. Again, the colonies should appear on the blood agar but the ordinary agar should remain sterile.

If only the first three tests are positive, and cultivation is unsuccessful or not attempted, the diagnosis is practically certain. But with the cultivation also giving a posititive result, Mr. Leathem thinks there would be no possible room for doubt about the identity of the organism. Unfortunately, in many cases of gonococcal infection gonococci cannot be detected—cases that have become chronic, and especially old cases in women in which the secretion is mucoid rather than purulent, and is crowded with all kinds of cocci and bacilli. In films from such cases very few pus-cells can be found and these do not as a rule contain any organism. Cultivation is not successful, the plates being overgrown by the numerous organisms present before the gonococci appear. A few non-Gram-staining diplococci are perhaps seen in films, but this, of course, is not sufficient evidence on which to base a diagnosis.

Drs. Gordon and Dunn ('Brit. Med. Journ.,' August 26th, 1905) advise that when a differential diagnosis is required between the various Gram-negative micrococci, a further test should be made as regards the power of the cocci to produce an acid reaction when cultivated in the lemco medium to which certain carbohydrates—viz. glucose, galactose, maltose, and saccharose—have respectively been added in the proportion of 1 per cent. Gonococci produce an acid reaction with the first two, but not with saccharose or maltose.

Wildholz ('Centralbl. f. Bakt.,' Feb. 14th, 1902) says that gonococci after culture on serum agar for four or five generations will grow on ordinary agar.

I now want to say something about the *complications*. Endometritis and metritis are not at all uncommon as complications. The gonococci will infect the endometrium and the patient gets a sensation of great pain and tenderness in the hypogastrium, and the discharge from the uterus becomes very profuse. Some have doubted whether gonococci really do penetrate the mucous membrane and get into the underlying tissue, but Wertheim says there is no doubt whatever that they do penetrate the mucous membrane into the submucous tissue, which in the case of the uterus is muscle. This explains why the uterus gets so very tender in many of these cases, and undoubtedly metritis actually does take place. Some people think that membranous dysmenorrhœa, where the entire membrane of the uterus is shed, is, in many cases, secondary to gonorrhœa. I do not think that is proved, however. If we find definite endometritis, the best treatment to prevent it going to the tubes is to seize hold of the uterus, under anæsthesia, with a volsellum, and dilate the cervix a little with bougies, and then apply strong iodine to the whole cavity. Some would curette, and that is not a bad plan, to curette at once and have done with it, and then apply strong iodide. In that way you will get down to any glands which by the curetting are left, and you may thereby save the patient from salpingitis and further complications. It is a good plan to keep the uterus a little open by gauze, for a week or two, by passing in on every second day a fresh piece of gauze dipped in iodine and glycerine, so as to get free drainage and an antiseptic application to the endometrium.

Another complication is salpingitis. That is merely a continuation of the inflammation in the endometrium. Sometimes it has no symptoms at all, sometimes it leads to a pyosalpinx being formed, and it will very often, if bilateral, lead to permanent sterility. Here are several good specimens. One shows inflammation of the tubes, with perimetric adhesions round them. It was of gonorrhœal origin. I do not know whether there was pus in that tube. Others of them are cases of pyosalpinx ; some are tubercular ; in others the condition is not stated, but they are very likely gonorrhœal. The treatment of salpingitis is the general treatment of inflammation, and keeping the vaginal passages antiseptic, insuring free drainage in case the tube wants to empty itself into the uterus. If a tube becomes adherent and distended, instead of the old plan of removing it by the abdomen, it is better and safer to incise it *per vaginam.* You simply do a posterior colpotomy—*i. e.* open the vagina posterior to the cervix and get into Douglas's pouch, feel the tube, and make a free incision into the tube and let the pus out. Then drain, or if you like apply some strong iodine to the cavity as I do. Then plug the opening which you have made in the tube with gauze, and leave it in for three or four days. After that you will find the tube will often quite recover itself. I remember a patient whose husband had gonorrhœal urethritis, and she became infected and as a consequence had double pyosalpinx. I opened both tubes through the vagina, and in less than a year she was pregnant again. And if the diagnosis was right, and I had opened both tubes, it showed that they had become again pervious. She miscarried at three or four months. Sänger found salpingitis in 33 per cent. of women who have had gonorrhœa. Ovarian abscesses have been described by many observers. The Fallopian tube becomes adherent to the ovary by means of lymph being thrown out, and it is easy for a Graafian follicle or corpus luteum to be infected and an abscess result there. Some observers believe that the present large number of tubal gestations which one comes across are due to gonorrhœa. But that, again, wants proving ; still, it confirms Lawson Tait's view, that purulent salpingitis was almost always present in tubal gestation. A further complication is perimetritis, which means that the inflammation has spread from the tubes to the peritoneum, and that lymph has been thrown out. And this, of course, is conservative. You very rarely indeed get a general peritonitis in these cases. Lymph is thrown out, the small intestines are matted together, roofing over the pelvis, and the general peritoneal cavity is shut off and saved from attack. Thus these cases rarely get general peritonitis.

Another complication is venereal warts, which are very troublesome and very infective. If a woman has a warty growth at the orifice of the vagina, a man is very apt, even if she has no gonococci present, to get warts on the penis. Much the best treatment for them is to snip them off and apply the actual cautery or the electric cautery to their bases, and then dust on powdered salicylic acid one part to two parts of oxide of zinc. That will prevent any recurrence. Buboes in the groin may occur if there is much vulvitis and ulceration of the vulva, and they should be treated on general principles. Urethritis is almost always present in gonorrhœa in women. You ascertain that fact by sponging or wiping away the discharge from the vulva and passing the finger into the vagina, bringing it back along the roof. You will then express pus through the urethra, and that should be tested for gonococci. Pure carbolic acid should be applied to the urethra. Cystitis very rarely follows gonorrhœa in women, partly because the urethra is so thoroughly washed out, as it is short and does not contain many glands and what glands there are, are in the floor. It is those glands which make the urethra feel so swollen and hard if you examine *per vaginam* in these cases. There are two main glands which you can sometimes see by everting the lips of the urethral orifice. These are Skene's ducts, which open just inside the urethra and run down into its floor. These are apt to become inflamed, and they remain inflamed after you have cured the urethra, and indeed they may reinfect the urethra, just as the endometrium may be reinfected after curetting if the tubes still contain gonococci. You very rarely get a periurethritis in these cases sufficient to produce retention of urine, and that is quite different to what happens in the male. I have seen a few cases of it in the female, but it occurs only very rarely. Proctitis, or inflammation of the rectum, is rare too. There are cases recorded, of course, in extremely depraved persons, of direct inoculation of the rectum by the disease. But in most cases of proctitis resulting from gonorrhœa it is due to a prolapsed pile becoming infected with the discharges from the genital canal. Again, infection of Bartholin's ducts and glands may supervene.

These glands become inflamed and may form suppurating retention cysts in consequence and they should be dissected out, because if you leave a piece of gland-tissue behind the inflammation will be restarted.

Ophthalmia is another complication of gonorrhœa, but we have not time to go into it to-day. Gonorrhœal rheumatism is another very important point. There is also the equally important and very interesting subject of gonococcal sepsis. Puerperal fever due to gonococci is one of the mooted points. There is a considerable diversity of opinion first of all as to the number of cases in which gonococci are found in a given series of cases of puerperal fever, and, secondly, when gonococci are found, as to their exact significance. Is it the fact that the gonococci produce puerperal fever, or does the gonococcus cause the suppuration and the pus thus produced form a suitable habitat for streptococci, staphylococci, and the other germs which are the causal factors in puerperal fever? I think this latter is the correct view. The presence of gonococci in the genital passages of a parturient woman is a serious matter; but they produce a local effect, and cause endometritis and salpingitis afterwards, and do not produce true puerperal fever or true general septicæmia. I think the other germs present are responsible for the general sepsis which is found associated with gonococci.

April 9th, 1906.

A BOOK of interest to the medical profession recently published is entitled ' On Leprosy and Fish-Eating,' by Jonathan Hutchinson. It comprises statements as to the history of leprosy, its nature, its prevalence in different countries, and the conditions under which it has disappeared from many. Facts are brought forward to show that it is not ordinarily contagious, and that its real cause is the use as food of badly cured fish. There are chapters on the influence of sex in relation to leprosy, of religious creed, and poverty. An account is given of the author's tours in South Africa and India, and the measures for the suppression of leprosy are fully discussed. The volume contains maps and illustrations, and is published by Archibald Constable and Co., Ltd.

SOME OF THE CLINICAL ASPECTS OF PNEUMONIA.

Being one of a series of Clinical Lectures delivered at the West London Hospital to the Post-Graduates.

By DONALD W. C. HOOD, C.V.O., M.D.,
F.R.C.P.,
Senior Physician to the Hospital.

GENTLEMEN,—On a former occasion [*] we discussed some of the varieties of the pneumonic process and your attention was called to those ambiguous conflicting symptoms which occasionally complicate an acute attack of inflammatory mischief within the chest—symptoms which from their character and local severity are apt to mislead us into thinking that the lesion is one of abdomen and not of chest. We have considered the peculiar nature of influenzal pneumonia and some of the complications which interfere with that critical fall of temperature so usual in cases of lobar pneumonia.

We will now discuss the anomalous symptoms principally met with in patients suffering from acute inflammation of the apex.

In many cases of pneumonia the general constitutional symptoms are of great severity. So intense, indeed, may they be that the true nature of the illness is in danger of being overlooked.

It is with pneumonia of the apex, especially when occurring amongst the young, that I have seen the most marked forms of constitutional disturbance. To some of these cases the words " brain fever" might be aptly applied—the brain fever of the novelist, and not that known to us as meningitis. The cerebral symptoms are paramount and may include headache, intolerance of light, vomiting, delirium, fits of screaming, retraction of the head, and restlessness.

To the superficial observer or one unacquainted with this peculiar phase of pneumonia these symptoms may readily be misleading, and the patient may be considered to be suffering from some form of cerebral disease.

You will find this interesting group of cases referred to by Henoch in his important work on diseases of children. He writes, when discussing the symptoms of pneumonia : " The latency of the physical symptoms, which may last from four to six

[*] ' Lancet,' December 30th, 1905.

days, along with the prominence of the cerebral and gastric symptoms, readily lead to the mistaken diagnosis of meningitis, or of typhoid fever, or even of intermittent fever, as I experienced in one case. Perhaps in such cases the pneumonia spreads gradually from the centre to the periphery, and only when it has reached this situation do the signs of consolidation appear distinctly. Whenever this does take place the gastric or cerebral symptoms which have hitherto been prominent usually now become less so, and the diagnosis at once becomes clear, but in some cases not until the fever is distinctly on the decline or may even have ended critically."

Ostler writes : " The disease may be entirely masked by the cerebral symptoms and the case mistaken for meningitis. It is remarkable in these cases how few indications there are of pulmonary trouble."

Personally I have often found that the severity of the cerebral symptoms have so completely effaced the ordinary clinical course of the pneumonia that the chest has not been carefully examined.

These cases may be grouped in three classes—those in which the cerebral symptoms precede consolidation by some days ; those in which the physical signs of pneumonia are concomitant with and easily to be detected at the period of excitement ; lastly, those in which the constitutional state is one of stupor and indifference, almost verging on coma. These cases, as regards diagnosis, may be of extreme difficulty, owing to the late development of physical signs in the lungs.

A child, æt. 2 years, was suddenly taken ill, with feverish symptoms, accompanied with intolerance of light, great restlessness, screaming, twitching of face and upper extremities. The temperature was 104·2° F. Meningitis had been diagnosed. On the fifth day of illness I first saw the child, and at this time there was distinct evidence of consolidation of the right apex. The temperature fell to below normal and all the nervous perturbation ceased. The cough gradually became less irritating, and as it lessened in frequency it began to assume paroxysmal characters, to be more pronounced at night, and to assume the symptoms of whooping-cough. The case resolved itself into one of that disease, commencing with an acute onset and complicated with a well-defined lobar

pneumonia. The prominent initial symptoms were certainly of cerebral type and concealed the true nature of the illness.

Within the past few months we have seen a similar case within our hospital. The patient, a child of five years, was admitted with apex pneumonia, accompanied by much excitement and constitutional disturbance. The local physical signs rapidly decreased, and whooping - cough gradually developed.

A child of nine years was brought to the hospital with a history of three days' cough, but advice was sought for symptoms which were more nervous than pulmonary : they were—delirium, screaming fits, sudden cries, restlessness, pain in head, intolerance of light, and rapid breathing. Evidence of lobar pneumonia was easily demonstrated, the inflammation being limited to the extreme upper lobe of the right lung. The attack speedily passed off, the third day after admission the temperature was subnormal and the physical signs less marked.

A very instructive case was one I saw with Dr. Elliot some years ago—a child of ten years, ill with fever, restlessness, wandering, and other constitutional symptoms of nerve type. We suspected pneumonia, but the local evidence of the inflammatory lesion did not appear until after the crisis had taken place.

Coma may be a symptom of apex pneumonia. A young girl was admitted under my care as a head case. She was apathetic, semi-conscious, lying in a drowsy condition, difficult to rouse. Her quick breathing and high temperature, which was 105° F., drew attention to the chest, where signs of apex pneumonia on the right side were clearly present. The inflammatory area was a very limited one, and the attack soon passed off, the temperature falling by crisis.

In any case, especially with children, it is important to bear well in mind that symptoms usually called cerebral, by which I mean twitching of muscles, headache, intolerance of light, vomiting, restlessness, delirium, stupor, may be symptomatic of pneumonia, just as they may, though far less frequently, initiate an attack of typhoid fever. These symptoms, when accompanied with a high temperature and quick inspiration, should always attract attention to the chest. Cough and expectoration may be very slight or entirely absent. You will find by experience that it is true that the more directly nervous the symptoms may be, the more violent the delirium, the more pronounced the constitutional excitement, the less likely it is that the patient is suffering from cerebral disease.

One is so accustomed to associate pneumonia with cough, rusty sputa, and easily defined physical signs, that cases in which for several days all these well-known symptoms are absent may prove both misleading and equivocal.

As one of the most common ordinary symptoms of pneumonia we recognise an expectoration of sputa coloured with blood. Every tint may be seen, from that which is but faintly rusty to a deep prune colour. We meet with varying amounts of hæmorrhage, and in some cases when the hæmorrhage is in large quantity the term " hæmorrhagic pneumonia " has been made use of.

Experience has taught me that occasionally a pneumonia of the apex may be accompanied by a sharp profuse hæmoptysis, and that, plus other symptoms, hæmoptysis may be symptomatic of pneumonia of the upper lobes. During the past twenty-four years I have paid special attention to conditions of apexpneumonia accompanied with hæmoptysis. Briefly, these cases group themselves under and are to be distinguished by the following symptoms : The patient in possession of ordinary health is taken ill with symptoms denoting a feverish chill. He spits up blood within a few hours of the first symptom of illness. The hæmoptysis may be of large or small quantity, and usually continues for four or six days, during which time the temperature is raised but is rarely or ever so high as that met with in ordinary lobar pneumonia. Usually under such conditions the chest cannot be thoroughly examined during the first few days of the attack, but when a careful complete examination is practicable very evident signs of consolidation can be found at the upper lobe of one or other lung. The physical signs are those ordinarily met with in lobar pneumonia. The period of consolidation is followed by the moist râles of crepitatio redux. The physical signs in the lung *completely clear up*, the patient regaining his usual strength.

The first case of this class occurred to me many many years ago, in the spring of 1881. I was hurriedly summoned to a patient staying at one of our large London hotels. The patient, a gentleman, æt. 35 years, was lying on his bed, and beside him was a basin containing about half a pint of blood, which he told me had been expectorated with cough. He had not been feeling well for a few days, but had not been prevented attending to his usual business in the City. He was on the point of starting for business when seized with the hæmorrhage, which commenced while at breakfast. During the meal he had a fit of coughing and noticed his handkerchief to be stained with blood. Retiring to the lavatory, he spat up much more, his handkerchief being soaked. I looked upon the case as one of ordinary hæmoptysis, and consequently did not wish to disturb the patient by a physical examination more than was absolutely necessary. Beyond noticing some fine crepitant râles under the left clavicle, I am in ignorance as to the condition of the lung at the time of my visit. One point, however, attracted my attention ; the temperature was high, being 101°. In all the previous cases of hæmoptysis that had been under my observation a depressed, usually subnormal, temperature had been invariably remarked. With regard to the previous history of this case, I learnt that three days before the attack of hæmorrhage, feeling out of sorts, he had consulted the late Sir William Gull, with whom I communicated, and was informed by him that he had carefully examined the patient's chest, and that at the time of the interview he considered it as being perfectly sound, the symptoms for which his advice was sought being those of an ordinary catarrh. Sir William Gull met me in consultation on the afternoon of the day on which the hæmoptysis occurred, and he suggested that the hæmorrhage was pneumonic, the area of inflammation being in the upper lobe of the left lung. The following day the chest was carefully examined. Posteriorly, on the left side, there was evident consolidation of the upper portion of the lung ; there was loss of resonance over the entire supra-spinous region, the dulness extending to a little below the spine of the scapula. The breath sounds over this area were loud and distinct, scarcely tubular, but when compared with the other side very markedly different. Vocal resonance was much increased. The constitutional symptoms remained the same, the temperature being from 101° to 102° ; the hæmorrhage had decreased. The illness lasted seven days, by the end of which time the temperature had fallen to normal and the expectoration had almost ceased. The latter had passed through various stages of colours, from bright crimson and frothy to a dark prune-juice-coloured sputum. The physical condition of the chest also showed improvement. There had been but slight increase in the total area affected; the dulness was not so marked, and by the time the patient was well there was but little, if any, trace left of the local mischief. From first to last I was extremely interested in the clinical phenomena presented by this patient. As I have before stated, it was new to me to find hæmoptysis accompanied by a high temperature, this increase of temperature being concomitant with the initial attack. Taken all in all, the case appeared to present many different aspects to those usually present with hæmorrhage arising from the pulmonary area, and I determined to pay special attention to all those instances of hæmoptysis which might subsequently come under my own observation, my intention being to try to ascertain if there was any connection, direct or indirect, between the inflammation of the upper lobe of the lungs and hæmoptysis.

Since the time when this patient came under my observation I have seen many cases of hæmoptysis, and I think I may affirm that scarcely a case has occurred with the symptoms alluded to without there being present physical symptoms of pneumonia of one of the upper lobes of the lung. The class of case to which my remarks refer is very fairly illustrated by the illness I have just described. Here was a patient presumably in good general health who within a few hours of the attack of hæmorrhage had been seen and carefully examined by one of the most astute clinical observers of the day. The patient's chest was considered normal, but within a short period of the examination he was suddenly seized with profuse hæmorrhage, the attack being accompanied with high temperature and all the physical symptoms pathognomonic of acute pneumonia of one lung. Moreover, in other respects the attack simulated in every particular the common ordinary symptoms of pneumonia. The consolidation passed away and as far as physical signs could help in giving us data for an opinion, the lung perfectly recovered from the inflammatory seizure. I say advisably that the physical signs denoted restoration of the normal texture of pulmonary tissue. I do not for a moment intend that my remarks should lead you to think that I do not attach the gravest import-

ance to such a marked symptom as hæmoptysis, whether it be caused, as I believe to be the case, by a hyperæmia accompanying pneumonic consolidation or arising as a consequence of a more decided tissue degeneration. Since the time of Hippocrates hæmoptysis has rightly been looked upon as a symptom of gravity. But I do consider that a hæmorrhage occurring in connection with pyrexia and accompanied with evident physical symptoms of pneumonic consolidation is not of such grave importance as are, undoubtedly, other cases of hæmoptysis. It may be argued that hæmoptysis is usually accompanied with fever, and further, that physical symptoms of consolidation are very usual in ordinary conditions of tuberculous disease, but with those patients whose symptoms I am describing the pyrexia does not precede the attacks of hæmorrhage, and the temperature, remaining raised for some days, falls to normal and remains so, an entirely different class of pyrexia to that so well known during the course of tubercular mischief. The physical symptoms of consolidation pass completely away; the lungs as regards physical signs of disease become absolutely normal.

I will now very briefly bring before you the clinical facts of importance which I believe are usually present in patients the subjects of pneumonic hæmoptysis.

A man æt. 21 years was admitted under my care into the North-West London Hospital on July 6th, 1887. The patient had been in good health up to two days before admission, when he considered he had caught cold and suffered from an irritating cough. The evening before admission he spat up blood and was admitted as a case of hæmoptysis. The hæmorrhage amounted to several ounces; it was mixed with sputa and was of a bright colour. The temperature on admission was 101·5° F. and remained above 100° F. till the eighth day of his illness; on the morning of that day it fell to 98° F.; rising again slightly for a few days more, it assumed its normal range. The hæmorrhage, rather profuse for the first forty-eight hours, gradually ceased and the colour of the blood darkened. A physical examination of the patient's chest disclosed consolidation of the right apex, which was looked upon as being pneumonic. It rapidly cleared up, and at the patient's discharge there was no appreciable difference, as far as auscultation and percussion assisted us in giving an opinion, between one side of the chest and the other. Two years later this patient applied to me at my house in reference to a life assurance. I examined him at that time and could detect nothing wrong with either lung. He was also examined by the medical officer attached to the insurance office and his life was accepted.

A man æt. 48 years was admitted into the North-West London Hospital on June 19th, 1890. He was then suffering from rather profuse hæmoptysis, which had commenced on the morning of admission and continued during the day, two ordinary spitoons being filled with sputum, mixed largely with bright blood. The temperature was noted as being 101·4° F. It remained high for the succeeding eight days. It gradually fell and remained normal till discharge. He was under observation in the hospital for twenty-eight days. During the first day or so of illness, in consequence of profuse hæmorrhage, no very exact physical examination of the chest was made. When the condition of the patient permitted it, the right upper lobe was found to be consolidated. There was marked dulness over and above the spine of the scapula, tubular breathing being heard over this region. A few days later all signs of consolidation were gone, and when the patient was discharged there was no appreciable difference between the two lungs.

A man æt. 35 years while at work spat up a large quantity of blood-stained sputum. On admission into the North-West London Hospital on May 28th, 1890, he was noted as being well-nourished and an apparently healthy man. He was coughing up blood, and the hæmoptysis continued for about forty-eight hours ; the blood was intimately mixed with sputa. The temperature on admission was 101·6° F. ; on the sixth day of illness it was normal, remaining so during the time the patient continued in hospital—nineteen days. There was dulness and tubular breathing at the right upper lobe of the lung, these symptoms being followed by moist râles, which gradually subsided. At the date of discharge there were no physical symptoms denoting pulmonary mischief.

R. W—, a man æt. 40 years, was admitted into the West London Hospital under my care on December 4th, 1898. The patient was suffering from hæmoptysis. He stated that during the previous night he woke up coughing and found that he was spitting up blood. He estimated the amount lost at that time at half a pint. He was expectorating blood while in the casualty-room. The man was well nourished and strong, but had stigmata on the face and a slight enlargement of the liver. He owned to be a hearty beer-drinker. During the first few days following admission it was not thought advisable to make any very thorough examination of the chest. The hæmorrage was severe; during the first few days of admission he had expectorated seventy ounces of blood.

On admission the temperature was 101° F. During the first few hours the hæmorrhage amounted to twenty-six ounces. On the fifth day the chest was carefully examined. There was evidence of consolidation of the upper lobe of the right lung ; there was no sign of disease in the left lung. Connected with this area of consolidation there were all the objective symptoms of a lobar pneumonia. The clinical condition was clear and unmistakable.

On the eighth day of illness the symptoms were still more difficult to interpret. The sputa was now barely blood-stained; it was muco-purulent and tenacious. Over the entire upper lobe of the affected lung large moist bubbling râles were to be heard. The evidence was strongly in favour of a rapid breaking down of lung-tissue. Gradually the moist sounds cleared up, and on the twenty-ninth of December—i. e. within one month of admission— there was no remaining lesion that could be discovered. The patient was kept under observation for twenty days after all lung symptoms had disappeared. His general health was good, temperature normal. There was no expectoration or night sweats. His appetite was healthy, his sleep undisturbed. The sputa had been examined on several occasions, but no trace of the tubercle bacillus could be found.

In the 'Lancet' in June, 1886, I published a series of cases in which a sharp hæmoptysis had been the initial symptom of an apex pneumonia.

In August, 1894, in a lecture published in the 'Lancet' in that month, I again alluded to several similar cases. The patients whose cases I have briefly described are typical instances of the class of hæmoptysis which I believe is almost invariably accompanied with pneumonia of the upper lobe of one or other lung, the hæmorrhage being often of large amount, occurring in a presumably healthy subject and coincident with well-marked physical symptoms of pneumonia. During the attack the temperature is raised, falling to normal and remaining so after all the lung symptoms have completely resolved.

I think it will be generally conceded that this is not the ordinary course followed by those patients in whom hæmoptysis is evidently of tubercular origin.

An old house physician wrote to me in May, 1889, from the Calcutta Hospital describing a severe case of hæmoptysis accompanied with pneumonia of the upper lobe. A sailor æt 26 years was admitted into hospital for profuse hæmoptysis and consolidation of left upper lobe, the temperature being 103° F. The hæmorrhage was large, a pint of blood being coughed on one occasion. The pneumonia gradually affected the entire left lung and the patient died. On examination after death the conditions found were those of an ordinary lobar pneumonia.

In February, 1892, I saw with Mr. Blackett a young woman who during the previous night had been suddenly seized with spitting blood. There was a raised temperature and the ordinary physical signs of consolidation of the left apex. Within a few days the physical symptoms had cleared up, the temperature fell to normal, and the patient made a complete recovery. A year or more later I heard of her as keeping perfectly well.

In February, 1901, I had under my care a patient suffering from pneumonia following a sharp attack of influenza. The pneumonia was limited to the left apex, and was ushered in with profuse hæmoptysis and a temperature of 104° F. The pneumonia finally subsided, and within a fortnight there was no apparent pulmonary lesion. A year later there was no symptom of chest mischief, recovery being complete. In this case the hæmorrhage continued for several days.

Another case was that of a man æt 43 years, admitted into hospital in December, 1902. He had been perfectly well up to three days before admission. His temperature was 103° F., and he was spitting up blood in rather large quantity. There was well-marked consolidation at upper part of left lung. Seven days after admission the temperature fell to normal. The general condition of the patient was in every way satisfactory. On January 6th I could detect no sign of disease in the chest, and the man was discharged apparently completely restored to health.

I have not myself seen any patient die while suffering from this form of hæmorrhagic pneumonia, but some years ago during an autumn absence from town a patient was admitted into my ward suffering from hæmoptysis and pyrexia. The patient succumbed to the attack and on making an examination after death the only discoverable lesion was that of pneumonia of the right apex.

April 9th, 1906.

A CASE OF
APPENDIX ABSCESS WITH PROFUSE HÆMORRHAGES; RECOVERY.

By JOHN D. MALCOLM, F.R.C.S.Ed.,
Surgeon to the Samaritan Free Hospital.

THE subject of the following history was an unmarried woman, æt. 36 years, who had a long record of indefinite discomfort, rather than pain, in the appendix region. The symptoms were always attributed to indigestion, and were for the most part made light of. In the summer of 1905, when it was noted that the patient was particularly well, she was suddenly seized with severe abdominal pain. The temperature rose, and after three days was 102·8° F., the pulse being about 100 at this time. The temperature then fell very gradually during six days to 101·6° F.

I saw the patient in consultation on the ninth day of the illness. She had then a tender swelling in the region of the vermiform appendix, with impaired resonance on firm percussion to the inner side of the right anterior superior iliac spine, but there was no complete dulness. The pulse was from 80 to 90, the general condition was good, the abdomen was not distended, and the bowels were easily evacuated by laxatives. I agreed with the diagnosis already made, that pus had formed around the vermiform appendix, and it was decided that an immediate operation for its evacuation should be undertaken. At noon I cut down upon the parts by an incision parallel to and about three quarters of an inch from the outer portion of Poupart's ligament. Although I separated the peritoneum deeply from its attachments and prolonged the incision towards the loin, I did not seem to get in touch with an abscess wall. The parts were everywhere soft, as if adherent bowel intervened between my fingers in the wound and the pus which I believed to be present. To make certain of the relations, I opened the abdominal cavity in the middle line and found that the head of the cæcum was everywhere surrounded by adhesions. Behind and rather to its inner side I made out a very soft fluctuating swelling about the size of a tennis-ball between a finger in the peritoneal cavity and one in my first wound. By pushing the cæcum further forwards and inwards I was able to insert a pair of forceps through the lateral incision into an abscess behind the bowel and to evacuate four or five ounces of exceedingly foul, thin, and rather dark-coloured pus. As the appendix was not at once felt, I did not make any search for it, but, after washing out the cavity with weak iodine and water solution, put in a rubber tube with a lumen of about half an inch in diameter and also a small sized one. The posterior part of the wound was closed by sutures. The median incision was sewn up also, it gave no trouble at any time, and although the bowels required laxatives and enemata there was never any cause for anxiety in connection with the peritoneum.

The patient's condition was satisfactory for three days, the temperature falling gradually, but the discharge continued to be very offensive. In the early morning of the third day, after sleeping off and on for nearly four hours, the patient felt something liquid running over her side, and, on examination, the dressings were found to be soaked with fresh blood. In a short time the temperature dropped a degree to $99 \cdot 4°$ F., and on changing the dressings it was obvious that there had been a very considerable hæmorrhage. Although the discharge was still foul the blood appeared quite healthy, and by means of a pair of forceps a complete cast of the smaller tube was withdrawn. Blood then welled up freely through this tube with a distinctly pulsating action, but it gradually ceased to flow. I padded the region to the inside of the wound very firmly, and the syringing with weak antiseptic solution, which had been performed twice daily, was discontinued. An oozing of dark blood continued, but the patient seemed fairly well. The temperature rose to $101 \cdot 4°$ F., and then gradually fell until the sixth day, when there was another hæmorrhage, so free that the patient fainted and became cold, her condition for a little while being very alarming. Strychnia and ergotin were injected before I arrived, and the condition of collapse was quickly recovered from.

The part of the side wound which had been sewn up had appeared to heal well until the fourth day, when some of the stitch-holes were red and inflamed and the sutures which caused the most irritation were then taken out. After the second hæmorrhage it was obvious that blood had been forced along the deep layers of the incision, and that all the scar-tissue was breaking down,

whilst some of the suture-holes were suppurating. It was also obvious that an attempt must be made to find and to tie the bleeding point. Before reopening the wound it was thought desirable that a consultation should be held and Mr. Clutton saw the patient. He agreed that the wound should be opened up, and it was conjectured that a sloughing appendix might be found in the abscess cavity and that the hæmorrhage arose from some vessels in its mesentery. On the seventh day I reopened the lateral wound and made a larger communication between the abscess cavity and the superficial parts by tearing the peritoneum freely. The deep cavity was distended by blood, and although there was still a very foul odour from the discharge, the clot was so firm that more than once I thought I might be pulling out the sloughed appendix. When all the clot was cleared away, however, no appendix was discovered. It was impossible to see the abscess walls, but some protruding tissues on their inner surface were removed and these were obviously appendices epiploicæ. My knowledge of the position of adhesions, obtained by having had my fingers in the peritoneal cavity at the first operation, enabled me to make a thorough exploration with safety. There was no fresh hæmorrhage and no bleeding point was discovered. On the new surface made by my incision there were several black, well-defined sloughs, of small size, not more than about one third of an inch in length and not extending deeply. The wound was lightly packed with gauze, and from this time convalescence was steadily progressive. In three days the discharge was not offensive, but there were still some sloughs to separate. When these came away union by granulation was very rapid. For a considerable time after the second operation there was a discharge of mucus, which must have come from the remains of the appendix, but the parts healed completely and the patient was able to leave London, with a practically closed wound, just over seven weeks from the date of the second operation. Six weeks later the incision was firmly healed and the scar was almost linear. The patient complained of a slight tenderness over the cæcal region, which might have been due to the condition of the appendix or possibly to the presence of adhesions. From the fact that the wound healed rapidly although there was a free discharge of mucus, it seemed certain that the communication between the appendix cavity and the cæcum was fairly free, whilst the flaccid condition of the abscess at the date of operation also favoured the view that a partial discharge was taking place through the appendix at that time. Its proximal part, and possibly the whole of the appendix, would therefore seem to be still in the body. The most recent account of this patient is that she has not suffered any pain, whilst the general health and the powers of digestion are improving

Hæmorrhage in connection with appendicitis is a rare complication, which may, however, occur in various ways.

Dr. Kelly and Dr. Hurdon * quote a case of fatal hæmorrhage from the epigastric artery which had been clamped, but not ligatured, in a child, and another in which six days after the resection of an appendix which was in a quiescent condition the patient passed an enormous quantity of blood *per rectum* and vomited between 300 and 400 c.c. of blood mixed with the contents of the stomach. The patient recovered with no more serious disturbance than the great fright.' The hæmorrhage in this case was attributed by the operator to slipping of a ligature.

The same authors, in describing the "symptoms of acute appendicitis," said that " Hæmatemesis has been described by Treves, by Dieulafoy, and by Matheson and others, and is attributed generally to a toxic degeneration of the gastric mucous membrane, with erosion of small blood-vessels." † They also stated that " in a few instances the erosion of a large blood-vessel occurring during the course of an appendicitis or as a post-operative complication has led to a fatal termination. Osler ('Montreal Hosp. Gaz.,' 1880) mentions an instance of fatal hæmorrhage into the intestine, Matheson *(loc. cit.)* a fatal hæmatemesis, and Lendet ('Arch. Gén. de Méd.,' vol. civ, p. 140) a case of hæmorrhage into the arachnoid space. The symptoms are those commonly produced by internal hæmorrhage and as a rule positive evidence is found in the passage of blood by the mouth or by the rectum." ‡

Mr. W. H. Battle and Mr. E. M. Corner des-

cribed hæmorrhage from the bowel in these cases as usually arising either near the site of the appendix or at the hepatic flexure of the colon. In the former situation they attributed the bleeding to causes arising within the bowel and in the latter to mischief coming from outside it. They said, however, that the connection between the appendix mischief and the hæmorrhage was not clear. * Three of the following cases are mentioned by these authors.

Dr. Charles B. Box and Mr. Cuthbert S. Wallace have published a case of " appendicitis with profuse hæmorrhage closely resembling typhoid fever." † After the patient had been ill for sixteen days there was a discharge of bright red blood from the bowel to the extent of half a pint. A similar discharge recurred twice, and on each occasion the bright blood was followed by some darker material. Death followed on the twenty-first day. An abscess round the appendix was found at the autopsy, with a secondary focus of suppuration in front of the right kidney and communicating with the adjacent colon.

A case resembling mine, but in which the hæmorrhage was a less urgent symptom, was published by Mr. Langton and Sir Dyce Duckworth.‡ A boy, æt. 16 years, had an appendix abscess opened six days after his illness began, two-thirds of the appendix being found gangrenous and the pus being very fœtid. The appendix with a concretion was removed and the parts were drained. On the eighth day after the appendix abscess was opened the patient complained of some pain and at the next dressing a large clot was found over the wound. The patient recovered and the hæmorrhage did not recur, although a secondary intra-peritoneal abscess formed on the left side of the abdomen and had to be evacuated and drained.

A much more severe case, as regards the hæmorrhage, has been recorded by Mr. F. Ramsay of Tasmania. The patient's age was 10 years, and about a month after the first symptoms occurred between three and four ounces of pus were evacuated from an appendix abscess and the cavity was drained by means of gauze and a rubber

---

* ' The Vermiform Appendix and its Diseases ' by Dr. Howard A. Kelly and Dr. E. Hurdon, p. 662.

† *Loc. cit.*, p. 391.

‡ *Loc. cit.*, p. 404.

---

* ' Diseases of the Vermiform Appendix and their Surgical Complications,' by Mr. W. H. Battle and Mr. E. M. Corner, p. 177.

† ' Lancet,' vol. i., 1903, p. 1588.

‡ ' Med.-Chir. Trans.,' vol. lxxii, p. 433.

tube. On the ninth and on the eleventh days after the operation there were severe hæmorrhages and the bleeding was not stopped until the external iliac artery was tied from the inside of the peritoneal sac and its distal end from inside the abscess, there being a large opening in this vessel. The patient recovered.*

Another, a fatal case, was put on record by Dr. John O'Connor of Buenos Ayres. A middle-aged man who refused to be operated on had his cæcal region poulticed for six weeks. No discharge took place, and the medical attendant was then allowed to make "a little cut just big enough to let out the matter." Toxic symptoms rapidly disappeared and the purulent discharge had almost ceased after ten days. The patient then felt wet, his dressings were found to be saturated with blood, and he "rapidly succumbed." There was no post-mortem examination.†

There can be little doubt that in the last three cases and in my own case the hæmorrhage was exactly comparable to that which we read about as "secondary hæmorrhage," and which was quite common before the days of antiseptics, being due to sloughing of the wall of some vessel.

In those pre-antiseptic days the infection was frequently carried from case to case on the hands or instruments of the surgeon or by his assistants, and it would appear that sometimes the atmosphere was so full of microbes that wounds became infected by exposure alone at the time of the operation or of the dressings.

But by modern methods of surgery this complication is almost unknown. My practice is to have all the instruments and swabs sterilised by heat, and I am careful that the instruments are quite clean before they are sterilised, a point which I think is not always sufficiently insisted upon, but which is of great importance, for even small particles of blood-clot or tissue of any kind may remain infective in spite of much heating. My hands, after the nails have been made as smooth and clean as possible by means of a penknife, are washed in a liberal quantity of methylated spirit, soap and water, a nail-brush, sterilised by heat and new for choice, being vigorously used. When the hands are as clean as I can make them they are thoroughly soaked in 1 in 1000 corrosive sublimate solution

* The 'Lancet,' vol. i, 1903, p. 1590.
† The 'Lancet' vol. ii, 1902, p. 428.

and again scrubbed in this with a nail-brush. The patient's skin is treated in a similar way, turpentine being also used, and, when there is time, it should be prepared the night before the operation, a compress soaked in 1 in 40 carbolic acid solution being applied and kept moist by some impervious material. A second thorough cleansing, as if the first had not been made, is desirable shortly before the operation. It is, of course, remembered that some skins are more delicate than others : some surgeons, for instance, find that 1 in 1000 corrosive sublimate solution makes the hands rough and harsh.

During dressings I am always careful not to expose the parts unnecessarily, as I believe that contamination by infection from the air is a possibility. Therefore an open wound, as soon as it is exposed, is covered by a sterilised swab wrung out of a weak antiseptic solution—1 in 60 carbolic or 1 in 3000 corrosive sublimate.

I state these details because the fact that, in all the cases of secondary hæmorrhage above referred to, the bleeding took place after the wounds had been repeatedly dressed—that is, from three to eleven days after the abscesses were opened—might be considered to point to infection from without as the cause of mischief. This view would be strengthened by the fact that in two of the cases I have quoted a month and six weeks elapsed between the onset of symptoms and the evacuation of pus, whilst in the other and in my own case there were respectively six and nine days, during the greater part of which suppuration had probably existed without causing hæmorrhage. Moreover, in the original accounts of the cases quoted, so far as I have seen them, I have not found it definitely stated in any that bleeding before an abscess was opened took place from within the abscess cavity.

The evidence that infection came from without would be of great importance if any ordinary, easily accessible infective organism could be held responsible for the mischief. But this was evidently not the case. There can be little doubt that the hæmorrhage depended on some peculiar micro-organism or some particularly virulent effect of one of the common forms of micro-organism. The precautions detailed having been taken, and the source of infection from within being so obvious, it may, I think, be regarded as certain that the particular micro-organism which caused the sloughing of tissues in the case under discussion developed in the abscess by infection from the colon. Hence, as in the pre-antiseptic days, it would appear that we may still, in connection with an appendix abscess, have a development of some "germ" which gives rise to a local sloughing of tissue, and it is exceedingly fortunate that this complication is a rare one.

It would seem that various pathogenic organisms may be found in the bowel, more than one of which may become the dominant factor controlling the phenomena which follow the development of an appendix abscess.

This accounts for the variety of consequences which may be observed. In one case a simple abscess forms, apparently with no tendency to spread, except by distension, and rapid healing follows if the pus finds vent either by rupture on to a surface or by incision. In another case there are hardly any defining walls to the abscess, and these are rapidly pushed away and replaced by others so that an indefinite extension of the pus cavity amongst the intestines takes place. In a third the abscess, whether localised or not, gives rise to secondary foci of suppuration, either in the immediate neighbourhood of the appendix, at some other part of the abdominal cavity, in the pleura, or elsewhere; and again, a sloughing effect, with or without hæmorrhage, may be produced.

Until I met with the case recorded above, I thought that a strictly localised, and especially a flaccid, abscess might be safely drained by means of tubes. It would appear, however, that the medical man and his patient are really to a great extent at the mercy of the dominant germ of each particular case; for, except perhaps in instances of colic of the appendix, and in some other rare conditions, certain cases of cancer, for example, septic complications always arise before professional aid is sought, on account of disease of this part. The surgeon, in deciding the treatment to be adopted, should therefore take into consideration that one of the more unusual micro-organisms may possibly be present and effective for mischief. It would be well to provide for such a contingency, and apparently it would be wise, as I understand is already the practice of some surgeons, not to use any sutures for the external wound in evacuating appendix abscesses, but to open the deeper parts as widely as is consistent with safety in other ways,

and always to pack the cavity with gauze. It is still possible, however, that hæmorrhage may arise under any method of treatment, and Mr. F. Ramsay's case above referred to was, in fact, drained by means of gauze and a rubber tube.

A defective power of clotting in the blood is sometimes put forward as a cause of hæmorrhage, and I would therefore again remark on the healthy, firm clots that were formed in my case.

It is to be regretted that a bacteriological investigation of the discharges was not made, but perhaps some member of this Society may be able to name the organism which appears to grow in the cæcum, which does not interfere with blood coagulation, which causes small black patches when enclosed between the raw surfaces of a wound after being exposed to the air and to weak antiseptic lotions, which may destroy the walls of a vessel and induce severe hæmorrhages, whilst the exposed parts of the wound are, to all appearances, healthy, which shows no tendency to induce secondary foci of suppuration, and which appears to grow freely when an abscess cavity is not fully drained, but ceases to be harmful if the wound is opened up thoroughly and packed with gauze.

April 9th, 1906.

MEDICINE AND THE PUBLIC. By S. SQUIRE SPRIGGE, M.A., M.D.Cantab. (London: William Heinemann).

THE importance of the public and the medical profession rightly understanding one another is very great, for, as Dr. Sprigge remarks in his preface, "The whole population of Great Britain is concerned in the quality of its medical service, and in the legislative and social conditions under which that service is rendered." In this book will be found an impartial discussion of many of the difficulties that exist and of some of the main grievances under which the members of the medical profession suffer, all set out in such a moderate manner that they cannot fail to impress those who read about them. Such burning questions as those of hospital abuse and other unfair charities are well considered, and very complete information is given about the careers open to men in the different services. The dominant note throughout is the necessity for loyal and thoughtful co-operation between the profession and the public, without which nothing satisfactory can result. This book should be a powerful aid towards a thorough understanding of many difficult questions, and we sincerely hope, both in the interest of medicine and the public, that it will be very widely read.

INDEX TO VOLUME XXVII.

Lightning Source UK Ltd.
Milton Keynes UK
UKHW011621160119
335572UK00012B/1019/P